J. W. Rohen
C. Yokochi
E. Lütjen-Drecoll

Color Atlas of Anatomy
A Photographic Study of the Human Body

Fifth Edition

Coeditions in 14 Languages

A Photographic Study
of the Human Body

Johannes W. Rohen
Chihiro Yokochi
Elke Lütjen-Drecoll

Color Atlas of Anatomy

Fifth Edition

with 1158 Figures,
1035 in Color and 123 CT and MRI Scans

LIPPINCOTT WILLIAMS & WILKINS
A **Wolters Kluwer** Company
Philadelphia · Baltimore · New York · London
Buenos Aires · Hong Kong · Sydney · Tokyo

Schattauer

IV

Prof. em. Dr. med. Dr. med. h. c. Johannes W. Rohen
Anatomisches Institut II der Universität Erlagen-Nürnberg
Universitätsstr. 19, D-91054 Erlangen, Germany

Chihiro Yokochi, M.D.
Professor Emeritus, Department of Anatomy
Kanagawa Dental College, Yokosuka, Kanagawa, Japan
Correspondence to:
Prof. Chihiro Yokochi, c/o Igaku-Shoin Ltd., 5-24-3 Hongo,
Bunkyo-ku, Tokyo 113-8719, Japan

Prof. Dr. med. Elke Lütjen-Drecoll
Anatomisches Institut II der Universität Erlangen-Nürnberg
Universitätsstr. 19, D-91054 Erlangen, Germany

Acknowledgements

We would like to express our great gratitude to all coworkers who helped to make the *Atlas* a success. We are particularly indebted to those who dissected new specimens with great skill and knowledge, particularly to Jeff Bryant (member of our staff) and Dr. Martin Rexer (now Klinikum Hof), who prepared most of the new specimens of the fifth edition. We would also like to thank Dr. K. Okamoto (now Nagasaki, Japan), who dissected many excellent specimens of the fourth edition, also included in this edition. Furthermore, we are greatly indebted to Prof. Winfried Neuhuber and his coworkers for their great efforts in supporting our work.

The specimens of the previous editions also depicted in this volume were dissected with great skill and enthusiasm by Prof. Dr. S. Nagashima (now Nagasaki, Japan), Dr. Mutsuko Takahashi (now Tokyo), Dr. Gabriele Lindner-Funk (Erlangen), Dr. P. Landgraf (Erlangen), and Miss Rachel M. McDonnell (now Dallas, Texas, USA).

We would also like to express our many thanks to Prof. W. Bautz (Institute of Diagnostic Radiology, University of Erlangen), who provided the newly included excellent CT and MRI scans.

We are also greatly indebted to Mr. Hans Sommer (SOMSO Co., Coburg), who kindly provided a number of excellent bone specimens.

Finally, we would like to express our great gratitude to our photographer, Mr. Marco Gößwein, who contributed the very excellent macrophotos. Excellent and untiring work was done by our secretaries, Mrs. Lis Köhler and Elisabeth Glas, as well by our artists, Mr. Jörg Pekarsky and Mrs. Annette Gack, who not only performed excellent new drawings but revised effectively the layout of the new edition.

Last but not least, we would like to express our sincere thanks to all scientists, students, and other coworkers, particularly to the ones at the publishing companies themselves.

J. W. Rohen, C. Yokochi, E. Lütjen-Drecoll

To purchase additional copies of this book, call our customer service department at **(800) 638-3030** or fax orders to **(301) 824-7390.** International customers should call **(301) 714-2324.**

Visit Lippincott Williams & Wilkins on the Internet:
http://www.LWW.com. Lippincott Williams & Wilkins customer service representatives are available from 8:30 am to 6:00 pm, EST.

Library of Congress Cataloging-in-Publication Data has been applied for.

Composing, printing, and binding:
Mayr Miesbach, Druckerei und Verlag GmbH,
Am Windfeld 15, D-83714 Miesbach, Germany
Printed in Germany

4 5 6 7 8 9 10

Preface to the Fifth Edition

Eighteen years after its first edition the *Atlas* was again thoroughly revised and modernized. Numerous new figures were incorporated. Nearly 40 new photographs taken from newly dissected specimens and several new drawings were added. To avoid an undesirable increase in volume size we omitted all figures of minor quality from the previous editions and revised thoroughly the layout of the book. To provide a more detailed outline on cross-sectional and regional anatomy which becomes increasingly important to clinical work, we added a number of CT and MRI scans taken with latest modern techniques.

Each chapter of this edition consists of two parts. The first part describes the anatomical structure of the organs in a systemic manner, e.g., in the case of an extremity: bones, joints, ligaments, muscles, blood vessels, and nerves. In the second part, the regional anatomy is depicted, so that the description of the superficial layers is followed by the deeper and deepest layers; thus the student in the lab can find the orientation needed for the dissection of the cadaver. When viewing the photographs, the use of a magnifier is strongly recommended in order to identify more precisely the three-dimensional structure of the tissues and organs depicted.

While preparing this new edition, the authors were reminded of how precisely, beautifully, and admirably the human body is constructed. If this book helps the student or medical doctor to appreciate the overwhelming beauty of the anatomical architecture of tissues and organs in the human, then it greatly fulfills its task. Deep interest and admiration of the anatomical structures may create the "love for man," which alone can be considered of primary importance for daily medical work.

We would like to express our great gratitude to all coworkers for their skilled work. Without their help the improvement of the *Atlas* would not have been possible. We would also like to express our sincere thanks to those at Schattauer GmbH, Stuttgart, Germany, Lippincott, Williams & Wilkins, Baltimore, Maryland, USA, and Igaku-Shoin, Tokyo, Japan, who always listened to our suggestions and invested again a great deal of their effort into improving this book.

Erlangen, January 2002   J. W. Rohen
C. Yokochi
E. Lütjen-Drecoll

Preface to the First Edition

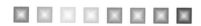

Today there exist any number of good anatomic atlases. Consequently, the advent of a new work requires justification. We found three main reasons to undertake the publication of such a book. First of all, most of the previous atlases contain mainly schematic or semischematic drawings which often reflect reality only in a limited way; the third dimension, i.e., the spatial effect, is lacking. In contrast, the photo of the actual anatomic specimen has the advantage of conveying the reality of the object with its proportions and spatial dimensions in a more exact and realistic manner than the "idealized", colored "nice" drawings of most previous atlases. Furthermore, the photo of the human specimen corresponds to the student's observations and needs in the dissection courses. Thus he has the advantage of immediate orientation by photographic specimens while working with the cadaver.

Secondly, some of the existing atlases are classified by systemic rather than regional aspects. As a result, the student needs several books each supplying the necessary facts for a certain region of the body. The present atlas, however, tries to portray macroscopic anatomy with regard to the regional and stratigraphic aspects of the object itself as realistically as possible. Hence it is an immediate help during the dissection courses in the study of medical and dental anatomy.

Another intention of the authors was to limit the subject to the essential and to offer it didactically in a way that is self-explanatory. To all regions of the body we added schematic drawings of the main tributaries of nerves and vessels, of the course and mechanism of the muscles, of the nomenclature of the various regions, etc. This will enhance the understanding of the details seen in the photographs. The complicated architecture of the skull bones, for example, was not presented in a descriptive way, but rather through a series of figures revealing the mosaic of bones by adding one bone to another, so that ultimately the composition of skull bones can be more easily understood.

Finally, the authors also considered the present situation in medical education. On one hand there is a universal lack of cadavers in many departments of anatomy, while on the other hand there has been a considerable increase in the number of students almost everywhere. As a consequence, students do not have access to sufficient illustrative material for their anatomic studies. Of course, photos can never replace the immediate observation, but we think the use of a macroscopic photo instead of a painted, mostly idealized picture is more appropriate and is an improvement in anatomic study over drawings alone.

The majority of the specimens depicted in the atlas were prepared by the authors either in the Dept. of Anatomy in Erlangen, Germany, or in the Dept. of Anatomy, Kanagawa Dental College, Yokosuka, Japan. The specimens of the chapter on the neck and those of the spinal cord demonstrating the dorsal branches of the spinal nerves were prepared by Dr. K. Schmidt with great skill and enthusiasm. The specimens of the ligaments of the vertebral column were prepared by Dr. Th. Mokrusch, and a great number of specimens in the chapter of the upper and lower limb was very carefully prepared by Dr. S. Nagashima, Kurume, Japan.

Once again, our warmest thanks go out to all of our co-workers for their unselfish, devoted and highly qualified work.

Erlangen, Spring 1983

J.W. Rohen
C. Yokochi

Contents

1 General Anatomy 1

Contents

2 Head and Neck 23

3 Trunk   184

4 Thoracic Organs   233

Contents

5 Abdominal Organs — 281

6 Retroperitoneal Organs — 311

■ 7 Upper Limb 356

■ 8 Lower Limb 417

List of Figures

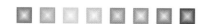

The schematic drawings have been performed by the following graphic designers:

General Anatomy

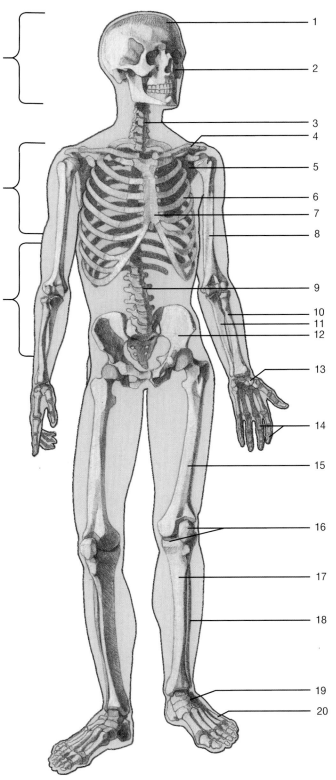

In contrast to most other mammals the human body is adapted for bipedal locomotion. Three general principles in the architecture of the human organism are recognizable:

1. The principle of **segmentation,** which dominates in the trunk. The vertebral column and the thorax consist of relatively equal, segmentally arranged elements.
2. The principle of **bilateral symmetry.** Both sides of the body are separated by a midsagittal plane and resemble each other like image and mirror-image.
3. The principle of **polarity** between the head at one end of the body and the lower extremities at the other. As the center of the information system the head contains the main sensory organs and the brain. The head has a predominantly spherical form, while the extremities consist of radially formed skeletal elements, the number of which increases distally.

A. The **skull** consists of two parts: 1. a **cranial part** containing mainly the brain and the sensory organs and 2. a **facial part** which contains the nasal and oral cavity and the chewing apparatus. The cranial cavity is continuous with the vertebral canal which contains the spinal cord.

B. The **thorax** contains the respiratory and circulatory organs (lung, heart, etc.) but also some of the abdominal organs which are located underneath the diaphragm.

C. The **abdominal cavity** contains the organs of metabolism such as the liver, the stomach and the intestinal tract as well as the excretory and genital organs (kidney, uterus, urinary bladder, etc.). The latter are located primarily in the **pelvic cavity** with the exception of the testes.

Structure of the human body and the skeleton. Blue = joints.
A Head (caput)   B   Thorax (thoracic cavity)   C   Abdominal and
pelvic cavities

1	Cranial part } of the skull	10	Radius } forearm
2	Facial part	11	Ulna
3	Vertebral column (cervical part)	12	Pelvis
4	Clavicle	13	Wrist (carpals) } hand
5	Scapula	14	Fingers (phalanges)
6	Ribs	15	Thigh (femur)
7	Sternum	16	Patella and knee joint
8	Arm (humerus)	17	Tibia } leg
9	Vertebral column (lumbar part)	18	Fibula
		19	Tarsals } foot
		20	Metatarsals

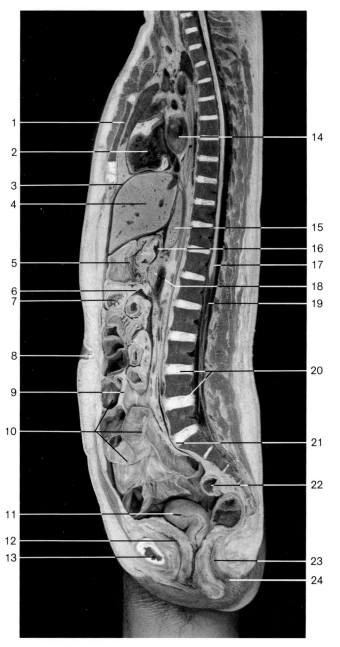

Median section through the trunk (female).

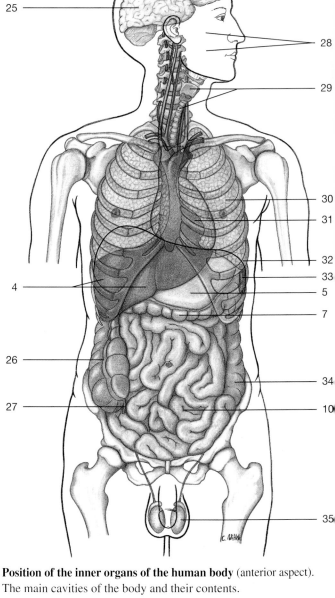

Position of the inner organs of the human body (anterior aspect).
The main cavities of the body and their contents.

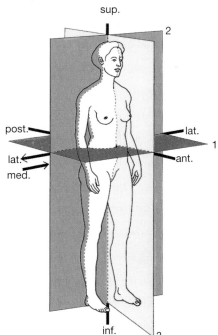

1	Sternum	21	Sacral promontory
2	Right ventricle of heart	22	Sigmoid colon
3	Diaphragm	23	Anal canal
4	**Liver**	24	Anus
5	**Stomach**	25	Head (neurocranium) with brain
6	Transverse mesocolon	26	Ascending colon
7	Transverse colon	27	Appendix
8	Umbilicus	28	Facial region (viscerocranium)
9	Mesentery		with oral and nasal cavities
10	**Small intestine**	29	Trachea and larynx
11	Uterus	30	Thorax with the lungs
12	Urinary bladder	31	**Heart**
13	Pubic symphysis	32	Surface projection of the diaphragm
14	Left atrium of heart	33	**Spleen**
15	Caudate lobe of liver	34	Descending colon
16	Omental bursa or lesser sac	35	Testis
17	Conus medullaris		
18	**Pancreas**		
19	Cauda equina		
20	Intervertebral discs		
	(lumbar vertebral column)		

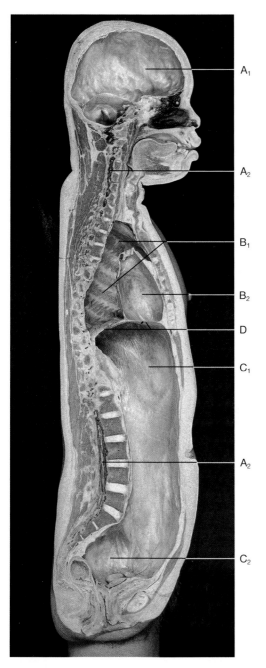

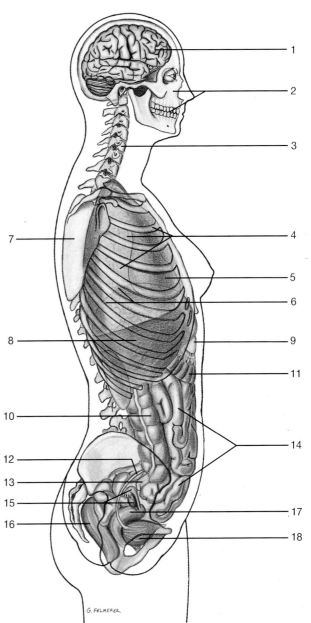

Sagittal section through the human body (female).
Demonstration of the main cavities of the body.
Internal organs are removed.

A₁ Cranial cavity
A₂ Vertebral canal
B₁ Thoracic cavity
B₂ Pericardial cavity
C₁ Abdominal cavity
C₂ Pelvic cavity
D   Diaphragm

Planes of the body
1 Transverse plane
2 Frontal plane
3 Sagittal plane (midsagittal)

Lines of direction
ant. = anterior
inf. = inferior
lat. = lateral
med. = medial
post. = posterior
sup. = superior

Position of the inner organs of the human body
(lateral aspect).
The three main cavities of the body and their contents.

1   Head (neurocranium) with the brain
2   Facial bones with oral and nasal cavities
3   Vertebral column (cervical part)
4   Thorax with the lungs
5   Heart
6   Surface projection of the diaphragm
7   Scapula
8   Liver
9   Stomach
10 Ascending colon
11 Transverse colon
12 Ureter
13 Appendix
14 Small intestine
15 Ovary, uterine tube
16 Rectum
17 Uterus
18 Urinary bladder

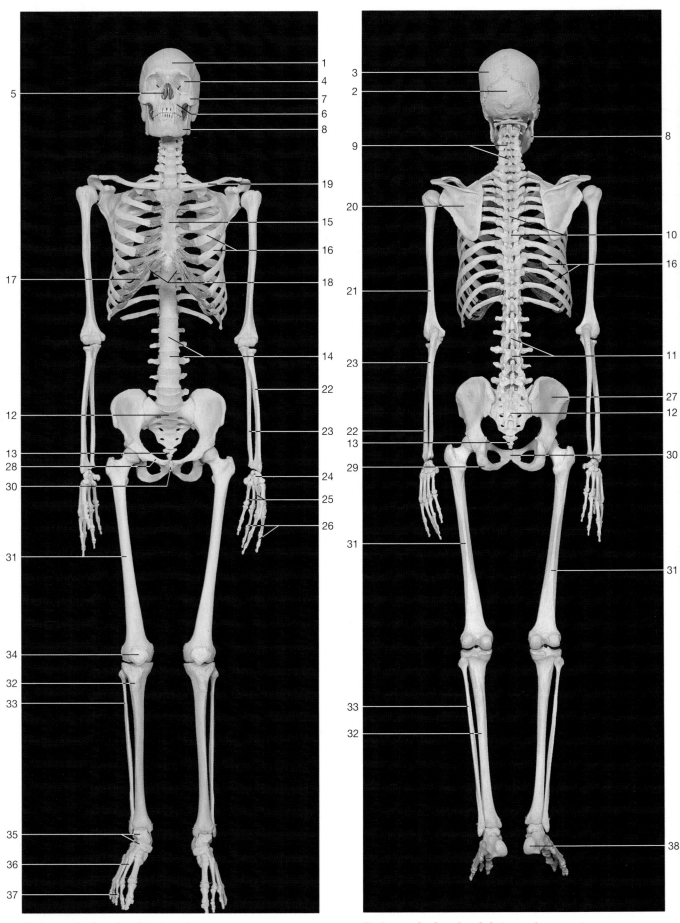

Skeleton of a female adult (anterior aspect).

Skeleton of a female adult (posterior aspect).

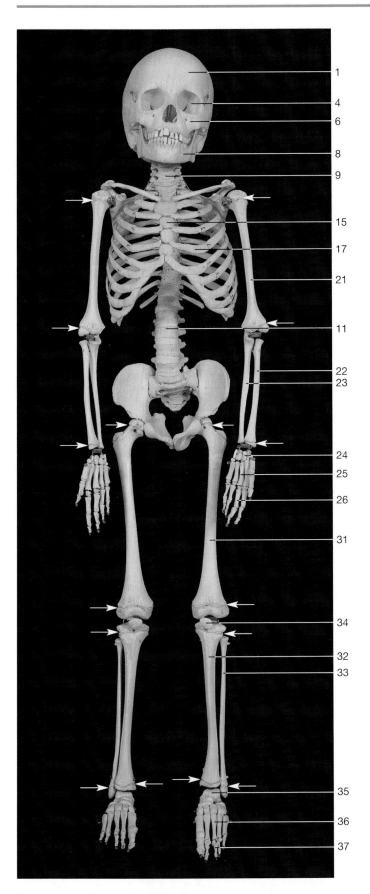

Axial skeleton
Head
1 Frontal bone
2 Occipital bone
3 Parietal bone
4 Orbit
5 Nasal cavity
6 Maxilla
7 Zygomatic bone
8 Mandible

Trunk and thorax
Vertebral column
9 Cervical vertebrae
10 Thoracic vertebrae
11 Lumbar vertebrae
12 Sacrum
13 Coccyx
14 Intervertebral discs

Thorax
15 Sternum
16 Ribs
17 Costal cartilage
18 Infrasternal angle

Appendicular skeleton
Upper limb and shoulder girdle
19 Clavicle
20 Scapula
21 Humerus
22 Radius
23 Ulna
24 Carpal bones
25 Metacarpal bones
26 Phalanges of the hand

Lower limb and pelvis
27 Ilium
28 Pubis
29 Ischium
30 Symphysis pubis
31 Femur
32 Tibia
33 Fibula
34 Patella
35 Tarsal bones
36 Metatarsal bones
37 Phalanges of the foot
38 Calcaneus

Skeleton of a 5-year-old child (anterior aspect).
The zones of the cartilaginous growth plates are seen (arrows).
In contrast to the adult, the ribs show a predominantly
horizontal position.

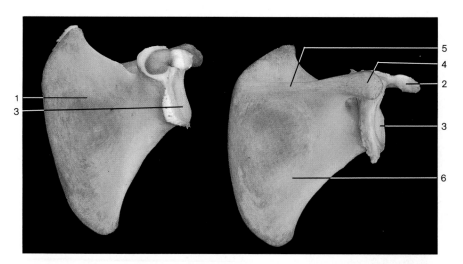

1 Subscapular fossa
2 Coracoid process
3 Glenoid fossa
4 Acromion
5 Spine of scapula
6 Infraspinous fossa

Ossification of the scapula
(left: anterior aspect, right: posterior aspect).

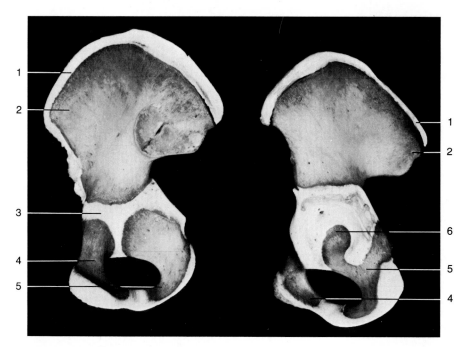

1 Cartilage of the iliac crest
2 Ilium
3 Cartilage
4 Pubis
5 Ischium
6 Acetabulum

Ossification of the hip bone
(left: medial aspect, right: lateral aspect).

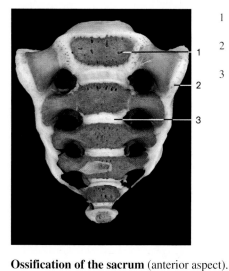

1 Bone tissue
  (vertebral body)
2 Cartilaginous tissue
  (lateral epiphysis)
3 Intervertebral discs

Ossification of the sacrum (anterior aspect).
Note the five vertebral bones, which are still separated
from each other.

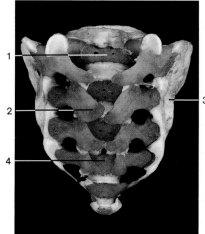
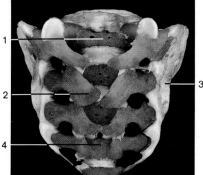

1 Bony tissue
  (center of
  ossification)
2 Vertebral arch
  (not completely
  united)
3 Cartilaginous
  tissue
  (lateral epiphysis)
4 Sacral canal

Ossification of the sacrum
(posterior aspect).

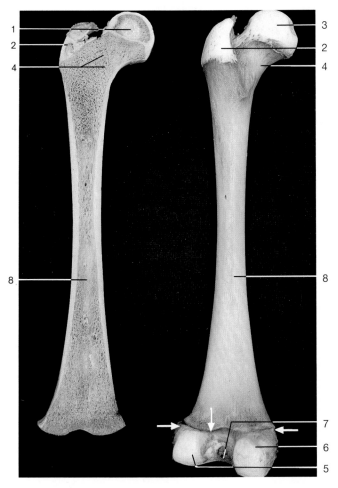

1 Ossification center in the head of the femur
2 Greater trochanter
3 Head of the femur
4 Neck of the femur
5 Lateral condyle
6 Medial condyle
7 Intercondylar notch
8 Diaphysis

Ossification of the femur (left: coronal section, right: posterior view of the femur). Arrows: distal epiphysis.

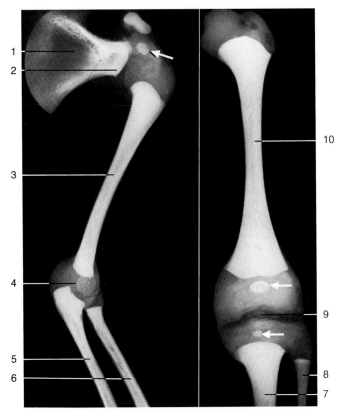

X-ray of the upper and lower limb of a newborn child.
Left: upper limb. Right: lower limb.
Arrows: ossification centers.

1	Scapula	4	Elbow joint	7	Tibia
2	Shoulder joint	5	Ulna	8	Fibula
3	Humerus	6	Radius	9	Knee joint
				10	Femur

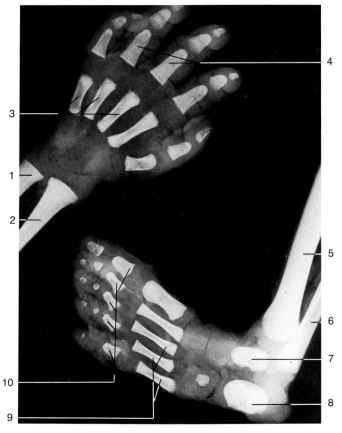

X-ray of hand and foot of a newborn.

1	Ulna	4	Phalanges	7	Talus
2	Radius	5	Tibia	8	Calcaneus
3	Metacarpals	6	Fibula	9	Metatarsals
				10	Phalanges

1	Metaphysis
2	Spongy bone
3	Medullary cavity in the diaphysis
4	Compact bone
5	Nutrient canal
6	Diaphysis
7	Epiphyseal line (remnants of the epiphyseal plate)
8	Epiphysis (head of the femur)
9	Fovea of head
10	Trabeculae of spongy bone
11	Neck of the femur
12	Greater trochanter
13	Lesser trochanter
14	Articular surface
15	Periosteum
16	Skin
17	Vastus medialis muscle
18	Sartorius muscle
19	Femoral artery and vein
20	Great saphenous vein
21	Gracilis muscle
22	Adductor longus muscle
23	Adductor magnus muscle
24	Semimembranosus muscle
25	Semitendinosus muscle
26	Rectus femoris muscle
27	Vastus lateralis muscle
28	Femur and medullary cavity
29	Vastus intermedius muscle
30	Sciatic nerve
31	Biceps femoris muscle
32	Spongy bone trabeculae containing bone marrow
33	Compact bone
34	Osteon with Haversian lamellae
35	Periosteum
36	Blood vessels and nerves for periosteum and bone

Femur of the adult. Left: the periosteum and the nutrient vessels are preserved. Right: coronal section of the proximal and distal epiphyses to display the spongy bone and the medullary cavity.

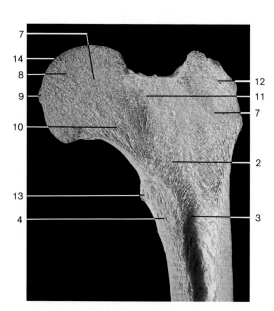

Coronal section through the proximal end of the adult femur, revealing the characteristic trajectorial structure of the spongy bone.

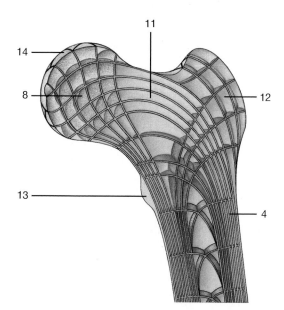

Three dimensional representation on the trajectorial lines of the femoral head (according to B. Kummer).

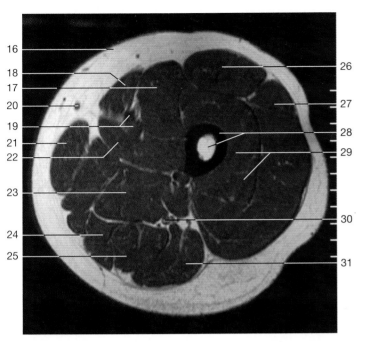

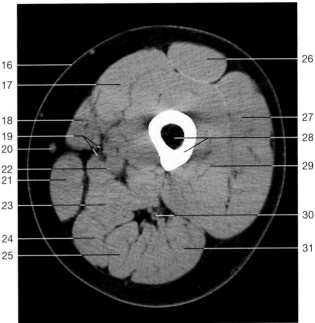

MRI scan of the thigh (axial section through the middle of the left thigh, the same level as the CT scan).

CT scan of the section through the middle of the left thigh (axial section). Note the differences between the CT and MRI scan (see text below).

The **bones** of the skeletal system consist of two different parts, the spongy and the compact bone. The spongy bone trabeculae are highly adapted to mechanical forces revealing a trajectorial structure. The intertrabecular spaces are filled with bone marrow, the site of blood formation. The appearance of bones, muscles and soft tissues is quite different in **CT** and **MRI scans.** The CT scans relate well to radiographs in that areas of great absorption such as bones are white, and those with little absorption such as fat appear black. In contrast, the intensity of signals in MRI scans, obtained without X-rays but by magnetic forces, is different so that dense areas of bones appear black and soft tissues such as bone marrow and fat appear white (for comparison see above figures).

A highly innervated **periosteum** is an essential structure for bone nutrition, blood supply, growth and bone repair.

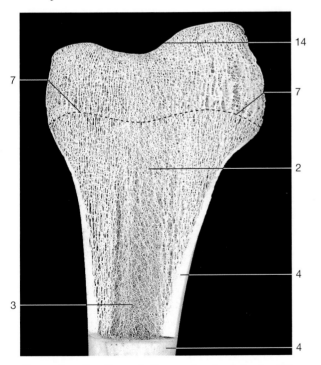

Coronal section through the proximal epiphysis of the adult tibia. Note the zone of dense bone at the site of the former epiphyseal plate (dotted line).

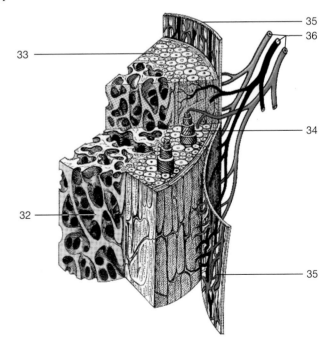

Structure of bones of the skeletal system (after Benninghoff). Note that the compact bone reveals a lamellar structure with Haversian lamellae and canals.

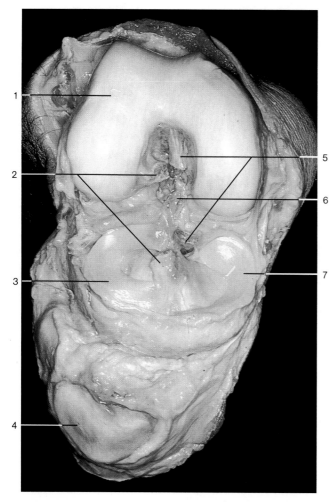

Knee joint. Anterior aspect, showing menisci and cruciate ligaments (cut). Quadriceps tendon cut and patella reflected distally.

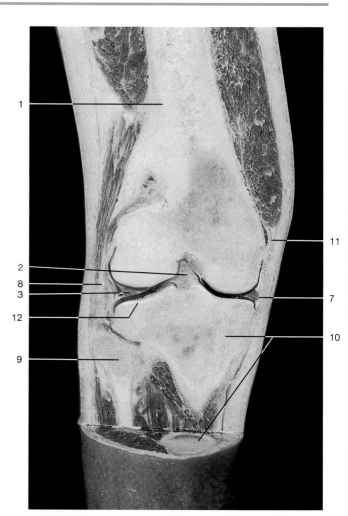

Coronal section through the knee joint.
Anterior aspect of the right joint in extension.

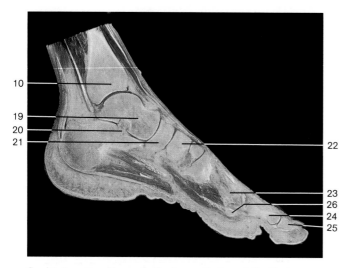

Sagittal section through the lower limb and the foot.

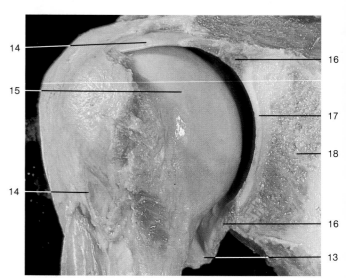

Shoulder joint (anterior view). The anterior part of the articular capsule has been removed.

1	Femur	10	Tibia
2	Anterior cruciate ligament	11	Tibial collateral ligament
3	Lateral meniscus	12	Articular cartilage
4	Patella	13	Articular capsule
5	Posterior cruciate ligament	14	Tendon of long head
6	Posterior meniscofemoral		of biceps brachii muscle
	ligament	15	Head of humerus
7	Medial meniscus	16	Glenoid labrum
8	Fibular collateral ligament	17	Articular cartilage of
9	Fibula		glenoid fossa

18	Scapula
19	Talus
20	Interosseous talocalcaneal ligament
21	Navicular bone
22	Medial cuneiform bone
23	First metatarsal bone
24	Proximal phalanx of the hallux (great toe)
25	Distal phalanx of the hallux
26	Sesamoid bone

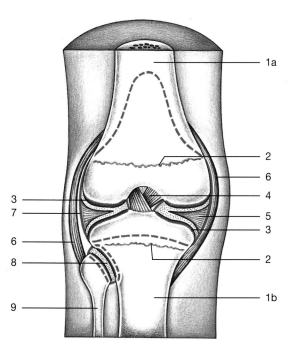

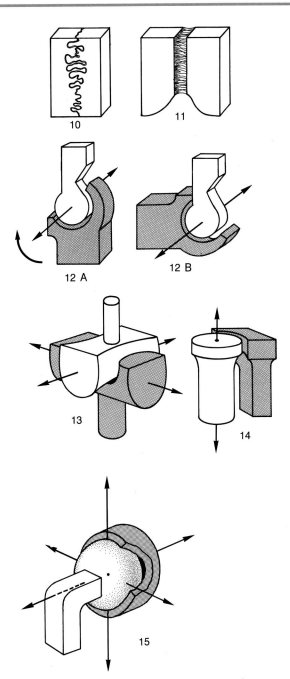

General architecture of a synovial joint with two articulating bones and a synovial cavity (right side, anterior view).
Coronal section through the knee joint.
Red line = Articular capsule with synovial membrane.
Dotted red line = extension of articular capsule (suprapatellar bursa).

1 Articulating bones: a) Femur, b) Tibia
2 Epiphysial line
3 **Articular cartilage**
4 Intraarticular ligaments (e.g., cruciate ligaments)
5 Fibrocartilaginous disk (e.g., meniscus)
6 Collateral ligaments
7 Articular capsule with synovial membrane
8 **Tibiofibular articulation** (example of gliding synovial joint)
9 Fibula

Main types of joints. Arrows: axes of movement.

Fibrous joints (synarthroses)
10 Serrate suture
11 Syndesmosis

Synovial joints (diarthroses)
12 Hinge joints (monaxial) ginglymus
    A Extension
    B Flexion
13 Saddle joint (biaxial)
14 Pivot joint (monaxial, rotation)
15 Ball-and-socket joint (multiaxial)

			Movement	Examples
A	**Fibrous joints**			
	1	Sutures	No movements	Sutures of the skull
	2	Syndesmoses	No movements	Distal tibiofibular joint
	3	Gomphosis	No movements	Roots of teeth in alveolar process
B	**Cartilaginous joints**			
	1	Synchondroses	No movements	Epiphyseal plates
	2	Symphyses	Slight movement	Symphysis pubis
				Intervertebral discs
C	**Synovial joints**			
	1	Gliding	Monaxial	Intercarpal joint
				Intertarsal joint
				Sacroiliacal joint
	2	Hinge	Monaxial	Interphalangeal joint
				Humeroulnar joint
				Talocrural joint
	3	Pivot	Monaxial	Atlantoaxial joint
				Radioulnar joint
	4	Ellipsoidal	Biaxial	Radiocarpal joint
	5	Saddle	Biaxial	Carpometacarpal joint of the thumb
	6	Ball-and-socket	Multiaxial	Shoulder and hip joint

An articulation or joint is the functional connection between two or more bones. Joints can be divided into two categories depending upon whether the articulating surfaces of the bones are separated by a real cavity (joint cavity) so that they are movable against each other **(synovial joints)** or whether the bones are firmly connected by fibrous or cartilaginous tissue and practically immovable **(fibrous joints, cartilaginous joints, symphysis, etc.).** Synovial joints always possess a joint capsule (with a vascularized synovial membrane), artic- ular cartilages, and a joint cavity. They are grouped according to the degree of movement they permit. A hinge joint (ginglymus) permits movement in only one plane about a single axis **(uniaxial or monaxial),** an ellipsoidal joint permits movements in two planes **(biaxial),** and ball-and-socket joints permit a range of movements around several axes **(multiaxial).** The following survey gives a few examples of these types of articulation.

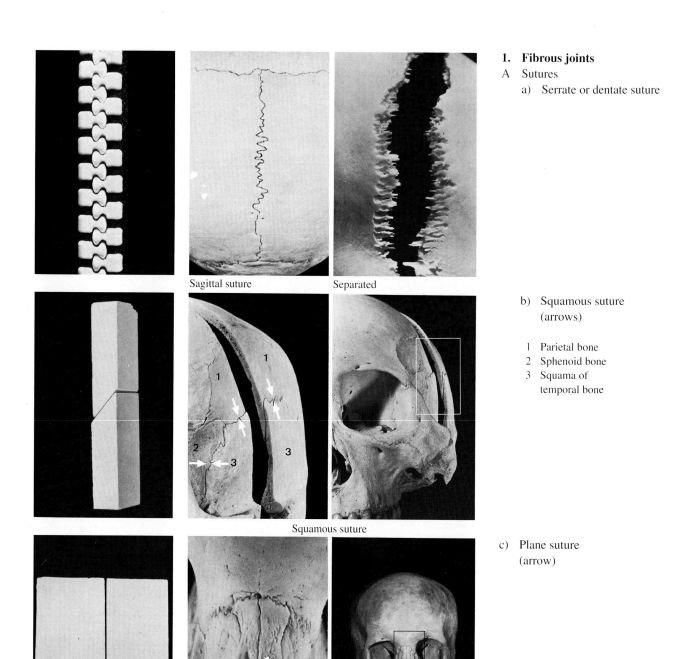

Sagittal suture   Separated

Squamous suture

Nasal bones

1. Fibrous joints
A Sutures
  a) Serrate or dentate suture

  b) Squamous suture
      (arrows)

      1 Parietal bone
      2 Sphenoid bone
      3 Squama of
         temporal bone

  c) Plane suture
      (arrow)

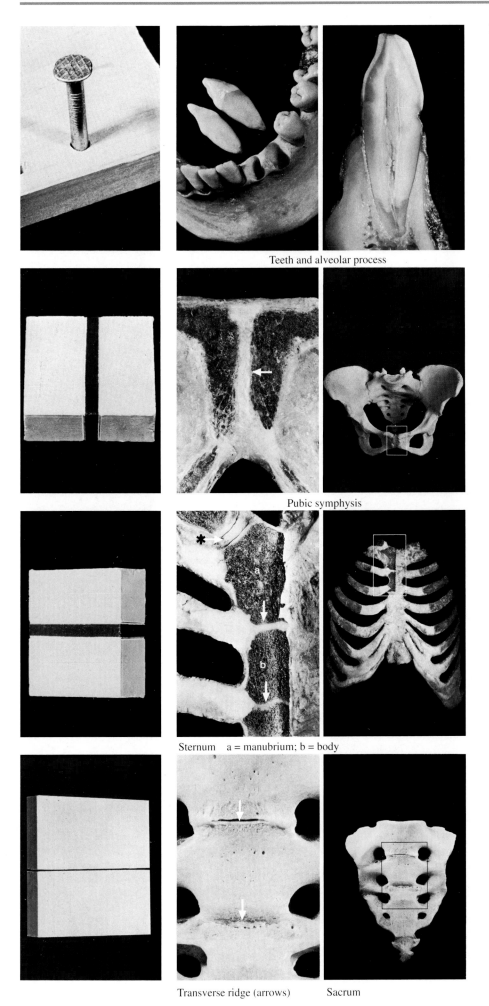

B   Peg suture
    (Gomphosis)

Teeth and alveolar process

2. **Cartilaginous joints**
   a) Symphysis
       (fibrocartilage)

Pubic symphysis

   b) Synchondrosis
       (hyaline cartilage)

Sternum   a = manubrium; b = body

*   Articular disc
    (sternoclavicular joint)

3. **Osseous joints**
   (synostosis)

Transverse ridge (arrows)   Sacrum

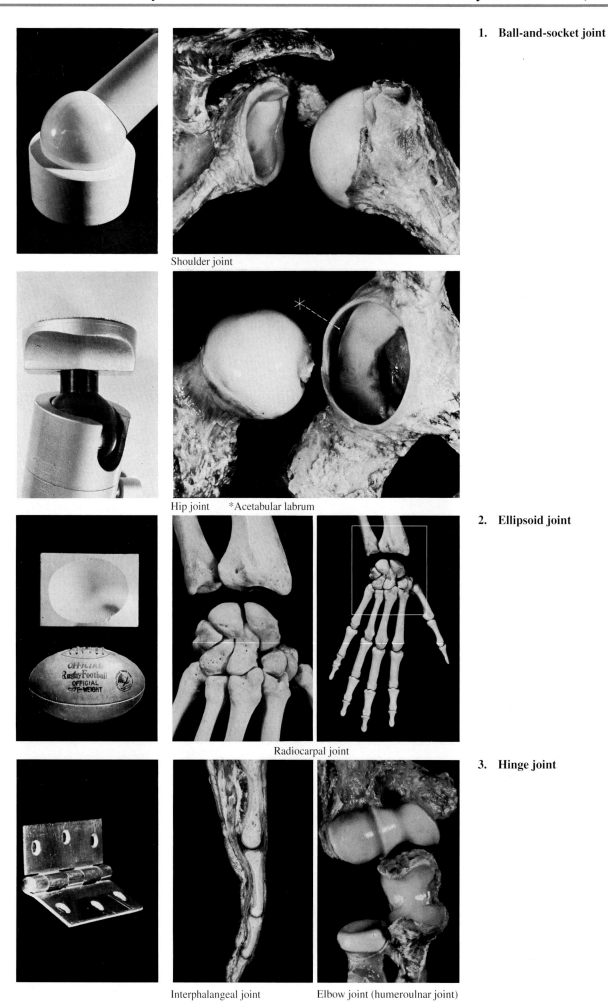

Shoulder joint

1. Ball-and-socket joint

Hip joint   *Acetabular labrum

2. Ellipsoid joint

Radiocarpal joint

3. Hinge joint

Interphalangeal joint   Elbow joint (humeroulnar joint)

4. Pivot joint

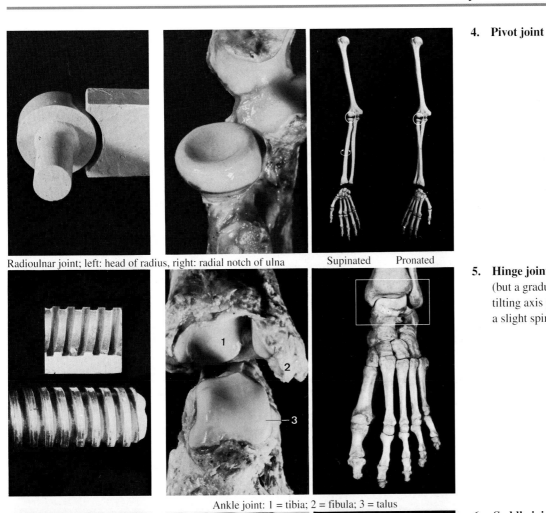

Radioulnar joint; left: head of radius, right: radial notch of ulna   Supinated   Pronated

Ankle joint: 1 = tibia; 2 = fibula; 3 = talus

5. Hinge joint
   (but a gradually
   tilting axis produces
   a slight spiral motion)

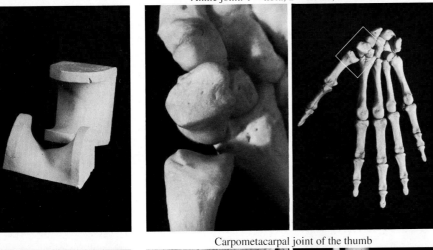

Carpometacarpal joint of the thumb

6. Saddle joint

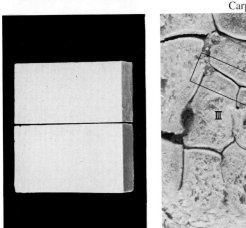

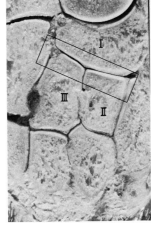

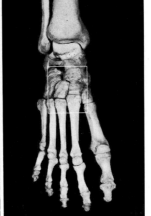

7. Plane joint

I = navicular; **II** = intermediate cuneiform; **III** = lateral cuneiform

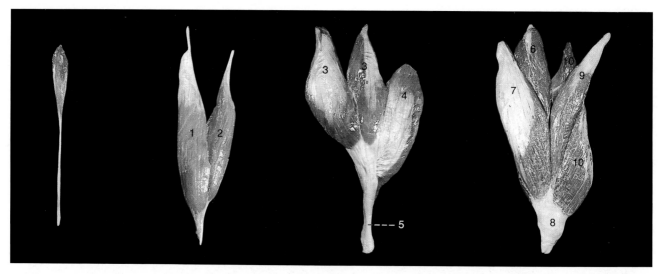

Fusiform
(palmaris longus muscle)

Bicipital
(biceps brachii muscle)

Tricipital
(triceps surae muscle)

Quadricipital
(quadriceps femoris muscle)

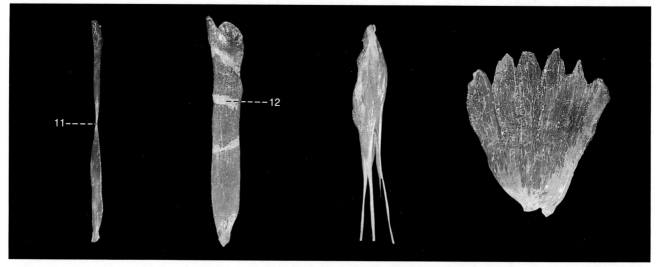

Digastric
(omohyoid muscle)

Multiventral
(rectus abdominis muscle)

Multicaudal
(flexor profundus muscle)

Serrated
(serratus anterior muscle)

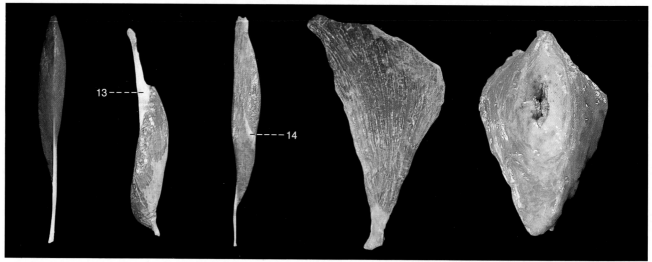

Bipennate
(tibialis anterior muscle)

Unipennate
(semimembranosus
muscle)

Semitendinous
(semitendinosus muscle)

Broad, flat muscle
(latissimus dorsi muscle)

Ring-like
(external anal sphincter Muscle)

1 Long head	4 Soleus muscle	8 Patella	12 Tendinous intersection
2 Short head	5 Achilles tendon	9 Rectus femoris muscle	13 Aponeurosis
3 Gastrocnemius muscle	6 Vastus intermedius muscle	10 Vastus medialis muscle	14 Tendinous intersection
(medial head, lateral head)	7 Vastus lateralis muscle	11 Intermediate tendon	

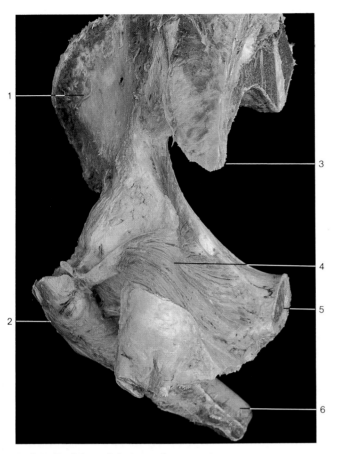

Left half of the pelvis (posterior aspect).
Obturator internus muscle as an example of a muscle, the tendon of which does not act in the direction of the main muscle fibers. Its fibers originate at the internal aspect of the obturator foramen, turn around the posterior rim of the ischium and insert at the greater trochanter of the femur. The ischium thereby serves as a pulley.

1	Ilium	3	Coccyx	5	Pubis
2	Greater trochanter	4	Obturator internus muscle	6	Femur

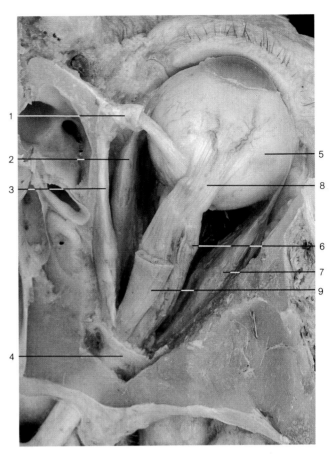

Superior oblique muscle of the eyeball, right eye (superior aspect). The tendon of this muscle bends over the trochlea, changing its direction so that it becomes attached to the posterior lateral quadrant of the eyeball.

1	Trochlea	6	Superior rectus muscle
2	Medial rectus muscle	7	Lateral rectus muscle
3	Superior oblique muscle	8	Superior rectus muscle (tendon)
4	Common annular tendon	9	Levator palpebrae superioris
5	Eyeball		muscle (divided)

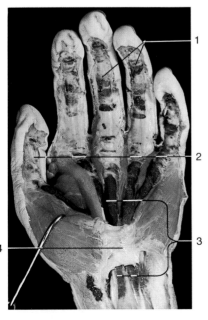

1 Digital synovial sheaths of the tendons of flexor digitorum superficialis and profundus muscles
2 Digital synovial sheaths of the tendon of long flexor pollicis longus muscle
3 Common flexor synovial sheaths of flexor digitorum superficialis and profundus muscles
4 Flexor retinaculum

The synovial sheaths of the tendons on the palmar aspect of the left wrist (colored fluid has been injected).

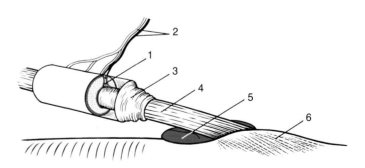

1 Mesotendon
2 Blood vessels
3 Synovial sheath
4 Tendon
5 Synovial bursa
6 Bone (tuberosity)

Structure of a tendon sheath. The synovial membrane, which also forms the mesotendon, is indicated in red. (Schematic drawing.)

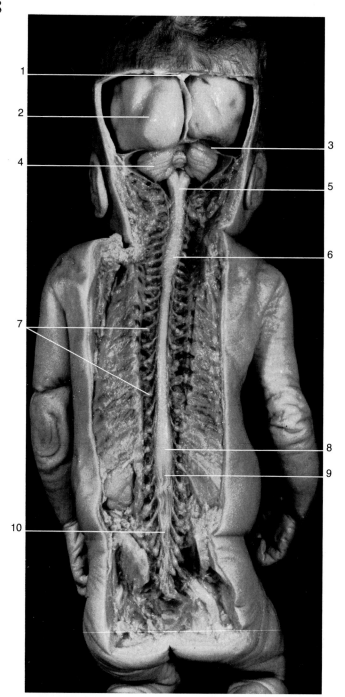

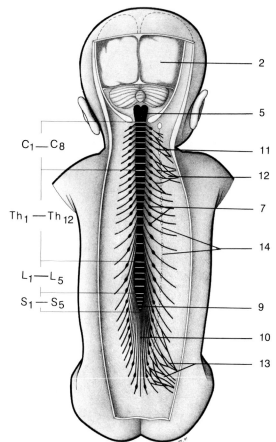

1 Falx cerebri
2 Cerebral hemispheres
3 Tentorium cerebelli
4 Cerebellum
5 Medulla oblongata
6 Spinal cord, cervical enlargement
7 Spinal ganglia
8 Spinal cord, lumbar enlargement
9 Conus medullaris
10 Cauda equina
11 Cervical plexus (formed from ventral rami of C_1–C_4)
12 Brachial plexus (formed from ventral rami of C_5–T_1)
13 Lumbosacral plexus (formed from ventral rami of L_1–S_4)
14 Sympathetic trunk

Brain, the **spinal cord** and the **spinal nerves** in the fetus (posterior aspect).

Schematic drawing to illustrate the three main parts of the nervous system in general.

The **nervous system** can be divided into three, functionally distinct parts:
1. The cranial part, which comprises the great sensory organs and the brain,
2. The spinal cord, which shows a segmental structure and serves predominantly as a reflex-organ, and
3. The autonomic nervous system, which controls the unvoluntary functions (subconscious control) of organs and tissues. The autonomic part of the nervous system forms many delicate plexus within the organs. At certain places these plexus contain aggregations of nerve cells (prevertebral and intramural ganglia).

The spinal nerves leave the spinal cord at regular intervals, forming the 8 cervical, 12 thoracic, 5 lumbar, 5 sacral and a varying number of coccygeal segments. The ventral rami of the first four cervical spinal nerves (C_1–C_4) form the cervical plexus (for innervation of the anterior neck), the ventral rami of the lower cervical spinal nerves (C_5–T_1) form the brachial plexus which innervates the upper extremity, and the ventral rami of the lumbar and sacral spinal nerves form the lumbosacral plexus (L_1–S_4) which innervates the pelvic and genital organs and the lower extremity.

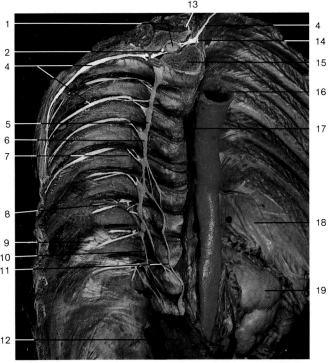

Posterior part of the thorax. Cross-section at the level of the 5th thoracic segment. Spinal nerves and their connections to the sympathetic trunk.

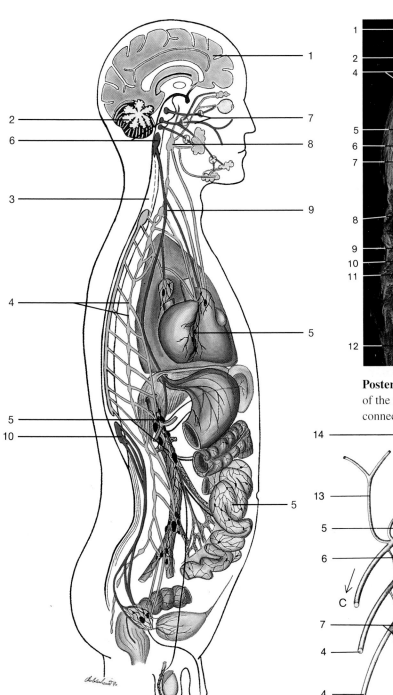

Diagram illustrating the localization of the
three functional portions of the **nervous system**
(brain, spinal cord and autonomic nervous system).
Yellow = sympathetic system; red = parasympathetic system.

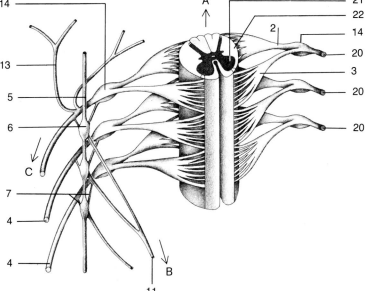

Organization of the spinal cord in structurally equal segments which form the paired spinal nerves. A = connections to the brain; B = connections to the autonomic nervous system; C = connections to the trunk and extremities (intercostal nerves and plexus). (Schematic drawing.)

1	Cerebrum		
2	Cerebellum		
3	Spinal cord		
4	Sympathetic trunk and ganglion		
5	Plexus and ganglia of the autonomic nervous system		
6	Cranial autonomic system		
7	Cranial nerves (n. III and n. VII)		
8	Superior cervical ganglion		
9	Vagus nerve (n. X)		
10	Sacral autonomic system		

1	Spinal cord	12	Inferior vena cava
2	**Dorsal root**	13	Dorsal ramus of spinal nerve
3	**Ventral root**	14	**Spinal (dorsal root) ganglion**
4	Intercostal nerves	15	Body of the vertebra
5	Sympathetic trunk	16	Aorta
6	Ganglia of the sympathetic trunk	17	Azygos vein
7	Rami communicantes	18	Diaphragm
8	Intercostal artery and vein	19	Left kidney
9	Subcostalis muscle	20	**Spinal nerve**
10	Lesser splanchnic nerve	21	Gray matter of the spinal cord
11	Greater splanchnic nerve	22	White matter of the spinal cord

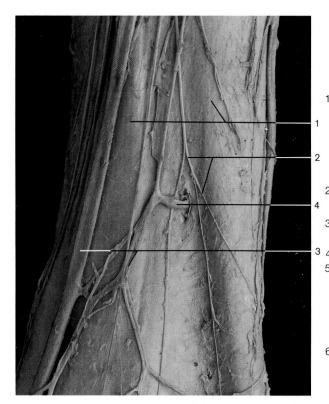

Superficial nerves and vessels of the lower leg, illustrating the structural differences between veins and nerves.

1 Crural fascia (fascia cruris)
2 Cutaneous nerves
3 Superficial cutaneous veins
4 Perforating vein

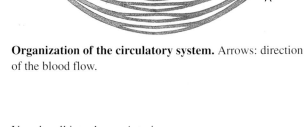

Organization of the circulatory system. Arrows: direction of the blood flow.

Vessel wall in red   = Arteries
Vessel wall in blue = Veins
Yellow   = Lymphatic vessels

A   Systemic circulation
B   Hepatic portal circulation
C   Pulmonary circulation

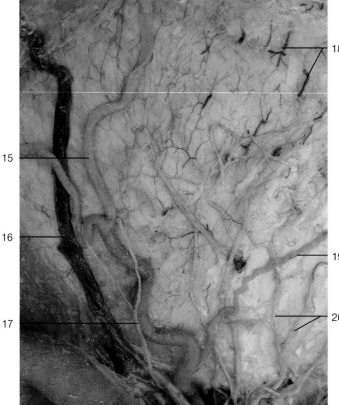
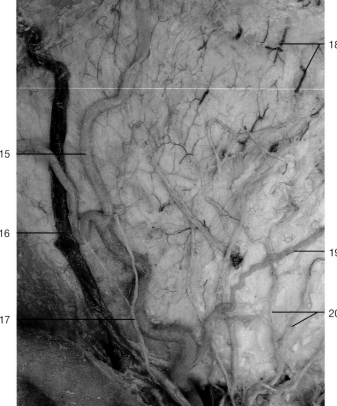

Superficial nerves and vessels. Temporal region. Note the differences between arteries, veins and nerves.

1 Pulmonary vein
2 Superior vena cava
3 Thoracic duct
4 Inferior vena cava
5 Hepatic vein
6 Liver
7 Lymph nodes and lymphatic vessels
8 Lung
9 Pulmonary artery
10 Aorta
11 Heart
12 Small intestine with capillary network
13 Portal vein
14 Mesenteric artery
15 Superficial temporal artery
16 Superficial temporal vein
17 Auriculotemporal nerve
18 Perforating veins for subcutaneous fatty tissue
19 Small artery
20 Small nerves (branches of facial nerve)

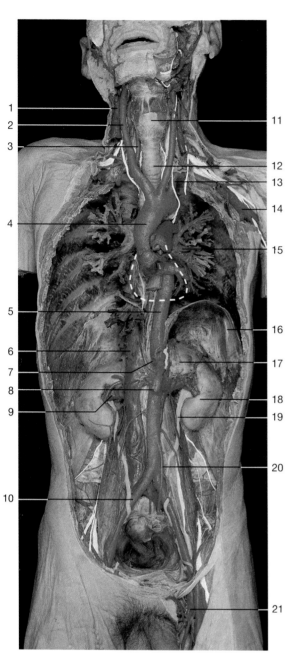

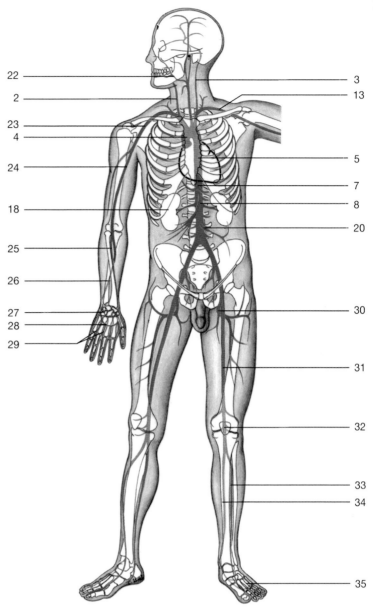

Major vessels of the trunk. The position of the heart is indicated by the dotted line.

Major arteries of the human body. (Schematic drawing.)

1	Internal jugular vein	18	Kidney
2	**Common carotid artery**	19	Ureter
3	Vertebral artery	20	Inferior mesenteric artery
4	**Ascending aorta**	21	**Femoral vein**
5	**Descending aorta**	22	Facial artery
6	**Inferior vena cava**	23	Axillary artery
7	Celiac trunk	24	Brachial artery
8	Superior mesenteric artery	25	Radial artery
9	Renal vein	26	Ulnar artery
10	**Common iliac artery**	27	Deep palmar arch
11	Larynx	28	Superficial palmar arch
12	Trachea	29	Common palmar digital arteries
13	Left subclavian artery	30	Profunda femoris artery
14	Left axillary vein	31	**Femoral artery**
15	**Pulmonary veins**	32	Popliteal artery
16	Diaphragm	33	Anterior tibial artery
17	Suprarenal gland	34	Posterior tibial artery
		35	Plantar arch

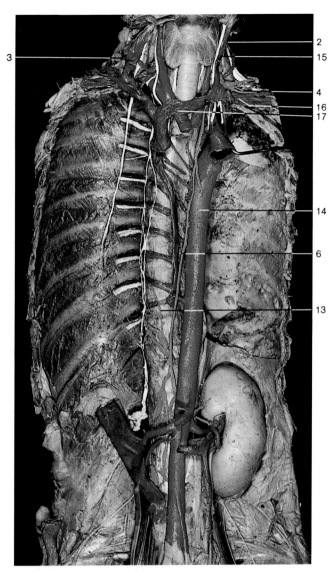

Major lymph vessels of the trunk.

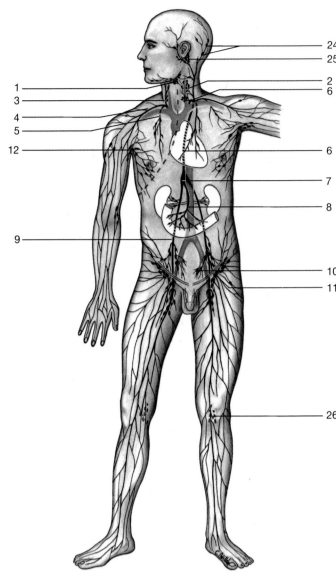

Lymphatic system. Course of the main lymphatic vessels and lymph nodes in the body. Dotted line = border between lymphatic vessels draining towards the right venous angle and towards the left.

1	Submandibular nodes	15	Internal jugular vein
2	Deep cervical nodes	16	Subclavian vein
3	Right jugular trunk	17	Left brachiocephalic vein
4	Subclavian trunk	18	Mandible
5	Right bronchomediastinal trunk	19	Larynx
6	Thoracic duct	20	Internal jugular vein
7	**Cisterna chyli**	21	**Deep cervical nodes**
8	**Intestinal trunk**	22	Cervical nerve plexus
9	Right **lumbar trunk**	23	Superficial layer of deep fascia
10	Internal iliac nodes	24	Occipital nodes
11	**Inguinal nodes**	25	Parotid nodes
12	**Axillary nodes**	26	Popliteal nodes
13	Descending trunk		
14	Descending aorta		

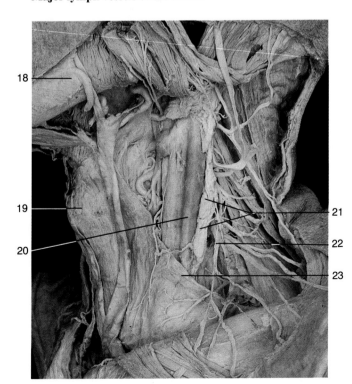

Deep cervical nodes, adjacent to the internal jugular vein.

Lymphatic vessels originate in the tissue spaces (lymph capillaries) and unite to form larger vessels (lymphatics). These resemble veins but have a much thinner wall, more valves and are interrupted by lymph nodes at various intervals. Large groups of lymph nodes are located in the inguinal and axillary regions, deep to the mandible and sternocleidomastoid muscle and within the root of the mesentery of the intestine.

Head and Neck

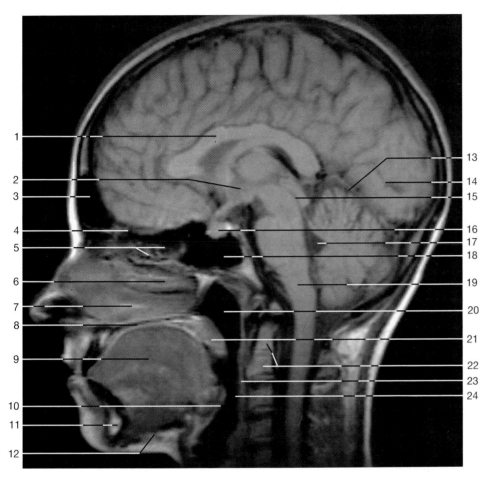

1 Corpus callosum
2 **Hypothalamus**
3 Frontal sinus
4 Cribriform plate
5 Ethmoidal air cells
6 Middle nasal concha
7 Inferior nasal concha
8 Hard palate
9 **Tongue**
10 Epiglottis
11 Mandible
12 Mylohyoid muscle
13 Tentorium of cerebellum
14 Calcarine fissure
15 Cerebral aqueduct
16 **Pituitary gland**
17 Fourth ventricle
18 **Sphenoidal sinus**
19 Medulla oblongata
20 Nasopharynx
21 Uvula
22 Dens of axis
23 Constrictor muscle of pharynx
24 Oral part of pharynx
25 **Cerebrum** (right hemisphere)
26 Calvaria
27 **Cerebellum**

Sagittal section through head and neck (MRI scan. 23-year-old female, courtesy of Prof. Dr. A. Heuck, Munich).

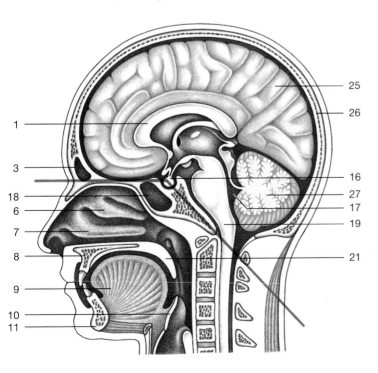

Sagittal section through the head (schematic drawing). The red line represents the border between the neurocranium and viscerocranium forming the clivus angle. The neural cavity contains the brain; the viscerocranium comprises the orbit, the nasal cavity and the oral cavity arranged one beneath the other.

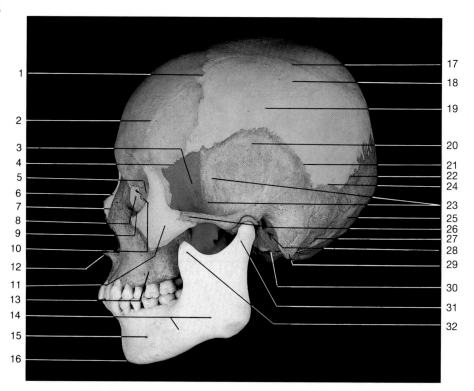

1	Coronal suture
2	**Frontal bone**
3	**Sphenoid bone**
4	Sphenofrontal suture
5	**Ethmoid bone**
6	**Nasal bone**
7	Nasomaxillary suture
8	**Lacrimal bone**
9	Lacrimomaxillary suture
10	Lacrimoethmoid suture
11	**Zygomatic bone**
12	Anterior nasal spine
13	**Maxilla**
14	**Mandible**
15	Mental foramen
16	Mental protuberance
17	Superior temporal line
18	Inferior temporal line
19	**Parietal bone**
20	**Temporal bone**
21	Squamous suture
22	Lambdoid suture
23	Temporal fossa
24	Parietomastoid suture
25	**Occipital bone**
26	Zygomatic arch
27	Occipitomastoid suture
28	External acoustic meatus
29	Mastoid process
30	Tympanic portion of temporal bone
31	Condylar process of mandible
32	Coronoid process of mandible

General architecture of the skull (lateral aspect). The different bones are indicated in color (numbers cf. table).

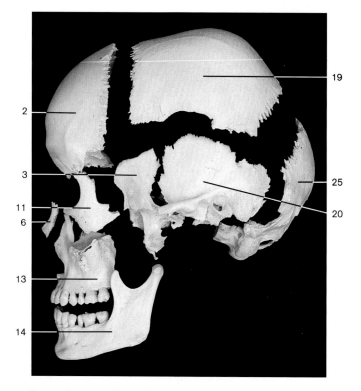

2 Frontal bone (orange)		
19 Parietal bone (light green)		
3 Greater wing of sphenoid bone (red)		Cranial bones
25 Squama of occipital bone (blue)		
20 Squama of temporal bone (brown)		
5 Ethmoid bone (dark green)		
3 Sphenoid bone (red)		
Temporal bone excluding squama (brown)		Base of skull
30 Tympanic portion of temporal bone (dark brown)		
Occipital bone excluding squama (blue)		
6 Nasal bone (white)		
8 Lacrimal bone (yellow)		
Inferior nasal concha		
Vomer		Facial bones
11 Zygomatic bone (light yellow)		
Palatine bone		
13 Maxilla (violet)		
14 Mandible (white)		
Malleus Incus Stapes	within petrous portion of temporal bone	Auditory ossicles
Hyoid		

Lateral aspect of the disarticulated skull (palatine bone, lacrimal bone, ethmoid bone and vomer are not depicted).

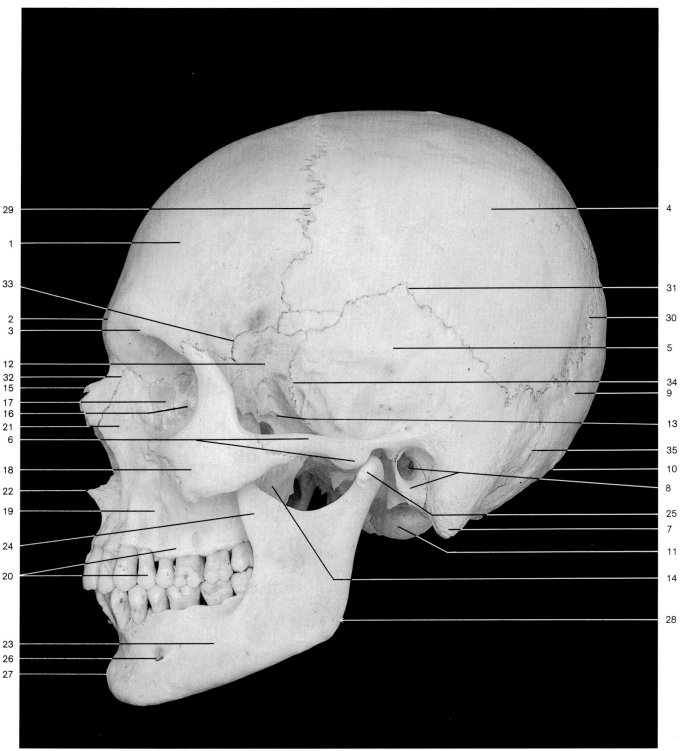

Lateral aspect of the skull.

1	**Frontal bone**
2	Glabella
3	Supraorbital margin
4	**Parietal bone**
5	**Temporal bone** (squamous part)
6	Zygomatic process (articular tubercle)
7	Mastoid process
8	Tympanic part (tympanic plate) and external acoustic meatus
9	**Occipital bone** (squamous part)
10	External occipital protuberance
11	Occipital condyle
12	**Sphenoid bone** (greater wing)
13	Infratemporal crest of sphenoid
14	Pterygoid process (lateral pterygoid plate)
15	**Nasal bone**
16	**Ethmoid bone** (orbital part)
17	**Lacrimal bone**
18	**Zygomatic bone**
19	**Maxilla** (body)
20	Alveolar process and teeth
21	Frontal process
22	Anterior nasal spine
23	**Mandible** (body)
24	Coronoid process
25	Condylar process
26	Mental foramen
27	Mental protuberance
28	Angle of the mandible

Sutures

29 Coronal suture
30 Lambdoid suture
31 Squamous suture
32 Nasomaxillary suture
33 Frontosphenoid suture
34 Sphenosquamosal suture
35 Occipitomastoid suture

26

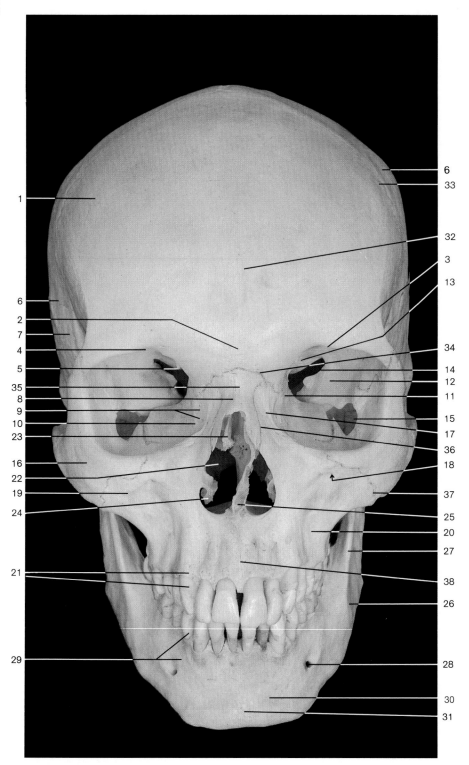

Anterior aspect of the skull.

1 **Frontal bone**
2 Glabella
3 Supraorbital margin
4 Supraorbital notch
5 Trochlear spine
6 **Parietal bone**
7 **Temporal bone**
8 **Nasal bone**

Orbit
9 Lacrimal bone
10 Posterior lacrimal crest
11 Ethmoid bone

Sphenoid bone
12 Greater wing of sphenoid bone
13 Lesser wing of sphenoid bone
14 Superior orbital fissure
15 Inferior orbital fissure
16 **Zygomatic bone**

Maxilla
17 Frontal process
18 Infraorbital foramen
19 Zygomatic process
20 Body of maxilla
21 Alveolar process with teeth

Nasal cavity
22 Anterior nasal aperture
23 Middle nasal concha
24 Inferior nasal concha
25 Nasal septum, vomer

Mandible
26 Body of mandible
27 Ramus of mandible
28 Mental foramen
29 Alveolar part with teeth
30 Base of mandible
31 Mental protuberance

Sutures
32 Frontal suture
33 Coronal suture
34 Frontonasal suture
35 Internasal suture
36 Nasomaxillary suture
37 Zygomaticomaxillary suture
38 Intermaxillary suture

The skull comprises a mosaic of numerous complicated bones which form the cranial cavity protecting the brain (**neurocranium**) and several cavities such as nasal and oral cavities in the facial region. The neurocranium consists of large bony plates which develop directly from the surrounding sheets of connective tissue (**desmocranium**). The bones of the skull base are formed out of cartilaginous tissue (**chondrocranium**) which ossifies secondarily. The **visceral skeleton** which, in fish, gives rise to the gills has, in higher vertebrates, been transformed into the bones of the masticatory and auditory apparatus (maxilla, mandible, auditory ossicles and hyoid bone).

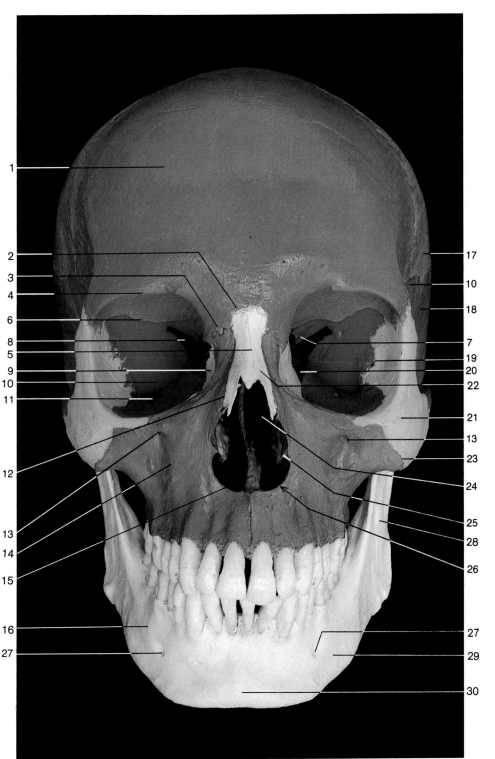

1	**Frontal bone**
2	Frontonasal suture
3	Frontomaxillary suture
4	Supraorbital margin
5	Internasal suture
6	Sphenofrontal suture
7	Optic canal in lesser wing of sphenoid bone
8	Superior orbital fissure
9	**Lacrimal bone**
10	**Sphenoid bone** (greater wing)
11	Inferior orbital fissure
12	Nasomaxillary suture
13	Infraorbital foramen
14	**Maxilla**
15	**Vomer**
16	Body of mandible
17	**Parietal bone**
18	**Temporal bone**
19	Sphenozygomatic suture
20	**Ethmoid bone**
21	**Zygomatic bone**
22	**Nasal bone**
23	Zygomaticomaxillary suture
24	Middle nasal concha
25	Inferior nasal concha
26	Anterior nasal aperture
27	Mental foramen
28	Ramus of mandible
29	Base of mandible
30	Mental protuberance

Bones
Frontal bone (brown)
Parietal bone (light green)
Temporal bone (dark brown)
Sphenoidal bone (red)
Zygomatic bone (yellow)
Ethmoid bone (dark green)
Lacrimal bone (yellow)
Vomer (orange)
Maxilla (violet)
Nasal bone (white)
Mandible (white)

Anterior aspect of the skull (individual bones indicated by color).

The following series of figures are arranged so that the mosaic-like pattern of the skull becomes understandable. It starts with the bones of the **skull base** (sphenoid and occipital) to which the other bones are added step by step. The facial skeleton is built up by the ethmoid bone to which the palatine bone and maxilla are attached laterally; the small nasal and lacrimal bones fill the remaining spaces. Cartilages remain only in the external part of the nose.

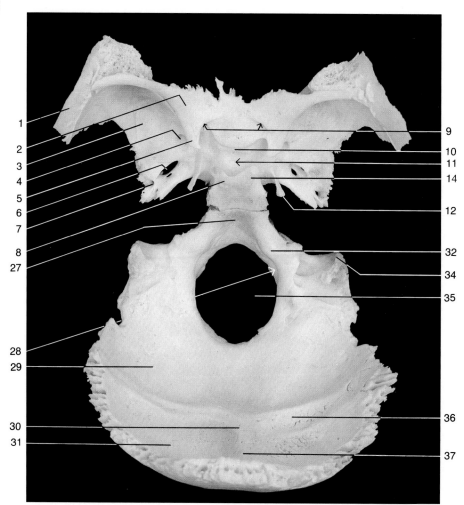

Sphenoid and occipital bone (from above).

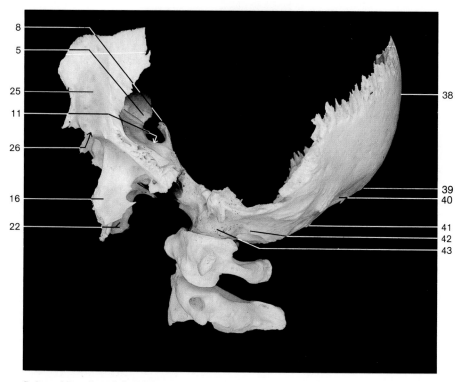

Sphenoid and occipital bone in connection with the atlas and axis
(1st and 2nd cervical vertebrae) (left lateral view).

Sphenoid bone
1 **Greater wing**
2 **Lesser wing**
3 Cerebral or superior surface of greater wing
4 **Foramen rotundum**
5 Anterior clinoid process
6 Foramen ovale
7 Foramen spinosum
8 Dorsum sellae
9 Optic canal
10 Chiasmatic groove (sulcus chiasmatis)
11 **Hypophysial fossa (sella turcica)**
12 Lingula
13 Opening of sphenoidal sinus
14 Posterior clinoid process
15 **Pterygoid canal**
16 Lateral pterygoid plate of **pterygoid process**
17 Pterygoid notch
18 Pterygoid hamulus
19 Orbital surface of greater wing
20 Sphenoid crest
21 Sphenoid rostrum
22 Medial pterygoid plate
23 Superior orbital fissure
24 Spine of sphenoid
25 Temporal surface of greater wing
26 Infratemporal crest

Occipital bone
27 **Clivus** with basilar part of occipital bone
28 **Hypoglossal canal**
29 Fossa for cerebellar hemisphere
30 Internal occipital protuberance
31 Fossa for cerebral hemisphere
32 Jugular tubercle
33 Condylar canal
34 Jugular process
35 **Foramen magnum**
36 Groove for transverse sinus
37 Groove for superior sagittal sinus
38 **Squamous part** of the occipital bone
39 External occipital protuberance
40 Superior nuchal line
41 Inferior nuchal line
42 Condylar fossa
43 **Condyle**
44 Pharyngeal tubercle
45 External occipital crest

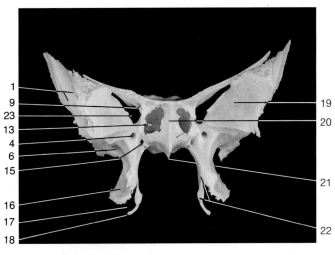

Sphenoid bone (anterior aspect).

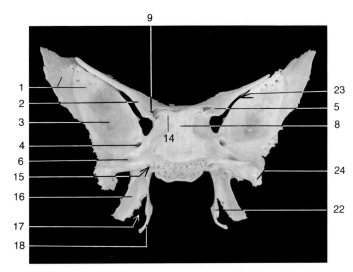

Sphenoid bone (posterior aspect).

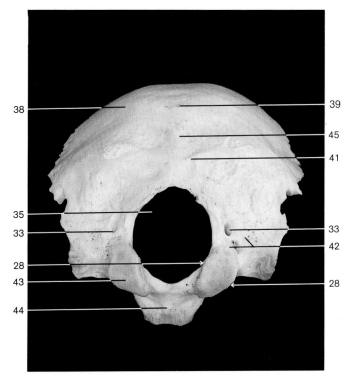

Occipital bone (from below).

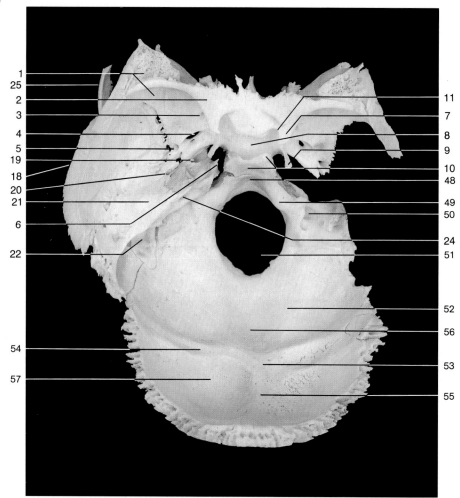

Sphenoid bone
1 **Greater wing**
2 **Lesser wing**
3 Foramen rotundum
4 **Foramen ovale**
5 Foramen spinosum
6 Foramen lacerum
7 Anterior clinoid process
8 Hypophysial fossa (**sella turcica**)
9 Lingula
10 Dorsum sellae and posterior clinoid process
11 **Optic canal**
12 Sphenoid rostrum
13 Medial pterygoid plate
14 Lateral pterygoid plate
15 Pterygoid hamulus
16 Infratemporal crest
17 Body of the sphenoid

Temporal bone
18 **Squamous part**
19 **Carotid canal**
20 Hiatus of facial canal (for the greater petrosal nerve)
21 Arcuate eminence
22 Groove for the sigmoid sinus
23 Mastoid foramen
24 **Internal acoustic meatus**
25 Zygomatic process
26 Mandibular fossa
27 Petrotympanic fissure
28 Canalis musculotubarius (bony part of auditory tube)
29 **External acoustic meatus**
30 Styloid process (remnant only)
31 Stylomastoid foramen
32 Mastoid canaliculus
33 Jugular fossa
34 **Mastoid process**
35 Mastoid notch

Sphenoid, occipital and left temporal bone (from above). Internal aspect of the base of the skull. The left temporal bone has been added to the preceding figure.

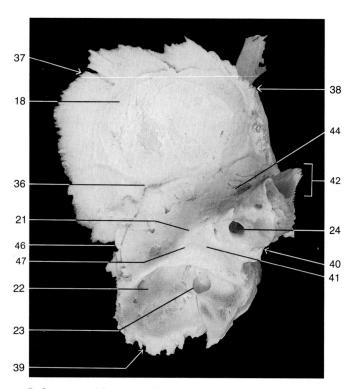

Left temporal bone (medial aspect).

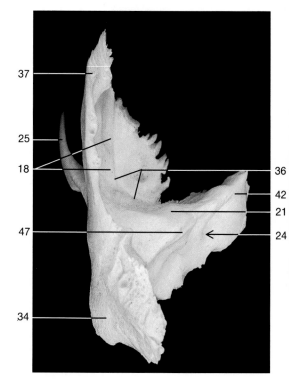

Left temporal bone (from above).

36 Groove for middle
    meningeal vessels
37 Parietal margin
38 Sphenoid margin
39 Occipital margin
40 Cochlear canaliculus
41 Aqueduct of the vestibule
42 Apex of the petrous part
43 **Tympanic part**
44 Trigeminal impression
45 **Articular tubercle**
46 Parietal notch
47 Groove for the superior
    petrosal sinus

Occipital bone
48 **Clivus**
49 Jugular tubercle
50 Condylar canal
51 **Foramen magnum**
52 Lower part of squamous
    occipital bone
    (cerebellar fossa)
53 Internal occipital protuberance
54 Groove for the transverse sinus
55 Groove for the superior sagittal sinus
56 Internal occipital crest
57 Upper part of squamous occipital
    bone (cerebral fossa)
58 **Condyle**
59 Nuchal plane
60 Superior nuchal line
61 **External occipital protuberance**
62 **Jugular foramen**
63 Inferior nuchal line
64 Pharyngeal tubercle
65 **Spheno-occipital synchondrosis**

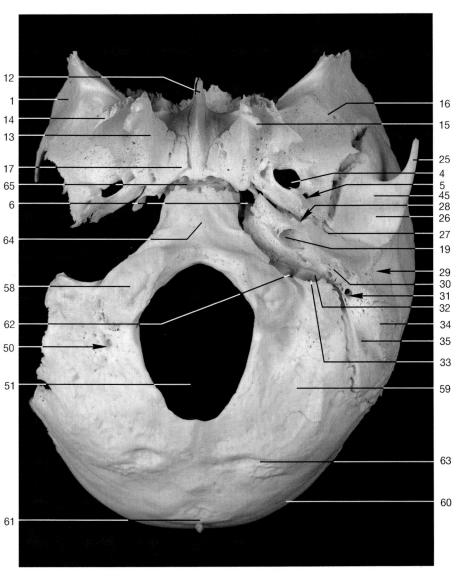

Sphenoid, occipital and left temporal bone. Base of the skull (external aspect).

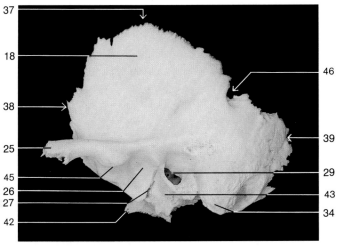

Left temporal bone (lateral aspect).

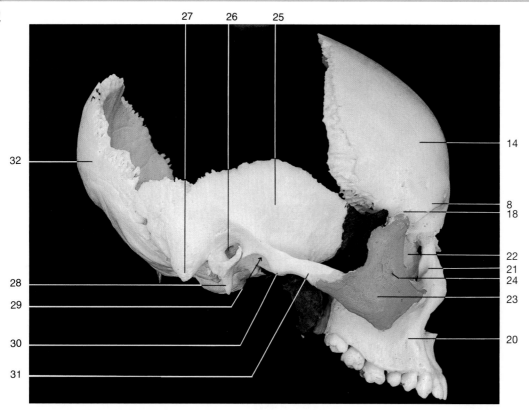

Part of a disarticulated skull (right lateral aspect). The **frontal bone** and the maxilla are connected with the temporal bone by the zygomatic bone (orange). Sphenoid bone (dark green), palatine bone (red), lacrimal bone (yellow).

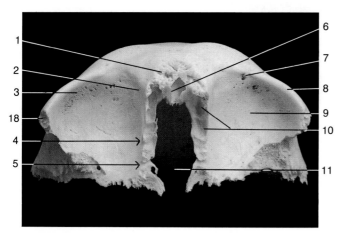

Frontal bone (inferior aspect). The ethmoidal foveolae cover the ethmoidal cavities of the ethmoid bone.

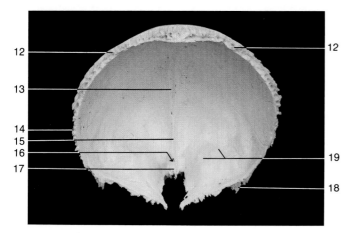

Frontal bone (posterior aspect).

Frontal bone
1 Nasal margin
2 Trochlear fossa
3 Fossa for lacrimal gland
4 Anterior ethmoidal foramen
5 Posterior ethmoidal foramen
6 Nasal spine
7 Supraorbital notch
8 Supraorbital margin
9 **Orbital plate**
10 Roofs of the ethmoidal air cells
11 Ethmoidal notch
12 Parietal margin
13 Groove for superior sagittal sinus
14 **Squamous part** of frontal bone
15 Frontal crest
16 Foramen cecum
17 Nasal spine
18 **Zygomatic process** of frontal bone
19 Juga cerebralia

Facial bones
20 **Maxilla**
21 Frontal process of maxilla
22 **Lacrimal bone** (yellow)
23 **Zygomatic bone** (orange)
24 Zygomaticofacial foramen

Temporal bone
25 Squamous part of temporal bone
26 External acoustic meatus
27 **Mastoid process**
28 **Styloid process**
29 **Mandibular fossa**
30 Articular tubercle
31 Zygomatic process

Occipital bone
32 Squamous part of occipital bone

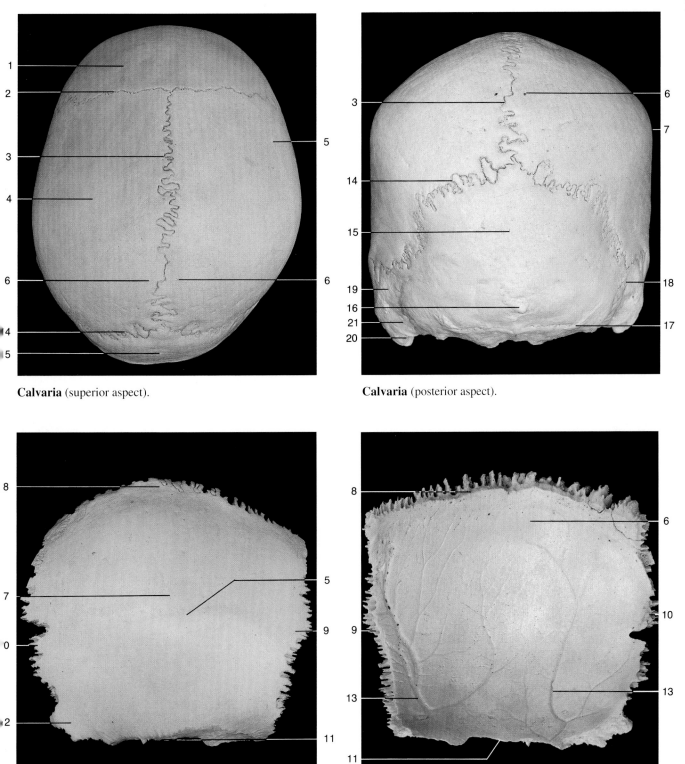

Calvaria (superior aspect).

Calvaria (posterior aspect).

Left parietal bone (external aspect).

Left parietal bone (internal aspect).

1	**Frontal bone**	8	Sagittal margin
2	Coronal suture	9	Occipital margin
3	Sagittal suture	10	Frontal margin
4	**Parietal bone**	11	Squamous margin
5	Superior temporal line	12	Sphenoidal angle
6	Parietal foramen	13	Groove for middle meningeal artery
7	Parietal tuber or eminence	14	Lambdoid suture

15	**Occipital bone**
16	External occipital protuberance
17	Inferior nuchal line
18	Occipitomastoid suture
19	**Temporal bone**
20	Mastoid process
21	Mastoid notch

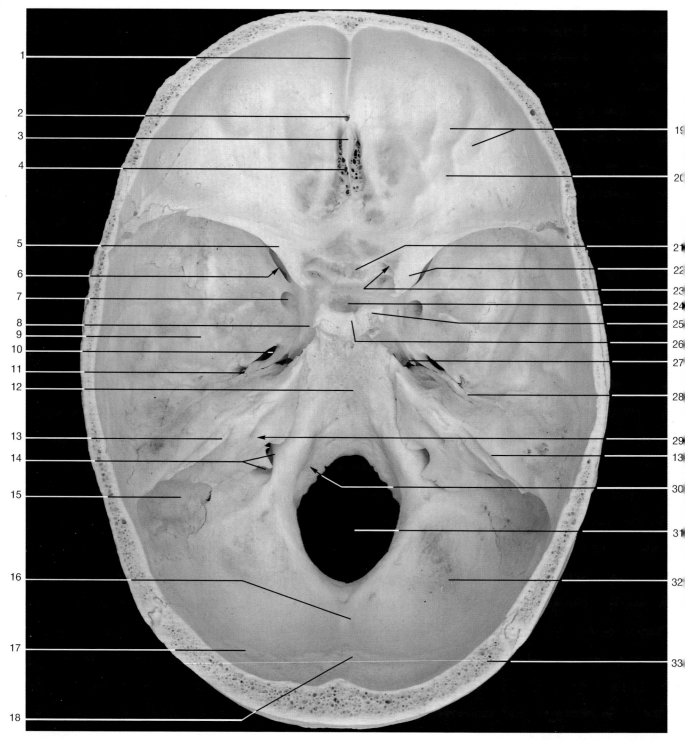

Base of the skull, calvaria removed (internal aspect).

1 Frontal crest
2 Foramen cecum
3 **Crista galli**
4 **Cribriform plate** of ethmoid bone
5 Lesser wing of sphenoid bone
6 Superior orbital fissure
7 **Foramen rotundum**
8 **Carotid sulcus**
9 Middle cranial fossa
10 **Foramen ovale**
11 Foramen spinosum

12 **Clivus**
13 Groove for superior petrosal sinus
14 **Jugular foramen**
15 Groove for sigmoid sinus
16 Internal occipital crest
17 Groove for transverse sinus
18 Internal occipital protuberance
19 Digitate impressions
20 Anterior cranial fossa
21 Chiasmatic sulcus
22 Anterior clinoid process
23 **Optic canal**

24 **Sella turcica** (hypophysial fossa)
25 Posterior clinoid process
26 Dorsum sellae
27 **Foramen lacerum**
28 Groove for greater petrosal nerve
29 Internal acoustic meatus
30 **Hypoglossal canal**
31 **Foramen magnum**
32 Posterior cranial fossa
33 Diploe

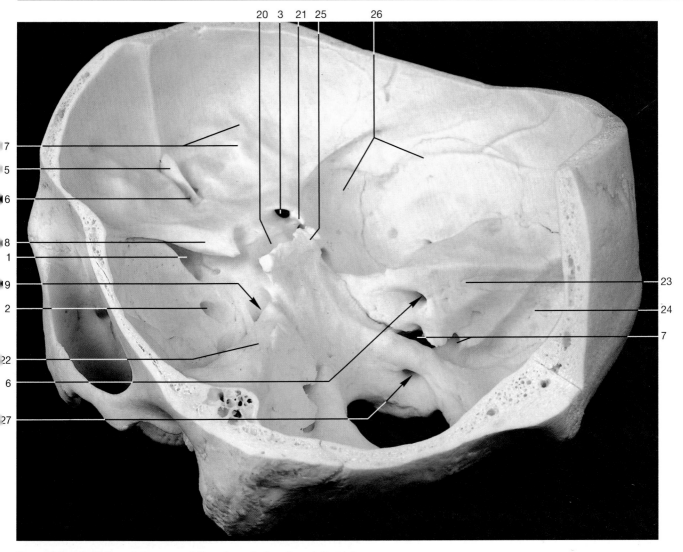

Base of the skull (internal aspect, oblique lateral view from left side).

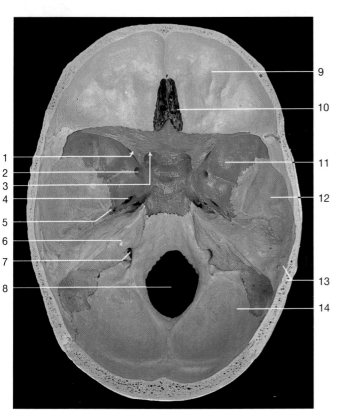

Canals, fissures and foramina of the base of the skull

1 Superior orbital fissure
2 Foramen rotundum
3 Optic canal
4 Foramen ovale
5 Foramen spinosum
6 Internal acoustic meatus
7 Jugular foramen
8 Foramen magnum

Bones

9 Frontal bone (orange)
10 Ethmoid bone (dark green)
11 Sphenoid bone (red)
12 Temporal bone (brown)
13 Parietal bone (yellow-green)
14 Occipital bone (blue)

Details of bones

15 Crista galli
16 Cribriform plate

17 Digitate impressions (frontal bone)
18 Lesser wing of sphenoid bone
19 Foramen lacerum
20 Hypophysial fossa (sella turcica)
21 Anterior clinoid process
22 Trigeminal impression
23 Petrous part of temporal bone
24 Groove for sigmoid sinus
25 Dorsum sellae (posterior clinoid process)
26 Greater wing of sphenoid bone, groove for middle meningeal artery
27 Hypoglossal canal

Base of the skull (internal aspect, superior view).
Individual bones indicated by color.

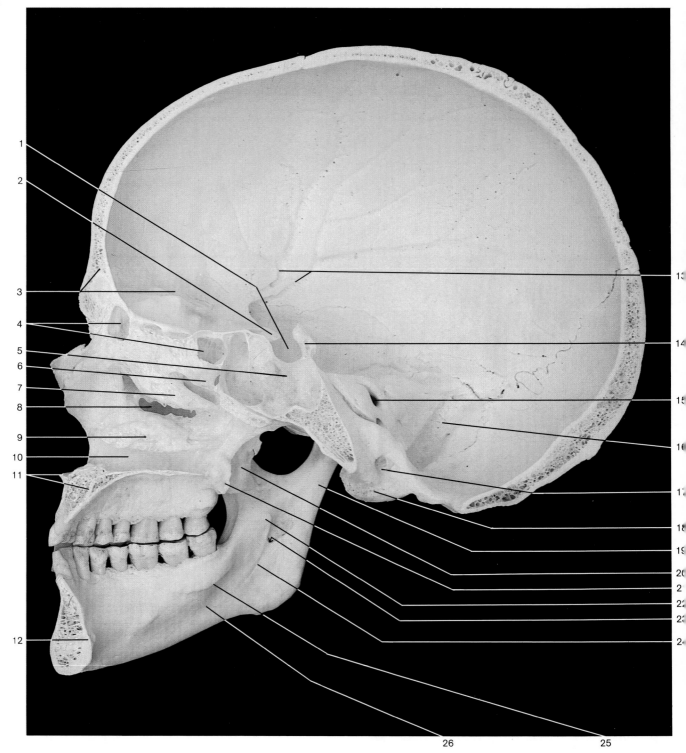

Median section through the skull, right half (internal aspect).

1	**Hypophysial fossa (sella turcica)**	
2	Anterior clinoid process	
3	**Frontal bone**	
4	**Ethmoidal air cells**	
5	**Sphenoidal sinus**	
6	Superior concha	
7	Middle concha	
8	**Maxillary hiatus**	
9	**Inferior concha**	
10	Inferior meatus	
11	Anterior nasal spine and maxilla	
12	Mental spine or genial tubercle	
13	Groove for middle meningeal artery	

14	Dorsum sellae	
15	Internal acoustic meatus	
16	Groove for sigmoid sinus	
17	**Hypoglossal canal**	
18	**Occipital condyle**	
19	Condylar process	
20	Lateral pterygoid plate	} of **pterygoid process**
21	Medial pterygoid plate	
22	Lingula of mandible	
23	**Mandibular foramen**	
24	Mylohyoid groove	
25	Mylohyoid line	
26	Submandibular fovea	

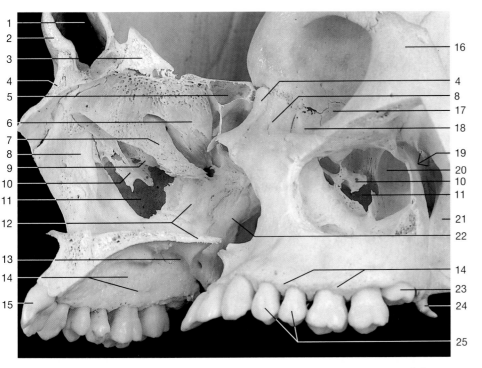

1 Frontal sinus
2 **Frontal bone**
3 Crista galli
4 **Nasal bone**
5 Sphenoidal sinus
6 **Superior concha** ⎱ of **ethmoid**
7 **Middle concha** ⎰ **bone**
8 Frontal process of maxilla
9 Ethmoidal bulla
10 **Uncinate process**
11 Maxillary hiatus
12 **Palatine bone**
13 Greater palatine foramen
14 **Alveolar process of maxilla**
15 Central incisor
16 Zygomatic bone
17 Ethmoid bone
18 **Lacrimal bone**
19 Pterygopalatine fossa
20 **Maxillary sinus**
21 Lateral pterygoid plate
22 Medial pterygoid plate
23 Third molar tooth
24 Pterygoid hamulus
25 Two premolar teeth

Facial part of the skull (viscerocranium), divided in two halves (lateral and medial aspect). Right inferior concha has been removed to show the maxillary hiatus. Left maxillary sinus opened.

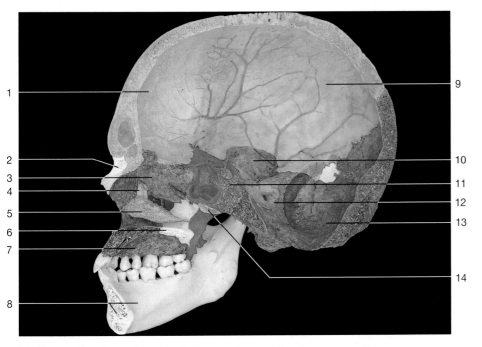

Bones (indicated by colors)
1 Frontal bone (yellow)
2 Nasal bone (white)
3 Ethmoid bone (dark green)
4 Lacrimal bone (yellow)
5 Inferior nasal concha (pink)
6 Palatine bone (white)
7 Maxilla (violet)
8 Mandible (white)
9 Parietal bone (light green)
10 Temporal bone (brown)
11 Sphenoid bone (red)
12 Petrous part of temporal bone (brown)
13 Occipital bone (blue)
14 Ala of vomer (light brown)

Median section through the skull. The nasal septum has been removed. Bones indicated by colors.

Because of the upright posture which the human developed in the course of evolution, the cranial cavity greatly increased in size, whereas the facial skeleton decreased. As a result, the base of the skull developed an angulation of about 120° between the clivus and the cribriform plate (see drawing on page 23). The hypophysial fossa containing the pituitary gland lies at the angle formed between these two planes.

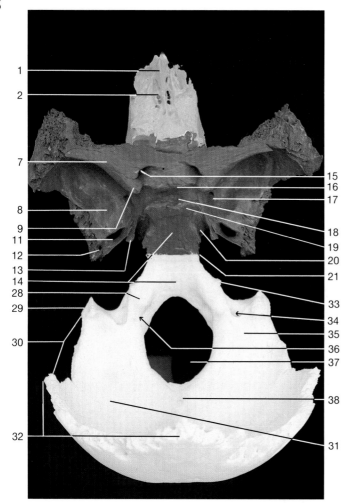

Ethmoid bone
1 Crista galli
2 Cribriform plate
3 Ethmoidal air cells
4 Middle concha
5 Perpendicular plate (part of nasal septum)
6 Orbital plate

Sphenoid bone
7 Lesser wing
8 Greater wing
9 Anterior clinoid process
10 Posterior clinoid process
11 Foramen ovale
12 Foramen spinosum
13 Lingula of the sphenoid
14 Clivus
15 Optic canal
16 Tuberculum sellae
17 Foramen rotundum (right side)
18 Hypophysial fossa (sella turcica)
19 Dorsum sellae
20 Carotid sulcus
21 Spheno-occipital synchondrosis
22 Lateral pterygoid plate
23 Greater wing of sphenoid bone (orbital surface)
24 Greater wing of sphenoid bone (maxillary surface)
25 Foramen rotundum (left side)
26 Superior orbital fissure
27 Infratemporal crest of the greater wing

Part of the disarticulated base of the skull.
Ethmoid, sphenoid and occipital bones (from above).
Green = sphenoid bone; yellow = ethmoid bone.

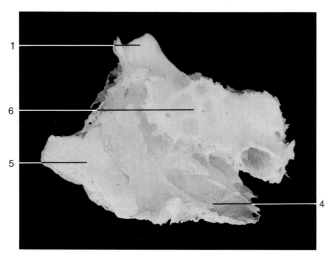

Ethmoid bone (lateral aspect), posterior portion to the right.

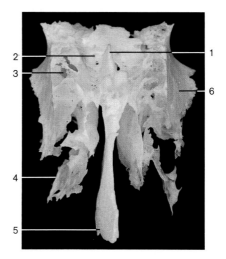

Ethmoid bone (anterior aspect).

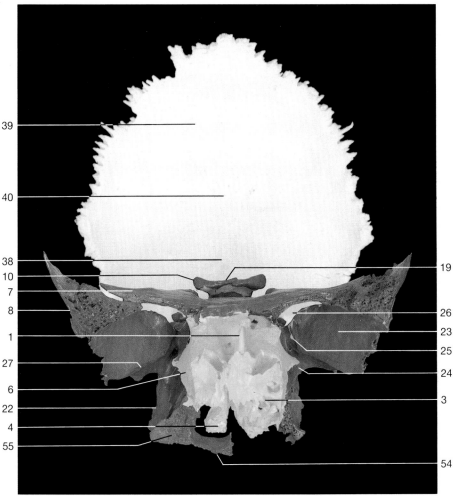

Occipital bone
28 Jugular tubercle
29 Jugular process
30 Mastoid margin
31 Posterior cranial fossa
32 Lambdoid margin
33 Intrajugular process
34 Condylar canal
35 Lateral part of occipital bone
36 Hypoglossal canal
37 Foramen magnum
38 Internal occipital crest
39 Squamous part of occipital bone
40 Internal occipital protuberance

Maxilla
41 Orbital surface
42 Infraorbital groove
43 Maxillary tuberosity with foramina
44 Frontal process
45 Nasolacrimal groove
46 Infraorbital margin
47 Anterior nasal spine
48 Zygomatic process
49 Alveolar process

Palatine bone
50 Orbital process
51 Sphenopalatine notch
52 Sphenoidal process
53 Perpendicular plate
54 Horizontal plate
55 Pyramidal process

Disarticulated base of the skull (anterior aspect).
Green = sphenoid bone; yellow = ethmoid bone; red = palatine bone.

Right maxilla, ethmoid and palatine bone (lateral aspect).

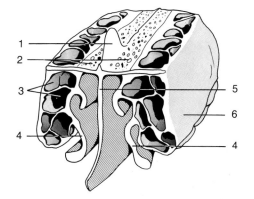

Ethmoid bone (oblique anterior aspect).
(Schematic drawing.)

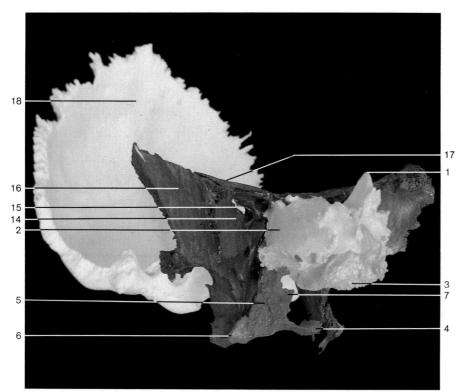

Part of a disarticulated skull base, similar to the foregoing figures, but with palatine bone. Green = sphenoid bone; yellow = ethmoid bone; red = palatine bone.

Ethmoid bone
1 Crista galli
2 Orbital plate
3 Middle concha

Palatine bone
4 Horizontal plate of palatine bone
5 Greater palatine canal
6 Pyramidal process
7 Maxillary process
8 Orbital process
9 Sphenopalatine notch
10 Perpendicular plate of palatine bone
11 Conchal crest
12 Nasal crest
13 Sphenoidal process

Sphenoid bone
14 Greater wing
15 Superior orbital fissure
16 Greater wing (orbital surface)
17 Lesser wing

Occipital bone
18 Squamous part of occipital bone

Maxilla
19 Maxillary tuberosity
20 Frontal process
21 Orbital surface
22 Infraorbital margin
23 Infraorbital groove
24 Zygomatic process
25 Alveolar process

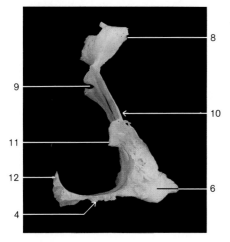

Left palatine bone (medial aspect, posterior aspect to the left).

Left palatine bone (anterior aspect).

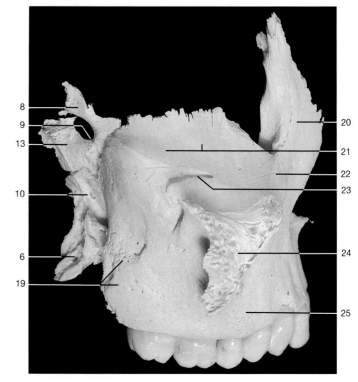

Right maxilla and right palatine bone (lateral aspect).

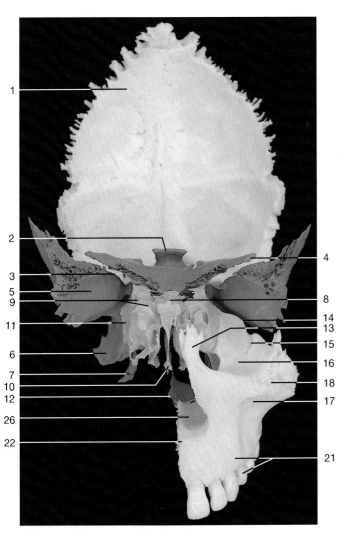

Occipital bone
1 Squamous part

Sphenoid bone
2 Dorsum sellae
3 Superior orbital fissure
4 Lesser wing
5 Greater wing (orbital surface)
6 Lateral pterygoid plate
7 Medial pterygoid plate

Ethmoid bone
8 Crista galli
9 Ethmoidal air cells
10 Perpendicular plate
11 Orbital plate

Palatine bone
12 Horizontal plate (nasal crest)

Maxilla
13 Frontal process
14 Inferior orbital fissure
15 Infraorbital groove
16 Orbital surface
17 Infraorbital foramen
18 Zygomatic process
19 Anterior lacrimal crest
20 Canine fossa
21 Alveolar process with teeth
22 Anterior nasal spine
23 Juga alveolaria (elevations formed by roots of teeth)
24 Lacrimal groove
25 Maxillary tuberosity with alveolar foramina
26 Palatine process of maxilla

Part of a disarticulated skull.
The left **maxilla** is added to the preceding specimen.

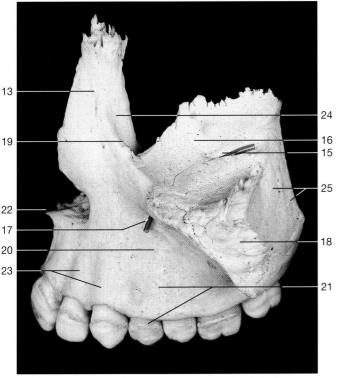

Left maxilla (lateral aspect). Probe = infraorbital canal.

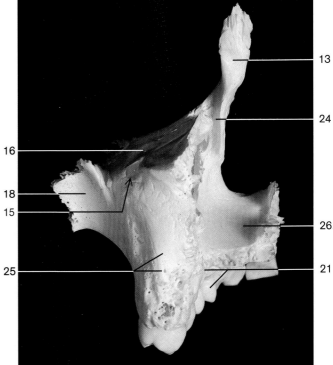

Left maxilla (posterior aspect).

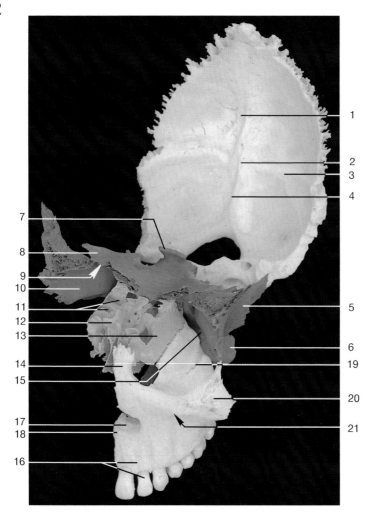

Part of a disarticulated base of skull. The mosaic of the facial bones [sphenoid bone (green), ethmoid bone (yellow), and palatine bone (red)] is seen from the anterior-lateral aspect.

Occipital bone
1 Groove for superior sagittal sinus
2 Internal occipital protuberance
3 Groove for transverse sinus
4 Internal occipital crest

Sphenoid bone
5 Greater wing (temporal surface)
6 Lateral pterygoid plate
7 Dorsum sellae
8 Lesser wing
9 Superior orbital fissure
10 Greater wing (orbital surface)

Ethmoid bone
11 Ethmoidal air cells
12 Crista galli
13 Orbital plate

Maxilla
14 Frontal process
15 Inferior orbital fissure
16 Alveolar process with teeth
17 Palatine process
18 Anterior nasal spine
19 Infraorbital groove
20 Zygomatic process
21 Location of infraorbital foramen
22 Middle nasal meatus
23 Inferior nasal meatus
24 Maxillary hiatus
     (leading to maxillary sinus)
25 Third molar
26 Lacrimal groove
27 Conchal crest
28 Body of maxilla (nasal surface)
29 Nasal crest
30 Incisive canal

Palatine bone
31 Orbital process
32 Sphenopalatine notch
33 Sphenoidal process
34 Perpendicular plate
35 Conchal crest
36 Horizontal plate
37 Pyramidal process

Frontal bone
38 Squamous part
39 Supraorbital foramen
40 Frontal notch
41 Frontal spine

Inferior nasal concha
42 Inferior nasal concha
     with maxillary process

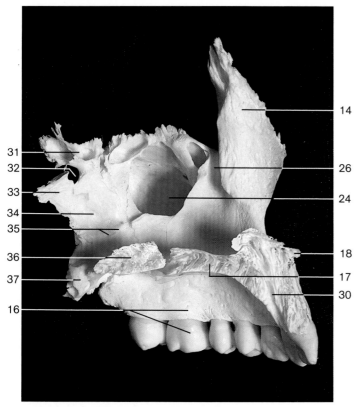

Left maxilla and palatine bone (medial aspect).

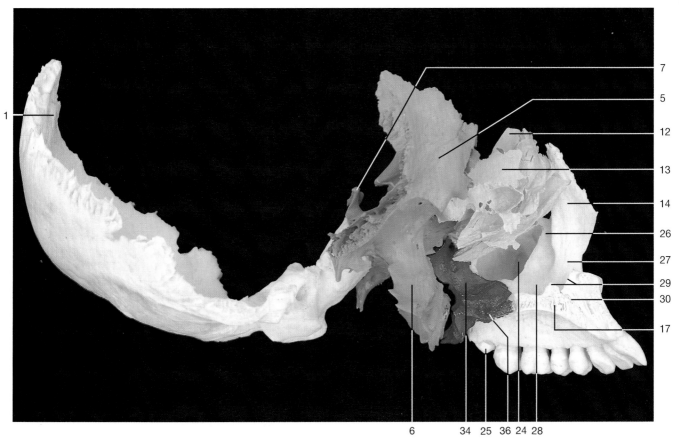

7
5
12
13
14
26
27
29
30
17

1

6   34   25   36 24 28

Part of a disarticulated base of skull (medial aspect). Green = sphenoid bone; yellow = ethmoid bone; red = palatine bone; natural colored = left maxilla.

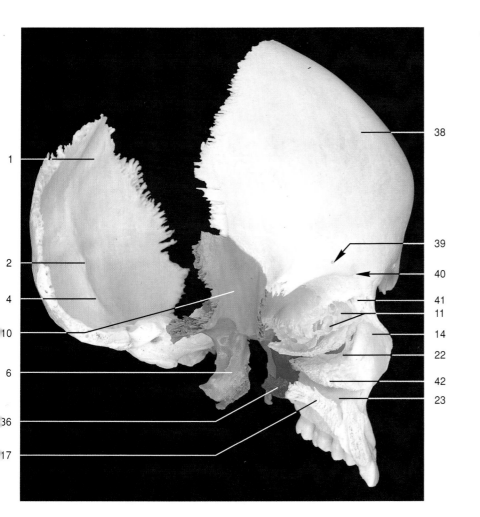

1

2

4

10

6

36

17

38

39

40

41
11

14

22

42

23

Part of a disarticulated base of skull. The same specimen as shown above but with frontal bone (oblique-lateral aspect).

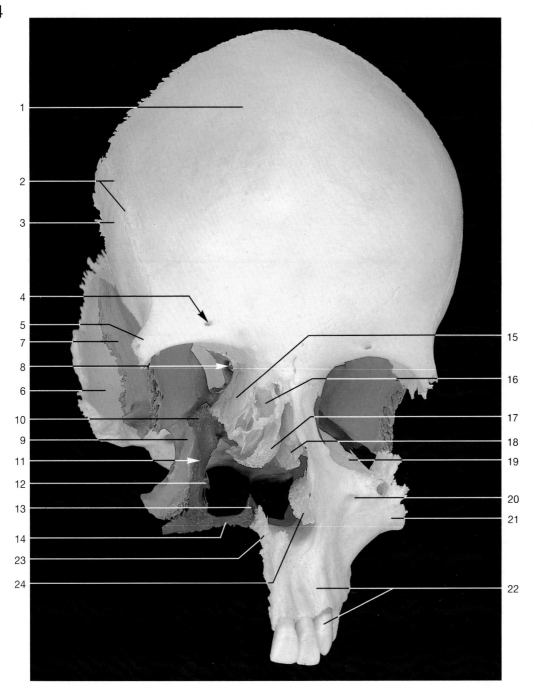

Part of a disarticulated skull, showing the connection of the palatine bone (red) and the maxilla with ethmoid bone (yellow) and sphenoid bone (light green) (anterior aspect).

Frontal bone
1 Squamous part
2 Inferior temporal line
3 Temporal surface
4 Supraorbital foramen
5 Zygomatic process

Occipital bone
6 Squamous part

Sphenoid bone
7 Greater wing (temporal surface)
8 Optic canal within the lesser wing
9 Lateral pterygoid plate

Palatine bone
10 Orbital process
11 Perpendicular plate
12 Conchal crest
13 Nasal crest
14 Horizontal plate

Ethmoid bone
15 Orbital plate
16 Ethmoidal air cell
17 Middle concha
18 Perpendicular plate
　 (part of bony nasal septum)

Maxilla
19 Infraorbital groove
20 Infraorbital foramen
21 Zygomatic process
22 Alveolar process with teeth
23 Palatine process

Left inferior nasal concha
24 Anterior part of
　 inferior concha

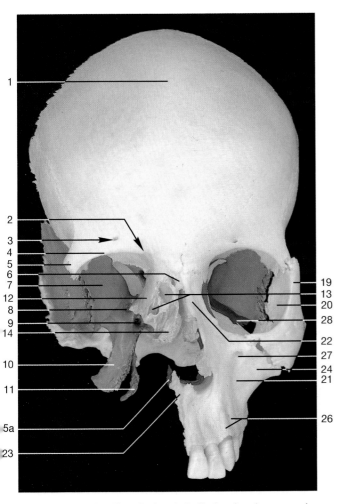

Frontal bone
1 Squamous part
2 Frontal notch
3 Supraorbital foramen
4 Supraorbital margin
5 Zygomatic process
6 Frontal spine

Sphenoid bone
7 Greater wing (orbital surface)
8 Foramen rotundum
9 Pterygoid or Vidian canal
10 Lateral pterygoid plate
11 Medial pterygoid plate

Ethmoid bone
12 Orbital plate
13 Ethmoidal air cells
14 Middle concha

Palatine bone
15 Horizontal plate
15a Nasal crest
16 Pyramidal process
17 Lesser palatine foramen
18 Greater palatine foramen

Zygomatic bone
19 Frontal process
20 Orbital surface

Maxilla
21 Canine fossa
22 Frontal process
23 Palatine process
24 Zygomatic process
25 Alveolar process and teeth
26 Juga alveolaria
27 Infraorbital foramen
28 Infraorbital groove
29 Anterior nasal aperture
30 Anterior nasal spine

Incisive bone
31 Central incisor and incisive bone or premaxilla
32 Incisive fossa

Vomer
33 Ala of the vomer

Sutures and choanae
34 Median palatine suture
35 Transverse palatine suture
36 Choanae

Anterior view of a disarticulated skull, showing the connection of the maxilla with the frontal and zygomatic bones. Yellow = ethmoid bone; red = palatine bone; green = sphenoid bone.

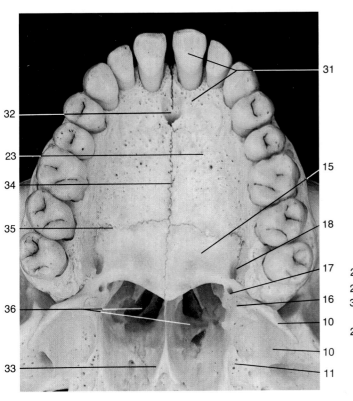

Bony palate and teeth of the maxillae (from below).

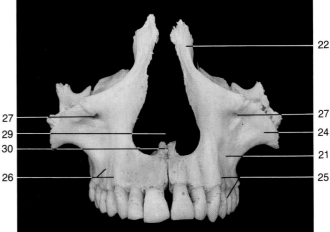

Anterior view of both maxillae, forming the anterior bony aperture of the nose.

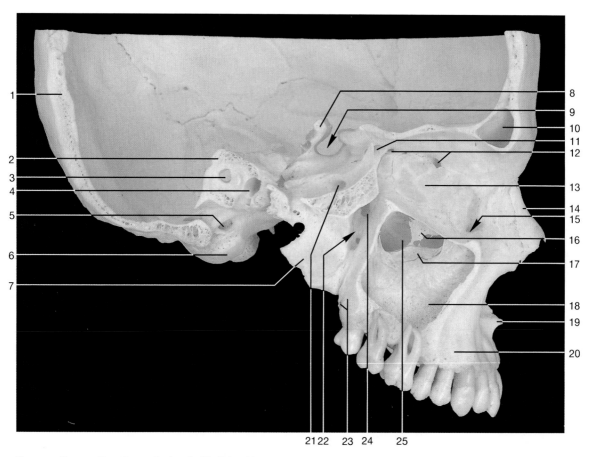

Paramedian section through the skull, right side (lateral aspect).
Frontal and maxillary sinus are opened.

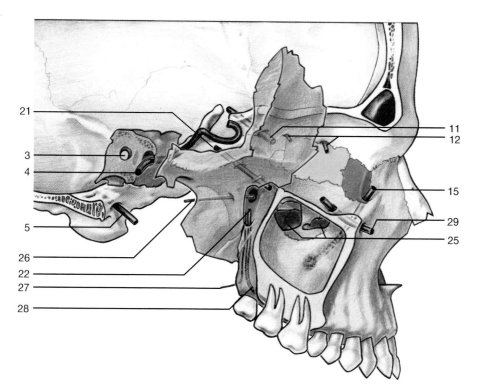

Illustration of canals and foramina connected with the right orbit and
pterygopalatine fossa (compare the above figure). The greater wing of sphenoid
bone (green) is shown as being transparent. Brown = temporal bone;
yellow = ethmoid bone; red = lacrimal bone; light red = inferior nasal concha;
violet = maxilla; orange = palatine bone.

1 Occipital bone
2 Temporal bone (petrous part)
3 **Internal acoustic meatus**
4 **Carotid canal**
5 **Hypoglossal canal**
6 Occipital condyle
7 Lateral plate of pterygoid process
8 Dorsum of sella turcica
9 Sella turcica
10 Frontal sinus
11 **Optic canal**
12 **Posterior** and **anterior**
    ethmoidal foramina
13 Orbital plate of ethmoidal bone
14 Nasal bone
15 **Nasolacrimal canal**
16 Uncinate process
17 Inferior nasal concha
    (maxillary process)
18 Maxillary sinus
19 Anterior nasal spine
20 Alveolar process of maxilla
21 **Foramen rotundum**
22 **Pterygopalatine fossa**
23 Tuberosity of maxilla
    with **alveolar foramina**
24 **Sphenopalatine foramen**
25 Maxillary hiatus
26 **Pterygoid** or Vidian **canal**
27 **Lesser palatine canal**
28 **Greater palatine canal**
29 **Infraorbital canal**

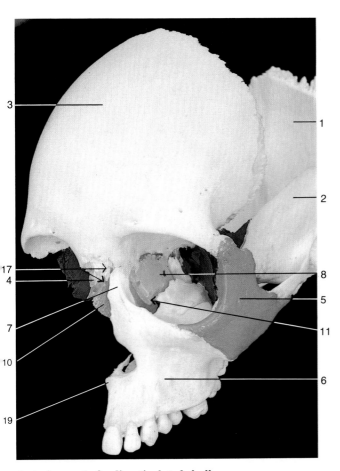

Anterior part of a disarticulated skull.
Orange = zygomatic bone; yellow = ethmoid bone;
green = sphenoidal bone. The arrows indicate the locations of
the lacrimal bone (11) and the nasal bone (17).

1 **Occipital bone**
2 **Temporal bone**
3 **Frontal bone**
4 Nasal spine of frontal bone
5 **Zygomatic bone**
6 **Maxilla**
7 Frontal process of maxilla
8 **Ethmoid bone**
9 Orbital plate of ethmoid bone
10 Perpendicular plate of ethmoid bone
11 Site of **lacrimal bone**
12 Lacrimal groove of lacrimal bone
13 Posterior lacrimal crest
14 Fossa for lacrimal sac
15 Lacrimal hamulus
16 Nasolacrimal canal
17 Site of **nasal bone**
18 Nasal foramina of nasal bone
19 Anterior nasal spine of maxilla
20 **Vomer**
21 Greater wing of sphenoid bone
22 Anterior and posterior ethmoidal foramina
23 Optic canal
24 Superior orbital fissure
25 Inferior orbital fissure
26 Infraorbital groove
27 Infraorbital foramen

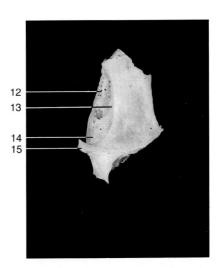

Left lacrimal bone (anterior aspect).

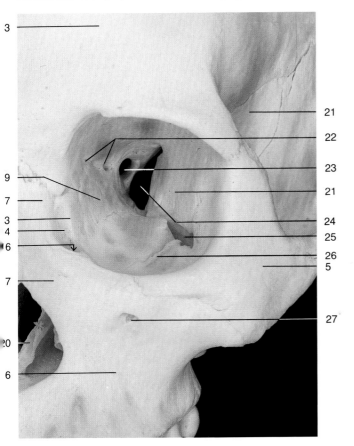

Left orbit (anterior aspect).

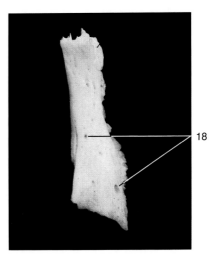

Left nasal bone (anterior aspect).

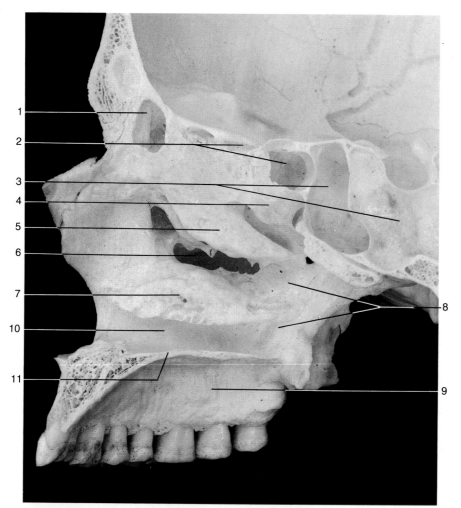

1 Frontal sinus
2 Ethmoidal air cells
3 Sphenoid sinus
4 Superior nasal concha
5 Middle nasal concha
6 Maxillary hiatus
7 Inferior nasal concha
8 Palatine bone
9 Maxilla
10 Inferior meatus
11 Palatine process of the maxilla

Lateral wall of the nasal cavity. Median section through the skull.

To page 49:

Blue = Occipital bone
Light green = Parietal bone
Light brown = Frontal bone
Dark brown = Temporal bone
Red = Sphenoid bone
Dark green = Ethmoid bone
Light blue = Nasal bone
Pink = Inferior concha
Orange = Vomer
Violet = Maxilla
White = Palatine bone
White = Mandible

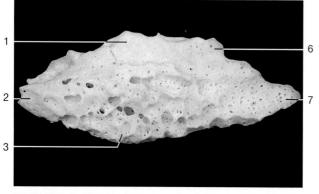

Right inferior nasal concha (medial aspect). Anterior part to the left.

Inferior Concha and Vomer
1 Ethmoidal process
2 Anterior part of concha
3 Inferior border
4 Ala of vomer
5 Posterior border of nasal septum
6 Lacrimal process
7 Posterior part of concha
8 Maxillary process

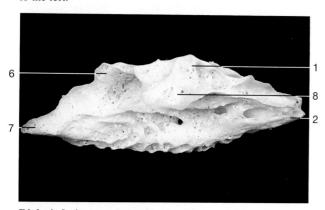

Right inferior nasal concha (lateral aspect). Anterior part to the right.

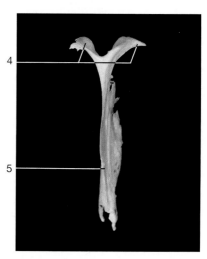

Vomer (posterior aspect).

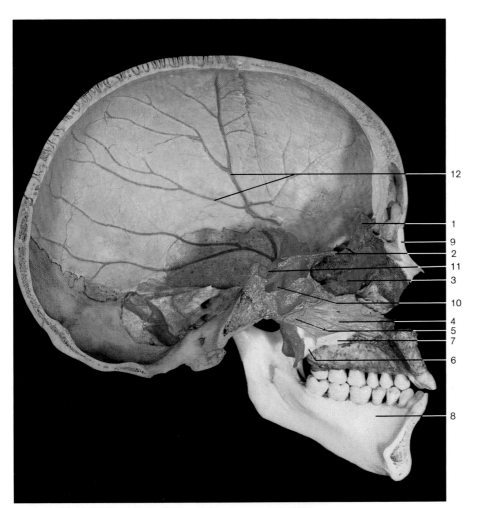

1 Crista galli
2 Cribriform plate
   of ethmoid bone
3 Perpendicular plate
   of ethmoid bone
4 Vomer
5 Ala of the vomer
6 Palatine bone
   (perpendicular process)
7 Palatine bone (horizontal plate)
8 Mandible
9 Nasal bone
10 Sphenoidal sinus
11 Hypophysial fossa (sella turcica)
12 Grooves for the middle
   meningeal artery

Cartilages of the nose
13 Lateral nasal cartilage
14 Greater alar cartilage
15 Lesser alar cartilages
16 Septal cartilage

17 Location of nasal bone

Paramedian sagittal section through the skull including the nasal septum.

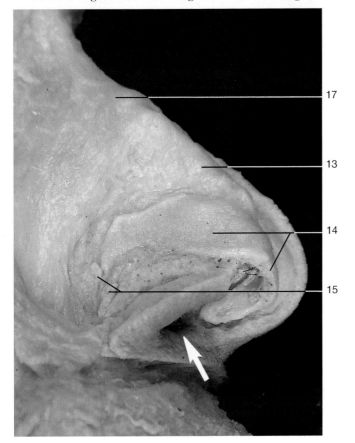

Cartilages of the nose (right anterior aspect). Arrow = nostril, framed by nasal wing.

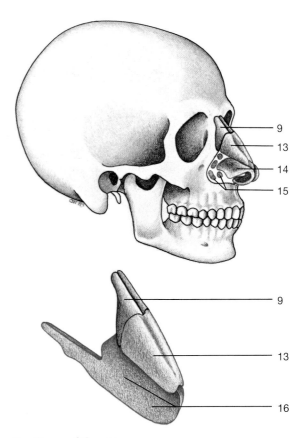

Cartilages of the nose.
Schematic diagram of the external nose.

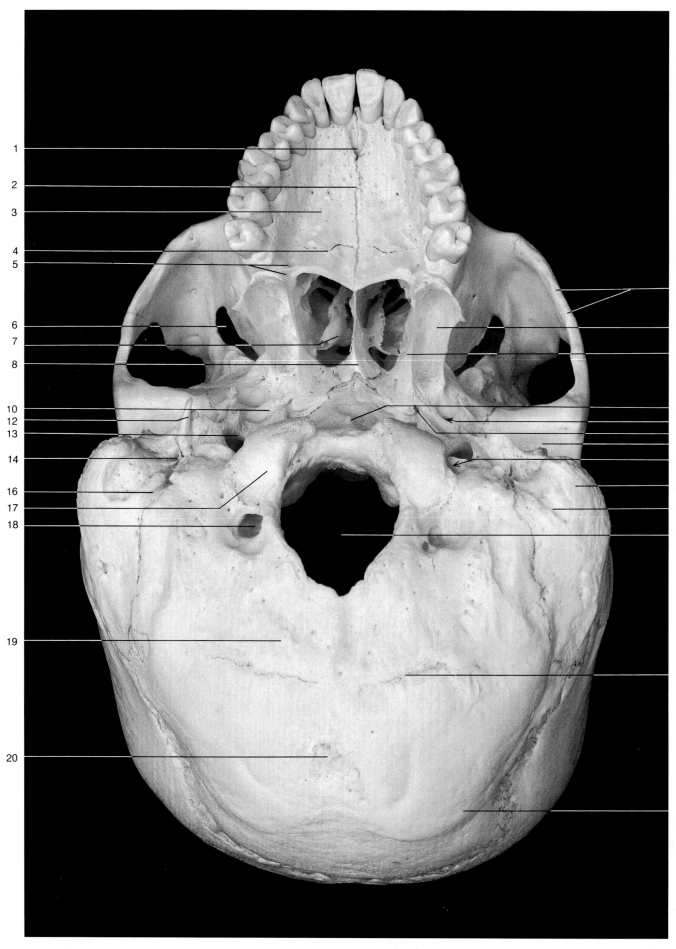

Base of the skull (inferior aspect).

A **Pterygoid canal**
B **Foramen ovale**
C Internal carotid artery within **carotid canal** and internal jugular vein within the venous part of jugular foramen
D **Stylomastoid foramen** (facial nerve)
E **Jugular foramen** (glossopharyngeal, vagus and accessory nerves)
F **Hypoglossal canal** (hypoglossal nerve)

1 Incisive canal
2 Median palatine suture
3 Palatine process of maxilla
4 Palatomaxillary suture
5 Greater and lesser palatine foramina
6 Inferior orbital fissure
7 Middle concha (process of ethmoid bone)
8 Vomer
9 Foramen ovale
10 Groove for auditory tube
11 Pterygoid canal
12 Styloid process
13 Carotid canal
14 Stylomastoid foramen
15 Jugular foramen
16 Groove for occipital artery
17 Occipital condyle
18 Condylar canal
19 Nuchal plane
20 External occipital protuberance
21 Zygomatic arch
22 Lateral pterygoid plate
23 Medial pterygoid plate
24 Mandibular fossa
25 Pharyngeal tubercle
26 Superior nuchal line
27 Mastoid process
28 Inferior nuchal line
29 Mastoid notch
30 Foramen magnum
31 **Incisive bone** or **premaxilla** (dark violet)
32 **Maxilla** (violet)
33 **Palatine bone** (white)
34 **Vomer** (orange)
35 **Sphenoid bone** (red)
36 **Zygomatic bone** (yellow)
37 **Temporal bone** (brown)
38 **Occipital bone** (blue)
39 Palatine process of maxilla
40 Vomer
41 Sphenoid bone
42 Petrous part of temporal bone
43 Basilar part ⎫
44 Lateral part ⎬ of occipital bone
45 Squamous part ⎭
46 Mandible
47 Zygomatic arch
48 Choana
49 Pterygoid process of sphenoid bone
50 Carotid canal
51 External acoustic meatus (tympanic annulus)
52 Sphenoidal fontanelle
53 Parietal bone
54 Mastoid fontanelle

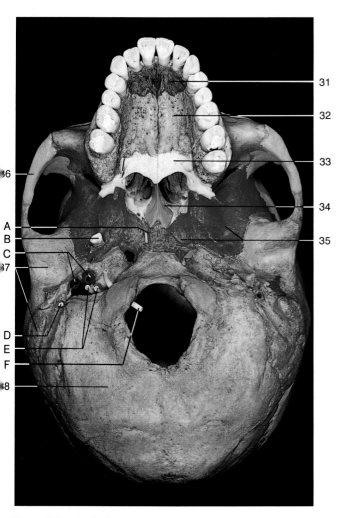

Base of the skull (from below). The individual bones are indicated by different colours.

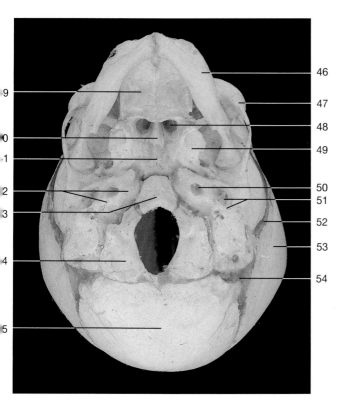

Skull of the newborn (inferior aspect).

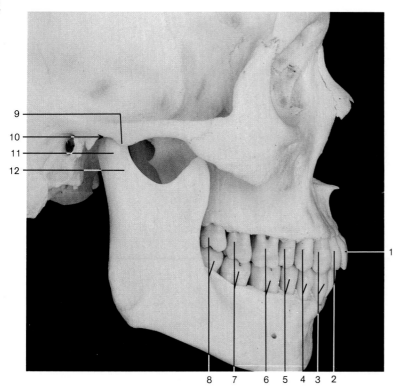

1	Central incisor
2	Lateral incisor
3	Canines
4	First premolars or bicuspids
5	Second premolars or bicuspids
6	First molars
7	Second molars
8	Third molars
9	Articular tubercle
10	Mandibular fossa
11	Head of mandible
12	Condylar process

Normal position of teeth. Dentition in centric occlusion (lateral view).

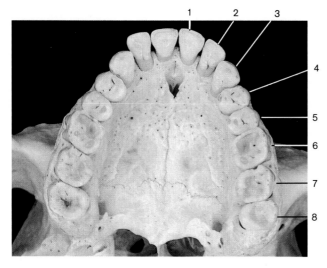

Upper teeth of the adult (inferior aspect).

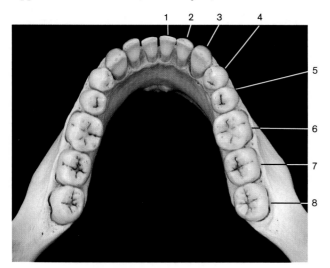

Lower teeth of the adult (superior aspect).

Table of dentition. Eruption of deciduous and permanent teeth (after C. Röse according to A. Kröncke).

Primary dentition (Deciduous teeth)	Maxilla months post partum	Mandible months
1. Central incisor	10.3	8.6
2. Lateral incisor	12.2	14.4
3. Cuspid incisor	19.5	20.1
4. First molar	15.5	16.5
5. Second molar	24.8	24.5

Secondary dentition (Permanent teeth)	years and months ♂	years and months ♀	years and months ♂	years and months ♀
1. Central incisor	7/8	7/5	6/10	6/7
2. Lateral incisor	8/11	8/6	7/11	7/7
3. Cuspid incisor	12/2	11/7	11/12	10/3
4. First premolar	10/5	10/1	11/3	10/8
5. Second premolar	11/4	11/1	12/0	11/7
6. First molar	6/7	6/6	6/5	6/3
7. Second molar	12/9	12/5	12/3	11/9

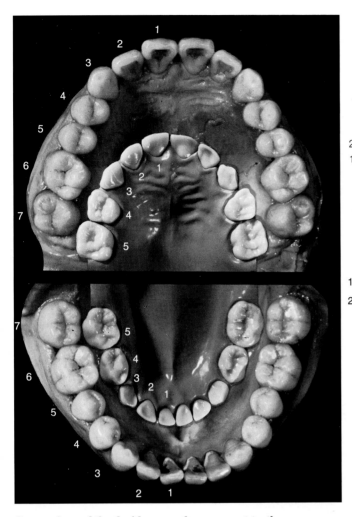

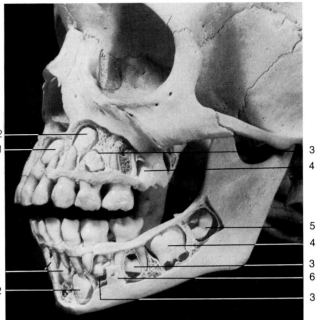

Deciduous teeth in child's skull. The developing crowns of the permanent teeth are displayed in their sockets in the maxilla and mandible.

△
1 Permanent incisors
2 Permanent cuspid (canine)
3 Premolars
4 First permanent molar
5 Second permanent molar
6 Mental foramen

Comparison of the deciduous and permanent teeth.
Notice that the breadth of the alveolar arch of the child's mandible and maxilla holding the deciduous teeth is nearly the same as the comparable portion in the jaws of the adult. Note the unerupted third molars.

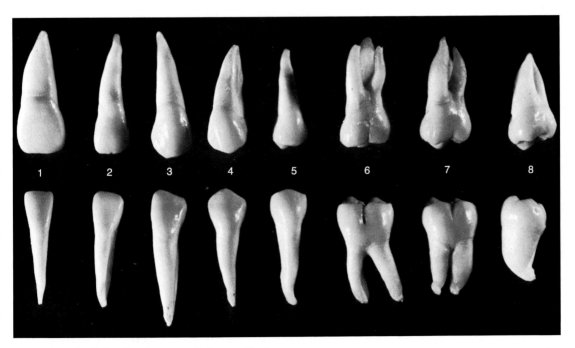

Isolated teeth of the alveolar part of the maxilla (top row) and the mandible (lower row), labial surface of the teeth.

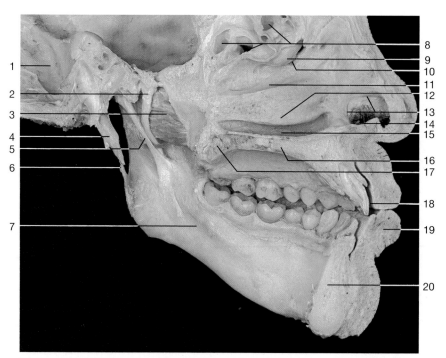

Ligaments of temporomandibular joint. Left half of the head (medial aspect).

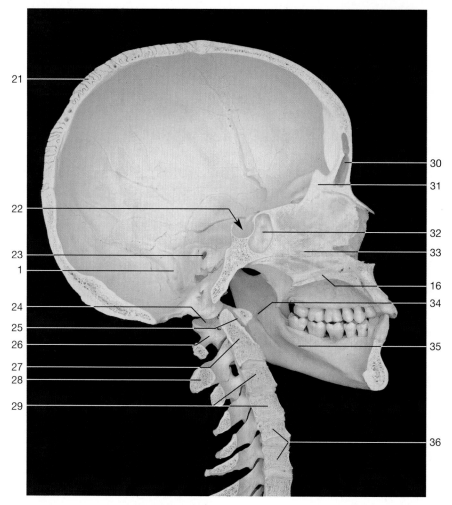

Head and cervical vertebral column (median section through skull and cervical vertebrae, medial aspect).

1 Groove for sigmoid sinus
2 Mandibular nerve
3 Lateral pterygoid muscle
4 Styloid process
5 **Sphenomandibular ligament**
6 **Stylomandibular ligament**
7 Mylohyoid groove
8 **Ethmoidal air cells**
9 Ethmoidal bulla
10 **Hiatus semilunaris**
11 Middle meatus
12 **Inferior nasal concha**
13 Limen nasi
14 Vestibule with hairs
15 Inferior meatus
16 Hard palate
17 Soft palate
18 Vestibule of oral cavity
19 Lower lip
20 Mandible
21 Calvaria with diploe
22 Sella turcica
23 Internal acoustic meatus
24 **Atlanto-occipital articulation**
25 Median atlanto-axial articulation
26 **Atlas** (C_1)
27 **Dens of axis** (C_2)
28 Spinous process of axis (C_2)
29 Cervical vertebrae (C_3, C_4)
30 Frontal sinus
31 Crista galli
32 Sphenoid sinus
33 Nasal septum
34 Mandibular foramen
35 Mylohyoid line
36 Bodies of cervical vertebrae (C_5, C_6)

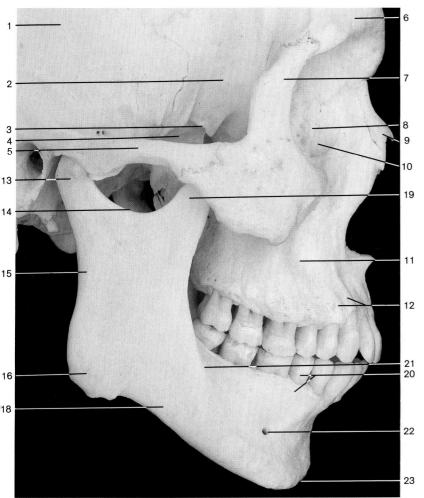

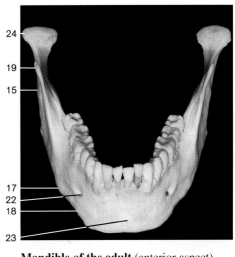

Mandible of the adult (anterior aspect).

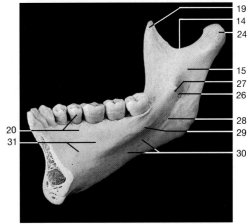

Right half of mandible (medial aspect).

Lateral aspect of the facial bones. Mandible and teeth in the position of occlusion. Upper and lower jaw occluded.

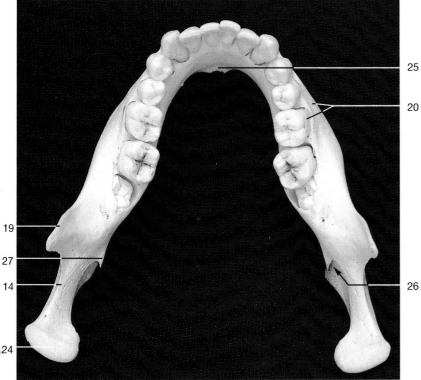

Mandible of the adult (superior aspect).

1 **Temporal bone**
2 Temporal fossa (greater wing of sphenoid bone)
3 Infratemporal crest
4 Infratemporal fossa
5 Zygomatic arch
6 **Frontal bone**

7 **Zygomatic bone** (frontal process)
8 **Lacrimal bone**
9 **Nasal bone**
10 Lacrimal groove
11 **Maxilla** (canine fossa)
12 Alveolar process of maxilla

Mandible
13 Condylar process
14 Mandibular notch
15 Ramus of the mandible
16 Masseteric tuberosity
17 Angle of the mandible
18 Body of the mandible
19 Coronoid process
20 Alveolar process including teeth
21 Oblique line
22 Mental foramen
23 Mental protuberance
24 Head of the mandible
25 Genial tubercle or mental spine
26 Mandibular foramen (entrance to mandibular canal)
27 Lingula
28 Mylohyoid sulcus
29 Mylohyoid line
30 Submandibular fossa
31 Sublingual fossa

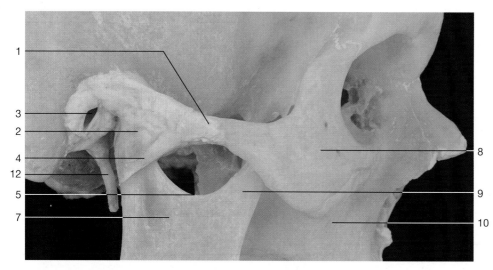

Temporomandibular joint with ligaments.

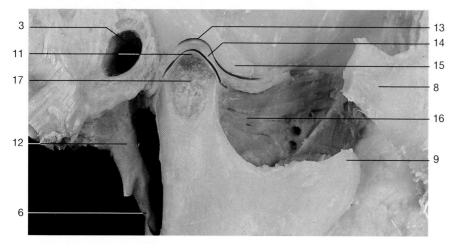

Temporomandibular joint, sagittal section.

1 Zygomatic arch
2 Articular capsule
3 External acoustic meatus
4 **Lateral ligament**
5 Mandibular notch
6 **Stylomandibular ligament**
7 Ramus of the mandible
8 Zygomatic bone
9 Coronoid process
10 Maxilla
11 Articular cartilage of
condylar process
12 Styloid process
13 Mandibular fossa
14 **Articular disc**
15 Articular tubercle
16 Lateral pterygoid muscle
17 Condylar process of mandible
18 Temporalis muscle
19 Digastric muscle, posterior belly
20 Masseter muscle
21 Medial pterygoid muscle
22 Parotid duct
23 Buccinator muscle
24 Mandible

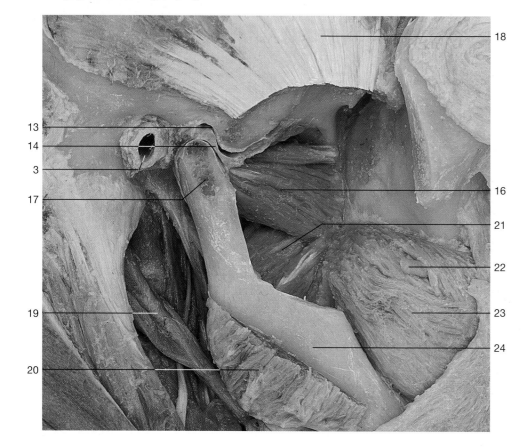

Temporomandibular joint.
Dissection of the articular
disk and the related muscles
(lateral aspect).

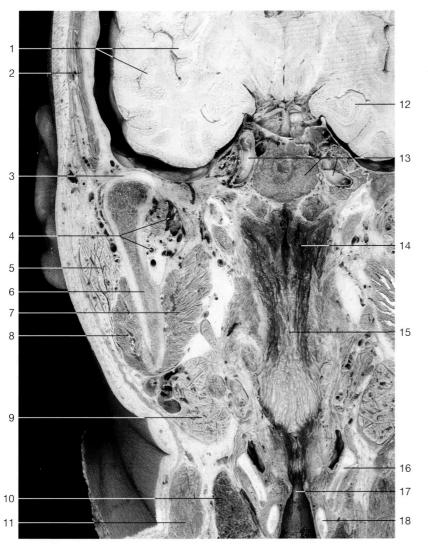

1   Insular lobe and temporal lobe
2   Temporalis muscle
3   **Articular disc of**
    temporomandibular joint
4   Maxillary artery and pterygoid
    venous plexus
5   Parotid gland
6   **Mandible**
7   **Medial pterygoid muscle**
8   **Masseter muscle**
9   Submandibular gland
10 Thyroid gland
11 Sternocleidomastoid muscle
12 Hippocampus
13 Internal carotid artery and
    sphenoid bone
14 Pharyngeal tonsil
15 Pharynx
16 Thyroid cartilage
17 Rima glottidis
18 Cricoid cartilage
19 **Hard palate** and palatine glands
20 **Oral cavity**
21 Upper molar
22 **Oral vestibule**
23 Lower molar
24 Platysma muscle
25 Maxillary sinus
26 Superior longitudinal muscle of tongue
27 **Transverse muscle of tongue**
28 Buccinator muscle
29 Inferior longitudinal muscle of tongue
30 Sublingual gland
31 **Genioglossus muscle**
32 Mastoid process
33 Styloid process
34 **Stylomandibular ligament**
35 Articular capsule
36 **Lateral ligament**
37 Zygomatic arch
38 **Sphenomandibular ligament**
39 Mandibular foramen

Coronal section through the head at the level of the temporomandibular joint (right side, anterior aspect).

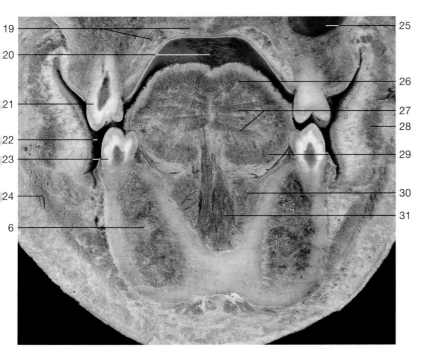

Coronal section through the oral cavity.

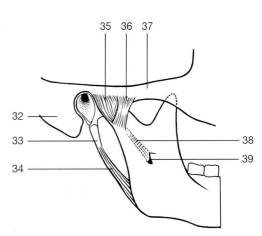

Ligaments related to the
temporomandibular joint.

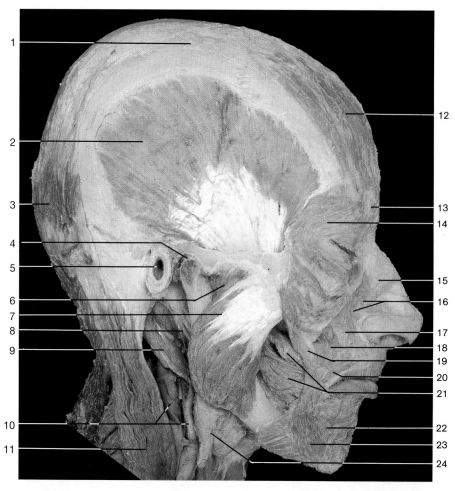

Temporalis and masseter muscles.
The temporal fascia has been removed, the temporomandibular joint severed and the zygomatic arch displayed.

1 Galea aponeurotica
2 **Temporalis muscle**
3 Occipital belly of occipitofrontalis muscle
4 **Temporomandibular joint**
5 External acoustic meatus
6 Deep layer of **masseter muscle**
7 Superficial layer of masseter muscle
8 Stylohyoid muscle
9 Posterior belly of **digastric muscle**
10 Internal jugular vein and external carotid artery
11 **Sternocleidomastoid muscle**
12 Frontal belly of occipitofrontalis muscle
13 Depressor supercilii muscle
14 **Orbicularis oculi muscle**
15 Transverse part of nasalis muscle
16 Levator labii superioris alaeque nasi muscle
17 Levator labii superioris muscle
18 Levator anguli oris muscle
19 **Zygomaticus major muscle**
20 **Orbicularis oris muscle**
21 **Buccinator muscle**
22 Depressor labii inferioris muscle
23 Depressor anguli oris muscle
24 **Submandibular gland**
25 Lateral nasal cartilage
26 Greater alar cartilage (lateral part)
27 Lesser alar cartilages
28 Greater alar cartilage (medial part)
29 Infraorbital nerve
30 Anterior belly of digastric muscle
31 Hypoglossal nerve and hyoglossus muscle
32 Superior thyroid artery
33 **Zygomatic arch**
34 Internal carotid artery
35 Common carotid artery

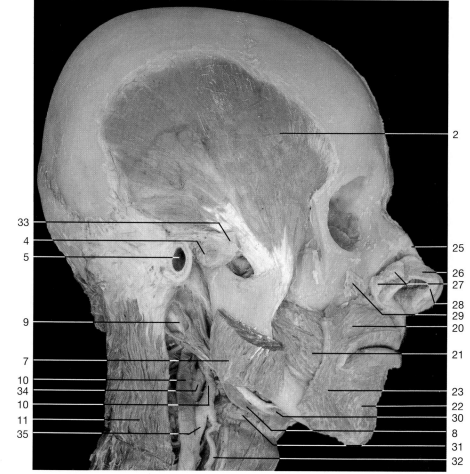

Temporalis muscle and temporomandibular joint. The zygomatic arch and the masseter muscle have been partially severed to display the insertion of the temporalis muscle.

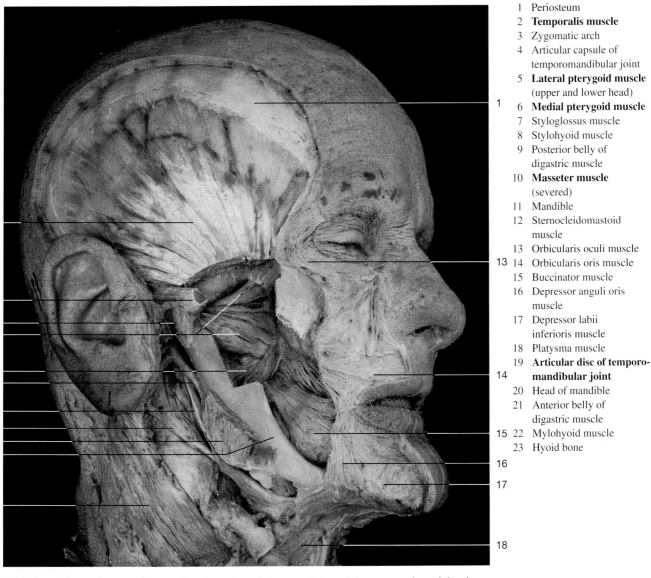

1   Periosteum
2   **Temporalis muscle**
3   Zygomatic arch
4   Articular capsule of
    temporomandibular joint
5   **Lateral pterygoid muscle**
    (upper and lower head)
6   **Medial pterygoid muscle**
7   Styloglossus muscle
8   Stylohyoid muscle
9   Posterior belly of
    digastric muscle
10 **Masseter muscle**
    (severed)
11 Mandible
12 Sternocleidomastoid
    muscle
13 Orbicularis oculi muscle
14 Orbicularis oris muscle
15 Buccinator muscle
16 Depressor anguli oris
    muscle
17 Depressor labii
    inferioris muscle
18 Platysma muscle
19 **Articular disc of temporo-**
    mandibular joint
20 Head of mandible
21 Anterior belly of
    digastric muscle
22 Mylohyoid muscle
23 Hyoid bone

Medial and lateral pterygoid muscles. A portion of the mandible and the zygomatic arch has been removed, revealing the pterygoid region or infratemporal fossa.

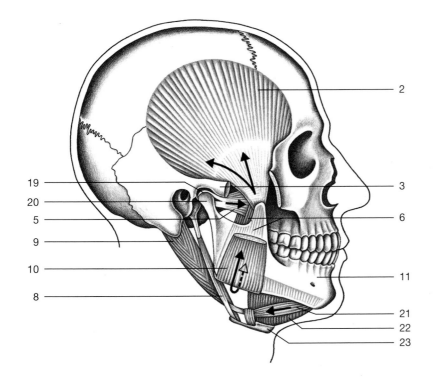

Effect of the muscles of mastication on the temporomandibular joint (arrows).

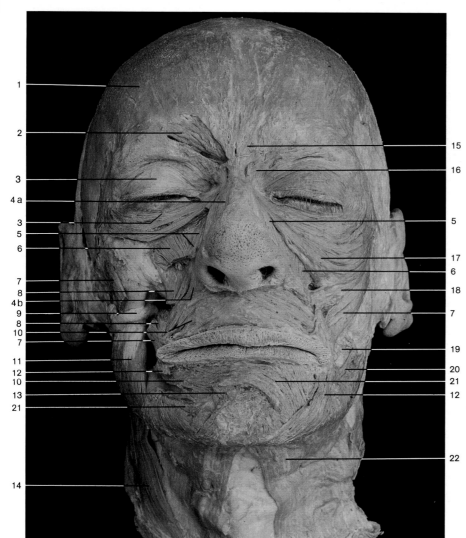

1 Frontal belly of **occipitofrontalis muscle**
2 **Corrugator supercilii muscle**
3 Palpebral part of orbicularis oculi muscle
4a Transverse part of nasalis muscle
4b Alar part of **nasalis muscle**
5 Levator labii superioris alaeque nasi muscle
6 **Levator labii superioris muscle**
7 **Zygomaticus major muscle**
8 Levator anguli oris muscle
9 Parotid duct
10 **Orbicularis oris muscle**
11 Masseter muscle
12 **Depressor anguli oris muscle**
13 **Mentalis muscle**
14 Sternocleidomastoid muscle
15 **Procerus muscle**
16 **Depressor supercilii muscle**
17 Orbital part of **orbicularis oculi muscle**
18 Zygomaticus minor muscle
19 **Buccinator muscle**
20 Risorius muscle
21 **Depressor labii inferioris muscle**
22 **Platysma muscle**
23 Galea aponeurotica
24 **Temporoparietalis muscle**
25 Occipital belly of occipitofrontalis muscle
26 Parotid gland with fascia
27 Temporal fascia
28 **Orbicularis oculi muscle**
29 Parotid duct, masseter muscle

Facial muscles (anterior aspect). Left side: superficial layer; right side: deeper layer.

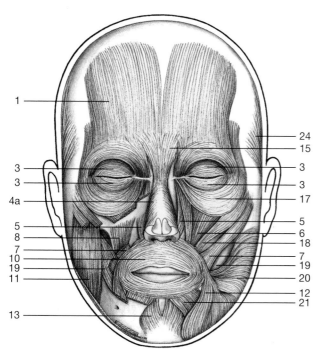

Facial muscles (schematic drawing).
Left side: superficial layer; right side: deeper layer.

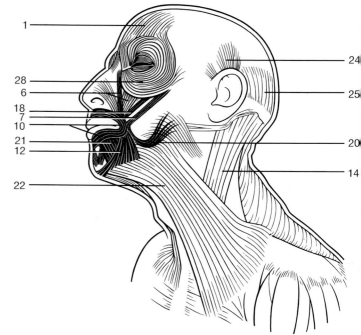

Facial muscles. Sphincter-like muscles surround the orifices of the head. Radially arranged muscles work as their antagonists.

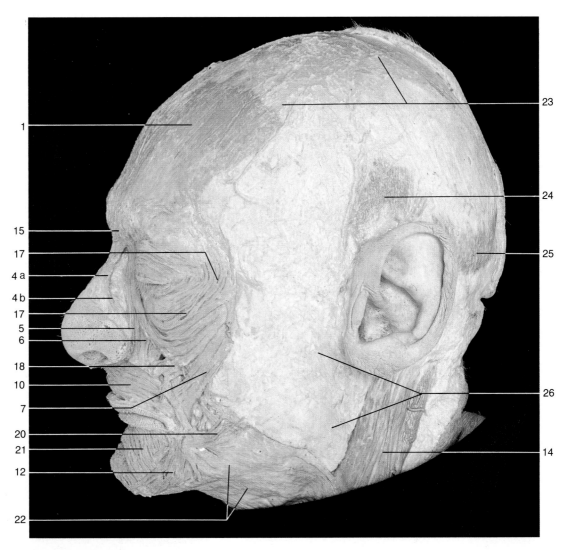

Facial muscles (lateral aspect).

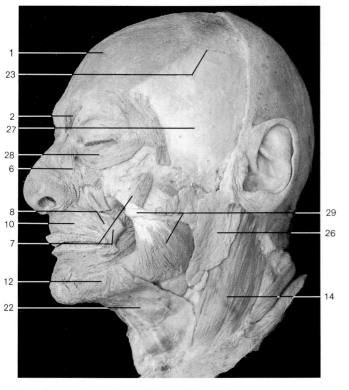

Facial muscles and parotid gland (lateral aspect).

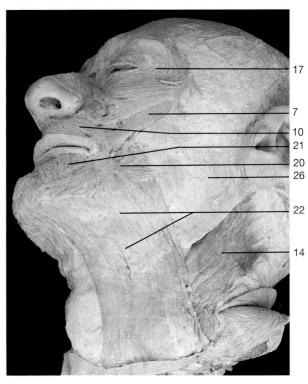

Platysma muscle (oblique lateral aspect). Superficial lamina of cervical fascia partly removed.

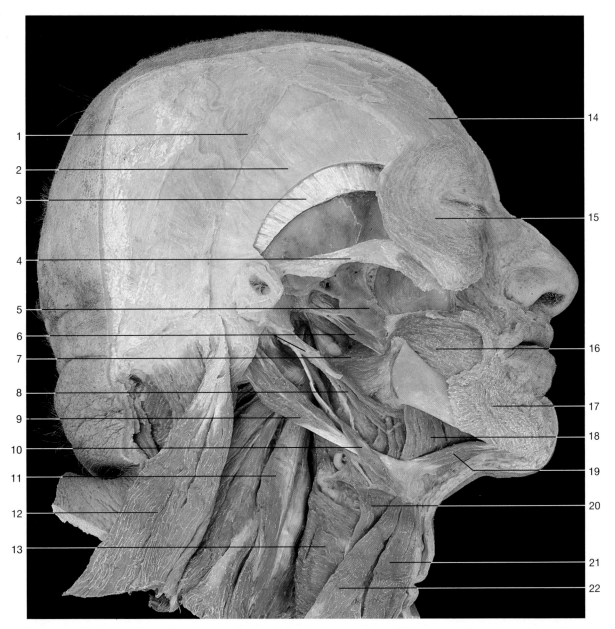

Supra- and infrahyoid muscles, pharynx I (lateral aspect). Ramus of mandible, pterygoid muscles and insertion of temporalis muscle removed.

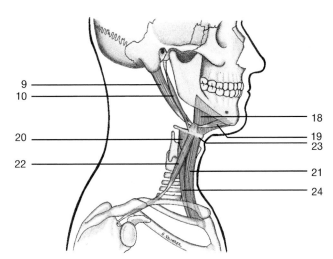

Supra- and infrahyoid muscles. (Schematic diagram.)

 1 Galea aponeurotica
 2 **Temporal fascia**
 3 Tendon of temporalis muscle
 4 Zygomatic arch
 5 Lateral pterygoid plate
 6 Tensor veli palatini muscle (styloid process)
 7 Superior constrictor muscle of pharynx
 8 **Styloglossus muscle**
 9 Posterior belly of digastric muscle
10 **Stylohyoid muscle**
11 Longus capitis muscle
12 Sternocleidomastoid muscle (reflected)
13 Inferior constrictor of pharynx
14 Frontal belly of occipitofrontalis muscle
15 Orbital part of orbicularis oculi muscle
16 **Buccinator muscle**
17 Depressor anguli oris muscle
18 **Mylohyoid muscle**
19 Anterior belly of digastric muscle
20 **Thyrohyoid muscle**
21 **Sternohyoid muscle**
22 **Omohyoid muscle**
23 Hyoid bone
24 Sternothyroid muscle

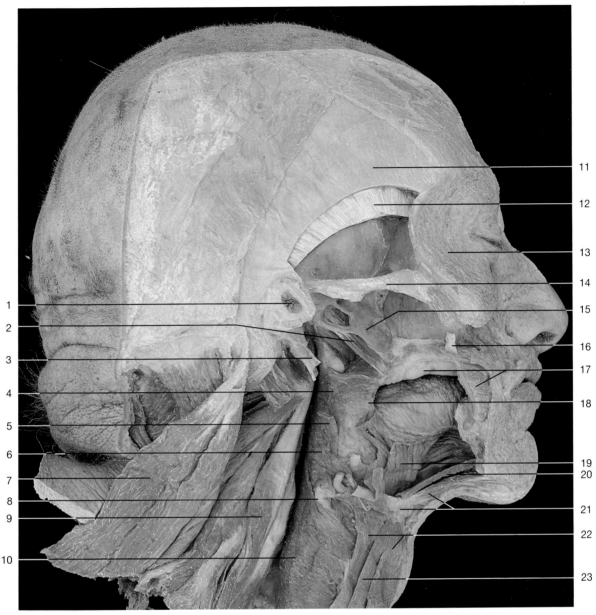

Supra- and infrahyoid muscles, pharynx II. Buccinator muscle removed; oral cavity opened.

1 External acoustic meatus
2 Tensor veli palatini muscle
3 Styloid process
4 **Superior constrictor muscle of pharynx**
5 Stylopharyngeus muscle (divided)
6 **Middle constrictor muscle of pharynx**
7 Sternocleidomastoid muscle
8 Greater horn of hyoid bone
9 Longus capitis
10 **Inferior constrictor muscle of pharynx**
11 Temporal fascia
12 Tendon of temporalis muscle
13 Orbicularis oculi muscle
14 Zygomatic arch
15 Lateral pterygoid plate
16 Parotid duct
17 Gingiva of upper jaw (without teeth),
    buccinator muscle (divided)
18 Pterygomandibular raphe
19 Hyoglossus muscle
20 Mylohyoid muscle
21 Anterior belly of digastric muscle (hyoid bone)
22 Sternohyoid and thyrohyoid muscles
23 Omohyoid muscle

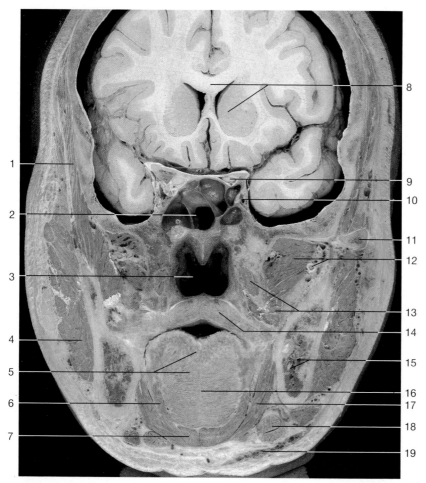

1 Temporalis muscle
2 **Sphenoidal sinus**
3 **Nasopharynx**
4 Masseter muscle
5 Superior longitudinal, transverse and vertical muscles of tongue
6 Hyoglossus muscle
7 Geniohyoid muscle
8 Corpus callosum (caudate nucleus)
9 Optic nerve
10 Cavernous sinus
11 Zygomatic arch
12 Cross section of lateral pterygoid muscle and maxillary artery
13 Section of medial pterygoid muscle
14 **Soft palate**
15 Mandible and inferior alveolar nerve
16 Septum of the tongue
17 **Mylohyoid muscle**
18 Submandibular gland
19 Platysma muscle
20 Foramen magnum, vertebral artery and spinal cord
21 Internal carotid artery
22 **Head of mandible**
23 Styloid process
24 Inferior alveolar nerve
25 Lingual nerve and chorda tympani nerve
26 **Medial pterygoid muscle**
27 Uvula
28 Anterior belly of digastric muscle (cut)
29 Condyle of occipital bone
30 Mastoid process
31 **Lateral pterygoid muscle**
32 Auditory tube and **levator veli palatini muscle**
33 **Tensor veli palatini muscle**

Coronal section through cranial, nasal and oral cavities at the level of sphenoidal sinus.

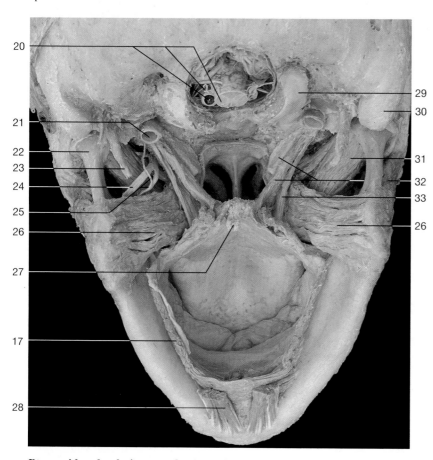

Pterygoid and palatine muscles (posterior aspect).

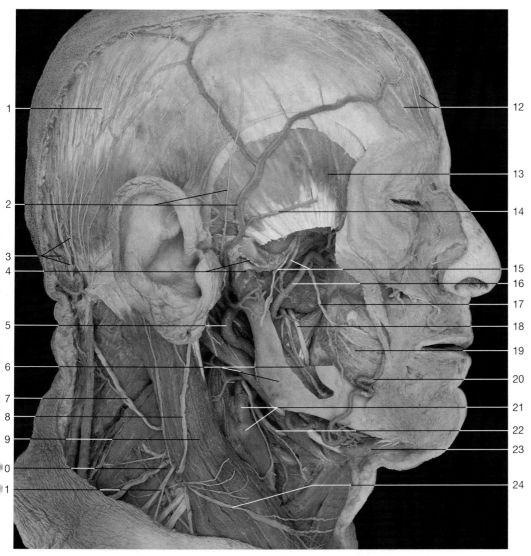

1	Galea aponeurotica
2	Superficial temporal artery and auriculotemporal nerve
3	**Occipital artery and greater occipital nerve** (C_2)
4	Temporomandibular joint (opened)
5	**External carotid artery**
6	Mandible and inferior mandibular artery and nerve
7	Accessory nerve (Var.)
8	Great auricular nerve
9	Sternocleidomastoideus muscle
10	Punctum nervosum
11	Supraclavicular nerves
12	Supraorbital nerves
13	Temporalis muscle
14	Transverse facial artery
15	Masseteric nerve and deep temporal branch of maxillary artery
16	**Maxillary artery**
17	Buccal nerve
18	Lingual nerve
19	Buccinator muscle
20	**Facial artery**
21	External carotid artery and sinus caroticus
22	Hypoglossal nerve
23	Digastric muscle
24	Transverse cervical nerves

Dissection of maxillary artery (lateral aspect, ramus mandibulae partly removed and canalis mandibulae opened).

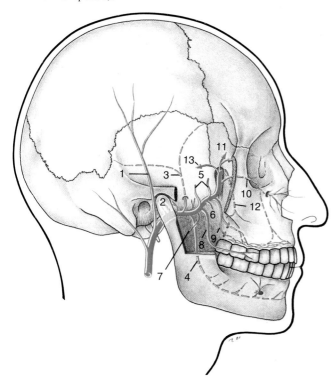

1 Superficial temporal artery

Branches of the first part
2 Deep auricular artery and anterior tympanic artery
3 Middle meningeal artery
4 Inferior alveolar artery

Branches of the second part
5 Deep temporal branches
6 Pterygoid branches
7 Masseteric artery
8 Buccal artery

Branches of the third part
9 Posterior superior alveolar artery
10 Infraorbital artery
11 Sphenopalatine artery and branches to the nasal cavity
12 Descending palatine artery
13 Artery of the pterygoid canal

Main branches of maxillary artery. (Schematic drawing.)

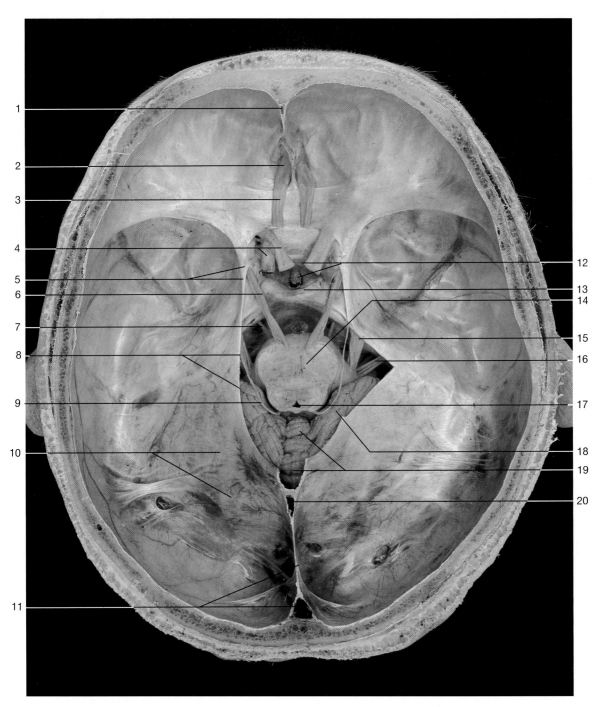

Base of the skull with cranial nerves (internal aspect). Both cerebral hemispheres and upper part of the brain stem removed. Incision on the right tentorium cerebelli to display the cranial nerves of the infratentorial space.

1 Superior sagittal sinus with falx cerebri
2 Olfactory bulb
3 **Olfactory tract**
4 **Optic nerve** and internal carotid artery
5 Anterior clinoid process and anterior attachment of tentorium cerebelli
6 **Oculomotor nerve** (n. III)
7 **Abducent nerve** (n. VI)
8 Tentorial notch (incisura tentorii)
9 **Trochlear nerve** (n. IV)
10 Tentorium cerebelli
11 Falx cerebri and confluence of sinuses

12 Hypophysial fossa, infundibulum, and diaphragma sellae
13 Dorsum sellae
14 Midbrain (divided)
15 **Trigeminal nerve** (n. V)
16 **Facial nerve** (n. VII), nervus intermedius, and **vestibulocochlear nerve** (n. VIII)
17 Cerebral aqueduct
18 Right hemisphere of cerebellum
19 Vermis of cerebellum
20 Straight sinus

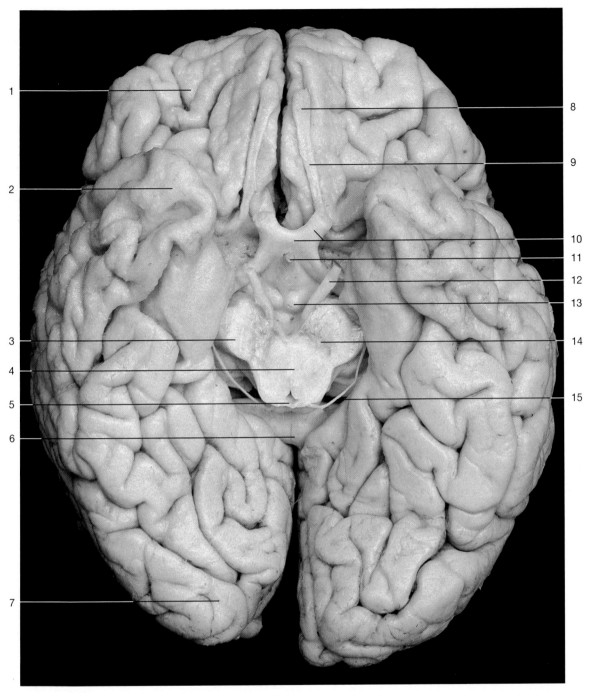

Inferior aspect of the brain with cranial nerves. Midbrain divided.

1 **Frontal lobe**
2 **Temporal lobe**
3 Pedunculus cerebri
4 **Midbrain** (divided)
5 Cerebral aqueduct
6 Splenium of corpus callosum
7 **Occipital lobe**
8 Olfactory bulb

9 Olfactory tract
10 **Optic nerve and optic chiasma**
11 Infundibulum
12 **Oculomotor nerve** (n. III)
13 Mamillary body
14 Substantia nigra
15 **Trochlear nerve** (n. IV)

Cranial nerves	
I = Olfactory nerves	VII = Facial nerve
II = Optic nerve	VIII = Vestibulocochlear nerve
III = Oculomotor nerve	IX = Glossopharyngeal nerve
IV = Trochlear nerve	X = Vagus nerve
V = Trigeminal nerve	XI = Accessory nerve
VI = Abducent nerve	XII = Hypoglossal nerve

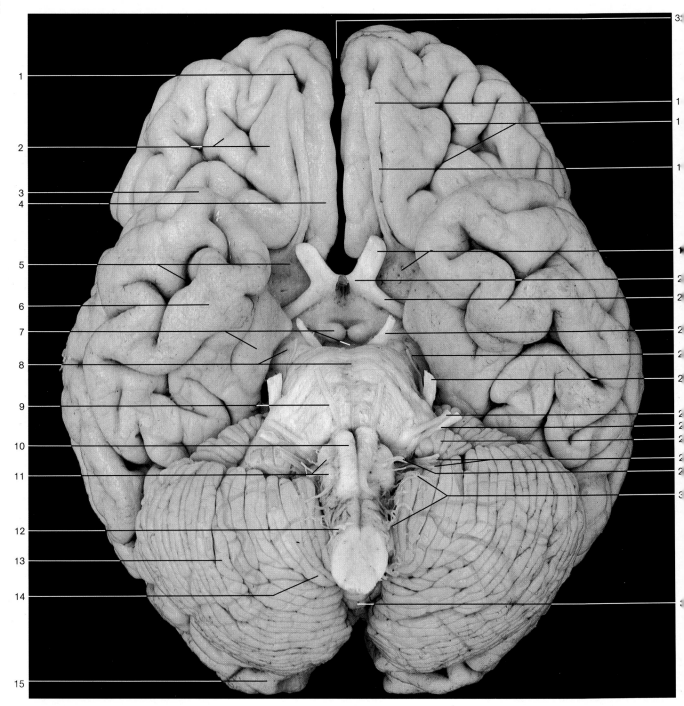

Cranial nerves. Brain (inferior aspect).

1 Olfactory sulcus (termination)
2 Orbital gyri
3 Temporal lobe
4 Straight gyrus
5 Olfactory trigone and inferior temporal sulcus
6 Medial occipitotemporal gyrus
7 Parahippocampal gyrus, mamillary body, and interpeduncular fossa
8 Pons and cerebral peduncle
9 **Abducent nerve** (n. VI)
10 Pyramid
11 Inferior olive
12 Cervical spinal nerves
13 Cerebellum
14 Tonsil of cerebellum
15 Occipital lobe (posterior pole)
16 Olfactory bulb
17 Orbital sulci of frontal lobe
18 **Olfactory tract**
19 **Optic nerve** (n. II) and anterior perforated substance
20 Optic chiasma
21 Optic tract
22 **Oculomotor nerve** (n. III)
23 **Trochlear nerve** (n. IV)
24 **Trigeminal nerve** (n. V)
25 **Facial nerve** (n. VII)
26 **Vestibulocochlear nerve** (n. VIII)
27 Flocculus of cerebellum
28 **Glossopharyngeal** (n. IX) and **vagus nerve** (n. X)
29 **Hypoglossal nerve** (n. XII)
30 **Accessory nerve** (n. XI)
31 Vermis of cerebellum
32 Longitudinal fissure

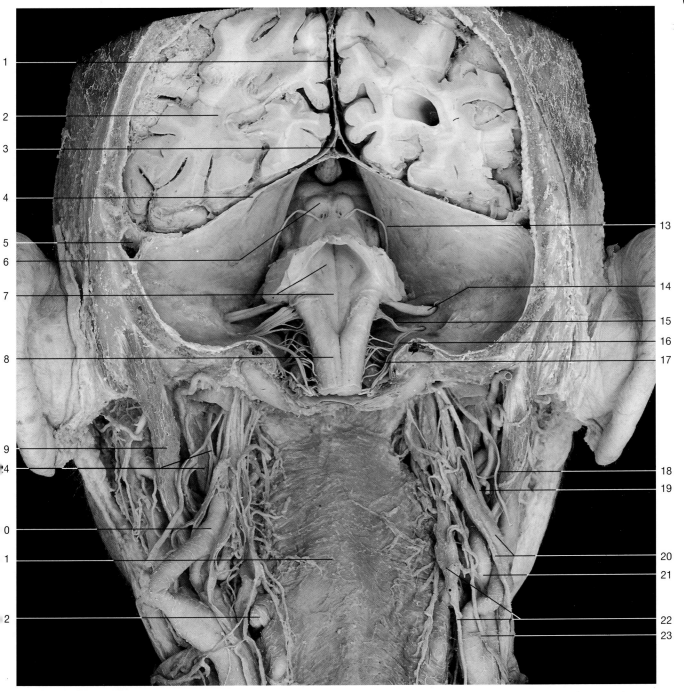

Brain stem and pharynx with cranial nerves (posterior aspect). Cranial cavity opened and cerebellum removed.

1   Falx cerebri
2   Occipital lobe
3   Straight sinus
4   Tentorium cerebelli
5   Transverse sinus
6   Inferior colliculus of midbrain
7   **Rhomboid fossa**
8   Medulla oblongata
9   Posterior belly of digastric muscle
10 Internal carotid artery
11 Pharynx (middle constrictor muscle)
12 Hyoid bone (greater horn)
13 **Trochlear nerve** (n. IV)
14 **Facial nerve** (n. VII),
    vestibulocochlear nerve (n. VIII)

15 **Glossopharyngeal nerve** (n. IX)
    and **vagus nerve** (n. X)
16 **Accessory nerve** (intracranial portion)
    (n. XI)
17 **Hypoglossal nerve** (intracranial portion)
    (n. XII)
18 **Accessory nerve** (n. XI)
19 **Hypoglossal nerve** (n. XII)
20 **Vagus nerve** (n. X) and internal carotid artery
21 External carotid artery
22 **Sympathetic trunk** and superior cervical ganglion
23 Ansa cervicalis (superior root of
    hypoglossal nerve)
24 **Glossopharyngeal nerve** (n. IX) and
    stylopharyngeus muscle

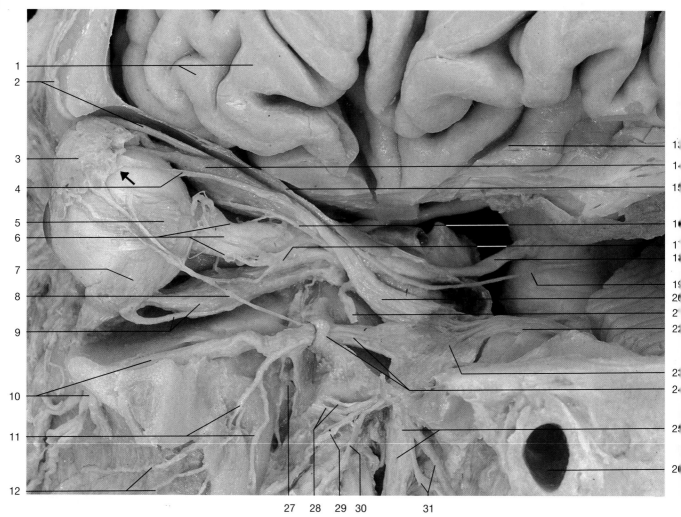

Cranial nerves of the orbit and pterygopalatine fossa. Left orbit (lateral aspect).
Note the zygomaticolacrimal anastomosis (arrow).

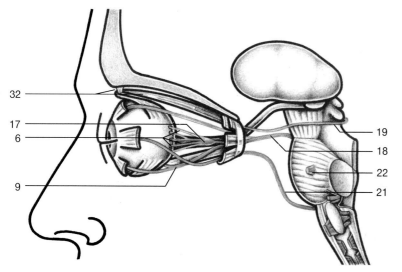

Cranial nerves innervating extraocular muscles (lateral aspect).
(Schematic drawing.)

1	Frontal lobe	7	Inferior oblique muscle
2	Supraorbital nerve	8	Zygomatic nerve
3	Lacrimal gland	9	Inferior branch of oculomotor nerve and
4	Lacrimal nerve		inferior rectus muscle
5	Lateral rectus muscle (divided)	10	Infraorbital nerve
6	**Optic nerve** and short ciliary nerves	11	Posterior superior alveolar nerves
		12	Branches of superior alveolar plexus adjacent to
			mucous membrane of maxillary sinus
		13	Central sulcus of insula
		14	Superior rectus muscle
		15	Periorbita (roof of orbit)
		16	Nasociliary nerve
		17	Ciliary ganglion
		18	**Oculomotor nerve** (n. III)
		19	**Trochlear nerve** (n. IV)
		20	**Ophthalmic nerve** (n. V_1)
		21	**Abducent nerve** (n. VI) (divided)
		22	**Trigeminal nerve** (n. V)
		23	Trigeminal ganglion
		24	**Maxillary nerve** (n. V_2) and foramen rotundum
		25	**Mandibular nerve** (n. V_3)
		26	External acoustic meatus
		27	Pterygopalatine nerves
		28	Deep temporal nerves
		29	Buccal nerve
		30	Masseteric nerve
		31	Auriculotemporal nerve
		32	Trochlea and superior oblique muscle

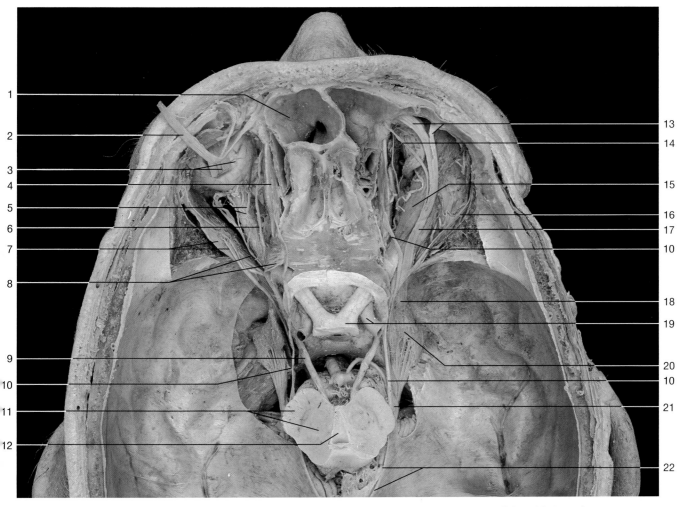

Cranial nerves of the orbit (superior aspect). Right side: superficial layer; left side: middle layer of the orbit (superior rectus muscle and frontal nerve divided and reflected). Tentorium and dura mater partly removed.

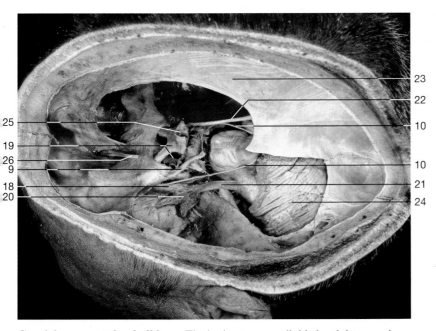

Cranial nerves at the skull base. The brain stem was divided and the tentorium fenestrated. Both hemispheres were removed.

1 Frontal sinus (enlarged)
2 Frontal nerve (divided and reflected)
3 Superior rectus muscle (divided) and eyeball
4 Superior oblique muscle
5 Short ciliary nerves and optic nerve (n. II)
6 Nasociliary nerve
7 **Abducent nerve** (n. VI) and lateral rectus muscle
8 Ciliary ganglion and superior rectus muscle (reflected)
9 **Oculomotor nerve** (n. III)
10 **Trochlear nerve** (n. IV)
11 Crus cerebri and midbrain
12 Inferior wall of the third ventricle connected with cerebral aqueduct
13 Lateral and medial branch of supraorbital nerve
14 Supratrochlear nerve
15 Superior rectus muscle
16 Lacrimal nerve
17 Frontal nerve
18 **Ophthalmic nerve** (n. V$_1$)
19 Optic chiasma and internal carotid artery
20 Trigeminal ganglion
21 **Trigeminal nerve** (n. V)
22 Tentorial notch
23 Falx cerebri
24 Cerebellum
25 Infundibulum
26 Olfactory tract

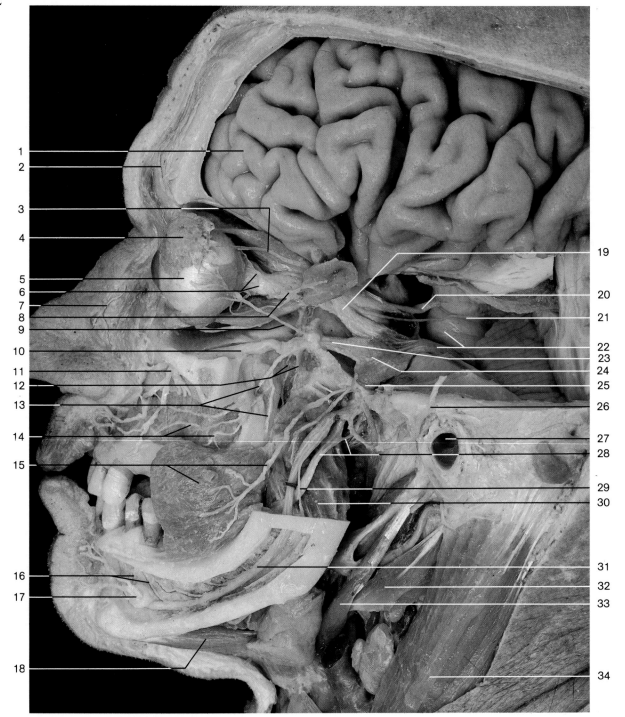

Dissection of the trigeminal nerve in its entirety. Lateral wall of cranial cavity, lateral wall of orbit, zygomatic arch and ramus of the mandible have been removed and the mandibular canal opened.

1 Frontal lobe of cerebrum	12 Pterygopalatine ganglion and pterygopalatine nerves
2 Supraorbital nerve	13 Posterior superior alveolar nerves
3 Lacrimal nerve	14 Superior dental plexus
4 Lacrimal gland	15 Buccinator muscle and buccal nerve
5 Eyeball	16 Inferior dental plexus
6 **Optic nerve** and short ciliary nerves	17 Mental foramen and mental nerve
7 External nasal branch of anterior ethmoidal nerve	18 Anterior belly of digastric muscle
8 Ciliary ganglion	19 **Ophthalmic nerve** (n. V$_1$)
9 Zygomatic nerve	20 **Oculomotor nerve** (n. III)
10 Infraorbital nerve	21 **Trochlear nerve** (n. IV)
11 Infraorbital foramen and terminal branches of infraorbital nerve	22 Trigeminal nerve and pons

23 **Maxillary nerve** (n. V$_2$)	
24 Trigeminal ganglion	
25 **Mandibular nerve** (n. V$_3$)	
26 Auriculotemporal nerve	
27 External acoustic meatus (divided)	
28 Lingual nerve and chorda tympani	
29 Mylohyoid nerve	
30 Medial pterygoid muscle	
31 Inferior alveolar nerve	
32 Posterior belly of digastric muscle	
33 Stylohyoid muscle	
34 Sternocleidomastoid muscle	

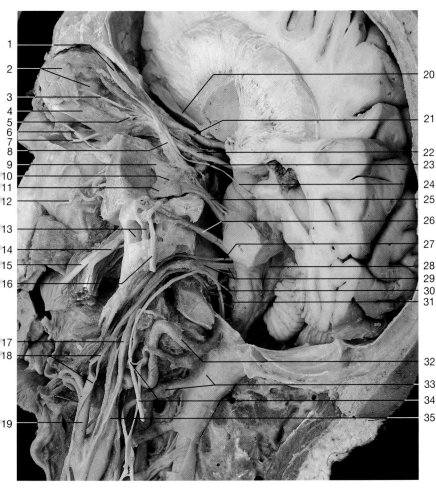

1 Frontal nerve
2 Lacrimal gland and eyeball
3 Lacrimal nerve
4 Lateral rectus muscle
5 **Ciliary ganglion** lateral to optic nerve
6 Zygomatic nerve
7 Inferior branch of oculomotor nerve
8 **Ophthalmic nerve** (n. V$_1$)
9 **Maxillary nerve** (n. V$_2$)
10 **Trigeminal ganglion**
11 **Mandibular nerve** (n. V$_3$)
12 Posterior superior alveolar nerves
13 Tympanic cavity, external acoustic meatus, and tympanic membrane
14 Inferior alveolar nerve
15 Lingual nerve
16 **Facial nerve** (n. VII)
17 **Vagus nerve** (n. X)
18 **Hypoglossal nerve** (n. XII) and superior root of ansa cervicalis
19 External carotid artery
20 **Olfactory tract** (n. I)
21 **Optic nerve** (n. II) (intracranial part)
22 **Oculomotor nerve** (n. III)
23 **Abducent nerve** (n. VI)
24 **Trochlear nerve** (n. IV)
25 **Trigeminal nerve** (n. V)
26 **Vestibulocochlear nerve** (n. VIII) and **facial nerve** (n. VII)
27 **Glossopharyngeal nerve** (n. IX) (leaving brain stem)
28 Rhomboid fossa
29 **Vagus nerve** (n. X) (leaving brain stem)
30 **Hypoglossal nerve** (n. XII) (leaving medulla oblongata)
31 **Accessory nerve** (n. XI) (ascending from foramen magnum)
32 Vertebral artery
33 Spinal ganglion and dura mater of spinal cord
34 Accessory nerve (n. XI)
35 Internal carotid artery
36 Lateral and medial branch of supraorbital nerve
37 Infratrochlear nerve
38 Infraorbital nerve
39 **Pterygopalatine ganglion** and middle superior alveolar nerve
40 Middle superior alveolar nerves (entering superior dental plexus)
41 Buccal nerve
42 Mental nerve and mental foramen
43 Auriculotemporal nerve
44 Otic ganglion (dotted line)
45 Chorda tympani
46 Mylohyoid nerve
47 Submandibular gland
48 Hyoid bone

Cranial nerves in connection with the brain stem. Left side (lateral superior aspect). Left half of brain and head partly removed. Notice the location of trigeminal ganglion.

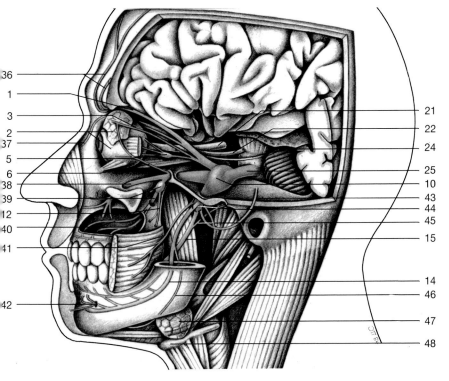

Main branches of trigeminal nerve. (Schematic drawing of figure on opposite page.)

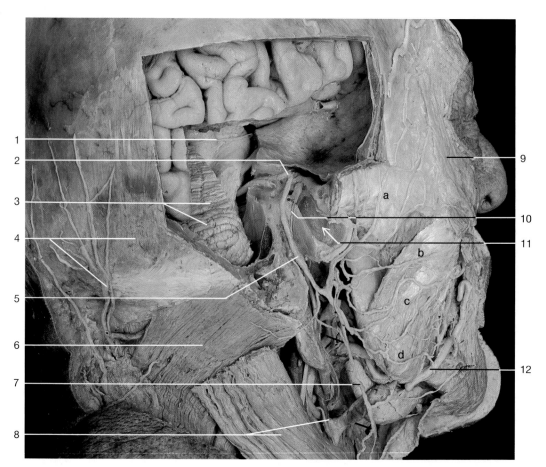

Dissection of facial nerve in its entirety. Cranial cavity fenestrated; temporal lobe partly removed. Facial canal and tympanic cavity opened, posterior wall of external acoustic meatus removed.
Branches of facial nerve: a = temporal branch; b = zygomatic branches; c = buccal branches; d = marginal mandibular branch.

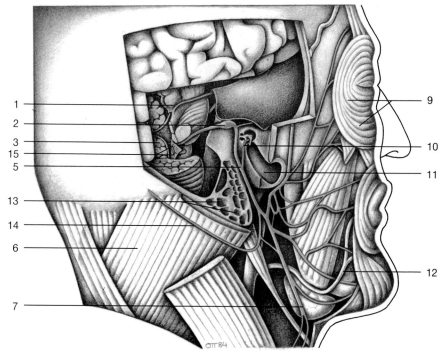

Facial nerve. (Schematic drawing of the dissection above.)

1 Trochlear nerve
2 Facial nerve with geniculate ganglion
3 Cerebellum (right hemisphere)
4 Occipital belly of occipitofrontalis and greater occipital nerve
5 Facial nerve at stylomastoid foramen
6 Splenius capitis muscle
7 Cervical branch of facial nerve
8 Sternocleidomastoid muscle and retromandibular vein
9 Orbicularis oculi muscle
10 Chorda tympani
11 External acoustic meatus
12 Facial artery
13 Mastoid air cells
14 Posterior auricular nerve
15 Nucleus and genu of facial nerve

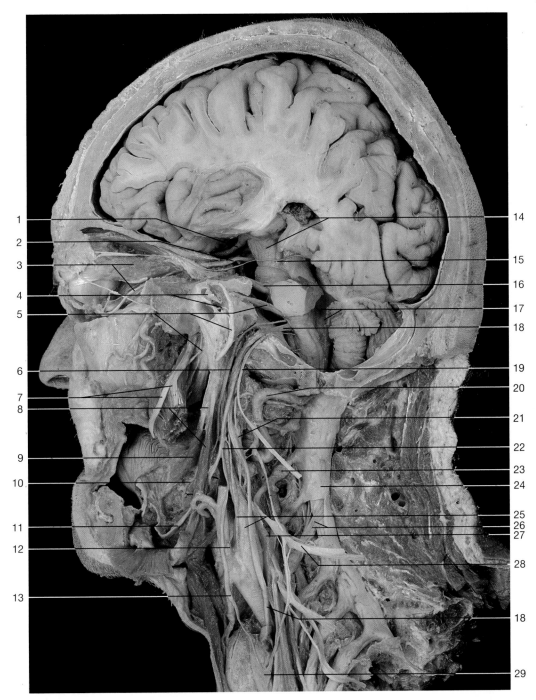

Cranial nerves in connection with the brain stem (oblique-lateral aspect). Lateral portion of the skull, brain, neck and facial structures, lateral wall of orbit and oral cavity have been removed. The tympanic cavity has been opened. The mandible has been divided and the muscles of mastication have been removed.

1 Optic tract
2 **Oculomotor nerve** (n. III)
3 Lateral rectus muscle and inferior branch of oculomotor nerve
4 Malleus and chorda tympani
5 Chorda tympani, **facial nerve** (n. VII), and **vestibulocochlear nerve** (n. VIII)
6 **Glossopharyngeal nerve** (n. XI)
7 Lingual nerve and inferior alveolar nerve
8 Styloid process and stylohyoid muscle
9 Styloglossus muscle
10 Lingual branches of glossopharyngeal nerve

11 Lingual branch of hypoglossal nerve
12 External carotid artery
13 Superior root of ansa cervicalis (branch of hypoglossal nerve)
14 Lateral ventricle with choroid plexus and cerebral peduncle
15 **Trochlear nerve** (n. IV)
16 **Trigeminal nerve** (n. V)
17 Fourth ventricle and rhomboid fossa
18 **Vagus nerve** (n. X)
19 **Accessory nerve** (n. XI)
20 Vertebral artery
21 Superior cervical ganglion

22 **Hypoglossal nerve** (n. XII)
23 Spinal ganglion with dural sheath
24 Dura mater of spinal cord
25 Internal carotid artery and carotid sinus branch of glossopharyngeal nerve
26 Dorsal roots of spinal nerve
27 Sympathetic trunk
28 Branch of cervical plexus (ventral primary ramus of third cervical spinal nerve)
29 Ansa cervicalis

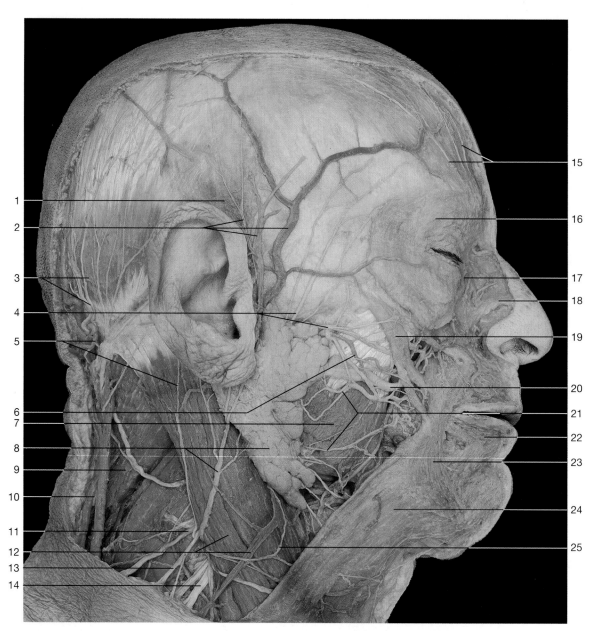

Lateral superficial aspect of the face. Peripheral distribution of facial nerve (n. VII).

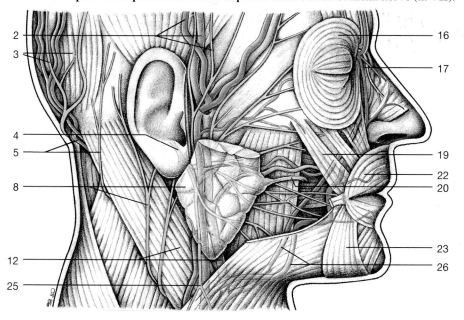

Superficial region of the face. Note the facial plexus within the parotid gland. (Semischematic drawing.)

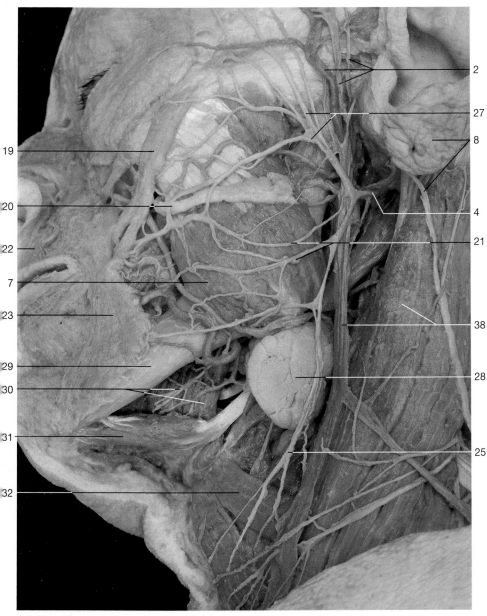

1 Temporoparietalis muscle
2 **Superficial temporal artery** and **vein** and **auriculotemporal nerve**
3 Occipital belly of occipitofrontalis muscle and **greater occipital nerve** (C$_2$)
4 **Facial nerve** (n. VII)
5 Lesser occipital nerve and **occipital artery**
6 Transverse facial artery
7 Masseter muscle
8 **Parotid gland** and great auricular nerve
9 Splenius capitis muscle
10 Trapezius muscle
11 **Punctum nervosum,** point of distribution of cutaneous nerves of cervical plexus
12 Sternocleidomastoid muscle and external jugular vein
13 Supraclavicular nerves
14 Brachial plexus
15 Supraorbital nerves
16 Orbicularis oculi muscle
17 Angular artery (terminal branch of facial artery)
18 Nasalis muscle
19 Zygomaticus major muscle
20 **Parotid duct**
21 Zygomatic and buccal branches of facial nerve
22 Orbicularis oris muscle
23 Depressor anguli oris muscle
24 **Platysma**
25 Cervical branch of facial nerve (anastomosing with transverse cervical nerve of cervical plexus)
26 Facial artery and vein
27 Temporal branches of facial nerve
28 **Submandibular gland**
29 Mandible
30 Mylohyoideus muscle and nerve
31 Digastricus muscle, anterior belly
32 Omohyoideus muscle
33 Greater petrosal nerve
34 Geniculate ganglion
35 Chorda tympani
36 Posterior auricular nerve
37 Stylomastoid foramen
38 Sternocleidomastoid muscle and retromandibular vein

Deep dissection of facial nerve. Retromandibular and submandibular region (lateral aspect, parotid gland has been removed).

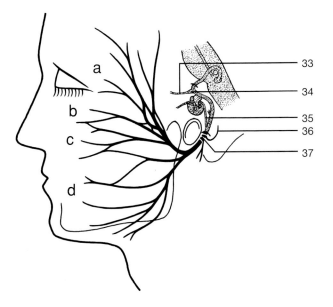

Main branches of facial nerve (schematic diagram).
a = temporal branches, b = zygomatic branches,
c = buccal branches, d = marginal mandibular branch.

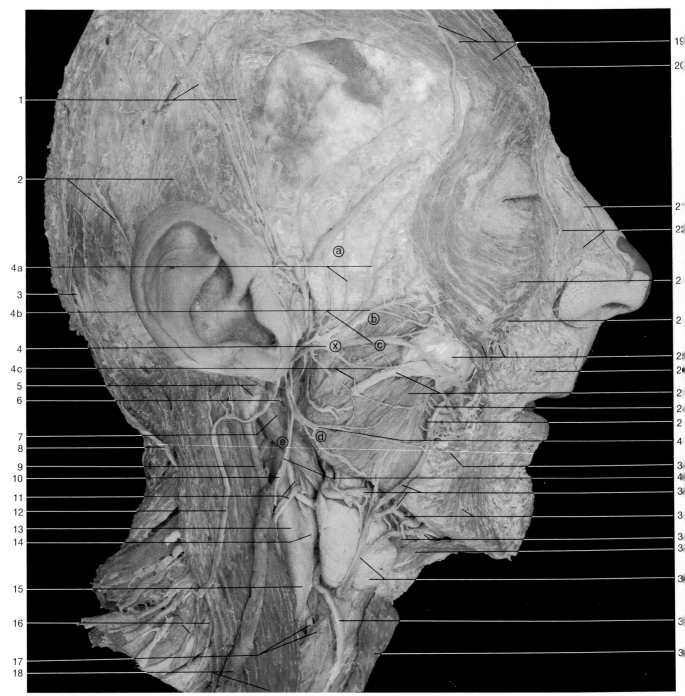

Lateral superficial aspect of the face. The parotid gland has been removed to display the parotid plexus of the facial nerve.
a–e = branches of facial nerve: a = temporal branch; b = zygomatic branches; c = buccal branches; d = marginal mandibular branch;
e = cervical branch.

1 Superficial temporal artery and auriculotemporal nerve
2 Posterior auricular artery and nerve and temporoparietalis muscle
3 Occipital artery
4 **Facial nerve (n. VII) (parotid plexus [×])**
  a Temporal branches
  b Zygomatic branches
  c Buccal branches
  d Marginal mandibular branch
  e Cervical branch
5 Posterior auricular nerve
6 Posterior auricular artery
7 Digastric muscle (posterior belly)
8 **Lesser occipital nerve**
9 Posterior auricular vein

10 Retromandibular vein
11 **Hypoglossal nerve** and sternocleidomastoid artery
12 **Great auricular nerve**
13 Internal carotid artery
14 External carotid artery
15 Common carotid artery
16 Branches of cervical plexus
17 Superior laryngeal artery and vein
18 External jugular vein and sternocleidomastoid muscle
19 Frontal branch of superficial temporal artery, lateral branch of supraorbital nerve, and frontal belly of occipitofrontalis muscle
20 Medial branch of supraorbital nerve
21 Dorsal nasal artery
22 Angular artery and nasalis muscle

23 **Orbicularis oculi muscle**
24 Zygomaticus minor muscle
25 Buccal fat pad, zygomaticus major muscle, and infraorbital nerve
26 **Orbicularis oris muscle**
27 **Parotid duct** and **masseter muscle**
28 Buccal artery and nerve
29 Buccinator muscle
30 Risorius muscle
31 **Facial artery** and **vein**
32 Submental artery and depressor anguli oris muscle
33 Mylohyoid nerve and mylohyoid muscle
34 Digastric muscle (anterior belly)
35 Facial vein and submandibular gland
36 **Superior thyroid artery**
37 Sternohyoid muscle

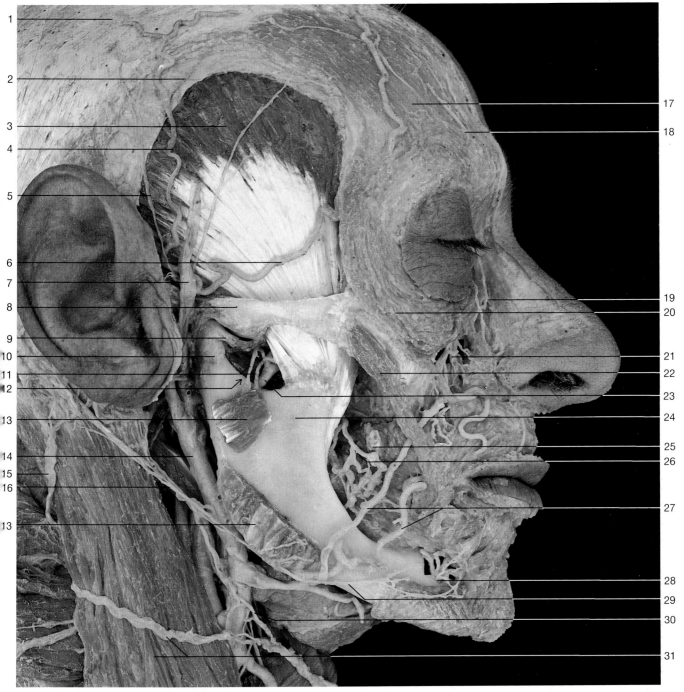

Lateral superficial aspect of the face. Masseter muscle and temporal fascia have been partly removed to display the masseteric artery and nerve.

1 Galea aponeurotica	10 **Head of mandible**	22 Zygomaticus major muscle
2 Temporal fascia	11 Masseteric artery and nerve	23 **Maxillary artery**
3 **Temporalis muscle**	12 Mandibular notch	24 **Coronoid process**
4 Parietal branch of **superficial temporal artery**	13 Masseter muscle (divided)	25 Parotid duct (divided)
5 **Auriculotemporal nerve**	14 **External carotid artery**	26 Buccal nerve
6 Frontal branch of superficial temporal artery	15 Great auricular nerve	27 **Facial artery** and **vein**
7 Superficial temporal vein	16 Facial nerve (reflected)	28 **Mental nerve**
8 **Zygomatic arch**	17 Frontal belly of occipitofrontalis muscle	29 Mandibular branch of facial nerve
9 **Articular disc of temporomandibular joint**	18 Medial branch of supraorbital nerve	30 Cervical branch of facial nerve
	19 **Angular artery**	31 Transverse cervical nerve (communicating branch with facial nerve) and sternocleidomastoid muscle
	20 Orbicularis oculi muscle	
	21 **Infraorbital nerve**	

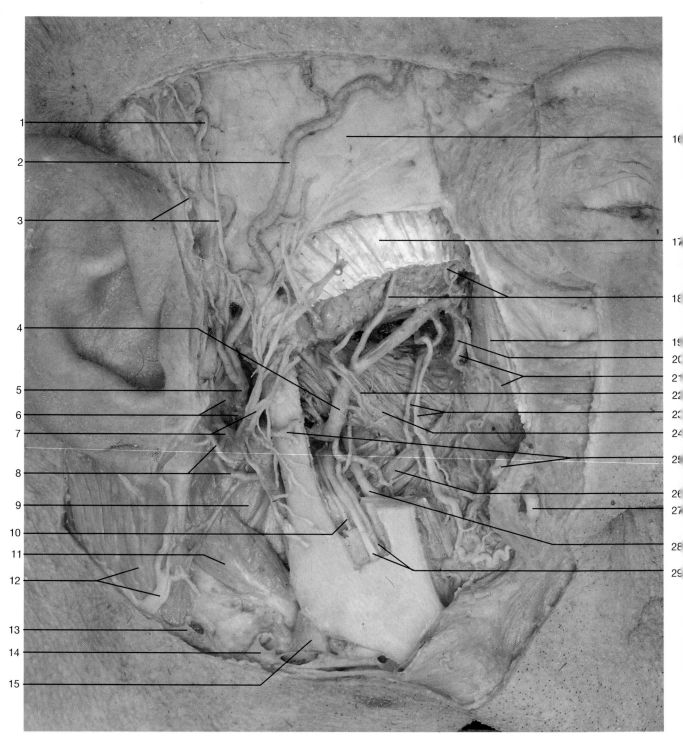

Deep dissection of facial and retromandibular regions. The coronoid process together with the insertions of temporalis muscle have been removed to display the maxillary artery. The upper part of the mandibular canal has been opened.

1 Parietal branch of the superficial temporal artery
2 Frontal branch of the superficial temporal artery
3 Auriculotemporal nerve
4 **Maxillary artery**
5 **Superficial temporal artery**
6 Communicating branches between facial and auriculotemporal nerves
7 **Facial nerve**
8 Posterior auricular artery and anterior auricular branch of superficial temporal artery
9 Internal jugular vein

10 Mylohyoid nerve
11 Posterior belly of digastric muscle
12 Great auricular nerve and sternocleidomastoid
13 External jugular vein
14 Retromandibular vein
15 Submandibular gland
16 Temporal fascia
17 **Temporalis tendon**
18 Deep temporal arteries
19 Posterior superior alveolar nerve
20 Sphenopalatine artery
21 Posterior superior alveolar arteries

22 Masseteric artery and nerve
23 **Buccal nerve and artery**
24 **Lateral pterygoid**
25 Transverse facial artery and parotid duct (divided)
26 Medial pterygoid
27 **Facial artery**
28 **Lingual nerve**
29 **Inferior alveolar artery and nerve** (mandibular canal opened)

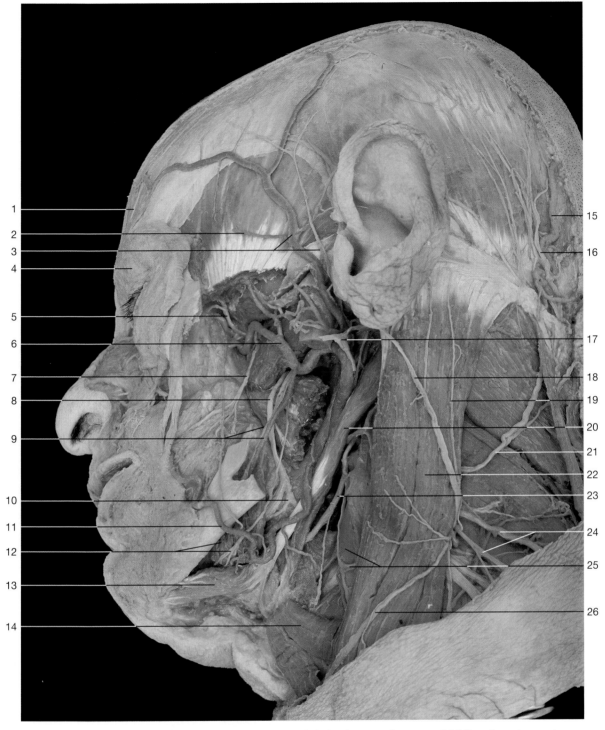

Peripharyngeal and retromandibular region. The mandible has been partly removed (oblique lateral aspect).

1   Supraorbital nerve (medial branch)
2   Temporalis muscle
3   Superficial temporal artery and
    auriculotemporal nerve
4   Orbicularis oculi muscle
5   Anterior deep temporal artery
6   **Maxillary artery**
7   Buccal nerve
8   **Lingual nerve**
9   Inferior alveolar nerve and artery

10 **Submandibular ganglion**
11 **Facial artery**
12 Mylohyoid muscle and nerve
13 Anterior belly of digastric muscle
14 Omohyoid muscle
15 Occipital artery
16 **Greater occipital nerve** (C$_2$)
17 Facial nerve (cut) (n. VII)
18 Great auricular nerve
19 Lesser occipital nerve

20 Posterior belly of digastric muscle
21 Accessory nerve (Var.)
22 Sternocleidomastoid muscle
23 Hypoglossus nerve (n. XII)
24 Supraclavicular nerves
    (lateral and intermedial branches)
25 Internal jugular vein and ansa
    cervicalis
26 Anterior supraclavicular nerve

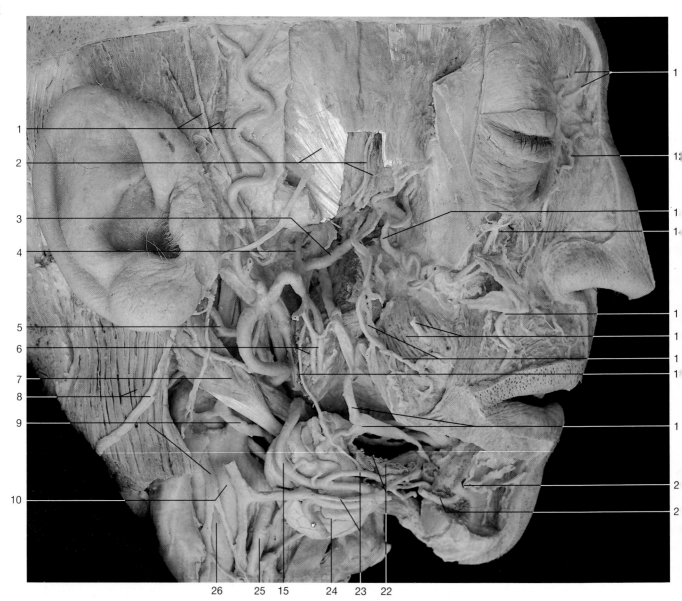

Dissection of deep facial and retromandibular regions after removal of mandible. Pterygoid muscles removed, temporalis muscle fenestrated.

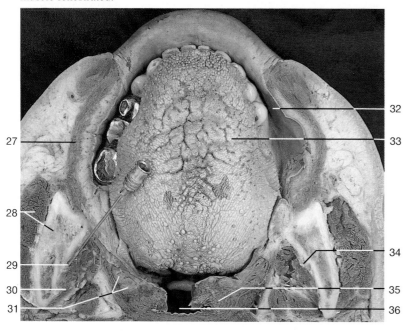

Transverse section through oral cavity and pharynx. The location of inferior alveolar nerve and artery is indicated by a needle.

1 Superficial temporal artery and vein and auriculotemporal nerve
2 Temporalis tendon, deep temporal nerves and artery
3 **Maxillary artery**
4 Middle meningeal artery
5 Occipital artery
6 Inferior alveolar artery and nerve
7 Posterior belly of digastric muscle
8 Great auricular nerve and sternocleidomastoid muscle
9 Hypoglossal nerve and superior root of ansa cervicalis
10 **External carotid artery**
11 Supratrochlear nerve and medial branch of supraorbital artery
12 Angular artery
13 Posterior superior alveolar artery
14 Infraorbital nerve
15 **Facial artery**
16 Parotid duct (divided) and buccinator muscle
17 Buccal artery and nerve

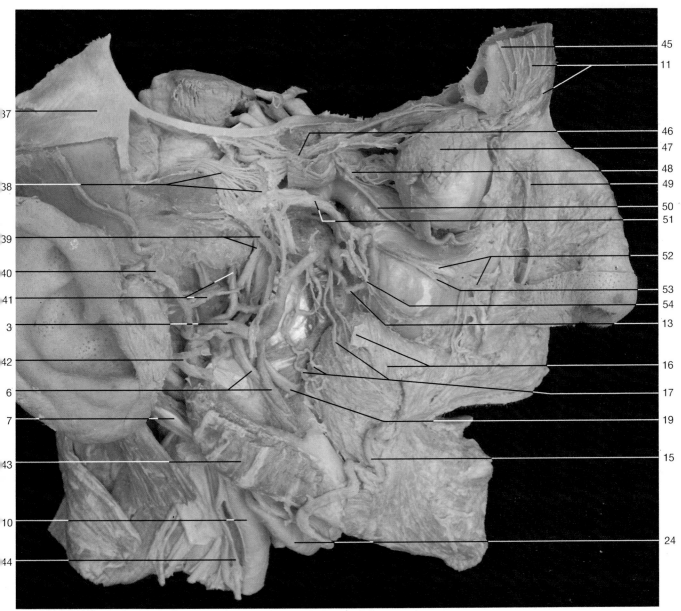

Para- and retropharyngeal regions. The mandible and the lateral wall of the orbit have been removed. The main branches of the trigeminal nerve and its ganglion are displayed.

18 Mylohyoid nerve
19 **Lingual nerve** and **submandibular ganglion**
20 Mental nerve and mental foramen
21 Inferior alveolar nerve
22 Mylohyoid muscle (divided) and hypoglossal nerve
23 Submental artery and vein
24 Submandibular gland
25 Superior thyroid artery
26 Common carotid artery
27 Buccinator muscle
28 Masseter muscle and mandible
29 Entrance of mandibular canal
30 Medial pterygoid muscle
31 Palatine tonsil
32 Oral vestibule
33 Tongue
34 Inferior alveolar nerve, artery and vein
35 Pharyngeal constrictor muscle

36 Pharynx
37 Tentorium of cerebellum
38 **Trigeminal nerve** and **ganglion**
39 **Mandibular nerve**
40 Superficial temporal artery
41 Auriculotemporal nerve and middle meningeal artery
42 Facial nerve (divided)
43 Masseter muscle
44 Superior root of ansa cervicalis
45 Lateral branch of supraorbital nerve
46 **Ophthalmic nerve**
47 Lacrimal gland
48 Ciliary ganglion and short ciliary nerves
49 Angular artery
50 Inferior branch of oculomotor nerve
51 **Maxillary nerve**
52 Infraorbital nerve
53 Anterior superior alveolar nerve
54 Posterior superior alveolar nerve

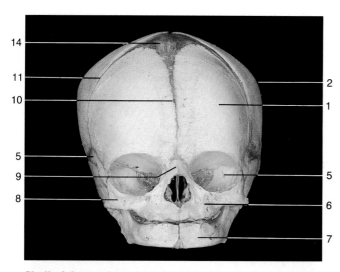

Skull of the newborn (anterior aspect).

Cranial skeleton
1 Frontal tuber or eminence
2 Parietal tuber or eminence
3 Occipital tuber or eminence
4 Squamous part of temporal bone
5 Greater wing of sphenoid bone

Facial skeleton
6 Maxilla
7 Mandible
8 Zygomatic bone
9 Nasal bone

Sutures and fontanelles
10 Frontal suture
11 Coronal suture
12 Sagittal suture
13 Lambdoid suture
14 Anterior fontanelle
15 Posterior fontanelle
16 Sphenoidal (anterolateral) fontanelle
17 Mastoid (posterolateral) fontanelle

Base of the skull
18 Frontal bone
19 Ethmoid bone
20 Sphenoid bone
21 Hypophysial fossa (sella turcica)
22 Dorsum sellae
23 Temporal bone
24 Mastoid (posterolateral) fontanelle
25 Occipital bone

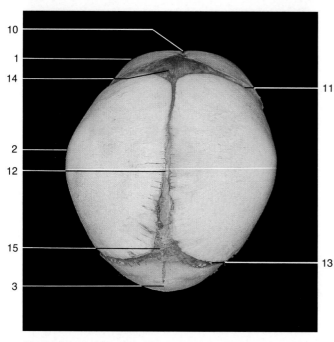

Skull of the newborn (superior aspect). Calvaria.

In the newborn the facial skeleton, in contrast to the cranial skeleton, appears relatively small. There are no teeth presenting. The bones of the cranium are separated by wide fontanelles.

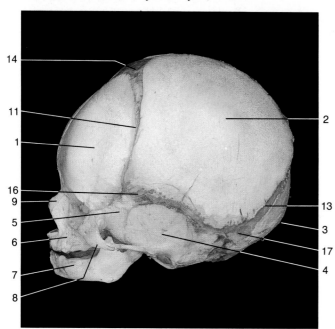

Skull of the newborn (lateral aspect).

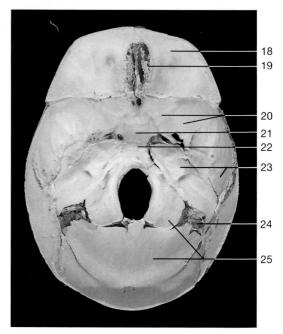

Base of the skull of the newborn (internal aspect).

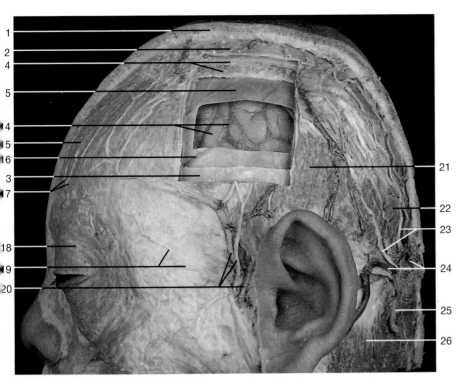

1   Skin
2   **Galea aponeurotica**
3   Pericranium (periosteum)
4   Skull with diploe
5   **Dura mater**
6   Subdural space
7   **Arachnoid mater**
8   **Subarachnoid space**
9   Arachnoid granulations
10 Superior sagittal sinus
11 **Pia mater** with cerebral vessels
12 Falx cerebri
13 Cerebral cortex
14 Arachnoid and pia mater with cortical vessels
15 Frontal belly of occipitofrontal muscle
16 Branch of middle meningeal artery
17 Lateral and medial branch of supraorbital nerve
18 Orbicularis oculi muscle
19 Zygomatico-orbital artery
20 **Auriculotemporal nerve, superficial temporal artery** and **vein**
21 Superior auricular muscle
22 Occipital belly of occipitofrontalis muscle
23 Branches of **greater occipital nerve**
24 **Occipital artery** and **vein**
25 Greater occipital nerve
26 Sternocleidomastoid muscle
27 Frontal lobe of left hemisphere
28 Chiasmatic cistern
29 Interpeduncular cistern
30 Corpus callosum
31 Cerebellum
32 **Cerebellomedullar cistern**

Nerves and blood vessels of the scalp. Scalp and meninges are demonstrated by a series of window-like openings.

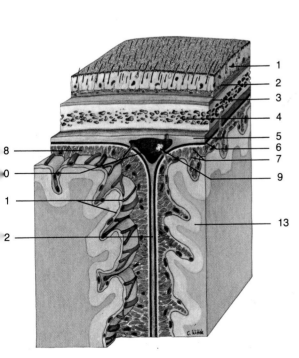

A coronal section through the vertex of the skull, showing the arrangement of the meninges and vessels of the brain. Together the arachnoid mater and the pia mater form the leptomeninx.

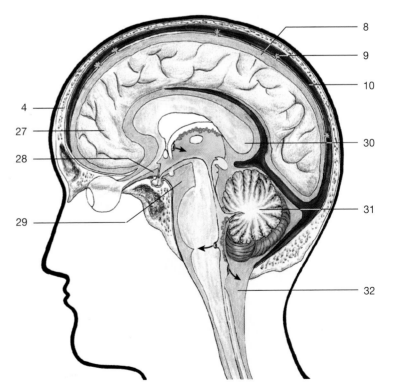

Subarachnoid cisterns of the brain (midsagittal section, green = cisterns; blue = dural sinus and ventricles; red = choroid plexus of third and fourth ventricles).

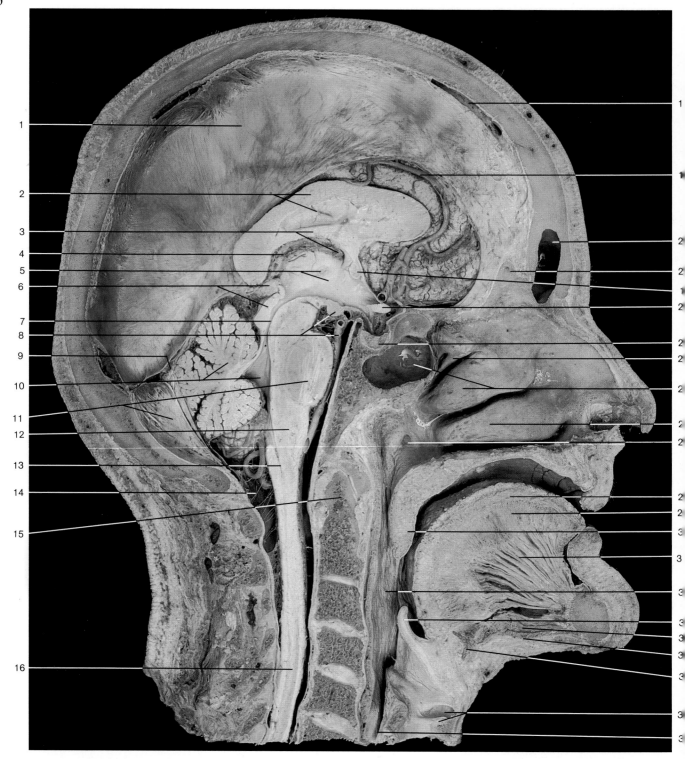

Median sagittal section through the head and neck.

1	Falx cerebri	14	**Cerebellomedullary cistern**
2	**Corpus callosum** and **septum pellucidum**	15	Dens of the axis (odontoid process)
3	Interventricular foramen and fornix	16	Spinal cord
4	Choroid plexus of third ventricle and	17	**Superior sagittal sinus**
	internal cerebral vein	18	**Anterior cerebral artery**
5	**Third ventricle** and interthalamic adhesion	19	Anterior commissure
6	**Pineal body** and **colliculi of the midbrain**	20	**Frontal sinus**
7	Cerebral aqueduct	21	Crista galli
8	Mamillary body and basilar artery	22	Optic chiasma
9	Straight sinus	23	Pituitary gland (hypophysis)
10	**Fourth ventricle** and **cerebellum**	24	Superior nasal concha
11	Pons and falx cerebelli	25	**Middle nasal concha** and **sphenoid**
12	**Medulla oblongata**		**sinus**
13	Central canal	26	**Inferior nasal concha**

27	**Pharyngeal opening of auditory tube**
28	Superior longitudinal muscle of
	tongue
29	Vertical muscle of the tongue
30	**Uvula**
31	Genioglossus muscle
32	Pharynx
33	**Epiglottis**
34	Geniohyoid muscle
35	Mylohyoid muscle
36	Hyoid bone
37	Vocal fold and sinus of larynx
38	Esophagus

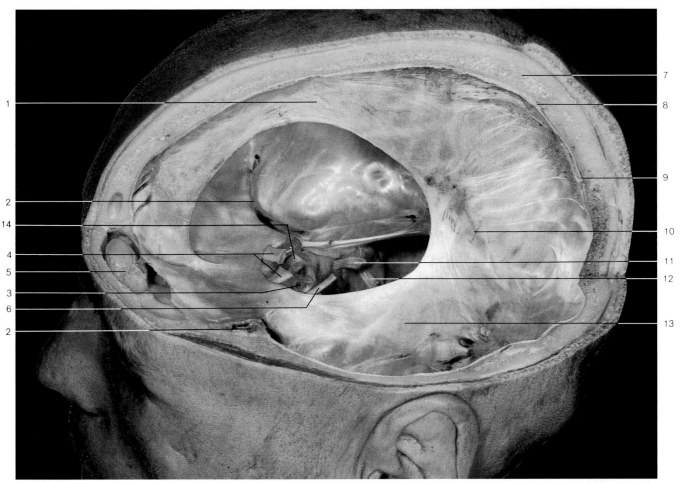

Dura mater and venous sinuses of the dura mater. The brain has been removed (oblique lateral aspect).

1 Falx cerebri
2 Position of middle meningeal
   artery and vein
3 Internal carotid artery
4 **Optic nerve** (n. II)
5 Frontal sinus
6 **Oculomotor nerve** (n. III)
7 Diploe
8 **Dura mater**
9 Superior sagittal sinus
10 Straight sinus
11 **Trigeminal nerve** (n. V)
12 Facial and vestibulocochlear nerve
   (n. VII and n. VIII)
13 **Tentorium cerebelli**
14 **Pituitary gland (hypophysis)**
15 Inferior sagittal sinus
16 Sigmoid sinus
17 Confluence of sinuses
18 Inferior petrosal sinus
19 Transverse sinus
20 Superior petrosal sinus
21 **Cavernous** and **intercavernous sinuses**

Dura mater and **venous sinuses**
(left lateral aspect). (Schematic drawing.)

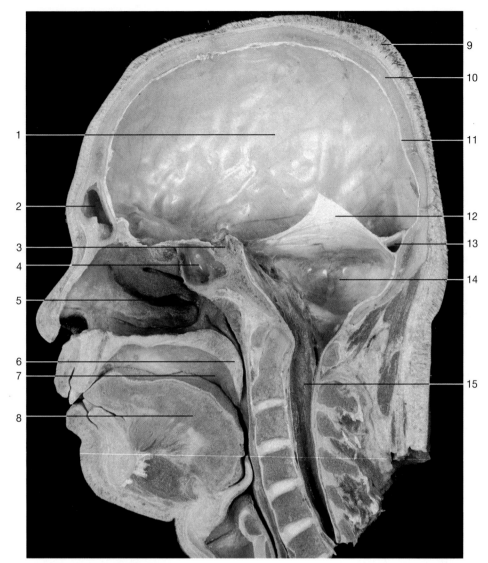

1 **Cranial cavity** with dura mater
   (the right cerebral hemisphere
   has been removed)
2 Frontal sinus
3 Hypophysial fossa with pituitary
   gland
4 Sphenoidal sinus
5 **Nasal cavity**
6 Soft palate (uvula)
7 **Oral cavity**
8 Tongue
9 Skin
10 Calvaria
11 Dura mater
12 Tentorium cerebelli
13 Confluence of sinuses
14 **Infratentorial space** (cerebellum
   and part of the brain stem have
   been removed)
15 Vertebral canal
16 Frontal branch of middle
   meningeal artery and veins
17 Middle meningeal artery
18 **Diploe**
19 Parietal branch of middle
   meningeal artery and vein
20 Occipital pole of left hemisphere
   covered with dura mater

Median section through the head. Demonstration of dura mater covering the cranial cavity. Brain and spinal cord are removed (right half of the head, as seen from medial).

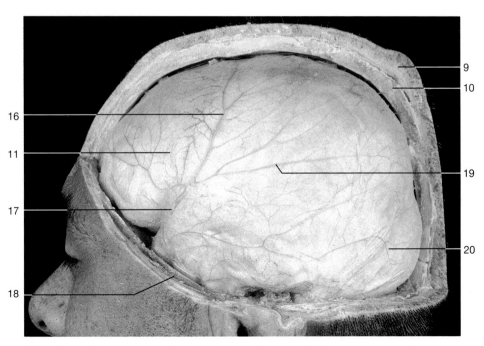

Dissection of dura mater and meningeal vessels. Left half of calvaria removed.

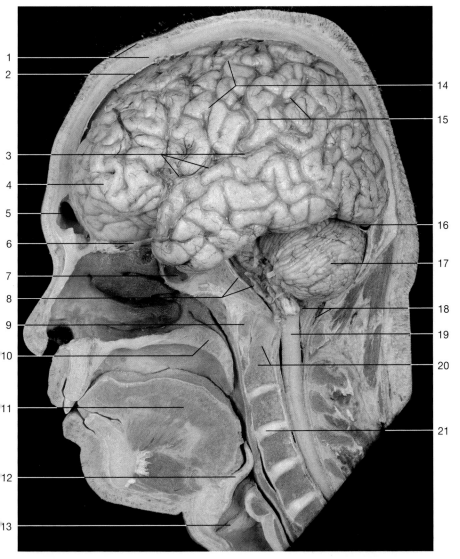

Dissection of the brain with pia mater and arachnoid in situ. The head is cut in half except for the brain, which is shown in its entirety.

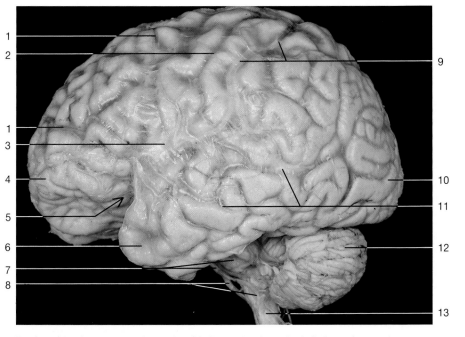

Brain with pia mater and arachnoid. Frontal pole to the left (lateral aspect).

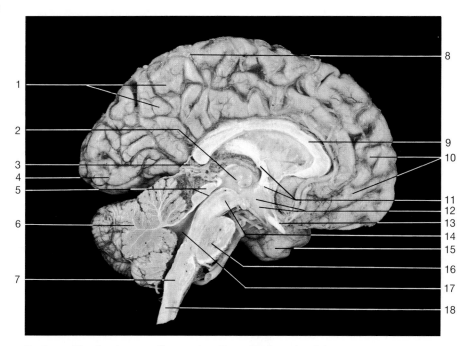

Brain and brain stem, median section. Frontal pole to the right.

1 Parietal lobe
2 Thalamus, **third ventricle** and intermediate mass
3 Great cerebral vein
4 **Occipital lobe**
5 Colliculi of the **midbrain** and **cerebral aqueduct**
6 Cerebellum
7 **Medulla oblongata**
8 Central sulcus
9 **Corpus callosum**
10 **Frontal lobe**
11 Fornix and anterior commissure
12 **Hypothalamus**
13 Optic chiasma
14 Midbrain
15 Temporal lobe
16 **Pons**
17 **Fourth ventricle**
18 Spinal cord
19 Inferior concha and nasal cavity
20 Alveolar process of maxilla
21 Tongue
22 Dens of axis
23 Oral part of pharynx
24 Alveolar process of mandible
25 Epiglottis

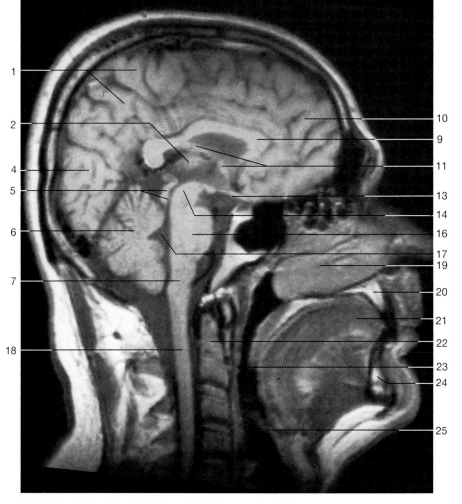

Median section through the head. (MRI scan, cf. section on opposite page.)

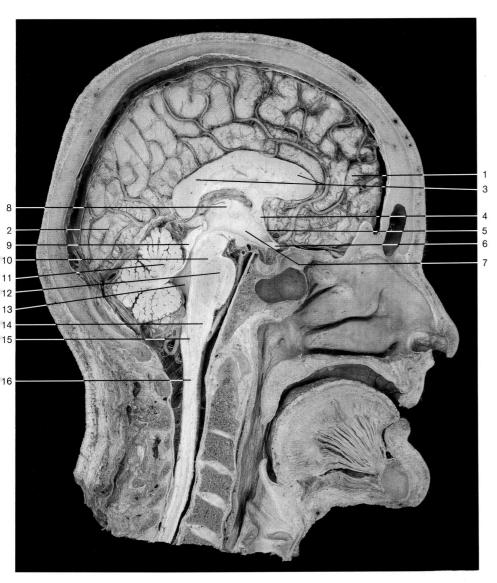

1 Frontal lobe of cerebrum
2 Occipital lobe of cerebrum
3 **Corpus callosum**
4 Anterior commissure
5 **Lamina terminalis**
6 Optic chiasma
7 **Hypothalamus**
8 Thalamus and third
    ventricle
9 **Colliculi of the midbrain**
10 Midbrain (inferior portion)
11 **Cerebellum**
12 Pons
13 **Fourth ventricle**
14 Medulla oblongata
15 Central canal
16 **Spinal cord**

Median section through the head. Regions of the brain. Falx cerebri removed.

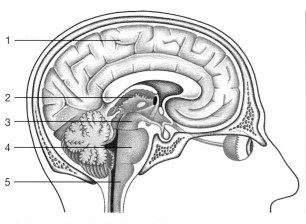

I. Prosencephalon (forebrain)	1. Telencephalon (cerebral hemispheres, striatum, etc.)
	2. Diencephalon (thalamus, metathalamus, hypothalamus, etc.)
II. Mesencephalon (midbrain)	3. Mesencephalon (colliculi, cerebral peduncles, tegmentum)
III. Rhombencephalon (hindbrain)	4. Metencephalon (pons, cerebellum)
	5. Myelencephalon (medulla oblongata)

Scheme of brain divisions (cf. table).
Red = choroidal plexus. (Schematic drawing.)
1 Telencephalon (yellow) with lateral ventricles
2 Diencephalon (orange) with IIIrd ventricle, optic nerve and retina
3 Mesencephalon (blue) with cerebral aqueduct
4 Metencephalon (green) with IVth ventricle
5 Myelencephalon (yellow-green)

Main divisions of the brain
I–III = primary brain vesicles; 1–5 = secondary brain vesicles

Diencephalon, midbrain, pons and medulla oblongata are collectively termed the **brain stem.**

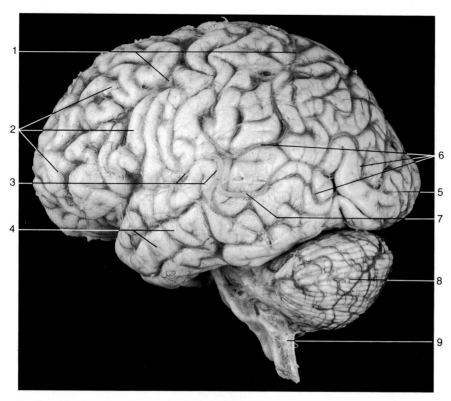

1 Superior cerebral veins and parietal lobe
2 Frontal lobe
3 Superficial middle cerebral vein and **cistern of lateral cerebral fossa**
4 Temporal lobe
5 Occipital lobe
6 Inferior cerebral veins and transverse occipital sulcus
7 Inferior anastomotic vein
8 Cerebellum
9 Medulla oblongata

Brain with pia mater. Cerebral veins (bluish). In the lateral sulcus the cistern of the lateral fossa is recognizable. Frontal lobe to the left.

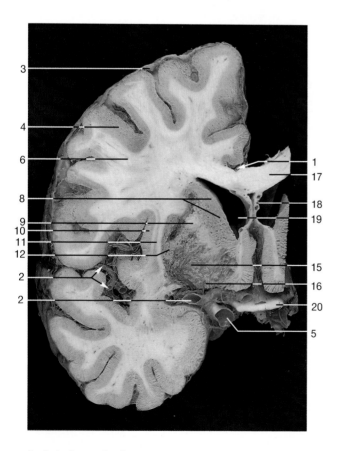

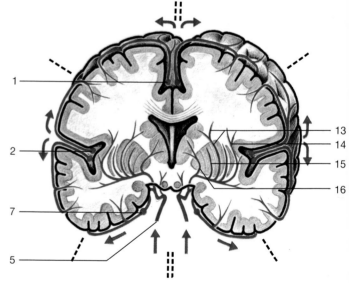

Arteries of the brain. Coronal section. Areas supplied by cortical and central arteries. Dotted lines indicate boundaries of arterial supply areas; arrows, direction of blood flow.

◁

Coronal section through the right hemisphere, showing arachnoid, pia mater, and the arterial blood supply (anterior aspect).

1 **Anterior cerebral artery**
2 **Middle cerebral arteries**
3 Arachnoid
4 Cortex
5 **Internal carotid artery**
6 Frontal lobe (white matter)
7 **Posterior cerebral artery**
8 Caudate nucleus
9 Internal capsule
10 Insular lobe
11 Claustrum
12 Putamen
13 Posterior striate branch
14 Insular artery
15 Pallidostriate artery
16 Thalamic artery
17 Corpus callosum
18 Septum pellucidum
19 Lateral ventricle
20 Optic chiasma

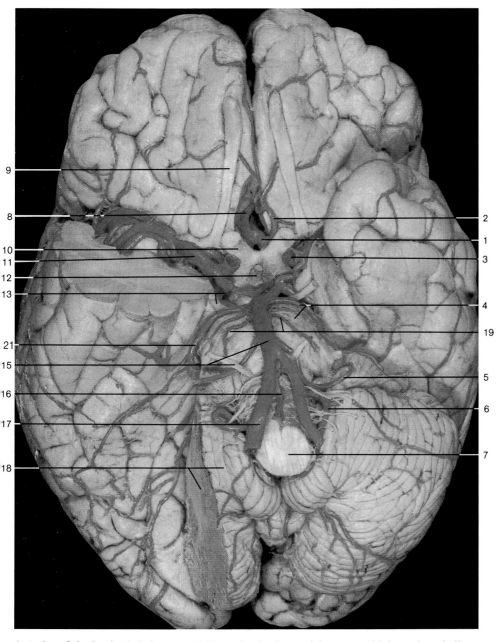

1 Anterior communicating artery
2 Left **anterior cerebral artery**
3 **Internal carotid artery**
4 Pons and left **superior cerebellar artery**
5 **Anterior inferior cerebellar artery**
6 **Posterior inferior cerebellar artery**
7 Medulla oblongata
8 **Right anterior cerebral artery**
9 Olfactory tract
10 Optic nerve
11 **Middle cerebral artery**
12 Infundibulum
13 Oculomotor nerve and **posterior communicating artery**
14 **Posterior cerebral artery**
15 **Basilar artery** and abducent nerve (n. VI)
16 Anterior spinal artery
17 **Vertebral artery**
18 Cerebellum
19 Labyrinthine arteries
20 Posterior spinal artery
21 Right **superior cerebellar artery**
22 Olfactory bulb

Arteries of the brain (inferior aspect). Frontal pole above; right temporal lobe and cerebellum partly removed.

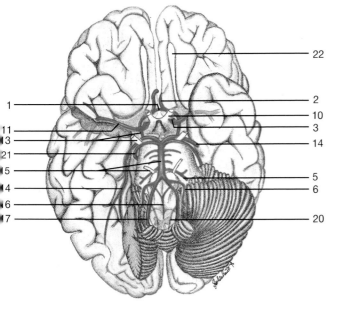

Arteries of the base of the brain, arterial circle of Willis. (Schematic drawing.)

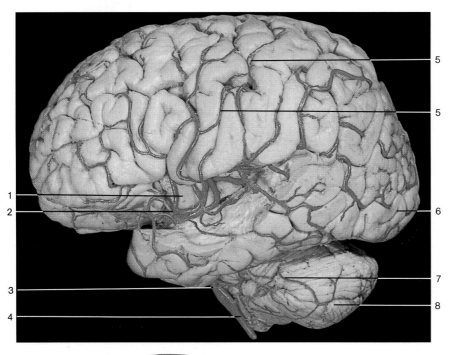

1 Insula
2 **Middle cerebral artery** (2 branches:
  a Parietal branches,
  b Temporal branches)
3 Basilar artery
4 **Vertebral artery**
5 Central sulcus
6 Occipital lobe
7 Superior cerebellar artery
8 Cerebellum
9 **Anterior cerebral artery**
10 Ethmoidal arteries
11 Ophthalmic artery
12 **Internal carotid artery**
13 Posterior communicating artery
14 **Posterior cerebral artery**
15 Anterior inferior cerebellar artery
16 Posterior inferior cerebellar artery

Cerebral arteries. Lateral aspect of the left hemisphere. The upper part of the temporal lobe has been removed to display the insula and cerebral arteries.

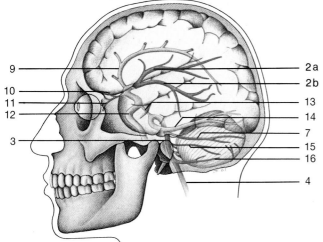

Arteries of the brain.

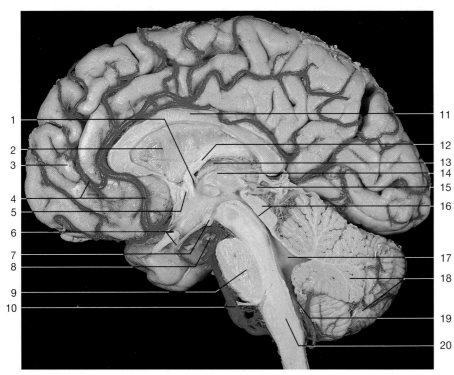

1 Interventricular foramen
2 Septum pellucidum
3 Frontal lobe
4 **Anterior cerebral artery**
5 Anterior commissure
6 Optic chiasma and infundibulum
7 Mamillary body
8 Oculomotor nerve (n. III)
9 Pons
10 **Basilar artery**
11 Corpus callosum
12 **Fornix**
13 **Choroid plexus**
14 **Third ventricle**
15 Pineal body
16 **Tectum** and **cerebral aqueduct**
17 **Fourth ventricle**
18 Cerebellum (arbor vitae, vermis)
19 Median aperture of Magendie
20 Medulla oblongata

Median section through the brain and brain stem. Cerebral arteries injected with red resin.

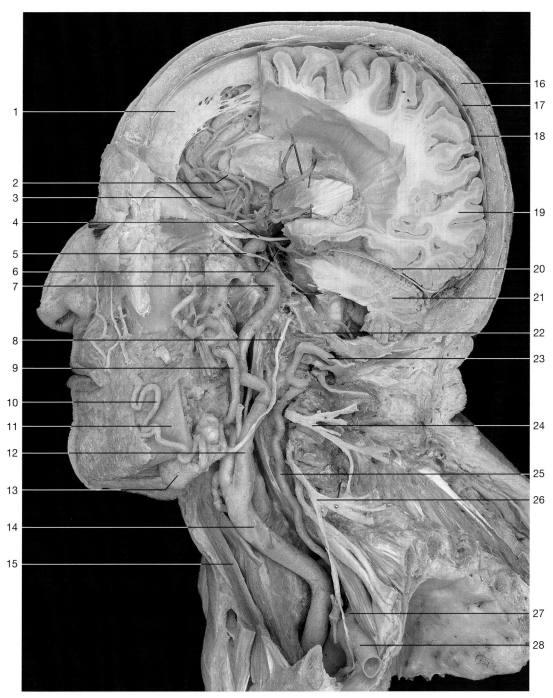

Dissection of the arteries of the brain and head (lateral aspect, superficial layers of facial region and left hemisphere and cerebellum partly removed).

1 Falx cerebri
2 **Anterior cerebral artery**
3 Frontal lobe
4 Oculomotor nerve (n. III)
5 Abducent nerve (n. VI)
6 **Posterior cerebral artery**
7 **Internal carotid artery,** entering sinus cavernosus
8 Hypoglossus nerve (n. XII)
9 Maxillary artery
10 Facial artery
11 Mandible
12 **External carotid artery**
13 Submandibular gland
14 **Common carotid artery**
15 Sternohyoid muscle

16 Calvaria
17 Dura mater
18 Subarachnoidal space
19 Occipital lobe
20 Tentorium of cerebellum
21 Cerebellum
22 Base of skull
23 **Vertebral artery** (on the posterior arch of the atlas)
24 Cervical plexus
25 Vertebral artery (removed from the cervical vertebrae)
26 Brachial plexus
27 Vertebral artery (branching from the subclavian artery)
28 Subclavian artery

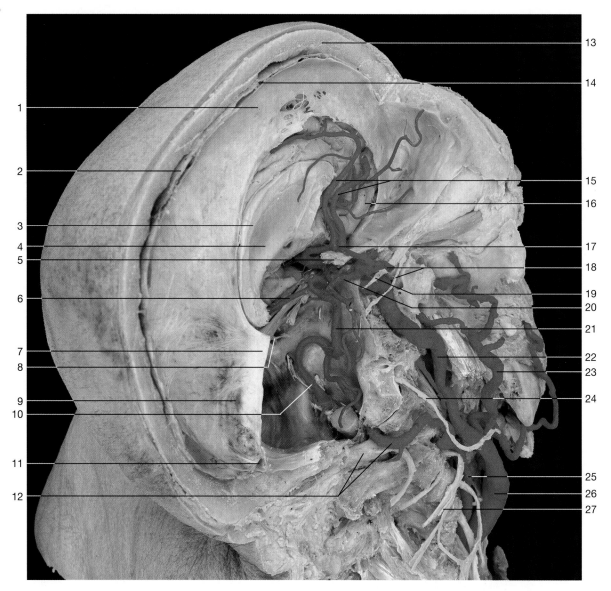

Dissection of the internal carotid artery and the arterial circle of Willis at the base of the skull (posterior lateral aspect, right hemisphere, cerebellum, and part of the deep facial regions have been removed).

1 Falx cerebri	15 Right and left **anterior cerebral artery**
2 Dura mater	16 Frontal lobe of the brain
3 Corpus callosum	17 Anterior communicating artery
4 Septum pellucidum	18 **Medial cerebral artery** and abducent nerve (n. VI)
5 Optic chiasma	19 Oculomotor nerve (n. III)
6 **Posterior cerebral artery**	20 **Arterial circle of Willis**
7 Tentorium of cerebellum	21 **Basilar artery**
8 Internal acoustic meatus	22 **Internal carotid artery**
9 Sinus sigmoideus	23 Maxillary artery
10 Left vertebral artery	24 Hypoglossal nerve (n. XII)
11 Confluens sinuum (continuing into the transverse sinus)	25 **Vertebral artery**
12 Atlas (posterior arch) with vertebral artery	26 Common carotid artery
13 Calvaria	27 Cervical plexus
14 Sinus sagittalis superior	

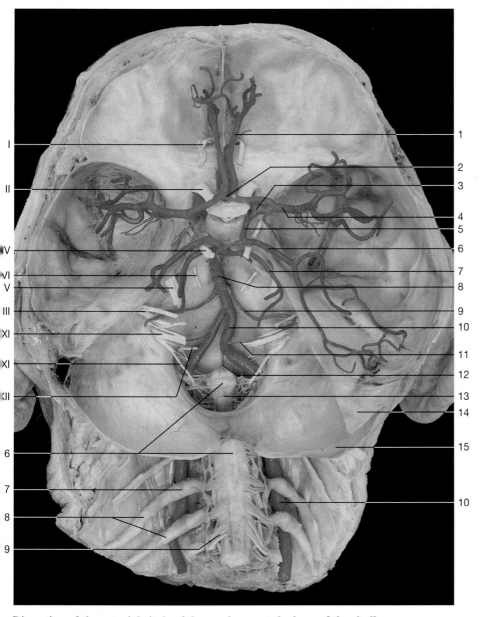

1	**Anterior cerebral artery**
2	Anterior communicating artery
3	Internal carotid artery
4	**Medial cerebral artery**
5	Posterior communicating artery
6	**Posterior cerebral artery**
7	Superior cerebellar artery
8	**Basilar artery**
9	Anterior inferior cerebellar artery with the artery of the labyrinth
10	**Vertebral artery**
11	Posterior inferior cerebellar artery
12	Anterior spinal artery
13	Pia mater of spinal cord
14	Tentorium cerebelli
15	Dura mater of the cranial cavity
16	Spinal cord
17	Spinal ganglion
18	Spinal nerves (C_3, C_4)
19	Posterior root filaments (fila radicularia post.)
20	Ophthalmic artery (within the orbit)
21	Internal carotid artery (within carotid canal)
22	Posterior spinal artery

I	Olfactory tract
II	Optic nerve
III	Oculomotor nerve
IV	Trochlear nerve
V	Trigeminal nerve
VI	Abducent nerve
VII	Facialis nerve
VIII	Vestibulocochlear nerve
IX	Glossopharyngeal nerve
X	Vagus nerve
XI	Accessory nerve
XII	Hypoglossus nerve

Dissection of the arterial circle of the cerebrum at the base of the skull
(from above; calvaria and brain have been removed; arteries are colored in red, cranial nerves (n. I – XII) in yellow).

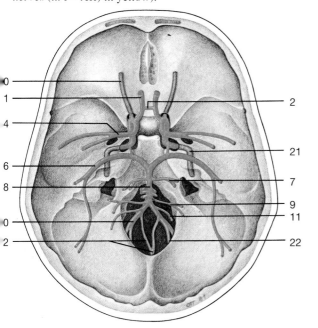

Arterial circle of Willis (superior aspect).
(Schematic drawing.)

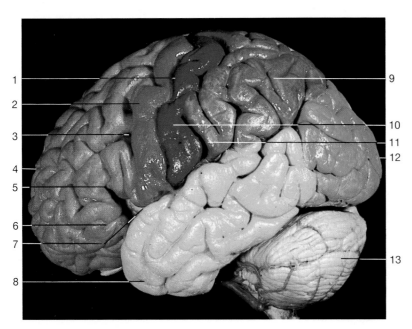

1 Central sulcus
2 Precentral gyrus
3 Precentral sulcus
4 **Frontal lobe**
5 Anterior ascending ramus of lateral sulcus
6 Anterior horizontal ramus of lateral sulcus
7 Lateral sulcus
8 **Temporal lobe**
9 **Parietal lobe**
10 Postcentral gyrus
11 Postcentral sulcus
12 **Occipital lobe**
13 Cerebellum
14 Superior frontal sulcus
15 Middle frontal gyrus
16 Lunate sulcus
17 Longitudinal fissure
18 Arachnoid granulations

Brain, left hemisphere (lateral aspect). Frontal pole to the left.

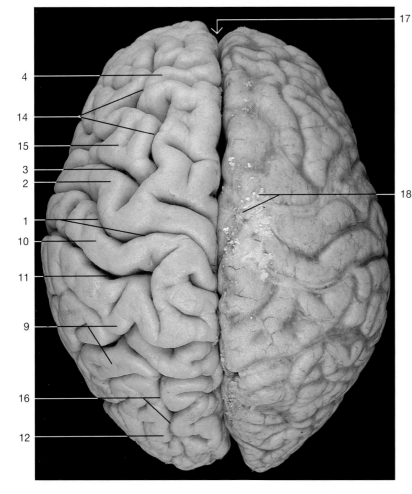

Pink   = Frontal lobe
Blue   = Parietal lobe
Green   = Occipital lobe
Yellow   = Temporal lobe
Dark red = Precentral gyrus
Dark blue = Postcentral gyrus

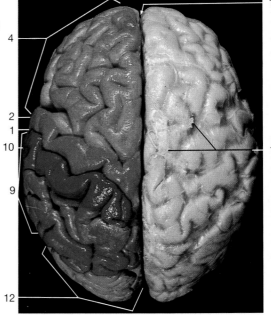

Brain (superior aspect). Right hemisphere with arachnoid and pia mater.

Brain (superior aspect). Lobes of the left hemisphere indicated by color; right hemisphere is covered with arachnoid and pia mater.

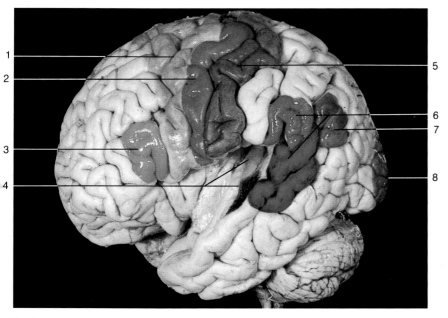

1 Premotor area
2 Somatomotor area
3 Motor speech area of Broca
4 Acoustic area
   (red: high tone; dark green: low tone)
5 Somatosensory area
6 Sensory speech area of Wernicke
7 Reading comprehension area
8 Visuosensory area

Brain, left hemisphere (lateral aspect). **Main cortical areas** are colored.
The lateral sulcus has been opened to display the insula and the inner surface of the
temporal lobe.

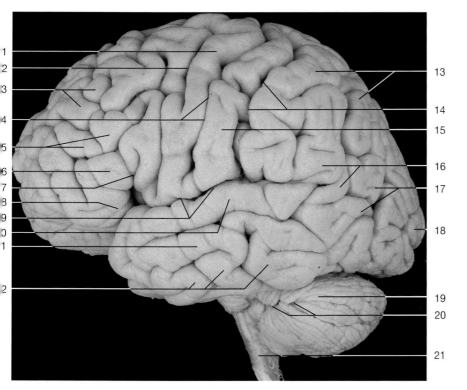

1 Precentral gyrus
2 Precentral sulcus
3 Superior frontal gyrus
4 **Central sulcus**
5 Middle frontal gyrus
6 Inferior frontal gyrus
7 Ascending ramus ⎫ of lateral
8 Horizontal ramus ⎬ sulcus
9 Posterior ramus ⎭
10 Superior temporal gyrus
11 Middle temporal gyrus
12 Inferior temporal gyrus
13 Parietal lobe
14 Postcentral sulcus
15 Postcentral gyrus
16 Supramarginal gyrus
17 Angular gyrus
18 **Occipital lobe**
19 **Cerebellum**
20 Horizontal fissure of cerebellum
21 Medulla oblongata

Brain, left hemisphere (lateral aspect). Frontal pole to the left.

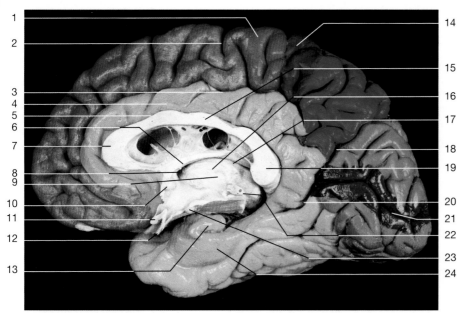

Brain, right hemisphere (medial aspect). Frontal pole to the left (midbrain divided, cerebellum and inferior part of brain stem removed).

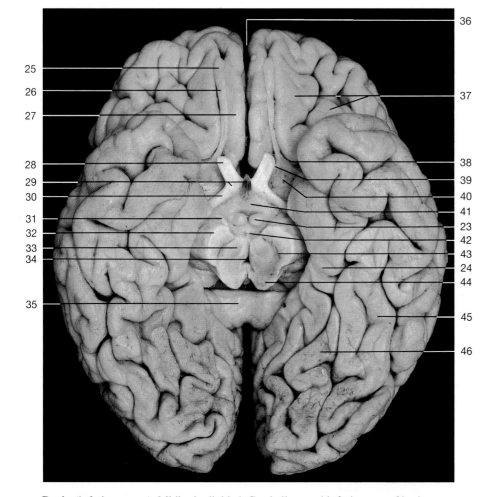

Brain (inferior aspect). Midbrain divided. Cerebellum and inferior part of brain stem removed. Frontal pole at the top.

1 **Precentral gyrus**
2 Precentral sulcus
3 Cingulate sulcus
4 **Cingulate gyrus**
5 Sulcus of corpus callosum
6 **Fornix**
7 Genu of **corpus callosum**
8 Interventricular foramen
9 Intermediate mass
10 Anterior commissure
11 **Optic chiasma**
12 **Infundibulum**
13 Uncus hippocampi
14 **Postcentral gyrus**
15 Body of corpus callosum
16 Third ventricle and thalamus
17 Stria medullaris
18 **Parieto-occipital sulcus**
19 Splenium of corpus callosum
20 Communication of calcarine and parieto-occipital sulcus
21 Calcarine sulcus
22 **Pineal body**
23 **Mamillary body**
24 **Parahippocampal gyrus**
25 **Olfactory bulb**
26 Olfactory tract
27 Gyrus rectus
28 **Optic nerve**
29 Infundibulum and optic chiasma
30 **Optic tract**
31 Oculomotor nerve
32 Pedunculus cerebri
33 **Red nucleus**
34 **Cerebral aqueduct**
35 Corpus callosum
36 Longitudinal fissure
37 Orbital gyri
38 Lateral root of olfactory tract
39 Medial root of olfactory tract
40 Olfactory tubercle and anterior perforated substance
41 Tuber cinereum
42 Interpeduncular fossa
43 **Substantia nigra**
44 Colliculi of the **midbrain**
45 Lateral occipitotemporal gyrus
46 Medial occipitotemporal gyrus

Pink = Frontal lobe
Blue = Parietal lobe
Green = Occipital lobe
Yellow = Temporal lobe
Dark red = Precentral lobe
Dark blue = Postcentral lobe
Orange = Limbic cortex (cingulate and parahippocampal gyri)

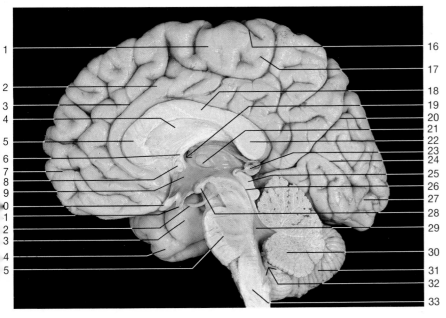

Brain (sagittal section). Frontal pole to the left.

1 Precentral gyrus
2 Cingulate gyrus
3 Cingulate sulcus
4 Septum pellucidum
5 Genu of corpus callosum
6 Fornix
7 **Frontal lobe**
8 Anterior commissure
9 **Hypothalamus**
10 Optic chiasma
11 Infundibulum
12 Oculomotor nerve
13 Uncus
14 **Temporal lobe**
15 Pons
16 Central sulcus
17 Postcentral gyrus
18 Body of corpus callosum
19 Interventricular foramen (arrow)
20 Parieto-occipital sulcus
21 Intermediate mass
22 Splenium of corpus callosum
23 Pineal body
24 Calcarine sulcus
25 Colliculi of midbrain
26 Cerebral aqueduct
27 **Occipital lobe**
28 Mamillary body
29 Fourth ventricle
30 Vermis of cerebellum
31 Right hemisphere of cerebellum
32 Median aperture of Magendie (arrow)
33 Medulla oblongata
34 Olfactory tract
35 Optic nerve
36 **Internal carotid artery**
37 Interpeduncular cistern
38 Superior cerebellar artery
39 Anterior inferior cerebellar artery
40 **Vertebral artery**
41 Posterior inferior cerebellar artery
42 **Basilar artery**
43 Trigeminal nerve (n. V)
44 Facial nerve (n. VII)
45 Accessory nerve (n. XI),
   hypoglossal nerve (n. XII)
46 Cerebellum

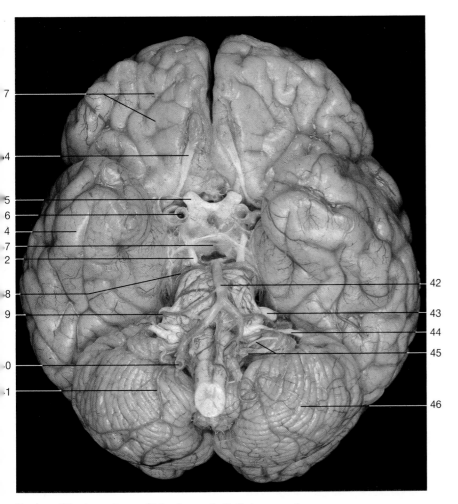

Brain, with pia mater and blood vessels (inferior aspect).

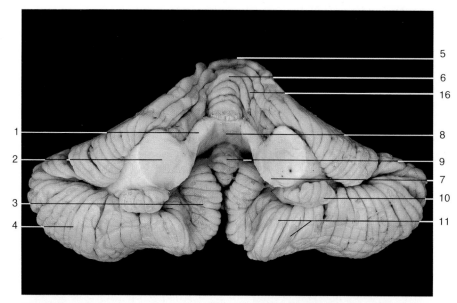

Cerebellum (inferior anterior aspect). The cerebellar peduncles have been severed.

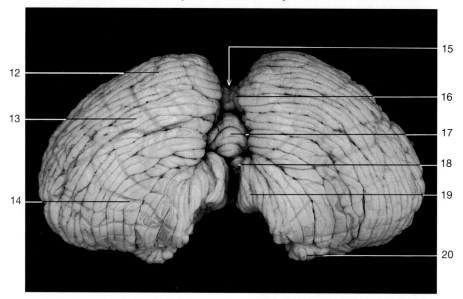

Cerebellum (inferior posterior aspect).

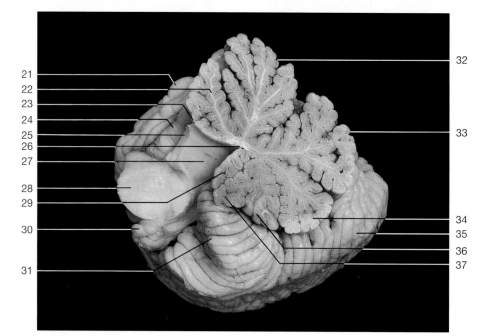

Median section through the cerebellum. Right cerebellar hemisphere and right half of vermis.

1 Superior cerebellar peduncle
2 Middle cerebellar peduncle
3 Cerebellar tonsil
4 Inferior semilunar lobule
5 **Vermis**
6 Central lobule of vermis
7 Inferior cerebellar peduncle
8 Superior medullary velum
9 **Nodule of vermis**
10 **Flocculus**
11 Biventral lobule
12 Left cerebellar hemisphere
13 Inferior semilunar lobule
14 Biventral lobule
15 Vermis of cerebellum
16 Tuber of vermis
17 Pyramid of vermis
18 Uvula of vermis
19 Tonsil of cerebellum
20 Floccule of cerebellum
21 Right cerebellar hemisphere
22 Vermis (central lobule)
23 Cerebellar lingula
24 Ala of central lobule
25 **Superior cerebellar peduncle**
26 Fastigium
27 **Fourth ventricle**
28 **Middle cerebellar peduncle**
29 Nodule of vermis
30 Flocculus of cerebellum
31 Cerebellar tonsil
32 Culmen of vermis
33 Declive of vermis
34 Tuber of vermis
35 Inferior semilunar lobule
36 Pyramid of vermis (cut)
37 Uvula of vermis

1 Olfactory bulb
2 **Olfactory tract**
3 Lateral olfactory stria
4 Anterior perforated substance
5 Infundibulum (divided)
6 **Mamillary body**
7 Substantia nigra
8 Pedunculus cerebri (cut)
9 **Red nucleus**
10 Decussation of superior cerebellar
   peduncle
11 **Cerebellar hemisphere**
12 Medial olfactory stria
13 **Optic nerve**
14 Optic chiasma
15 Optic tract
16 Posterior perforated substance
17 Interpeduncular fossa
18 **Superior cerebellar peduncle**
   and cerebellorubral tract
19 **Dentate nucleus**
20 **Vermis of cerebellum**
21 Cingulate gyrus
22 **Corpus callosum**
23 Stria terminalis
24 Septum pellucidum
25 **Columna fornicis**
26 Cerebral peduncle at midbrain level
27 Pons
28 Inferior olive
29 Medulla oblongata with lateral
   pyramidal tract
30 Occipital lobe
31 Calcarine sulcus
32 **Thalamus**
33 Inferior colliculus with brachium
34 **Medial lemniscus**
35 **Superior cerebellar peduncle**
36 **Inferior cerebellar peduncle**
37 **Middle cerebellar peduncle**
38 Cerebellar hemisphere

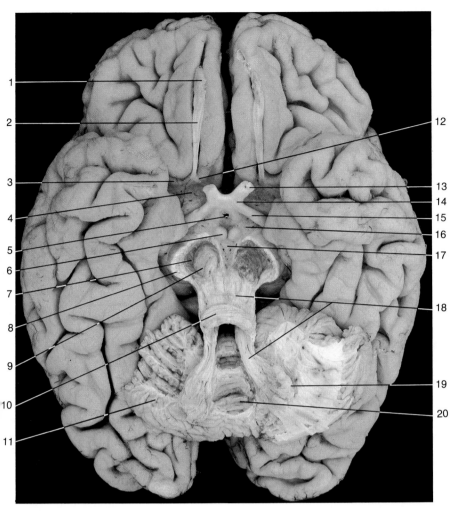

Brain and cerebellum (inferior aspect). Parts of the cerebellum have been removed to display the dentate nucleus and the main pathway to the midbrain (cerebellorubral tract).

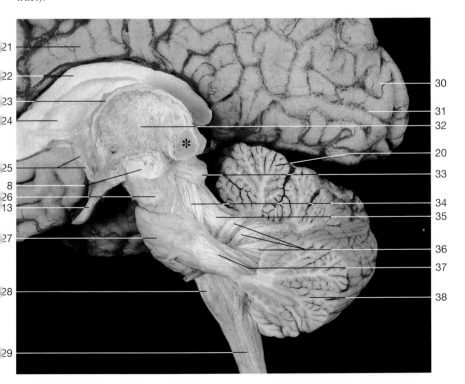

Dissection of the cerebellar peduncles and their connection with midbrain and diencephalon. A small part of pulvinar thalami (∗) has been cut to show inferior brachium.

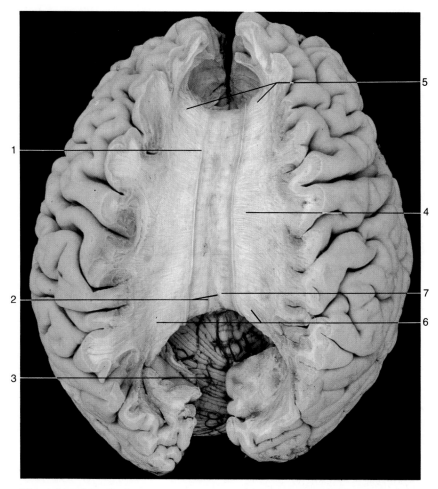

1 Lateral longitudinal stria
   of indusium griseum
2 Medial longitudinal stria
   of indusium griseum
3 Cerebellum
4 Radiating fibers of the corpus callosum
5 Forceps minor of corpus callosum
6 Forceps major of corpus callosum
7 Splenium of corpus callosum

Dissection of the brain I. The fiber system of the corpus callosum has been displayed by removing the cortex lying above it. Frontal pole at the top.

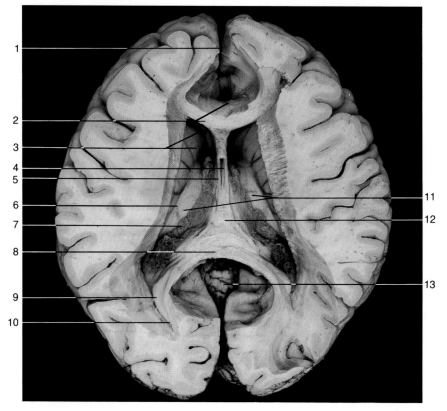

1 Longitudinal cerebral fissure
2 Genu of corpus callosum
3 Head of **caudate nucleus** and
   anterior horn of lateral ventricle
4 Cavum of septum pellucidum
5 **Septum pellucidum**
6 Stria terminalis
7 **Choroid plexus** of **lateral ventricle**
8 Splenium of **corpus callosum**
9 Calcar avis
10 Posterior horn of lateral ventricle
11 **Thalamus** (lamina affixa)
12 Commissure of fornix
13 Vermis of cerebellum

Dissection of the brain II. The lateral ventricles and subcortical nuclei of the brain are dissected. The corpus callosum has been partly removed. Frontal pole at the top.

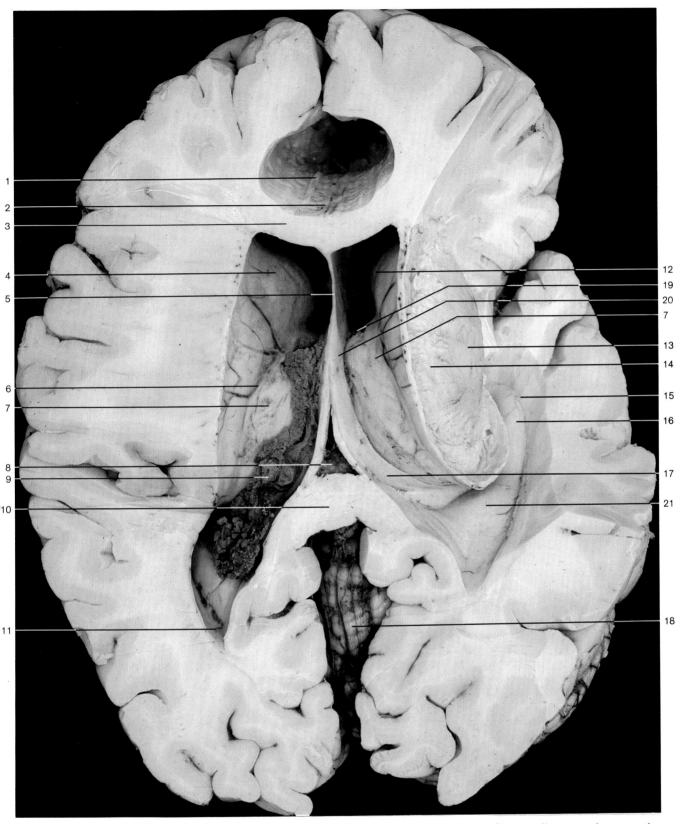

Dissection of the brain III (superior view of lateral ventricle and subcortical nuclei of the brain). Corpus callosum partly removed. At right, the entire lateral ventricle has been opened, the insula with claustrum and the extreme and external capsules have been removed, exposing the lentiform nucleus and the internal capsule.

1	Lateral longitudinal stria	9	**Choroid plexus of lateral ventricle**	16	**Pes hippocampi**
2	Medial longitudinal stria	10	Splenium of corpus callosum	17	**Crus of fornix**
3	Genu of corpus callosum	11	Posterior horn of lateral ventricle	18	Vermis of cerebellum with arachnoid and
4	Head of **caudate nucleus**	12	Anterior horn of lateral ventricle		pia mater
5	**Septum pellucidum**		(head of caudate nucleus)	19	Interventricular foramen
6	Stria terminalis	13	**Putamen** of **lentiform nucleus**	20	Right column of fornix
7	**Thalamus** (lamina affixa)	14	**Internal capsule**	21	Collateral eminence
8	Choroid plexus of third ventricle	15	Inferior horn of lateral ventricle		

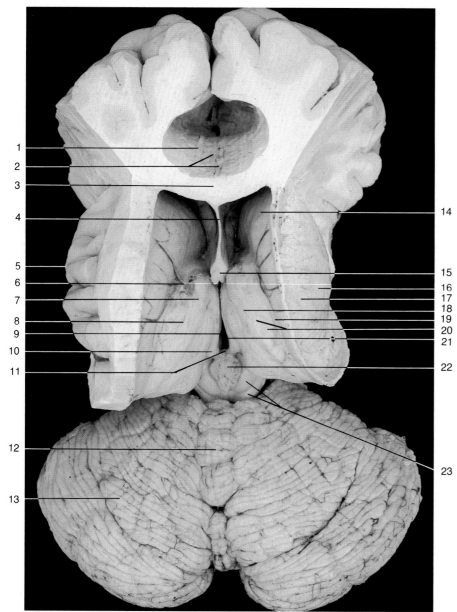

1	Lateral longitudinal stria
2	Medial longitudinal stria
3	**Corpus callosum**
4	Septum pellucidum
5	Insular gyri
6	Thalamostriate vein
7	Anterior tubercle of thalamus
8	**Thalamus**
9	Medullary stria of thalamus
10	Habenular trigone
11	Habenular commissure
12	**Vermis of the cerebellum**
13	**Left hemisphere of cerebellum**
14	**Head of caudate nucleus**
15	**Columns of fornix**
16	Putamen of lentiform nucleus
17	**Internal capsule**
18	Taenia of choroid plexus
19	Stria terminalis and thalamostriate vein
20	Lamina affixa
21	**Third ventricle**
22	**Pineal body**
23	Superior and inferior colliculus of midbrain

Dissection of the brain IVa. Temporal lobe, fornix and the posterior corpus callosum have been removed (this part of the specimen is depicted below). Frontal pole at top (superior aspect).

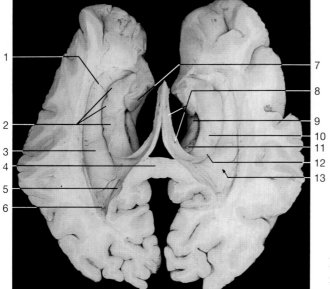

1	Inferior horn of lateral ventricle
2	**Hippocampal digitations**
3	Collateral eminence
4	Splenium of corpus callosum
5	Calcar avis
6	Posterior horn of lateral ventricle
7	**Uncus** of parahippocampal gyrus
8	Body and crus of **fornix**
9	**Parahippocampal gyrus**
10	**Pes hippocampi**
11	Dentate gyrus
12	Hippocampal fimbria
13	Lateral ventricle

Dissection of the brain IVb. Depicted is the portion of the brain removed from the specimen above. **Temporal lobe and limbic system** (superior aspect). Columns of fornix are cut.

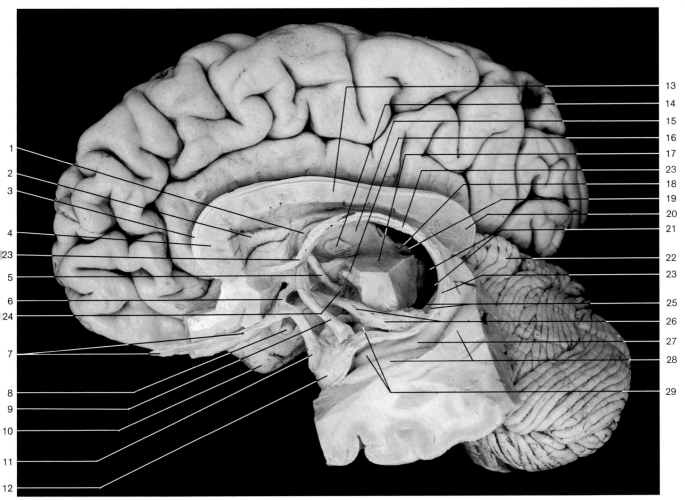

Dissection of the limbic system. Left side, lateral aspect. Corpus callosum has been cut in the median plane. The left thalamus and the left hemisphere have been partly removed.

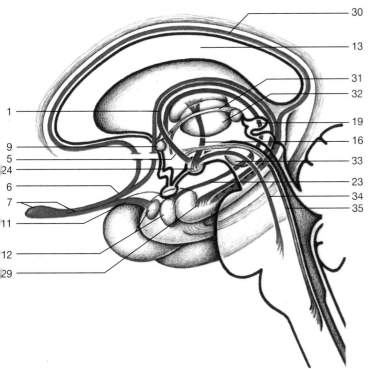

1	**Body of fornix**	20	Splenium of corpus
2	Septum pellucidum		callosum
3	**Lateral longitudinal stria**	21	Colliculi of midbrain
4	Genu of corpus callosum	22	Vermis of cerebellum
5	**Column of fornix**	23	**Stria terminalis**
6	Medial olfactory stria	24	**Mamillary body**
7	**Olfactory bulb and**	25	Fimbria of hippocampus
	olfactory tract		and pes hippocampi
8	Optic nerve	26	Left optic tract and
9	Anterior commissure		lateral geniculate body
	(left half)	27	Lateral ventricle and
10	Right temporal lobe		**parahippocampal gyrus**
11	**Lateral olfactory stria**	28	Collateral eminence
12	**Amygdala**	29	Hippocampal digitations
13	Body of **corpus callosum**	30	**Supracallosal gyrus**
14	Interthalamic adhesion		(longitudinal stria)
15	Third ventricle and right	31	Stria medullaris thalami
	thalamus	32	Thalamus
16	**Mamillothalamic tract**	33	Red nucleus
17	Part of the thalamus	34	Mamillotegmental tract
18	Habenular commissure	35	Dorsal longitudinal
19	Pineal body		fasciculus (Schütz)

Main pathways of **limbic and olfactory system.** (Schematic drawing.) Blue = afferent pathways; red = efferent pathways.

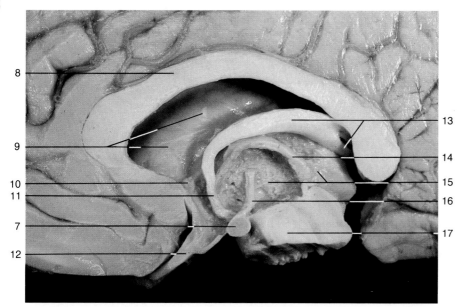

Median section through the diencephalon. Medial part of the thalamus and septum pellucidum have been removed to show the fornix and mamillothalamic tract.

1   Paraventricular nucleus ⎫
2   Preoptic nucleus   ⎪
3   Ventromedial nucleus   ⎬ **Hypothalamic**
4   Supraoptic nucleus   ⎪ **nuclei**
5   Posterior nucleus   ⎪
6   Dorsomedial nucleus   ⎭
7   **Mamillary body**
8   **Corpus callosum**
9   Lateral ventricle (showing caudate nucleus)
10 Anterior commissure
11 **Column of fornix**
12 Optic chiasma
13 **Crus of fornix**
14 Medullary stria of thalamus
15 Thalamus and interthalamic adhesion
16 **Mamillothalamic tract** of Vicq d'Azyr
17 Cerebral peduncle
18 **Pineal body**
19 Tectum of midbrain
20 Lamina terminalis

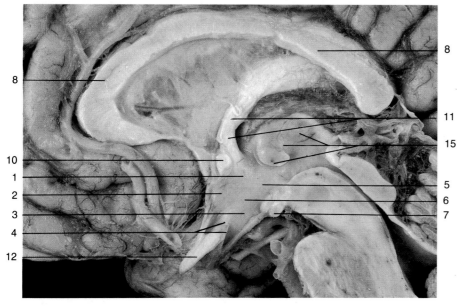

Median section through the diencephalon and midbrain; location of hypothalamic nuclei.

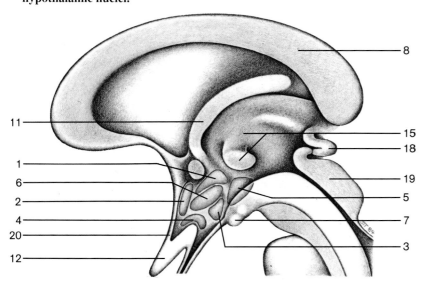

Position of main hypothalamic nuclei. (Schematic diagram.)

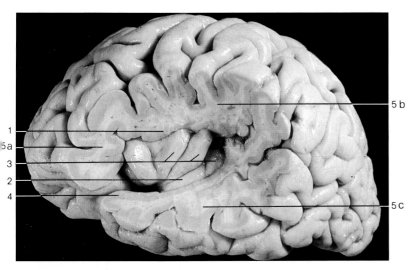

Insula (Reili). The opercula of the frontal, parietal and temporal lobes have been removed to display the insular gyri. Left hemisphere.

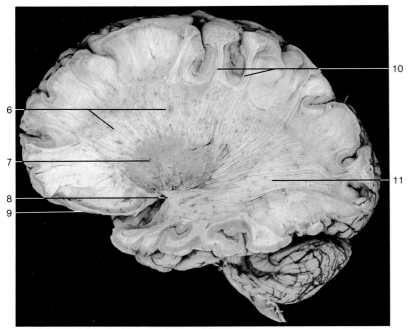

Dissection of the corona radiata, left hemisphere. Frontal pole on the left.

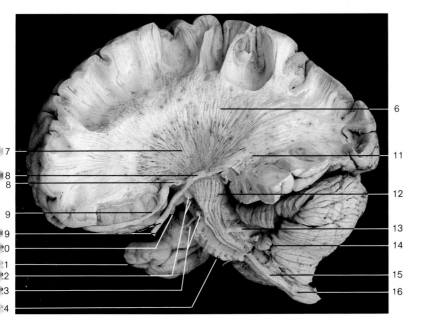

1 Circular sulcus of insula
2 Long gyrus of insula
3 Short gyri of insula
4 Limen insulae
5 Opercula (cut)
  a Frontal operculum
  b Frontoparietal operculum
  c Temporal operculum
6 **Corona radiata**
7 **Lentiform nucleus**
8 **Anterior commissure**
9 Olfactory tract
10 Cerebral arcuate fibers
11 Optic radiation
12 Cerebral peduncle
13 Trigeminal nerve (n. V)
14 Flocculus of cerebellum
15 **Pyramidal tract**
16 Decussation of pyramidal tract
17 Internal capsule
18 Optic tract
19 Optic nerve (n. II)
20 Infundibulum
21 Temporal lobe (right side)
22 Mamillary bodies
23 Oculomotor nerve (n. III)
24 Transverse fibers of pons

◁ **Corona radiata and internal capsule,**
  left hemisphere. Lentiform nucleus
  removed (frontal pole to the left).

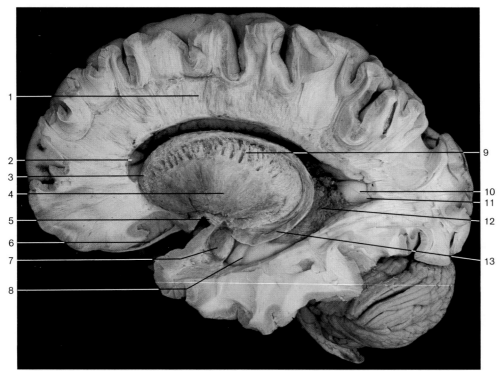

1 Corona radiata
2 Anterior horn of lateral
   ventricle
3 Head of **caudate nucleus**
4 **Putamen**
5 Anterior commissure
6 Olfactory tract
7 **Amygdala**
8 Hippocampal digitations
9 **Internal capsule**
10 Calcar avis
11 Posterior horn of lateral
   ventricle
12 Choroid plexus of lateral
   ventricle
13 Caudal extremity of caudate
   nucleus
14 **Thalamus**
15 Cerebral arcuate fibers
16 Globus pallidus (remnants)

Dissection of the subcortical nuclei and internal capsule, left hemisphere (lateral aspect).
Frontal pole to the left. The lateral ventricle has been opened, and the insular gyri and
claustrum have been removed, revealing the lentiform nucleus and the internal capsule.

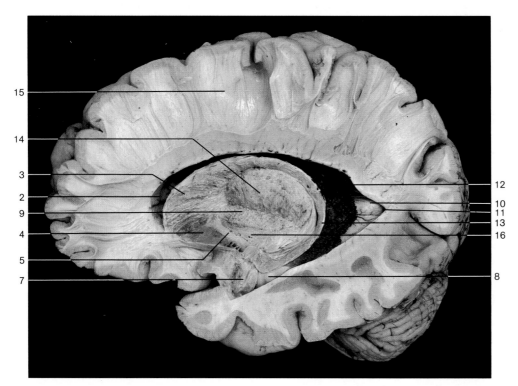

Dissection of the subcortical nuclei (lateral aspect). Lentiform nucleus removed, frontal pole
to the left.

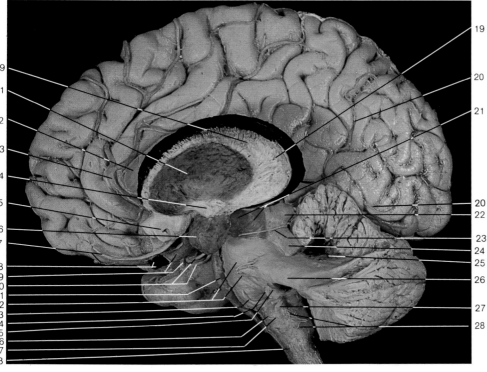

Brain stem and the connections with the cerebellum. Internal capsule (lateral aspect). Red = pyramidal tract; yellow = middle cerebellar peduncle; green = inferior cerebellar peduncle; pink = superior cerebellar peduncle.

1 **Putamen**
2 Genu of corpus callosum
3 Anterior cerebral artery
4 Anterior commissure
5 Subcallosal area
6 Amygdala
7 Olfactory tract
8 Optic nerve (n. II)
9 Internal carotid artery and infundibulum
10 Oculomotor nerves (right and left nerve, n. III)
11 **Basilar artery**
12 Pons and trigeminal nerve (n. V)
13 Abducent nerve (n. VI)
14 Facial nerve (n. VII)
15 Vestibulocochlear nerve (n. VIII)
16 Hypoglossal nerve (n. XII)
17 Olive
18 Pyramidal tract
19 **Internal capsule**
20 Posterior cerebral artery
21 Cerebral peduncle
22 **Colliculi of midbrain**
23 Trochlear nerve (n. IV)
24 Superior cerebellar peduncle
25 Inferior cerebellar peduncle
26 **Middle cerebellar peduncle**
27 Glossopharyngeal nerve (n. IX)
28 Vagus (n. X) and accessory nerves (n. XI)
29 **Corpus callosum**
30 Lateral ventricle (anterior horn)
31 Caudate nucleus
32 Internal capsule (anterior limb)
33 Insula
34 **Claustrum**
35 **Thalamus**
36 Superior and inferior colliculus of midbrain
37 Cerebellum
38 Middle peduncle of cerebellum (efferent tracts)
39 Medulla oblongata (afferent tracts)
40 Putamen of lentiform nucleus
41 **Globus pallidus** of lentiform nucleus
42 Genu and posterior limb of internal capsule

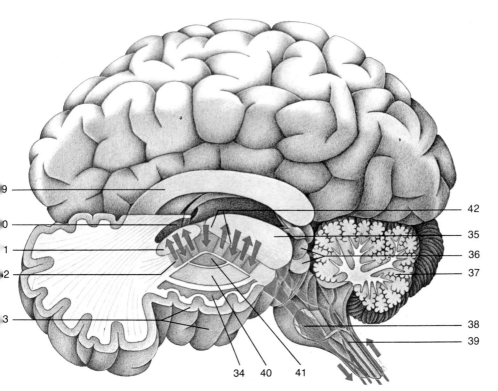

Internal capsule and subcortical nuclei. Left brain, frontal pole to the left, horizontal section. (Semischematic drawing.) Blue = afferent tracts; red = efferent tracts.

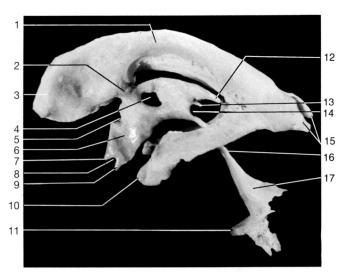

Cast of ventricular cavities of the brain (lateral aspect), frontal pole to the left.

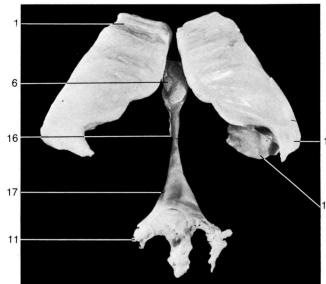

Cast of ventricular cavities (posterior aspect).

1 Central part of the **lateral ventricle**
2 **Interventricular foramen** of Monro
3 Anterior horn of the lateral ventricle
4 Site of interthalamic adhesion
5 Notch for anterior commissure
6 **Third ventricle**
7 Optic recess
8 Notch for optic chiasma
9 Infundibular recess
10 Inferior horn of lateral ventricle with indentation of amygdaloid body
11 Lateral recess and lateral aperture of Luschka
12 Suprapineal recess

13 Pineal recess
14 Notch for posterior commissure
15 Posterior horn of lateral ventricle
16 **Cerebral aqueduct**
17 **Fourth ventricle**
18 Median aperture of Magendie
19 **Cerebellomedullary cistern**
20 Superior sagittal sinus
21 Inferior sagittal sinus
22 Intervaginal space of optic nerve
23 Arachnoid granulations of Pacchioni
24 Straight sinus

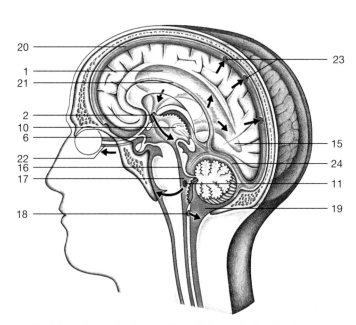

Position of ventricular cavities. (Schematic drawing.)
The direction of flow of cerebrospinal fluid is indicated by arrows.
Green = right lateral ventricle;
red = choroidal plexus.

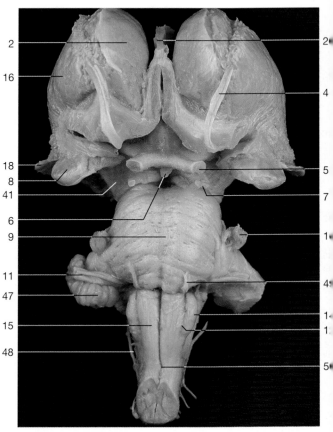

Brain stem (ventral aspect). (Numbers see p. 113)

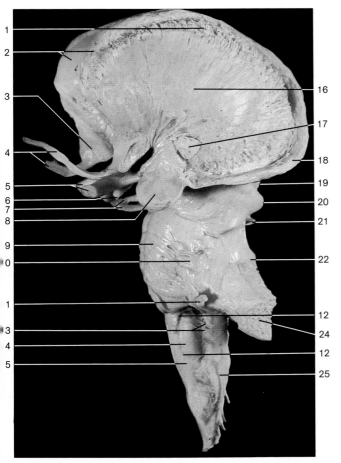

1 Internal capsule
2 Head of the caudate nucleus
3 Olfactory trigone
4 Olfactory tracts
5 Optic nerves
6 Infundibulum
7 Oculomotor nerve
8 **Amygdaloid body**
9 **Pons**
10 Trigeminal nerve
11 Facial and vestibulocochlear nerves
12 Hypoglossal nerve
13 Glossopharyngeal and vagus nerves
14 **Olive**
15 Medulla oblongata
16 **Lentiform nucleus**
17 **Anterior commissure**
18 Tail of caudate nucleus
19 Superior colliculus
20 Inferior colliculus
21 Trochlear nerve
22 Superior cerebellar peduncle
23 Inferior cerebellar peduncle
24 **Middle cerebellar peduncle**
25 Accessory nerve (n. XI)
26 Columns of fornix (divided)
27 Lamina affixa
28 **Third ventricle**
29 Pulvinar of thalamus
30 Inferior brachium
31 Frenulum veli
32 Superior medullary velum
33 Facial colliculus
34 Striae medullares and rhomboid fossa
35 Hypoglossal triangle
36 Stria terminalis and thalamostriate vein
37 Habenular trigone
38 Choroid plexus of lateral ventricle
39 **Pineal body**
40 Medial geniculate body
41 Cerebral peduncle
42 Choroid plexus of fourth ventricle
43 Clava
44 Dorsal root of cervical nerve
45 Cuneate tubercle
46 Lateral geniculate body
47 Flocculus
48 Accessory nerve (n. XI)
49 Abducent nerve (n. VI)
50 Decussation of the pyramids

Brain stem (left lateral aspect). Cerebellar peduncles have been severed, cerebellum and cerebral cortex have been removed.

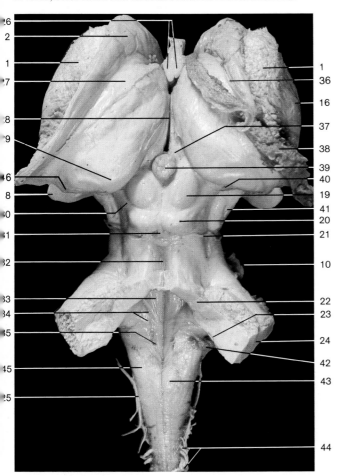

Brain stem (dorsal aspect). Cerebellum removed.

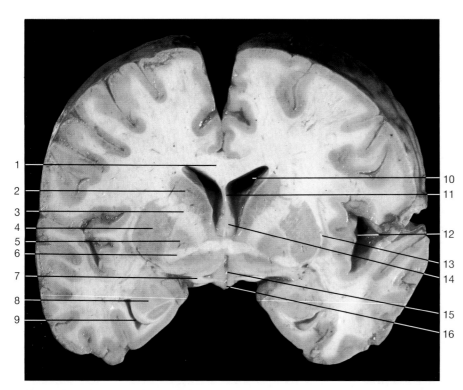

Coronal section through the brain at the level of the anterior commissure. Section 1.

1 Corpus callosum
2 Head of **caudate nucleus**
3 **Internal capsule**
4 **Putamen**
5 **Globus pallidus**
6 Anterior commissure
7 Optic tract
8 Amygdaloid body
9 Inferior horn of lateral ventricle
10 **Lateral ventricle**
11 Septum pellucidum
12 Lobus insularis (insula)
13 External capsule
14 Column of fornix
15 Optic recess
16 Infundibulum
17 **Thalamus**
18 Claustrum
19 Lenticular ansa
20 **Third ventricle** and **hypothalamus**
21 Basilar artery and pons
22 Cortex of temporal lobe
23 Inferior colliculus
24 Superior colliculus
25 Cerebral aqueduct
26 Red nucleus
27 Substantia nigra
28 Cerebral peduncle
29 Trochlear nerve (n. IV)
30 Gray matter
31 Nucleus of oculomotor nerve
32 Fibers of oculomotor nerve (n. III)
33 Vermis of cerebellum
34 Fourth ventricle
35 Reticular formation
36 Pons and transverse pontine fibers
37 Emboliform nucleus
38 Dentate nucleus
39 Middle cerebellar peduncle
40 Choroid plexus
41 Hypoglossal nucleus at rhomboid fossa
42 Medial longitudinal fasciculus
43 Trigeminal nerve (n. V.)
44 Inferior olivary nucleus
45 Corticospinal fibers and arcuate fibers
46 Fourth ventricle with choroid plexus
47 Vestibular nuclei
48 Nucleus and tractus solitarius
49 Inferior cerebellar peduncle
    (restiform body)
50 Reticular formation
51 Medial lemniscus
52 Cuneate nucleus of Burdach
53 Central canal
54 **Pyramidal tract**
55 Flocculus of cerebellum
56 Cerebellar hemisphere with pia mater
57 "Arbor vitae" of cerebellum
58 Nucleus gracilis of Goll
59 Lateral recess of choroid plexus
    of IVth ventricle
60 Posterior inferior cerebellar artery
61 Choroid plexus of lateral ventricle

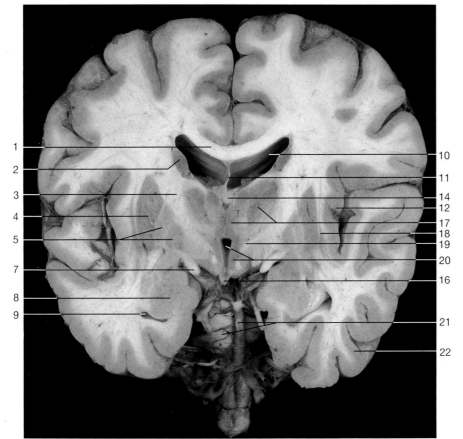

Coronal section through the brain at the level of the third ventricle and the interthalamic adhesion. Section 2.

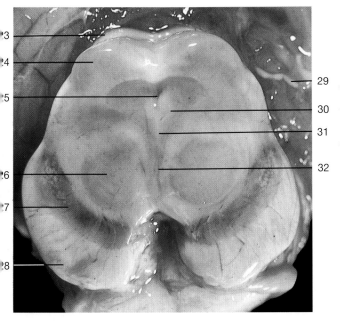

3
4
5
6
7
8

29
30
31
32

Cross section of the midbrain (mesencephalon) at the level of the superior colliculus (superior aspect). Section 4.

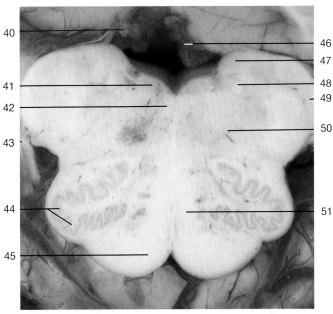

40
41
42
43
44
45

46
47
48
49
50
51

Cross section of the rhombencephalon at the level of the olive (inferior aspect). Section 6.

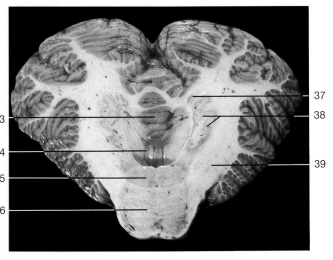

33
34
35
36

37
38
39

Cross section through the rhombencephalon at the level of pons (inferior aspect). Section 5.

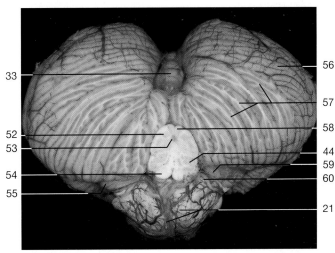

33
52
53
54
55

56
57
58
44
59
60
21

Cross section through medulla oblongata and cerebellum (inferior aspect). Section 7.

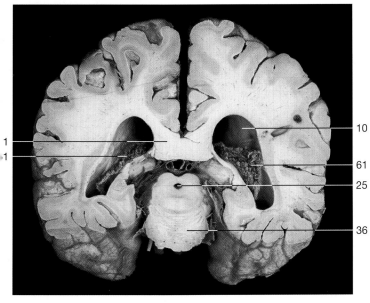

1
11

10
61
25
36

Coronal section at the level of **inferior colliculus** (posterior aspect). Section 3.

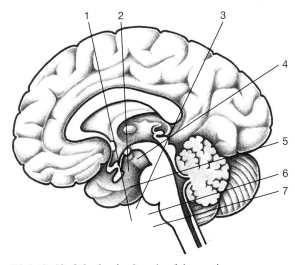

1 2   3
4
5
6
7

Right half of the brain. Levels of the sections are indicated.

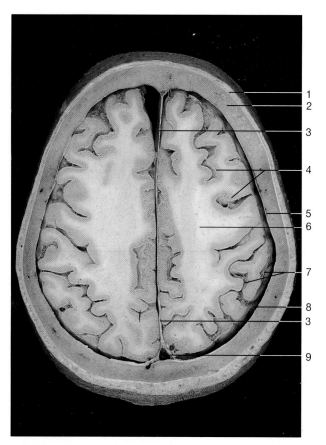

Horizontal section through the head.
Section 1.

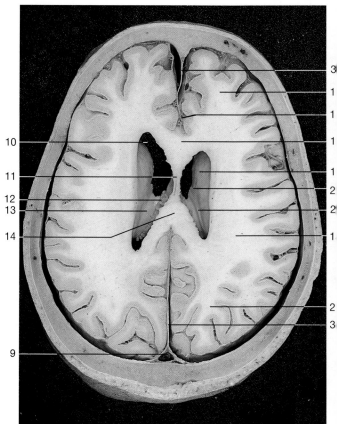

Horizontal section through the head.
Section 2.

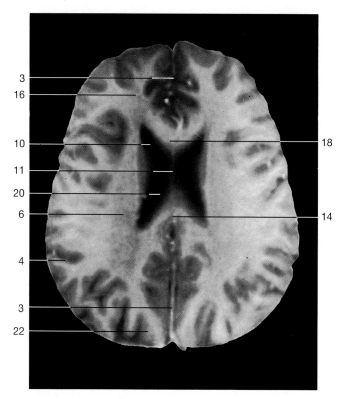

MRI scan of the human head at the level of section 2.

1   Skin of scalp
2   Calvaria (diploe of the skull)
3   **Falx cerebri**
4   Gray matter of brain (cortex)
5   Dura mater
6   **White matter of brain**
7   Arachnoid and pia mater with vessels
8   Subdural space (slightly expanded due to shrinkage of the brain)
9   Superior sagittal sinus
10 Anterior horn of lateral ventricle
11 **Septum pellucidum**
12 Choroid plexus
13 Thalamus
14 Splenium of corpus callosum
15 Parietal lobe
16 Frontal lobe
17 Anterior cerebral artery
18 Genu of corpus callosum
19 Caudate nucleus
20 **Central part of lateral ventricle**
21 Stria terminalis
22 Occipital lobe

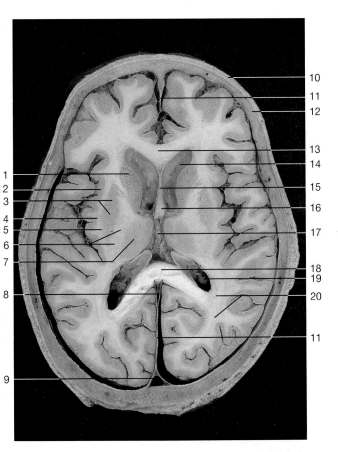

1 **Caudate nucleus**
2 Lobus insularis (insula)
3 **Lentiform nucleus**
4 Claustrum
5 External capsule
6 Internal capsule
7 **Thalamus**
8 Straight sinus (sinus rectus)
9 Superior sagittal sinus
10 Skin of scalp
11 Falx cerebri
12 Calvaria (diploe of skull)
13 Genu of corpus callosum
14 Anterior horn of lateral ventricle
15 **Septum pellucidum**
16 Column of fornix
17 Choroid plexus of third ventricle
18 Splenium of corpus callosum
19 Entrance to inferior horn of lateral ventricle with
   choroid plexus
20 Optic radiation
21 **Third ventricle**

**Horizontal section through the head at the level of third
ventricle** of internal capsule and neighboring nuclei.
Section 3.

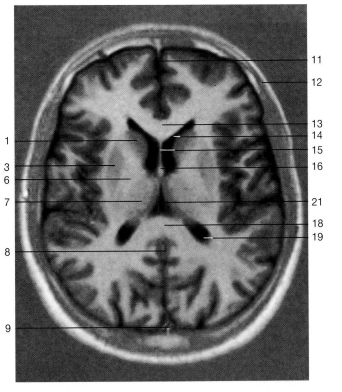

MRI scan at the corresponding level to the above figure.
Section 3.

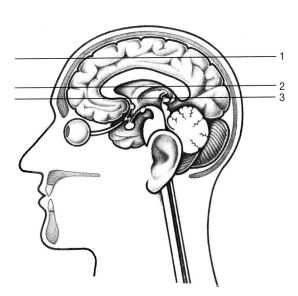

Sagittal sections through the head. Levels of the
horizontal sections are indicated.

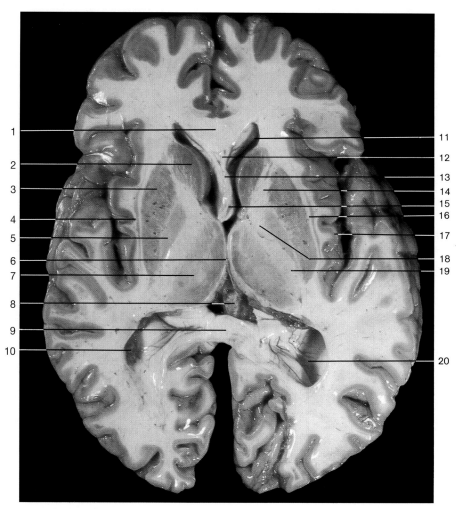

Horizontal section through the brain, showing the subcortical nuclei and internal capsule. Section 1.

1 Genu of corpus callosum
2 **Head of caudate nucleus**
3 **Putamen**
4 **Claustrum**
5 **Globus pallidus**
6 Third ventricle
7 Thalamus
8 **Pineal body**
9 Splenium of corpus callosum
10 Choroid plexus of the lateral ventricle
11 Anterior horn of lateral ventricle
12 Cavity of septum pellucidum
13 **Septum pellucidum**
14 Anterior limb of internal capsule
15 Column of fornix
16 External capsule
17 **Lobus insularis** (insula)
18 Genu of **internal capsule**
19 Posterior limb of internal capsule
20 Posterior horn of lateral ventricle
21 Anterior commissure
22 Optic radiation
23 Falx cerebri
24 **Maxillary sinus**
25 Position of auditory tube
26 Tympanic cavity
27 External acoustic meatus
28 **Medulla oblongata**
29 Fourth ventricle
30 Cerebellum (left hemisphere)
31 Temporomandibular joint
32 Tympanic membrane
33 Base of cochlea
34 Mastoid air cells
35 Sigmoid sinus
36 Vermis of cerebellum
37 Intermediate mass

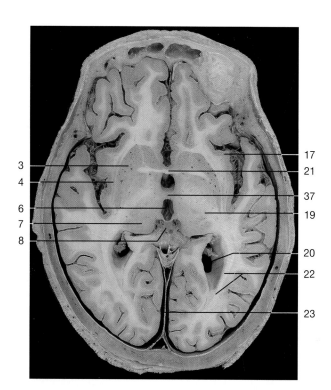

Horizontal section through the head. Section 2.

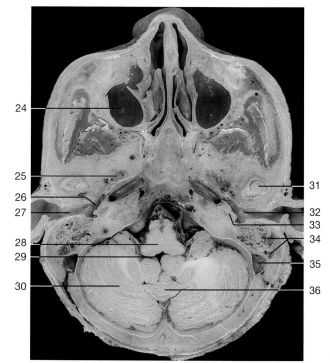

Horizontal section through the head. Section 4.

1 Upper lid (tarsal plate)
2 Lens
3 Ethmoidal sinus
4 **Optic nerve** (n. II)
5 Internal carotid artery
6 Infundibulum and **pituitary gland**
7 Temporal lobe
8 Basilar artery
9 Pons (cross section of brain stem)
10 **Cerebral aqueduct** (beginning of fourth ventricle)
11 Vermis of cerebellum
12 Straight sinus
13 Transverse sinus
14 Nasal septum
15 **Eyeball** (sclera)
16 Nasal cavity
17 Lateral rectus muscle
18 Sphenoidal sinus
19 Oculomotor nerve (n. III)
20 **Tentorium of cerebellum**
21 Skin of scalp
22 Calvaria
23 Occipital lobe
24 Striate cortex (visual cortex)

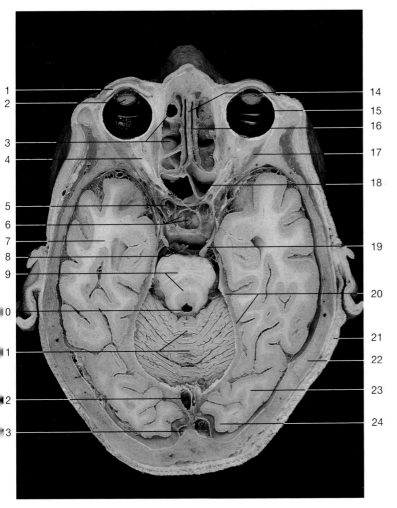

Horizontal section through the head. Section 3.

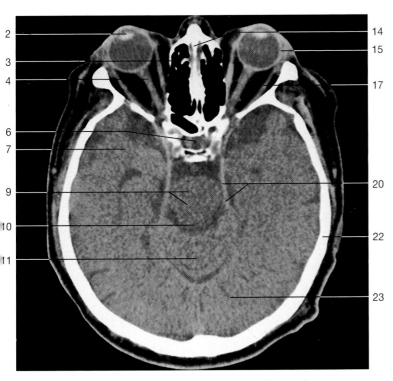

Horizontal section through the head. (CT scan.) Section 3.

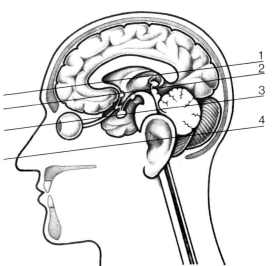

Sagittal section through the head.
Levels of the horizontal sections are indicated.

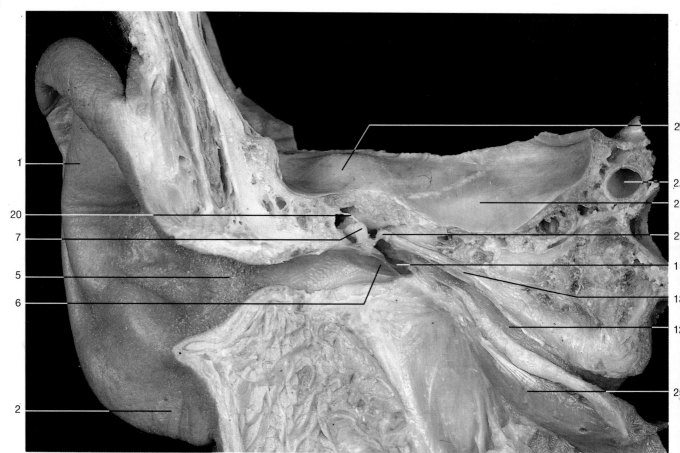

Longitudinal section through the right temporal bone I. The outer and middle ear and auditory ossicles and tube are shown (anterior aspect).

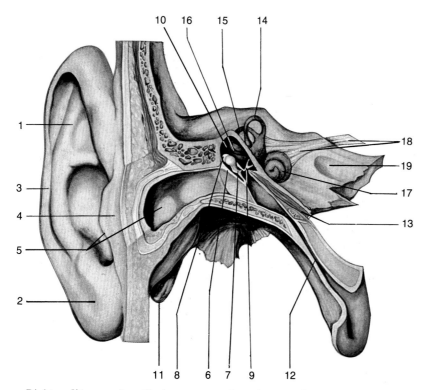

Right **auditory and vestibular** apparatus (anterior aspect). (Schematic drawing.)

Outer ear

1 Auricle
2 Lobule of auricle
3 Helix
4 Tragus
5 External acoustic meatus

Middle ear

6 Tympanic membrane
7 Malleus
8 Incus
9 Stapes
10 Tympanic cavity
11 Mastoid process
12 Auditory tube
13 Tensor tympani muscle

Inner ear

14 Anterior semicircular duct
15 Posterior semicircular duct
16 Lateral semicircular duct
17 Cochlea
18 Vestibulocochlear nerve
19 Petrous part of the temporal bone

Additional structures

20 Superior ligament of malleus
21 Arcuate eminence
22 Internal carotid artery
23 Anterior surface of pyramid with dura mater
24 Stapes
25 Levator veli palatini muscle

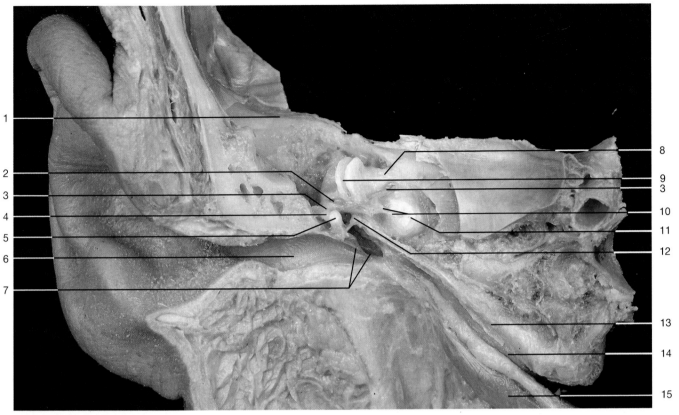

Longitudinal section through the right outer, middle and inner ear II. The cochlea and semicircular canals have been further dissected (anterior aspect).

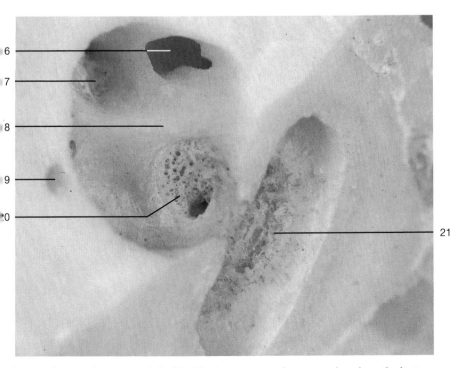

Internal acoustic meatus, left side. The bone was partly removed to show the bottom of the meatus.

1 Roof of tympanic cavity
2 **Lateral osseous semicircular canal**
3 **Facial nerve**
4 Incus
5 **Malleus**
6 External acoustic meatus
7 **Tympanic cavity** and **tympanic membrane**
8 Vestibulocochlear nerve
9 Anterior osseous semicircular canal
10 Geniculate ganglion and greater petrosal nerve
11 **Cochlea**
12 **Stapes**
13 Tensor tympani muscle
14 **Auditory tube**
15 Levator veli palatini muscle
16 Area of facial nerve
17 Superior vestibular area
18 Transverse crest
19 Foramen singulare
20 Foraminous spiral tract (outlet of cochlear part of vestibulocochlear nerve)
21 Base of cochlea

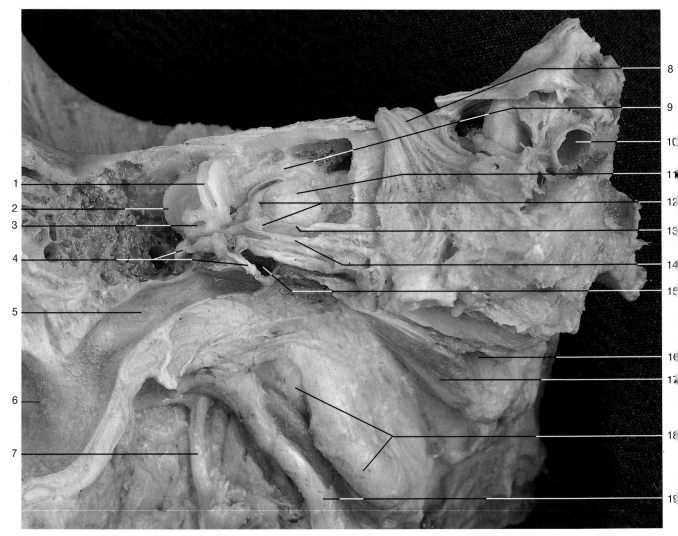

Longitudinal section through the outer, middle and inner ear III. Deeper dissection to display facial nerve and lesser and greater petrosal nerves (anterior aspect).

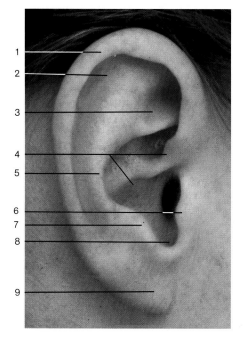

Right auricle (lateral aspect).

1 Helix
2 Scaphoid fossa
3 Triangular fossa
4 Concha
5 Antihelix
6 Tragus
7 Antitragus
8 Intertragic notch
9 Lobule

△ 1 **Anterior osseous semicircular canal** (opened)
   2 **Posterior osseous semicircular canal**
   3 **Lateral osseous semicircular canal** (opened)
   4 Facial nerve and chorda tympani
   5 External acoustic meatus
   6 Auricle
   7 **Facial nerve**
   8 Trigeminal nerve
   9 Bony base of internal acoustic meatus
  10 Internal carotid artery within cavernous sinus
  11 **Cochlea**
  12 **Facial nerve** with **geniculate ganglion**
  13 Greater petrosal nerve
  14 Lesser petrosal nerve
  15 **Tympanic cavity**
  16 Auditory tube
  17 Levator veli palatini muscle
  18 Internal carotid artery, internal jugular vein
  19 Styloid process

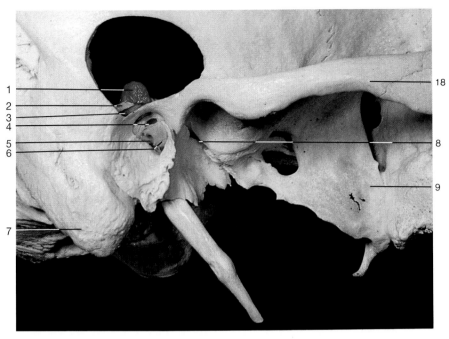

1   Anterior semicircular canal (red)
2   Posterior semicircular canal (yellow)
3   Lateral or horizontal semicircular canal (green)
4   **Fenestra vestibuli**
5   **Fenestra cochleae**
6   Tympanic cavity
7   Mastoid process
8   **Petrotympanic fissure** (red probe: **chorda tympani**)
9   Lateral pterygoid plate
10 Mastoid air cells
11 **Facial canal** (blue)
12 Foramen ovale
13 **Carotid canal** (red)
14 **Tympanic ring**
15 Petromastoid part of temporal bone
16 Squamous part of temporal bone
17 Squamomastoid suture
18 Zygomatic process of temporal bone
19 Incisure of tympanic ring
20 **Promontory**
21 Apex of cochlea (cupula)
22 Spiral canal of cochlea at base of cochlea
23 Epitympanic recess
24 Auditory ossicles and tympanic cavity
25 Hypotympanic recess
26 Canaliculus chordae tympani (green probe)
27 Mastoid process
28 Canaliculus for stapedius nerve (red)
29 **Cochlea**
30 Canaliculus mastoideus (red probe)

Right temporal bone (lateral aspect). Petrosquamous portion has been partly removed to display the semicircular canals.

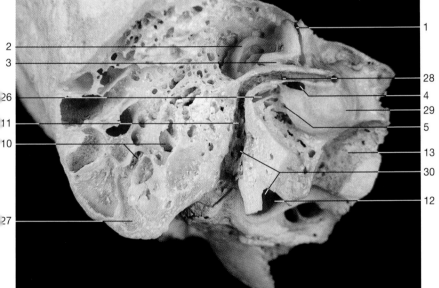

Right temporal bone (lateral aspect). Mastoid air cells and facial canal had been opened. The three semicircular canals were dissected.

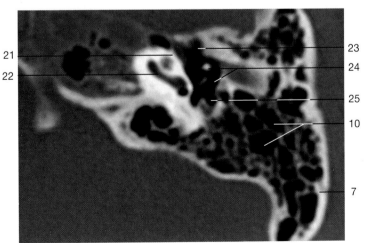

Right temporal bone of the newborn (lateral aspect).

Frontal section through petrous part. (CT scan.)

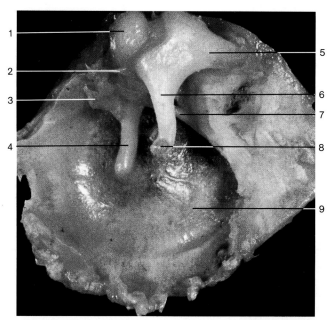

1 Head of malleus
2 Anterior ligament of malleus
3 Tendon of tensor tympani muscle
4 Handle of **malleus**
5 Short crus of incus
6 Long crus of **incus**
7 Chorda tympani
8 Lenticular process
9 **Tympanic membrane**

Tympanic membrane with malleus and incus (internal aspect; right side).

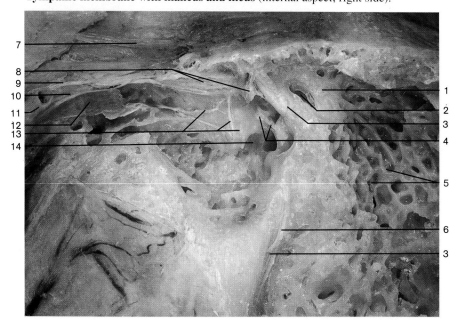

1 Tympanic antrum
2 Lateral semicircular canal (opened)
3 **Facial canal**
4 Stapes with tendon of stapedius
5 Mastoid air cells
6 Chorda tympani (intracranial part)
7 Greater petrosal nerve
8 Tensor tympani muscle (processus cochleariformis)
9 Lesser petrosal nerve
10 Anterior tympanic artery
11 Middle meningeal artery
12 **Auditory tube**
13 **Promontory with tympanic plexus**
14 Fenestra cochleae

Tympanic cavity, medial wall. External auditory meatus and lateral wall of tympanic cavity together with incus. Malleus and tympanic membrane have been removed; mastoid air cells are opened (left side).

1 **Tympanic membrane**
2 Chorda tympani (intracranial part)
3 Floor of the external acoustic meatus
4 **Facial nerve** and facial canal
5 Incus
6 Head of malleus
7 Mandibular fossa
8 Spine of sphenoid
9 **Chorda tympani** (extracranial part)
10 Styloid process

Tympanic membrane (lateral aspect). External acoustic meatus and facial canal have been opened to expose the chorda tympani (magn. ~1.5×) (left side).

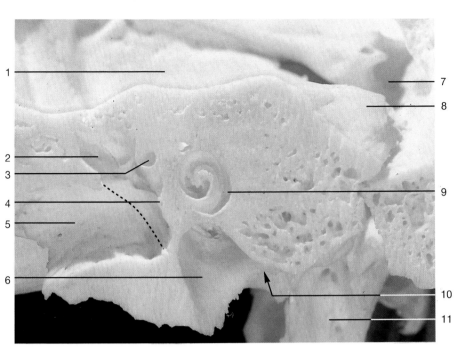

Frontal section through the petrous part of the left temporal bone at the level of the cochlea (posterior aspect). Position of tympanic membrane indicated by dotted line.

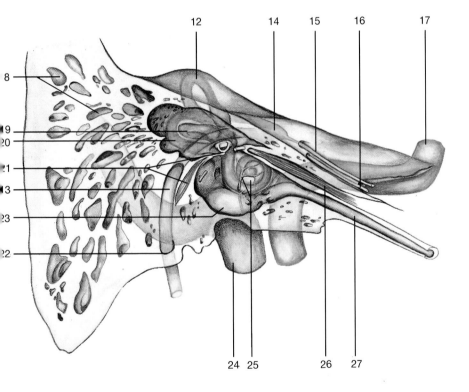

Medial wall of tympanic cavity and its relation to neighboring structures of the inner ear, facial nerve, and blood vessels. (Schematic drawing.) Frontal section through the right temporal bone (anterior aspect).

1 Anterior surface of the pyramid	10 Carotid canal	20 Posterior semicircular duct
2 Mastoid antrum	11 Pterygoid process	21 Stapes with stapedius muscle
3 Lateral semicircular canal	12 Anterior semicircular duct	22 Stylomastoid foramen
4 Cochleariform process	13 **Facial nerve**	23 Inferior recess of tympanic cavity
5 External acoustic meatus	14 Geniculate ganglion	(hypotympanon)
6 **Jugular fossa**	15 Greater petrosal nerve	24 **Internal jugular vein**
7 Foramen lacerum	16 Lesser petrosal nerve	25 Promontory with tympanic plexus
8 Apex of petrous part	17 **Internal carotid artery**	(position of cochlea)
9 Position of **cochlea** (modiolus with	18 Mastoid air cells	26 Tensor muscle of tympanum
crista spiralis ossea)	19 Lateral semicircular duct	27 **Auditory tube**

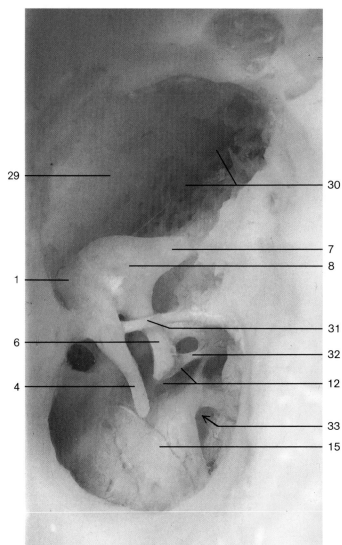

Tympanic cavity with malleus, incus and stapes, left side (lateral aspect). Tympanic membrane removed, mastoid antrum opened.

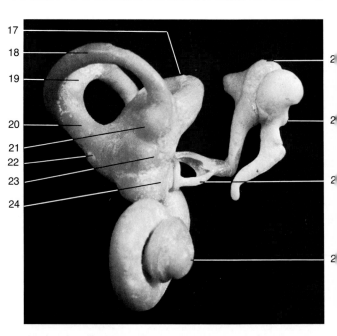

Chain of auditory ossicles in connection with the inner ear, left side (anterior-lateral aspect).

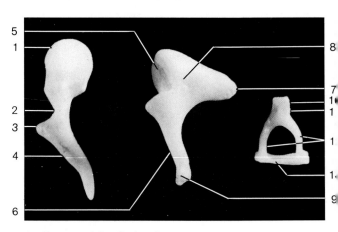

Auditory ossicles (isolated).

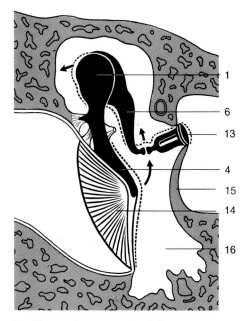

Position and movements of the auditory ossicles. (Schematic diagram.)

Malleus
1 Head
2 Neck
3 Lateral process
4 Handle

Incus
5 Articular facet for malleus
6 Long crus
7 Short crus
8 Body
9 Lenticular process

Stapes
10 Head
11 Neck
12 Anterior and posterior crura
13 Base

Walls of tympanic cavity
14 Tympanic membrane
15 Promontory
16 Hypotympanic recess of tympanic cavity

Internal ear (labyrinth)
17 Lateral semicircular duct
18 Anterior semicircular duct
19 Posterior semicircular duct
20 Common crus
21 Ampulla
22 Beginning of endolymphatic duct
23 Utricular prominence
24 Saccular prominence
25 Incus
26 Malleus
27 Stapes
28 Cochlea

Tympanic cavity
29 Epitympanic recess
30 Mastoid antrum
31 Chorda tympani
32 Tendon of stapedius muscle
33 Round window (fenestra cochleae)

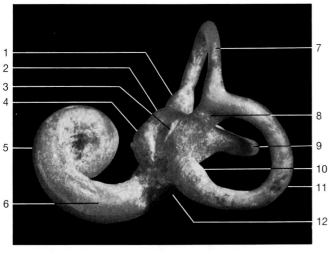

Cast of the right labyrinth (postero medial aspect).

1 Ampulla (anterior semicircular canal)
2 Elliptical recess
3 Aqueduct of the vestibule
4 Spherical recess
5 **Cochlea**
6 Base of cochlea
7 **Anterior semicircular canal**
8 Crus commune or common limb
9 **Lateral semicircular canal**
10 Posterior bony ampulla
11 **Posterior semicircular canal** (posterior canal)
12 **Fenestra cochleae**
13 Bony ampulla
14 **Fenestra vestibuli**
15 Cupula of cochlea
16 External acoustic meatus
17 Mastoid air cells
18 Tympanic cavity and fenestra cochleae (probe)
19 External acoustic meatus
20 Facial canal
21 Base of cochlea and canalis musculotubarius
22 Malleus and incus
23 Stapes
24 Tympanic membrane
25 Tympanic cavity
26 Aqueduct of cochlea
27 Saccus endolymphaticus
28 Ductus endolymphaticus
29 Macula of utricle
30 Macula of saccule

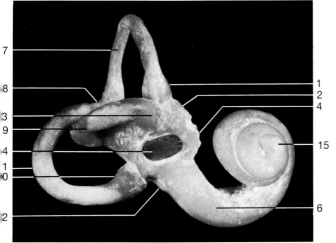

Cast of the right labyrinth (lateral aspect).

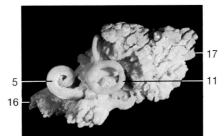

Cast of the labyrinth and mastoid cells.
Life size (posterior aspect).

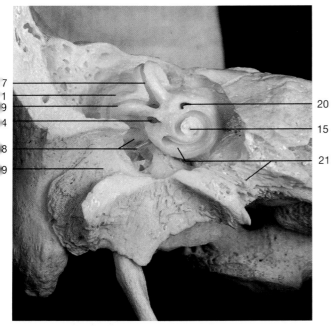

Dissection of bony labyrinth in situ. Semicircular canals and cochlear duct opened.

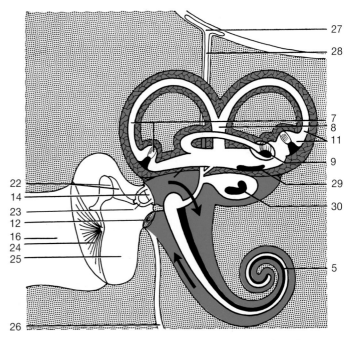

Auditory and vestibular apparatus. Arrows: direction of sound waves; blue = perilymphatic ducts. (Schematic diagram.)

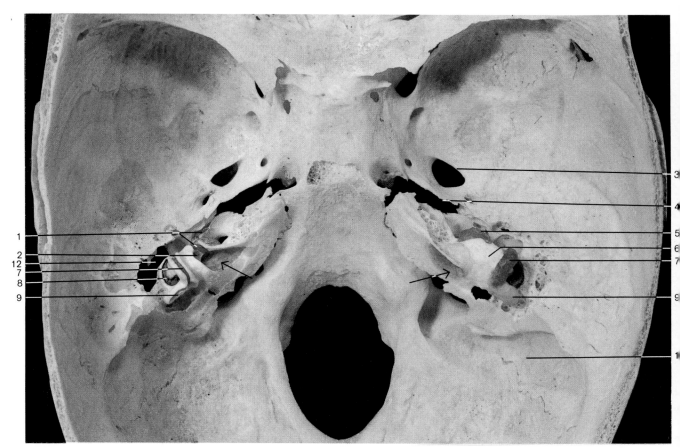

Bony labyrinth, petrous part of the temporal bone (from above). At left: semicircular canals opened; at right, closed. Arrows: internal acoustic meatus.

1 Facial canal and semicanal of auditory tube
2 Superior vestibular area
3 Foramen ovale
4 Foramen lacerum
5 Cochlea
6 Vestibule
7 Anterior semicircular canal
8 Lateral semicircular canal

9 Posterior semicircular canal
10 Groove for sigmoid sinus
11 Sigmoid sinus
12 Tympanic cavity
13 Auditory tube
14 Mastoid air cells
15 Facial and vestibulocochlear nerves
16 Temporal fossa

17 Fenestra vestibuli
18 Promontory
19 Zygomatic process
20 Fenestra cochleae
21 Mastoid process

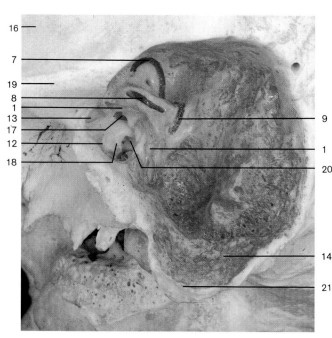

Bony labyrinth (left lateral aspect). Temporal and tympanic bone partly removed, semicircular canals opened.

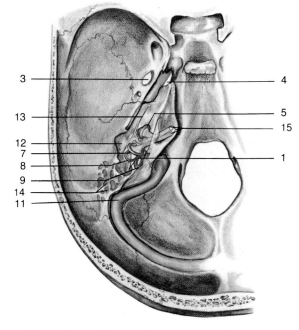

Internal ear. Diagram showing the position of the membranous labyrinth and the tympanic cavity.

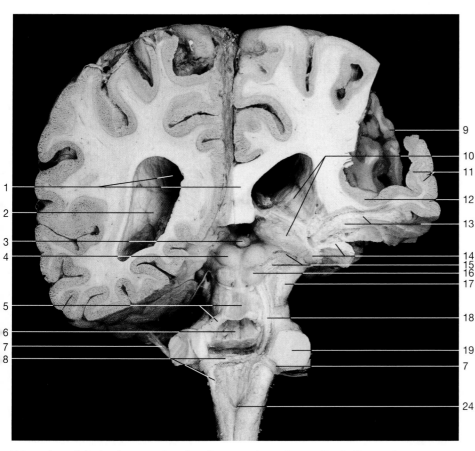

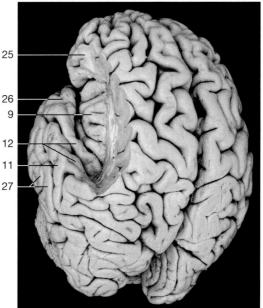

1   Left lateral ventricle
    and corpus callosum
2   Thalamus
3   Pineal gland (epiphysis)
4   Superior colliculus
5   Superior medullary velum and
    superior cerebellar peduncle
6   Rhomboid fossa
7   **Vestibulocochlear nerve** (n. VIII)
8   **Dorsal acoustic striae** and
    inferior cerebellar peduncle
9   Insular lobe
10 Caudate nucleus and thalamus
11 Temporal lobe (superior temporal
    gyrus) (area of **acoustic centers**)
12 Transverse temporal gyri of
    Heschl (area of **primary
    acoustic centers**)
13 Acoustic radiation of internal
    capsule
14 Lateral geniculate body and
    optic radiation (cut)
15 **Medial geniculate body** and
    brachium of inferior colliculus
16 **Inferior colliculus**
17 Cerebral peduncle
18 **Lateral lemniscus**
19 Middle cerebellar peduncle
20 Dorsal (posterior) cochlear
    nucleus
21 Ventral (anterior) cochlear
    nucleus
22 Inferior olive with tractus olivo-
    cochlearis of Rasmussen (red)
23 Ganglion spirale
24 Obex
25 Frontal lobe
26 Temporal lobe
27 Middle temporal gyrus (area of
    tertiary acoustic centers)
28 Trapezoid body

Dissection of the brain stem showing the acoustic pathway. Cerebellum and posterior part of the two hemispheres have been removed (dorsal aspect).

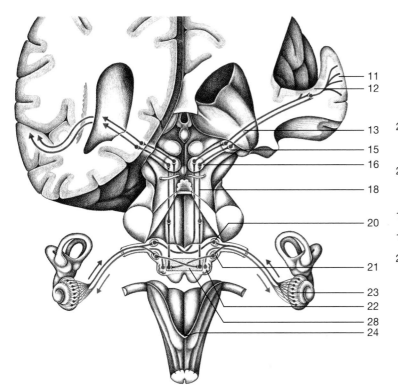

Acoustic pathway (schematic drawing, compare with figure above).

Acoustic areas in the left hemisphere (superior lateral aspect). Parts of the frontal and parietal lobe have been removed.

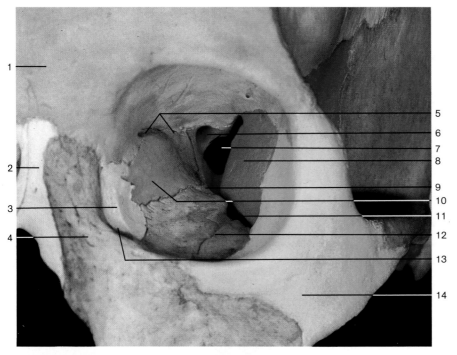

Bones of the left orbit (indicated by different colors).

1 Frontal bone
2 Nasal bone
3 Lacrimal bone
4 Maxilla (frontal process)
5 Ethmoidal foramina
6 Lesser wing of sphenoid bone
and optic canal
7 Superior orbital fissure
8 Greater wing of sphenoid bone
9 Orbital process of palatine bone
10 Orbital plate of ethmoid bone
11 Inferior orbital fissure
12 Infraorbital sulcus
13 Nasolacrimal canal
14 Zygomatic bone
15 Frontal sinus
16 **Superior rectus muscle**
17 Orbital fatty tissue
18 **Optic nerve**
19 **Sclera**
20 **Inferior rectus muscle**
21 Periorbita and maxilla
22 Maxillary sinus
23 Levator palpebrae superioris
muscle
24 **Superior conjunctival fornix**
25 Superior tarsal plate
26 Inferior tarsal plate
27 **Inferior conjunctival fornix**
28 **Inferior oblique muscle**
29 **Lateral rectus muscle**
30 **Medial rectus muscle**
31 **Superior oblique muscle**
32 Nasal septum
33 Middle nasal concha
34 Inferior nasal concha
35 Tenon's space
36 Ophthalmic artery
37 **Cornea**
38 **Lens**

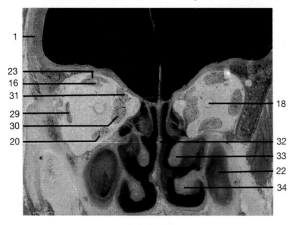

Frontal section through the posterior part of the orbit.

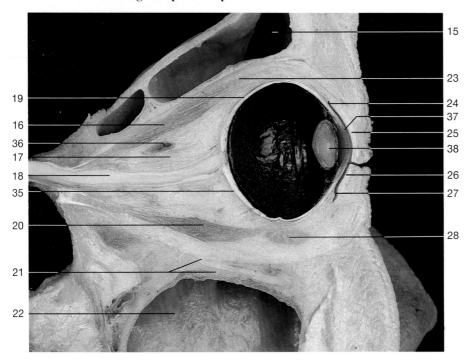
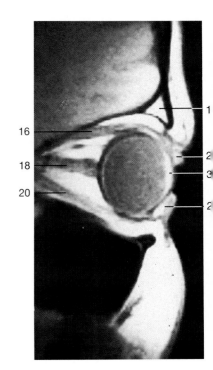

Sagittal section through orbit and eyeball. (Right: MRI scan.)

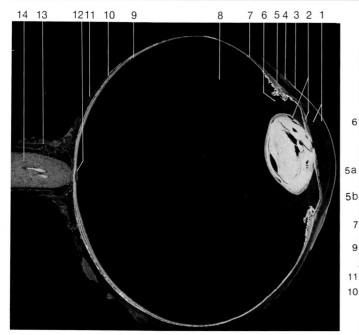

14 13 12 11 10 9   8   7 6 5 4 3 2 1

Horizontal section through the human eye (2×).

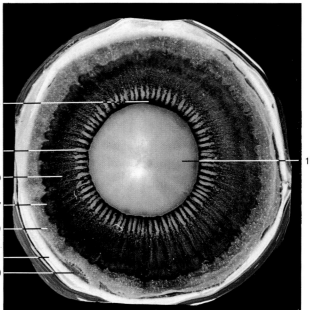

6
5a
5b
7
9
11
10
15

Anterior segment of the eyeball (posterior aspect). The opacity of the lens is an artifact.

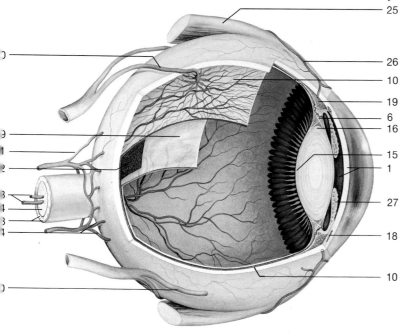

25
26
10
19
6
16
15
1
27
18
10

Organization of the eyeball. Demonstration of vascular tunic of bulb. (Schematic drawing.)

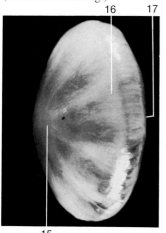

16   17

15

Lens (equatorial aspect), anterior pole to the right.

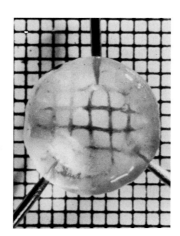

Lens (frontal aspect). Note the magnification effect.

1 **Cornea** and anterior chamber
2 Iris and lens
3 Transitional zone between corneal and conjunctival epithelium
4 Conjunctiva of the eyeball
5 **Ciliary body**
   a Ciliary processes (pars plicata)
   b Ciliary ring (pars plana)
6 Zonular fibers
7 **Ora serrata**
8 Vitreous body
9 **Retina**
10 **Choroid**
11 **Sclera**
12 Optic disc
13 Dura mater and subarachnoid space
14 **Optic nerve** (n. II)
15 Lens (posterior pole)
16 Equator of lens
17 **Lens** (anterior pole)
18 Canal of Schlemm
19 Ciliary muscle
20 Vena vorticosa
21 Long posterior ciliary artery
22 Retinal pigmented epithelium
23 Central retinal artery and vein
24 Short posterior ciliary arteries
25 External ocular muscle
26 Anterior ciliary artery
27 **Iris**

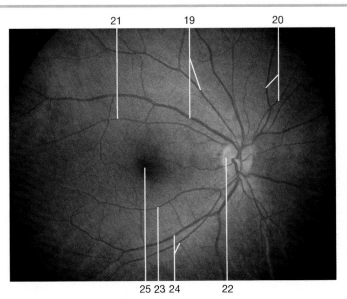

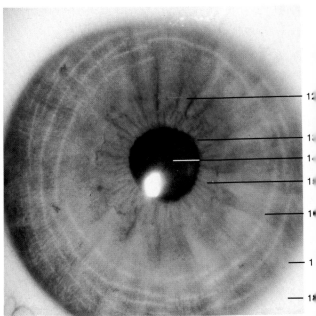

Fundus of a normal right eye (courtesy of Prof. Dr. R. Okamura, Univ. Eye Dept., Kumamoto, Japan). Notice, the arteries are smaller and lighter than the veins.

Anterior segment of the human eye (courtesy of Prof. Dr. G. O. H. Naumann, Eye Dept., University of Erlangen, Germany). Note the colored iris (16) and the location of the lens behind the iris (14).

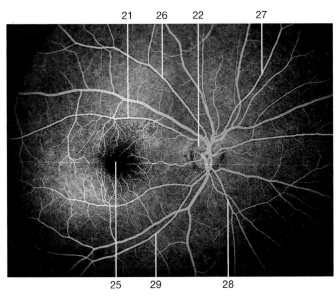

Fluorescent angiography of the right eye; retinal vessels. The same eye as above. (Courtesy of Prof. Dr. R. Okamura, Univ. Eye Dept., Kumamoto, Japan.)

1	Posterior and anterior ethmoidal arteries
2	Long and short **posterior ciliary arteries**
3	Optic nerve and **ophthalmic artery**
4	Central retinal artery
5	Retinal arteries
6	Supratrochlear artery
7	Supraorbital artery
8	Dorsal nasal artery
9	**Anterior ciliary artery**
10	Iridial arteries
11	Circulus arteriosus major of iris
12	Iridial fold
13	Pupillary margin of iris
14	Anterior pole of lens
15	Lesser circle of **iris**
16	Greater circle of iris
17	Margin of cornea or limbus
18	Sclera
19	Superior temporal artery and vein of retina
20	Superior nasal artery and vein of retina
21	Superior macular artery
22	**Optic disc**
23	Inferior macular artery
24	Inferior temporal artery and vein
25	**Fovea centralis** and **macula lutea**
26	Superior temporal artery ⎫
27	Superior nasal artery ⎬ of retina
28	Inferior nasal artery ⎪
29	Inferior temporal artery ⎭

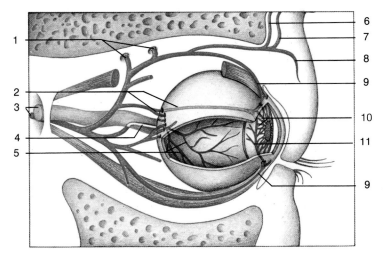

Diagram of the ophthalmic artery and its branches.

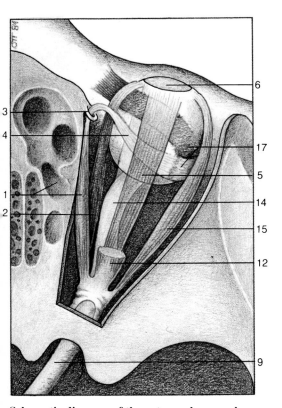

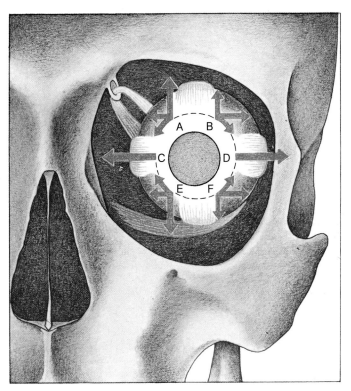

Schematic diagram of the extraocular muscles.
Right orbit (from above). Levator palpebrae
superioris muscle has been severed.

The action of the extraocular muscles.
Left orbit (anterior aspect).

A   Superior rectus muscle   D   Lateral rectus muscle
B   Inferior oblique muscle   E   Inferior rectus muscle
C   Medial rectus muscle   F   Superior oblique muscle

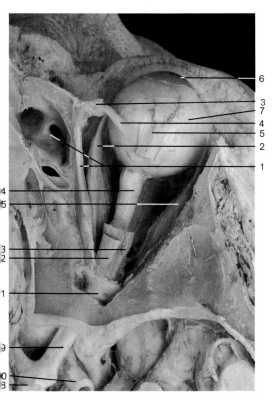

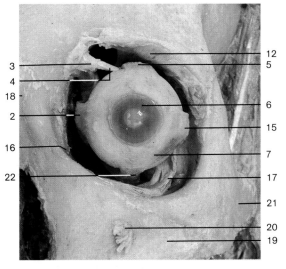

Left orbit with eyeball and extraocular muscles
(anterior aspect). Lids, conjunctiva and lacrimal
apparatus have been removed.

**Right orbit with eyeball and extraocular
muscles** (from above). The roof of the orbit has
been removed, the superior rectus muscle and the
levator palpebrae superioris muscle have been
severed.

1 **Superior oblique muscle** and ethmoid air cells	12 Levator palpebrae superioris muscle
2 **Medial rectus muscle**	13 **Superior rectus muscle**
3 Trochlea	14 Optic nerve (extracranial part)
4 Tendon of superior oblique muscle	15 **Lateral rectus muscle**
5 **Superior rectus muscle**	16 Nasolacrimal duct
6 Cornea	17 **Inferior oblique muscle**
7 Eyeball	18 Nasal bone
8 Optic chiasma	19 Maxilla
9 Optic nerve (intracranial part)	20 Infraorbital foramen and nerves
10 Internal carotid artery	21 Zygomatic bone
11 **Common annular tendon**	22 **Inferior rectus muscle**

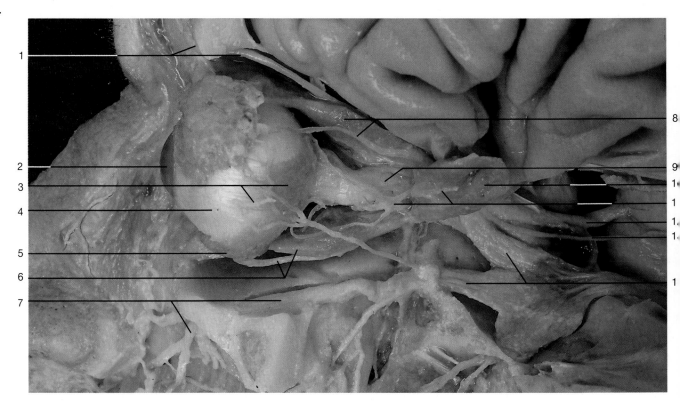

Extraocular muscles and their nerves (lateral aspect of left eye). Lateral rectus divided and reflected.

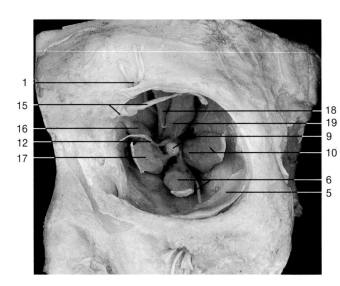

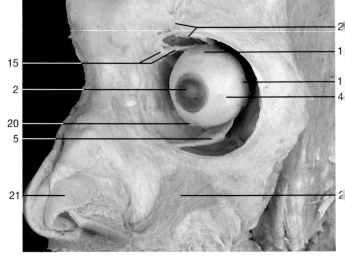

Left orbit with extraocular muscles (anterior aspect). Eyeball removed.

Extraocular eye muscles (anterior-lateral aspect).

1 Supraorbital nerve
2 Cornea
3 Insertion of lateral rectus muscle
4 Eyeball (sclera)
5 **Inferior oblique muscle**
6 **Inferior rectus muscle** and inferior branch of oculomotor
   nerve
7 Infraorbital nerve
8 Superior rectus muscle and lacrimal nerve
9 Optic nerve
10 **Lateral rectus muscle**
11 Ciliary ganglion and abducens nerve (n. VI)
12 Oculomotor nerve (n. III)

13 Trochlear nerve (n. IV)
14 Ophthalmic nerve (n. V_1) and maxillary nerve (n. V_2)
15 Trochlea and tendon of superior oblique muscle
16 **Superior oblique muscle**
17 **Medial rectus muscle**
18 Levator palpebrae superioris muscle
19 **Superior rectus muscle**
20 **Inferior rectus muscle**
21 Greater alar cartilage
22 Supraorbital nerve and levator palpebrae superioris muscle
23 Levator labii superioris muscle

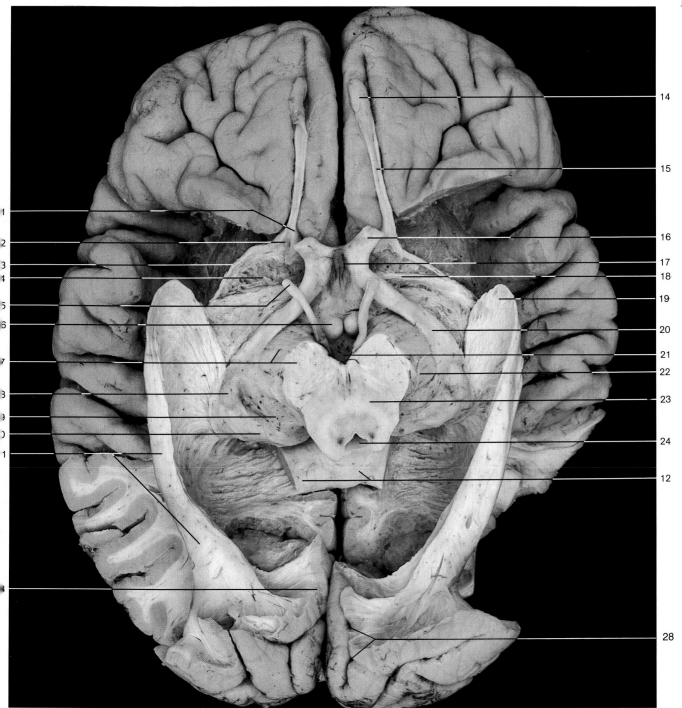

14
15
16
17
18
19
20
21
22
23
24
12
28

1
2
3
4
5
6
7
8
9
10
11
28

Dissection of the visual pathway (inferior aspect). Frontal pole at top, midbrain divided.

1	Medial olfactory stria
2	Olfactory trigone
3	Lateral olfactory stria
4	Anterior perforated substance
5	Oculomotor nerve (n. III)
6	Mamillary body
7	Cerebral peduncle
8	**Lateral geniculate body**
9	Medial geniculate body
10	**Pulvinar of thalamus**
11	Optic radiation
12	Splenium of the corpus callosum (commissural fibers)
13	Cuneus
14	Olfactory bulb

15	Olfactory tract
16	**Optic nerve** (n. II)
17	Infundibulum
18	Anterior commissure
19	**Genu of optic radiation**
20	**Optic tract**
21	Interpeduncular fossa and posterior perforated substance
22	Trochlear nerve (n. IV)
23	Substantia nigra
24	Cerebral aqueduct
25	**Visual cortex**
26	Line of Gennari
27	Gyrus of striate cortex
28	**Calcarine sulcus**

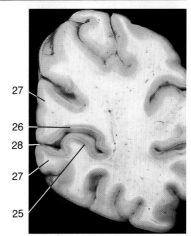

27
26
28
27
25

Frontal section of the striate cortex at the level of the striate area in the occipital lobe.

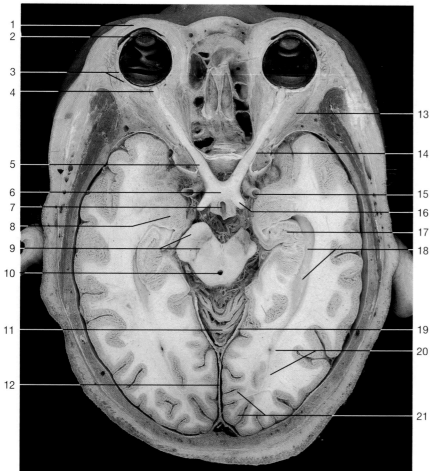

Horizontal section through the head at the level of optic chiasma and striate cortex (superior aspect). Note the relationship of hypothalamic infundibulum to optic chiasma.

1   Upper lid
2   Cornea
3   **Eyeball** (sclera, retina)
4   Head of optic nerve
5   Optic nerve
6   **Optic chiasma**
7   Infundibular recess of hypothalamus
8   Amygdaloid body
9   Substantia nigra and crus cerebri
10 Cerebral aqueduct
11 Vermis of cerebellum
12 Falx cerebri
13 Lateral rectus muscle
14 Optic canal
15 Internal carotid artery
16 **Optic tract**
17 Hippocampus
18 Inferior horn of lateral ventricle
19 Tentorium cerebelli
20 **Optic radiation** of Gratiolet
21 **Visual cortex (area calcarina, striate cortex)**
22 Lens
23 **Eyeball**
24 Ethmoidal cells
25 Optic nerve with dura sheath
26 Cerebral peduncle
27 Aqueduct of mesencephalon
28 Vermis of cerebellum

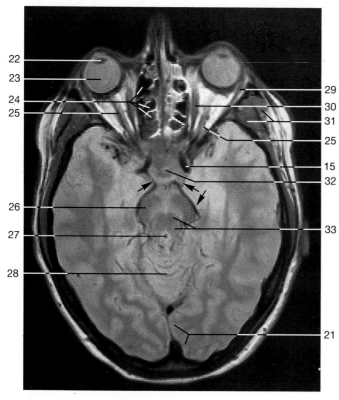

Horizontal section through the human head
(MRI scan, courtesy of Prof. W. J. Huk, Erlangen, Germany).
Arrows = branches of arterial circle of Willis.

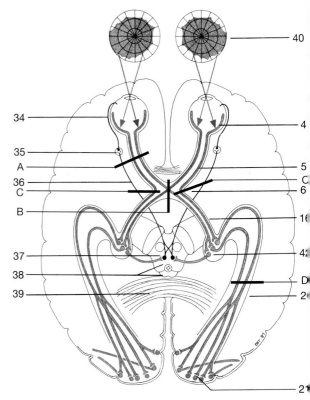

Diagram of the visual pathway and path of the light reflex.

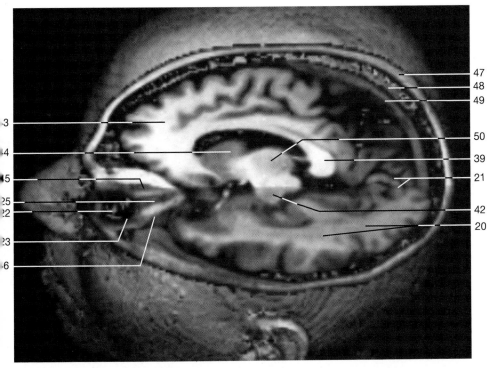

3-D reconstruction of the human visual system (MRI scan flash 40°, courtesy of Prof. W. J. Huk, University of Erlangen, Germany).

29	Lateral rectus muscle
30	Medial rectus muscle
31	Temporalis muscle
32	Hypophysis (pituitary gland)
33	Midbrain
34	Ciliary nerves (long and short)
35	Ciliary ganglion
36	Oculomotor nerve
37	Accessory oculomotor nucleus
38	Colliculi of midbrain
39	Corpus callosum
40	Visual field
41	Retina
42	**Lateral geniculate body**
43	Frontal lobe
44	**Caudate nucleus**
45	Medial rectus muscle
46	Lateral rectus muscle
47	Skin
48	Diploë (skull)
49	Dura mater
50	**Thalamus**
51	**Anterior cerebral artery**
52	Caudate nucleus
53	Frontal sinus
54	**Internal capsule**
55	Lentiform nucleus (putamen)
56	**Hippocampus**
57	Temporal lobe of left hemisphere

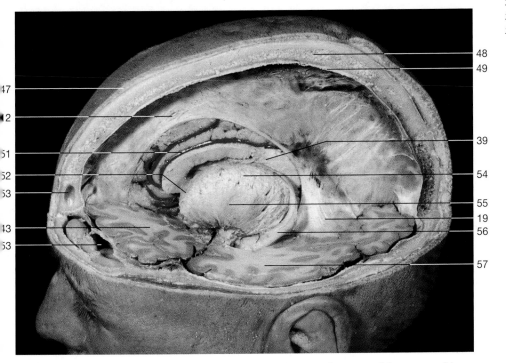

Dissection of brain stem in situ. Left hemisphere has been partly removed (compare with MRI scan above).

In **binocular vision** the visual field (40) is projected upon portions of both retinae (blue and red in the drawing). In the chiasma the fibers from the two retinal portions are combined to form the left optic tract. The fibers of the two eyes remain separated from each other throughout the entire visual pathway up to their final termination in the calcarine cortex (21). **Injuries** on the optic pathway produce visual defects whose nature depends on the location of the injury. Destruction of one optic nerve (A) produces blindness in the corresponding eye with loss of pupillary light reflex. If lesions of the **chiasma** destroy the crossing fibers of the nasal portions of the retina (B), both temporal fields of vision are lost (bitemporal hemianopsia). If both lateral angles of the chiasma are compressed (C), the nondecussating fibers from the temporal retinae are affected, resulting in loss of nasal visual fields (binasal hemianopsia). Lesions posterior to the chiasma (D) (i.e., optic tract, lateral geniculate body, optic radiation or visual cortex) result in a loss of the entire opposite field of vision (homonymous hemianopsia).

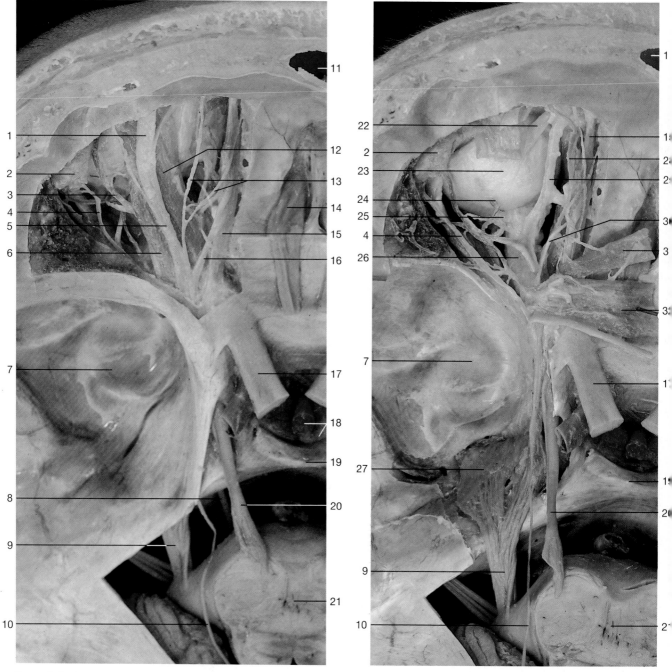

Superficial layer of the left orbit (superior aspect). The roof of the orbit and a portion of the left tentorium have been removed.

Middle layer of the left orbit (superior aspect). The roof of the orbit has been removed and the superior extraocular muscles have been divided and reflected.

1 Lateral branch of frontal nerve	10 **Trochlear nerve** (intracranial part) (n. IV)	19 Dorsum sellae
2 Lacrimal gland	11 Frontal sinus	20 **Oculomotor nerve** (n. III)
3 Lacrimal vein	12 Levator palpebrae superioris muscle	21 Midbrain
4 Lacrimal nerve	13 Branches of supratrochlear nerve	22 Tendon of superior oblique muscle
5 **Frontal nerve**	14 Olfactory bulb	23 Eyeball
6 Superior rectus	15 Superior oblique muscle	24 Vena vorticosa
7 Middle cranial fossa	16 **Trochlear nerve** (intraorbital part) (n. IV)	25 Short ciliary nerves
8 **Abducent nerve** (n. VI)	17 **Optic nerve** (intracranial part)	26 Optic nerve (extracranial part)
9 Trigeminal nerve (n. V)	18 Pituitary gland and infundibulum	27 **Trigeminal ganglion**

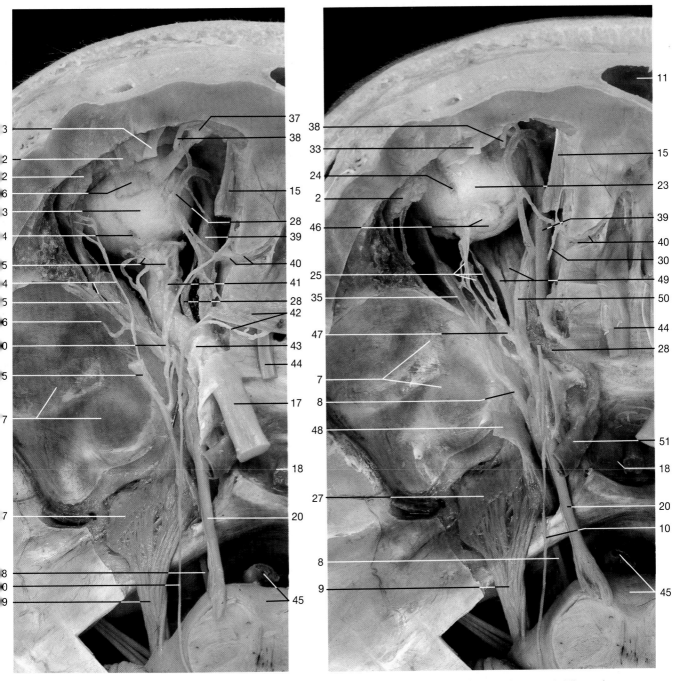

Middle layer of the left orbit (superior aspect). The roof of the orbit and the superior extraocular muscles have been removed.

Deeper layer of the left orbit (superior aspect). The optic nerve has now been removed.

28 **Ophthalmic artery**	37 Trochlea	45 Basilar artery and pons
29 Superior ophthalmic vein	38 Medial branch of supraorbital nerve	46 Optic nerve (external sheath of optic
30 **Nasociliary nerve**	39 Medial rectus muscle	nerve, divided)
31 Levator palpebrae superioris muscle	40 Anterior ethmoidal artery and nerve	47 **Ciliary ganglion**
(reflected)	41 Long ciliary nerve	48 Ophthalmic nerve (divided, reflected)
32 Superior rectus muscle (reflected)	42 Superior oblique muscle and trochlear	49 Inferior branch of oculomotor nerve
33 Lateral branch of supraorbital nerve	nerve	and inferior rectus muscle
34 Lacrimal nerve and artery	43 Common tendinous ring	50 Superior branch of oculomotor nerve
35 Lateral rectus muscle	44 Olfactory tract	51 Internal carotid artery
36 Meningolacrimal artery (anastomosing		
with middle meningeal artery)		

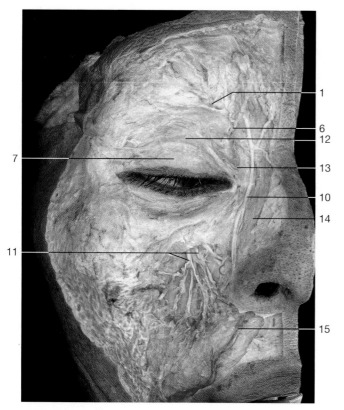

Eyelids (superficial layer, right side).

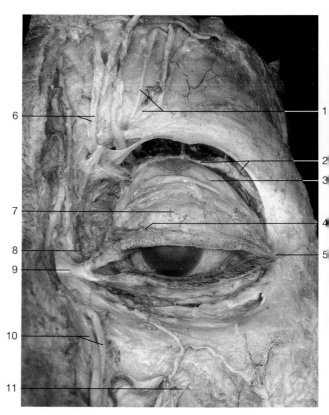

Eyelids (deeper layer, left side).

1   Supraorbital artery, supraorbital nerve, lateral branch
2   **Lacrimal gland**
3   Aponeurosis of levator palpebrae superioris muscle
4   Arterial arch of upper eyelid
5   Lateral palpebral ligament
6   Supratrochlear artery, supratrochlear nerve
7   Upper eyelid, superior tarsal plate (tarsus)
8   Lacrimal sac
9   **Medial palpebral ligament**
10 Angular artery and vein
11 Infraorbital artery, vein and nerve
12 Orbital septum

13 Infratrochlear nerve
14 Levator labii superioris alaeque nasi muscle
15 Facial artery and vein
16 **Superior lacrimal canaliculus**
17 **Inferior lacrimal canaliculus**
18 Lacrimal papilla and punctum
19 Lacrimal bone
20 **Nasolacrimal duct**
21 Mucous membrane of nasal cavity
22 Palpebral conjunctiva of lower eyelid
23 Lacrimal sac and superior lacrimal canaliculus
24 Lateral fixation of levator aponeurosis
25 Infraorbital foramen

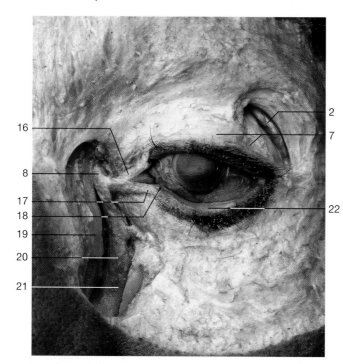

Lacrimal apparatus of left eye (anterior aspect).

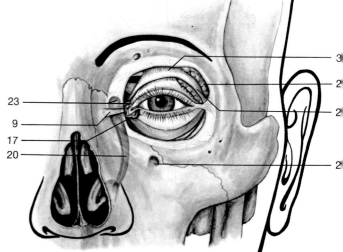

Lacrimal apparatus of left eye (anterior aspect).

1 Crista galli
2 Pituitary gland and sella turcica
3 **Sphenoidal sinus** (relatively large)
4 Tubal elevation
5 Pharyngeal opening of the **auditory tube**
6 Pharyngeal recess
7 Atlas (anterior arch)
8 Soft palate
9 Frontal sinus
10 Perpendicular plate of ethmoid
11 **Cartilage of nasal septum**
12 Vomer
13 Hard palate
14 Nasal branch of anterior ethmoidal artery and anterior ethmoidal nerve
15 Nasopharynx
16 Nasal septum
17 **Olfactory nerves**
18 Septal artery
19 Crest of nasal septum
20 Incisive canal
21 Anterior ethmoidal artery
22 Olfactory bulb
23 Olfactory tract
24 Internal carotid artery
25 Posterior nasal and septal arteries
26 Nasopalatine nerve
27 **Choana** (arrow)
28 Tongue

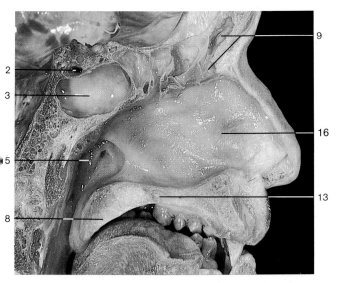

Nasal septum, covered by a mucous membrane.

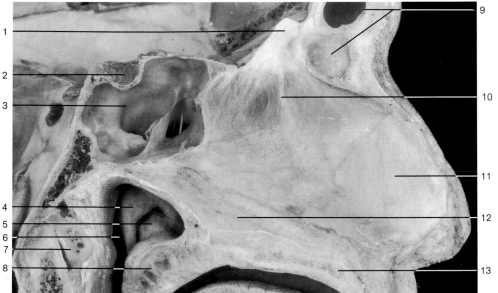

Nasal septum. Mucous membrane removed.

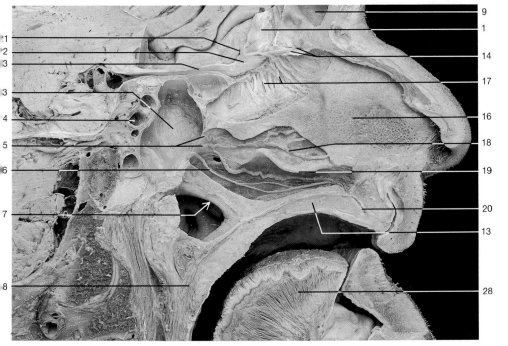

Nasal septum. Dissection of nerves and vessels.

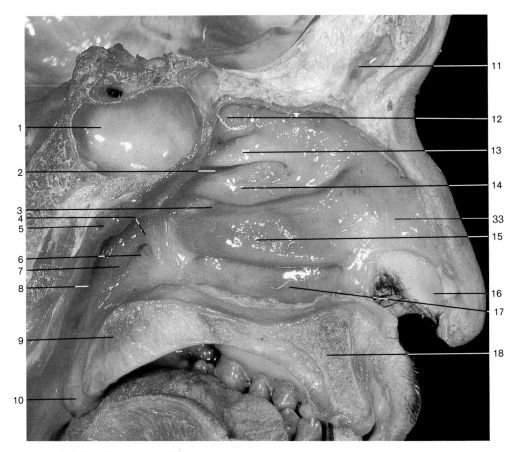

1 Sphenoidal sinus
2 Superior meatus
3 Middle meatus
4 Tubal elevation
5 Pharyngeal tonsil
6 Pharyngeal orifice of
   auditory tube
7 Salpingopharyngeal fold
8 Pharyngeal recess
9 **Soft palate**
10 **Uvula**
11 Frontal sinus
12 Sphenoethmoidal recess
13 **Superior nasal concha**
14 **Middle nasal concha**
15 **Inferior nasal concha**
16 Vestibule
17 Inferior meatus
18 **Hard palate**
19 Grooves for the middle
   meningeal artery and
   parietal bone (light green)
20 **Maxillary hiatus**
21 Perpendicular process of
   palatine bone
22 Openings of ethmoidal air
   cells
23 Opening of frontal sinus
24 Medial pterygoid plate (red)
25 Horizontal plate of palatine
   process
26 **Ethmoidal air cells**
27 **Maxillary sinus**
28 Nasal septum
29 Pterygoid hamulus
30 Nasal bone (white)
31 Frontal process of maxilla
   (violet)
32 Palatine process of maxilla
   (violet)
33 Nasal atrium

Lateral wall of the nasal cavity. Septum removed.

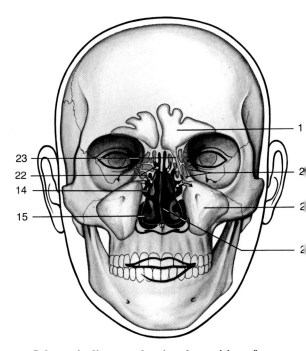

Bones of left nasal cavity, medial aspect.

Schematic diagram showing the position of paranasal sinuses. Openings indicated by arrows.

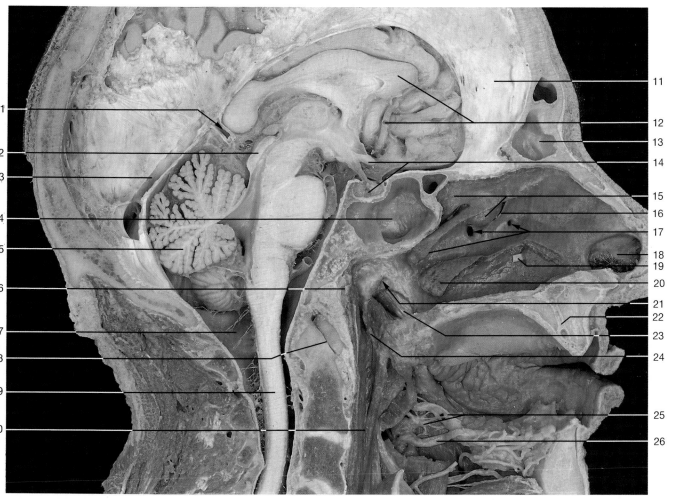

Median section through the head with nasal and oral cavity. The middle and inferior nasal conchae have been partly removed to show the openings of paranasal sinuses.

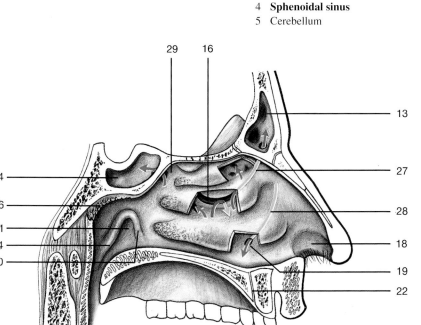

Lateral wall of nasal cavity. Openings indicated by red arrows. (Schematic drawing.)

1 Great cerebral vein (Galen's vein)
2 **Tectum of midbrain**
3 Straight sinus
4 **Sphenoidal sinus**
5 Cerebellum
6 **Pharyngeal tonsil**
7 **Cerebellomedullary cistern**
8 Median atlantoaxial joint
9 Spinal cord
10 Oral part of pharynx
11 Falx cerebri
12 Corpus callosum and anterior cerebral artery
13 **Frontal sinus**
14 Optic chiasm and pituitary gland
15 Superior nasal concha and ethmoidal bulla
16 **Semilunar hiatus**
17 Accessory **openings to maxillary sinus** and cut edge of middle nasal concha
18 Vestibule
19 **Opening of nasolacrimal duct**
20 Inferior nasal concha (cut)
21 **Opening of auditory tube**
22 Incisive canal
23 Levator veli palatini muscle
24 Salpingopharyngeal fold
25 Lingual nerve and submandibular ganglion
26 Submandibular duct
27 **Nasofrontal duct**
28 **Nasolacrimal duct**
29 Sphenoethmoidal recess (of Rosenmüller)
30 Salpingopalatine fold

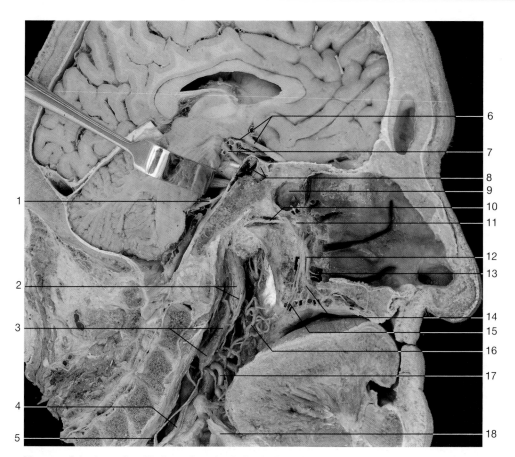

Nerves of the lateral wall of nasal cavity I. Sagittal section through the head. Mucous membranes partly removed, pterygoid canal opened.

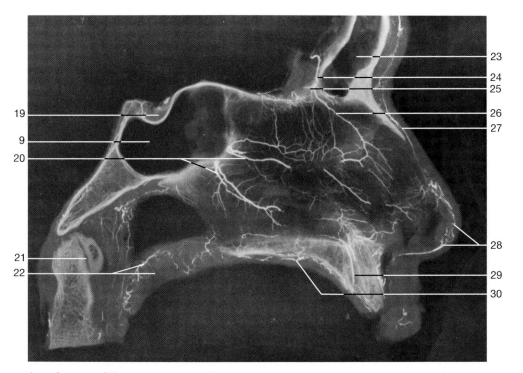

Arteriogram of the nasal septum, left side (lateral aspect).

1   Facial nerve
2   **Internal carotid artery** and **internal carotid plexus**
3   **Superior cervical ganglion**
4   Vagus nerve
5   Sympathetic trunk
6   Optic nerve and ophthalmic artery
7   Oculomotor nerve
8   Internal carotid artery and cavernous sinus
9   Sphenoidal sinus
10   Nerve of the pterygoid canal
11   **Pterygopalatine ganglion**
12   **Descending palatine artery**
13   Lateral inferior posterior nasal branches and lateral posterior nasal and septal arteries
14   Greater palatine nerves and artery
15   Lesser palatine nerves and arteries
16   Branches of ascending pharyngeal artery
17   Lingual artery
18   Epiglottis
19   **Sella turcica**
20   **Posterior lateral nasal and septal arteries** (branches of sphenopalatine artery)
21   Median atlanto-axial joint
22   Soft palate and lesser palatine arteries (branches of descending palatine artery)
23   Frontal sinus
24   Anterior meningeal artery
25   Anterior ethmoidal artery (branch of ophthalmic artery)
26   **Septal branch of anterior ethmoidal artery**
27   Dorsal nasal artery
28   Nasal branches of anterior ethmoidal artery
29   Incisive canal with nasopalatine artery
30   Hard palate and greater palatine artery (branch of descending palatine artery)
31   Tentorium cerebelli
32   Trochlear nerve
33   **Trigeminal nerve** with motor root
34   **Internal carotid plexus**
35   **Lingual nerve with chorda tympani**
36   Medial pterygoid muscle and medial pterygoid plate
37   **Inferior alveolar nerve**
38   **Sympathetic trunk**
39   Oculomotor nerve
40   **Palatine nerves**
41   Tongue
42   **Trigeminal ganglion**
43   Trigeminal nerve (n. V)
44   **Facial nerve** (n. VII)
45   Geniculate ganglion
46   Stylomastoid foramen
47   Medial pterygoid muscle

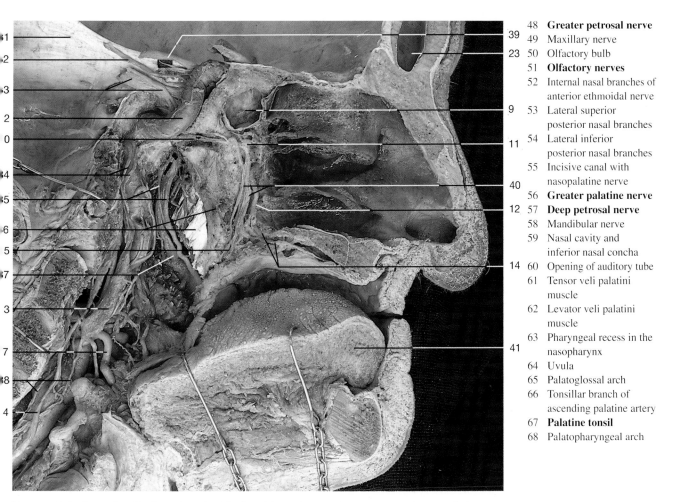

48 **Greater petrosal nerve**
49 Maxillary nerve
50 Olfactory bulb
51 **Olfactory nerves**
52 Internal nasal branches of anterior ethmoidal nerve
53 Lateral superior posterior nasal branches
54 Lateral inferior posterior nasal branches
55 Incisive canal with nasopalatine nerve
56 **Greater palatine nerve**
57 **Deep petrosal nerve**
58 Mandibular nerve
59 Nasal cavity and inferior nasal concha
60 Opening of auditory tube
61 Tensor veli palatini muscle
62 Levator veli palatini muscle
63 Pharyngeal recess in the nasopharynx
64 Uvula
65 Palatoglossal arch
66 Tonsillar branch of ascending palatine artery
67 **Palatine tonsil**
68 Palatopharyngeal arch

Nerves of the lateral wall of nasal cavity II. Carotid canal opened, mucous membranes of pharynx and nasal cavity partly removed.

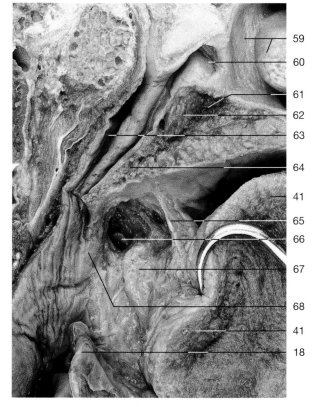

Dissection of palatine tonsil located in the lateral wall of the nasopharynx (left side). Root of tongue reflected.

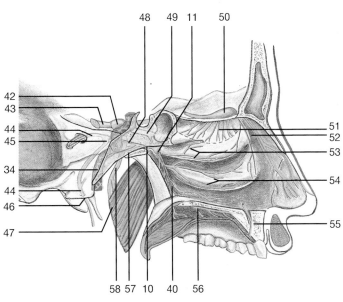

Nerves of the lateral wall of nasal cavity. Body of sphenoid bone appears transparent (schematic drawing).

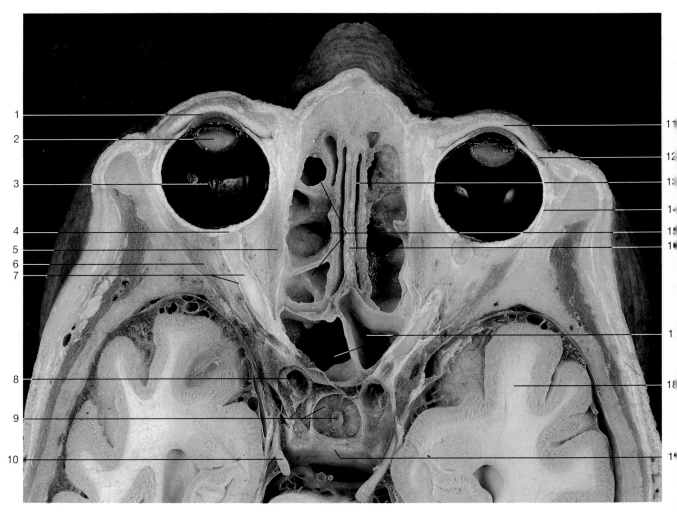

Horizontal section through the nasal cavity, the orbits and temporal lobes of the brain at the level of pituitary gland.

1 Cornea	4 Head of optic nerve	7 **Optic nerve** with dural sheath
2 Lens	5 Medial rectus muscle	8 Internal carotid artery
3 Vitreous body **(eyeball)**	6 Lateral rectus muscle	9 **Pituitary gland** and **infundibulum**

10 **Oculomotor nerve**
11 Superior tarsal plate of eyelid
12 Fornix of conjunctiva
13 **Nasal cavity**
14 Sclera
15 Ethmoidal sinus
16 **Nasal septum**
17 **Sphenoidal sinus**
18 Temporal lobe
19 Clivus
20 Middle cranial fossa
21 External acoustic meatus
22 Superior sagittal sinus
23 Falx cerebri
24 Superior rectus and levator
   palpebrae superioris muscles
25 Eyeball and lacrimal gland
26 Inferior rectus and inferior oblique muscle
27 Zygomatic bone
28 **Maxillary sinus**
29 Inferior nasal concha
30 Hard palate
31 Superior longitudinal muscle of tongue
32 Lingual septum

Horizontal section through the head. CT scan. Bar = 2 cm.
Arrow: fracture.

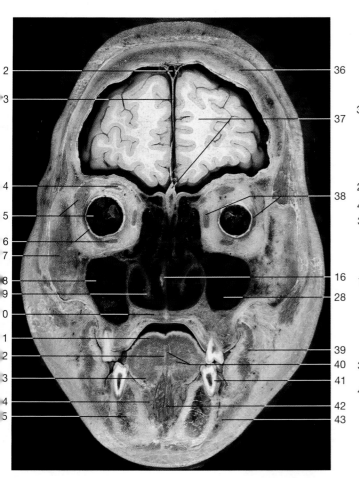

Coronal section through the head at the level of the second premolar of the mandible.

Coronal section through the head (MRI scan, courtesy of Prof. Dr. A. Heuck, Munich, Germany). Note the situation of the head cavities.

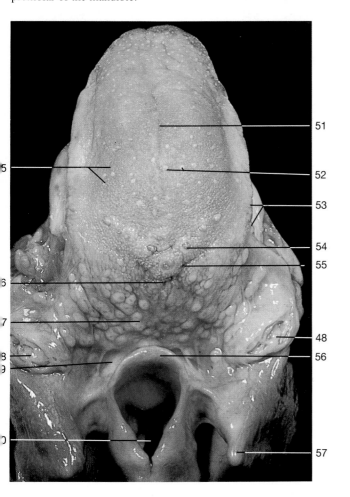

33 Inferior longitudinal muscle of tongue
34 **Sublingual gland**
35 Mandible
36 Calvaria
37 Frontal lobe of brain and crista galli
38 Lateral and medial rectus muscles
39 Buccinator muscle
40 Vertical and transverse muscles of tongue
41 Second premolar of mandible
42 Genioglossus muscle
43 Platysma muscle
44 **Orbit** and **optic nerve**
45 Filiform papillae
46 **Foramen cecum**
47 **Root of tongue** (lingual tonsil)
48 **Palatine tonsil**
49 Vallecula of epiglottis
50 Vestibule of larynx
51 Median sulcus of tongue
52 Fungiform papillae
53 Foliate papillae
54 **Circumvallate papilla**
55 Sulcus terminalis
56 Epiglottis
57 Greater cornu of hyoid bone

Dorsal surface of the tongue and laryngeal inlet.

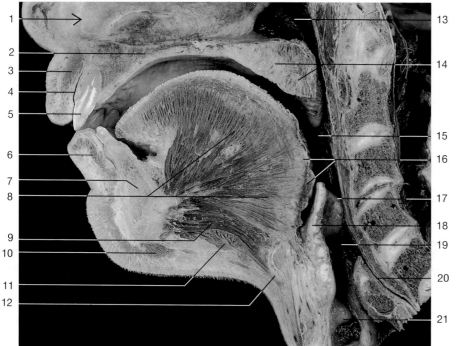

1 Nasal cavity
2 **Hard palate**
3 Upper lip and orbicularis oris muscle
4 Vestibule of oral cavity
5 First incisor
6 Lower lip and orbicularis oris muscle
7 Mandible
8 Genioglossus muscle
9 Geniohyoid muscle
10 Anterior belly of diagastric muscle
11 Mylohyoid muscle
12 **Hyoid bone**
13 **Nasopharynx**
14 **Soft palate** and **uvula**
15 **Oropharynx**
16 Root of tongue and lingual tonsil
17 **Laryngopharynx**
18 Epiglottis
19 Aryepiglottic fold
20 Laryngopharynx continuous with esophagus
21 Larynx

Median sagittal section through the oral cavity and pharynx.

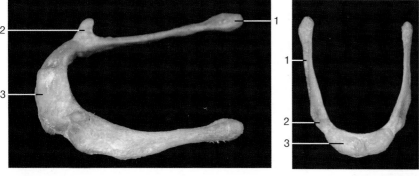

1 Greater cornu ⎫
2 Lesser cornu ⎬ of hyoid bone
3 Body ⎭

Hyoid bone (oblique lateral aspect).

Hyoid bone (anterior aspect).

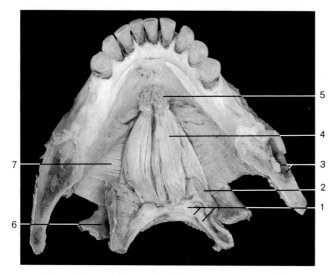

Muscles of the floor of the oral cavity (superior aspect).

1 Lesser cornu and body of hyoid bone
2 Hyoglossus muscle (divided)
3 Ramus of mandible and inferior alveolar nerve
4 **Geniohyoid muscle**
5 Genioglossus muscle (divided)
6 Stylohyoid muscle (divided)

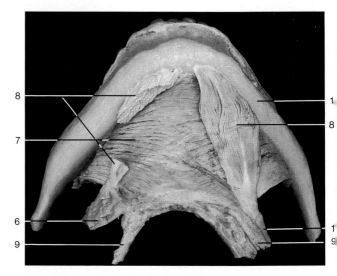

Oral diaphragm, muscles (inferior aspect). Cut on the base.

7 **Mylohyoid muscle**
8 Anterior belly of **digastric muscle**
9 Hyoid bone
10 Mandible
11 Intermediate tendon of digastric muscle

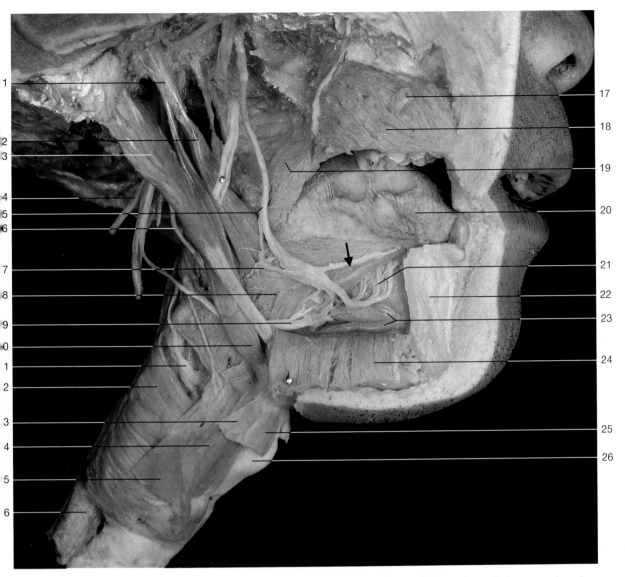

Parapharyngeal and sublingual regions. Innervation of the tongue. Lateral part of face and mandible removed, oral cavity opened. Arrow: submandibular duct.

1 Styloid process	4 Vagus nerve (n. X)	7 Submandibular ganglion
2 Styloglossus muscle	5 **Lingual nerve** (n. V₃)	8 Hyoglossus muscle
3 Digastric muscle (posterior belly)	6 **Glossopharyngeal nerve** (n. IX)	9 **Hypoglossal nerve** (n. XII)

10 Stylohyoid muscle
11 Internal branch of superior laryngeal nerve (branch of vagus nerve, not visible)
12 Middle constrictor muscle of pharynx
13 Omohyoid muscle (divided)
14 Thyrohyoid muscle
15 Sternothyroid muscle
16 Esophagus
17 Parotid duct (divided)
18 Buccinator
19 Superior constrictor muscle of pharynx
20 Tongue
21 Terminal branches of lingual nerve
22 Mandible (divided)
23 Genioglossus and geniohyoid muscles
24 Mylohyoid muscle (divided and reflected)
25 Sternohyoid muscle (divided)
26 Thyroid cartilage
27 Anterior belly of digastric muscle
28 Hyoid bone

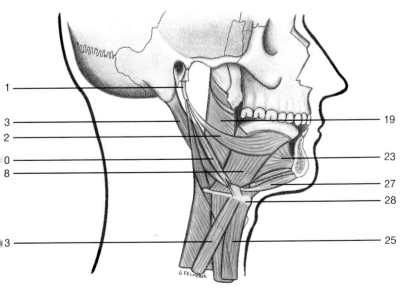

Supra- and infrahyoid muscles and pharynx (schematic drawing).

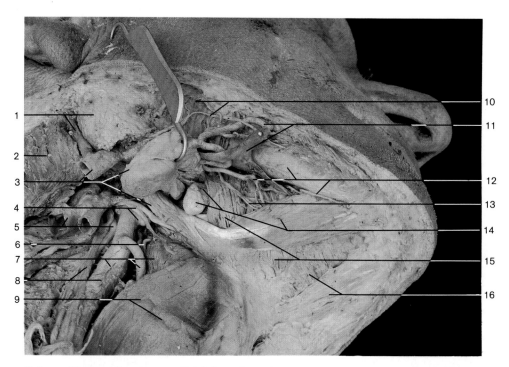

Submandibular triangle, superficial dissection. Right side (inferior aspect). Submandibular gland has been reflected.

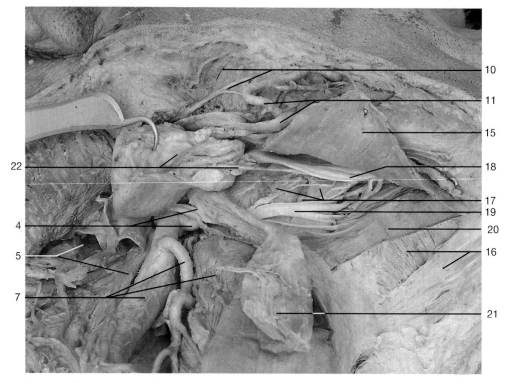

Submandibular triangle, deep dissection. Right side. Mylohyoid muscle has been severed and reflected to display the lingual and hypoglossal nerves.

1 Parotid gland and retromandibular vein
2 Sternocleidomastoid muscle
3 Retromandibular vein, submandibular gland and stylohyoid muscle
4 Hypoglossal nerve and lingual artery
5 Vagus nerve and internal jugular vein
6 Superior laryngeal artery
7 **External carotid artery,** thyrohyoid muscle, and superior thyroid artery
8 Common carotid artery and superior root of ansa cervicalis
9 Omohyoid and sternohyoid
10 Masseter and marginal mandibular branch of facial nerve
11 **Facial artery and vein**

12 Mandible and submental artery and vein
13 Mylohyoid nerve
14 Submandibular duct, sublingual gland, and anterior belly of digastric muscle
15 Mylohyoid (right side)
16 Left mylohyoid and anterior belly of left digastric muscle
17 Hyoglossus muscle and lingual artery
18 **Lingual nerve**
19 **Hypoglossal nerve**
20 Geniohyoid muscle
21 Anterior belly of right digastric muscle
22 Submandibular gland and duct

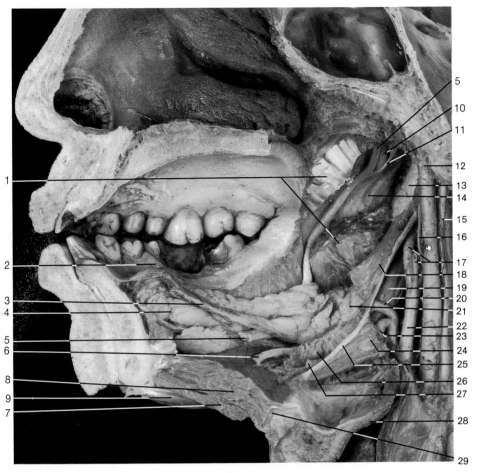

1   Medial pterygoid muscle
2   Sublingual papilla
3   **Submandibular duct**
4   **Sublingual gland**
5   **Lingual nerve**
6   Hypoglossal nerve
7   Mylohyoid muscle
8   Geniohyoid muscle
9   Anterior belly of digastric
    muscle
10 Inferior alveolar nerve
11 **Chorda tympani**
12 Internal carotid artery
13 Parotid gland
14 Sphenomandibular ligament
15 Vagus nerve
16 Glossopharyngeal nerve
17 Superficial temporal artery and
    ascending pharyngeal artery
18 Styloglossus muscle
19 Posterior belly of digastric
    muscle
20 **Facial artery**
21 Submandibular gland
22 **External carotid artery**
23 Lingual artery
24 Middle pharyngeal constrictor
    muscle
25 **Stylohyoid ligament**
26 Hyoglossus muscle
27 Deep lingual artery
28 Epiglottis
29 Hyoid bone
30 Buccinator muscle
31 Tongue
32 Mandible (divided)
33 **Parotid duct**
34 Masseter muscle
35 Right and left sublingual papillae

Oral cavity (internal aspect). Tongue and pharyngeal wall removed.

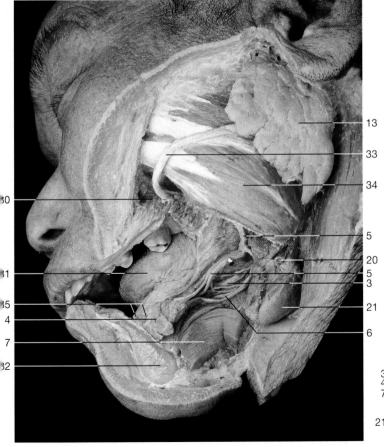

Dissection of major salivary glands. Left mandible and buccinator muscle partly removed to view the oral cavity (inferior lateral aspect).

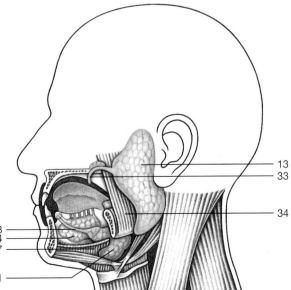

Location of the major salivary glands in relation to the oral cavity.

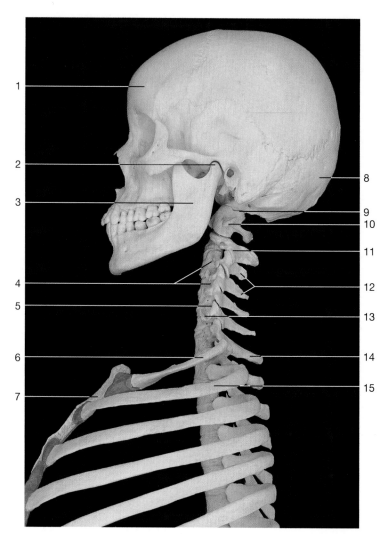

Cervical spine between skull and upper thorax (lateral aspect).

1 Frontal bone
2 Temporomandibular joint
3 **Mandible**
4 Bodies of the third and fourth cervical vertebrae (C₃, C₄)
5 Intervertebral foramen
6 First rib
7 Manubrium of the sternum
8 Occipital bone
9 Atlanto-occipital joint
10 **Atlas**
11 **Axis**
12 Spinous processes of the third and fourth **cervical vertebrae**
13 Transverse process with groove for spinal nerve
14 Vertebra prominens (seventh cervical vertebra)
15 Second rib

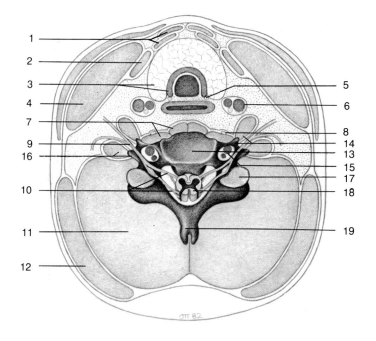

Cervical vertebra and the **organization of the neck.** (Schematic drawing.)

1 Sternohyoid and sternothyroid muscles
2 Omohyoid muscle
3 Thyroid gland and trachea
4 Sternocleidomastoid muscle
5 Recurrent laryngeal nerve
6 Internal jugular vein, common carotid artery and vagus
7 Longus colli and longus capitis muscles
8 Sympathetic trunk
9 Spinal nerve
10 Ventral and dorsal root of spinal nerve
11 True muscles of the neck
12 Trapezius muscle
13 Body of cervical vertebra
14 Anterior tubercle of transverse process and origin of scalenus anterior muscle
15 Vertebral artery and foramen transversarium
16 Posterior tubercle of transverse process and origin of scalenus medius and posterior muscles
17 Superior facet of articular process
18 Spinal cord
19 Spinous process

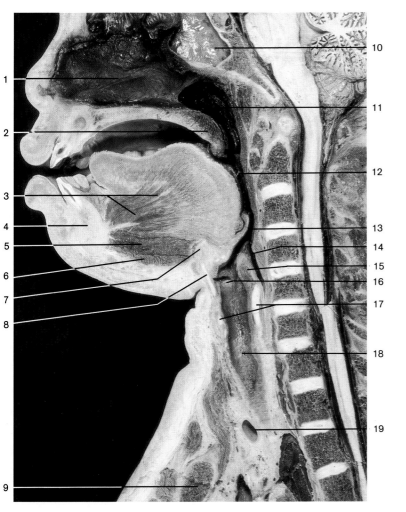

1 Nasal septum
2 Uvula
3 Genioglossus muscle
4 Mandible
5 Geniohyoid muscle
6 Mylohyoid muscle
7 **Hyoid bone**
8 Thyroid cartilage
9 Manubrium sterni
10 Sphenoidal sinus
11 **Nasopharynx**
12 **Oropharynx**
13 **Epiglottis**
14 **Laryngopharynx**
15 Arytenoid muscle
16 **Vocal fold**
17 Cricoid cartilage
18 **Trachea**
19 Left brachiocephalic vein
20 Thymus
21 Esophagus
22 Occipital lobe
23 Cerebellum and fourth ventricle
24 Medulla oblongata
25 Dens of axis
26 Intervertebral discs
   of cervical vertebral column

Median section through adult head and neck. Note the low position of the adult larynx when compared with that of the neonate (cf. with figure below).

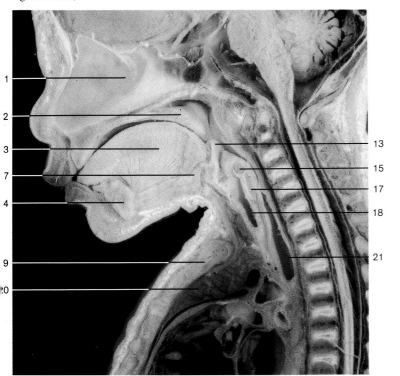

Median section through neonate head and neck. Note the high position of the larynx permitting the epiglottis nearly to reach the uvula (cf. with the figure above).

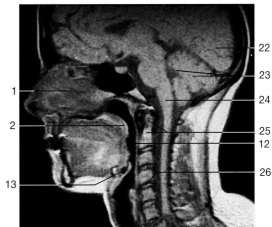

Sagittal section through the head. (MRI scan.)

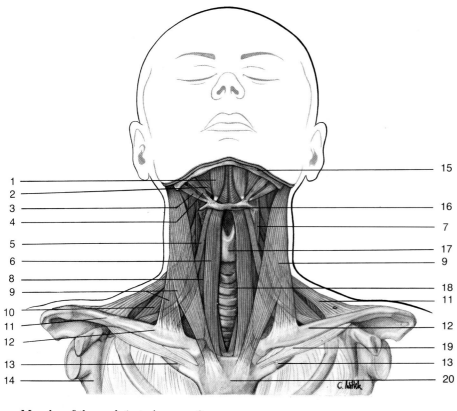

Muscles of the neck (anterior aspect).

Suprahyoid muscles
1 Anterior belly of digastric muscle
2 Mylohyoid muscle
3 Posterior belly of digastric muscle
4 Stylohyoid muscle

Infrahyoid muscles
5 Omohyoid muscle
6 Sternohyoid muscle
7 Thyrohyoid muscle
8 Sternothyroid muscle

Other structures
9 Sternocleidomastoid muscle
10 Scalenus muscles
11 Trapezius muscle
12 Clavicle
13 First rib
14 Scapula
15 Mandible
16 Hyoid bone
17 Larynx (thyroid cartilage)
18 Trachea
19 Subclavius muscle
20 Manubrium sterni
21 Mucous membrane of larynx (conus elasticus)
22 Cricoid cartilage
23 Inferior horn of thyroid cartilage
24 Esophagus
25 Body of cervical vertebra
26 Posterior root ganglion
27 Spinal cord
28 Spinous process
29 Internal jugular vein, common carotid artery, and vagus nerve
30 True muscles of the neck (semispinalis cervicis and capitis muscles)

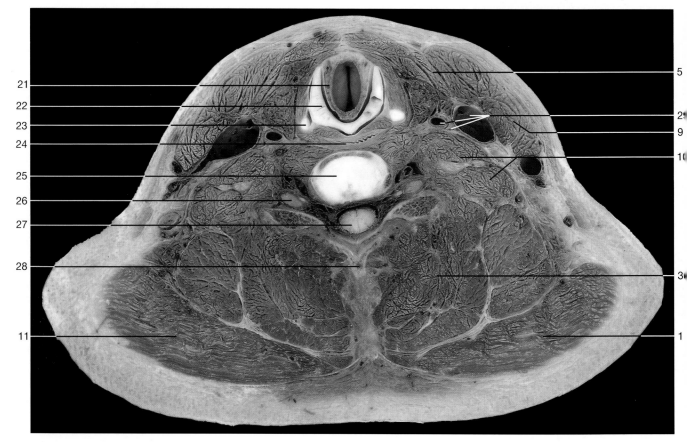

Cross section of the neck at the level of the intervertebral disc between the 5th and 6th cervical vertebra (inferior aspect).

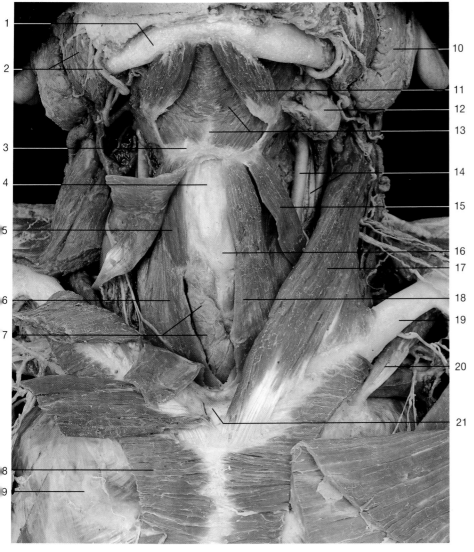

1	Mandible
2	Masseter muscle and facial artery
3	**Hyoid bone**
4	Median thyrohyoid ligament
5	**Thyrohyoid muscle**
6	**Sternothyroid muscle**
7	Thyroid gland (pyramidal lobe)
8	Pectoralis major muscle
9	Second rib
10	Parotid gland
11	Anterior belly of **digastric muscle**
12	Submandibular gland (divided)
13	**Mylohyoid muscle** and mylohyoid raphe
14	External carotid artery and vagus nerve
15	**Omohyoid muscle**
16	Thyroid cartilage
17	Sternocleidomastoid muscle
18	**Sternohyoid muscle**
19	Clavicle
20	Subclavius muscle
21	Jugular fossa and interclavicular ligament

Muscles of the neck (anterior aspect). Sternocleidomastoid and sternohyoid muscles on the right have been divided and reflected.

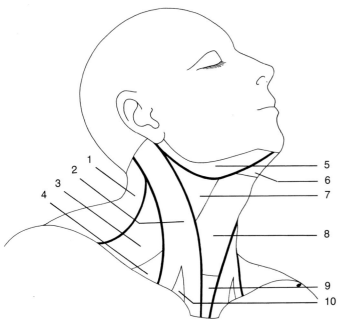

Regions and triangles of the neck.

1	Trapezius muscle
2	Sternocleidomastoid muscle
3	Lateral cervical triangle
4	Supraclavicular triangle
5	Submandibular triangle
6	Submental triangle
7	Carotid triangle
8	Muscular triangle
9	Jugular fossa
10	Lesser supraclavicular fossa

Posterior triangle (3, 4)

Anterior triangle (5, 6, 7)

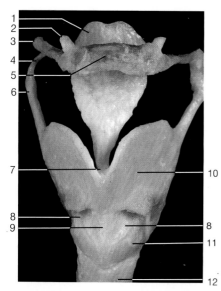

Cartilages of the larynx and the hyoid bone (anterior aspect).

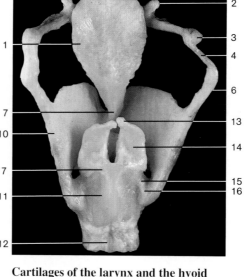

Cartilages of the larynx and the hyoid bone (posterior aspect).

1 **Epiglottis**
2 Lesser cornu of hyoid bone
3 Greater cornu of hyoid bone
4 Lateral thyrohyoid ligament
5 Body of **hyoid bone**
6 Superior cornu of thyroid cartilage
7 Thyroepiglottic ligament
8 Conus elasticus
9 Cricothyroid ligament
10 **Thyroid cartilage**
11 **Cricoid cartilage**
12 Trachea
13 Corniculate cartilage
14 **Arytenoid cartilage**
15 Posterior cricoarytenoid ligament
16 **Cricothyroid joint**
17 **Cricoarytenoid joint**

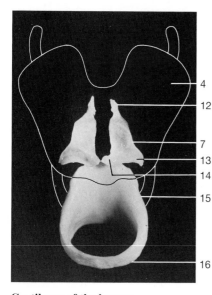

Cartilages of the larynx (anterior aspect). Thyroid cartilage is indicated by the outline.

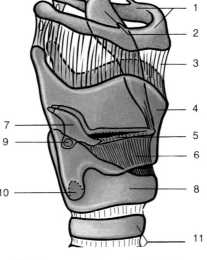

Cartilages and ligaments of the larynx (lateral aspect). (Schematic drawing.)

1 Hyoid bone
2 Epiglottis
3 Thyrohyoid membrane
4 **Thyroid cartilage**
5 **Vocal ligament**
6 Conus elasticus
7 Arytenoid cartilage
8 **Cricoid cartilage**
9 **Cricoarytenoid joint**
10 **Cricothyroid joint**
11 Tracheal cartilages
12 Corniculate cartilage
13 Muscular process of arytenoid cartilage
14 Vocal process of arytenoid cartilage
15 Lamina of cricoid cartilage
16 Arch of cricoid cartilage

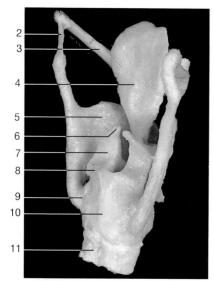

Cartilages of the larynx (oblique posterior aspect).

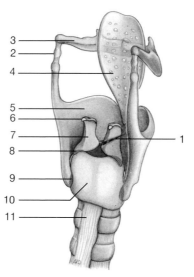

Cartilages of the larynx (oblique-posterior aspect).

1 **Vocal ligament** (red)
2 Lateral thyrohyoid ligament
3 Greater cornu of hyoid bone
4 **Epiglottis**
5 **Thyroid cartilage**
6 Corniculate cartilage
7 **Arytenoid cartilage**
8 **Cricoarytenoid joint**
9 **Cricothyroid joint**
10 **Cricoid cartilage**
11 Trachea

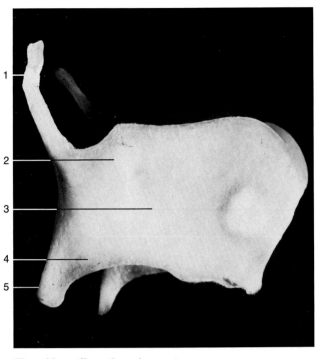

Thyroid cartilage (lateral aspect).

1 Superior cornu
2 Superior thyroid tubercle
3 Lamina of thyroid cartilage

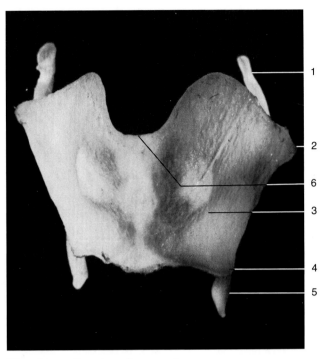

Thyroid cartilage (anterior aspect)

4 Inferior thyroid tubercle
5 Inferior cornu
6 Superior thyroid notch

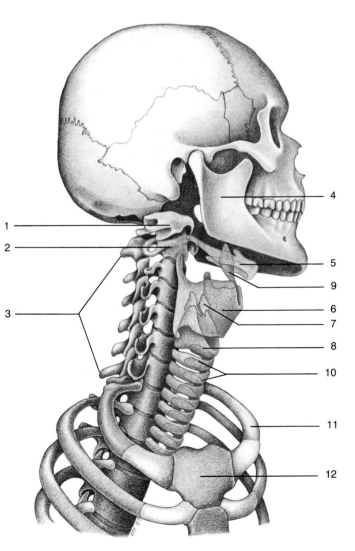

1 Atlas
2 Axis
3 Cervical vertebrae (C_2–C_7)
4 Mandible
5 **Hyoid bone**
6 **Thyroid cartilage**
7 Arytenoid cartilage
8 **Cricoid cartilage**
9 Epiglottis
10 **Tracheal cartilages**
11 First rib
12 Manubrium sterni

Position of the larynx in the neck (oblique lateral aspect).
(Schematic drawing.)

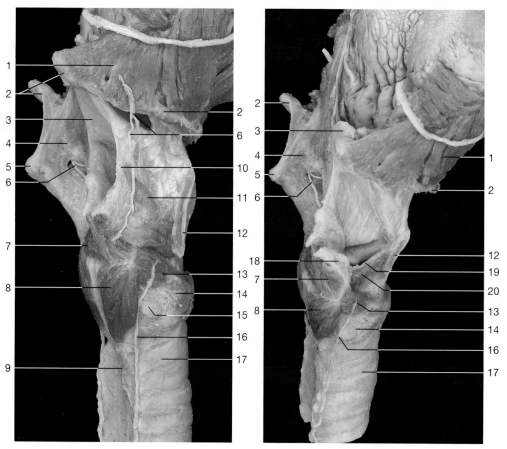

1 Hyoglossus muscle
2 Hyoid bone
· 3 **Epiglottis**
4 Thyrohyoid membrane
5 Superior cornu of thyroid cartilage
6 Superior laryngeal nerve
7 **Transverse arytenoid muscle**
8 **Posterior cricoarytenoid muscle**
9 Transverse muscle of trachea
10 Aryepiglottic fold
11 Thyroepiglottic muscle
12 Thyroid cartilage
13 **Lateral cricoarytenoid muscle**
14 Cricoid cartilage
15 Articular facet for thyroid cartilage
16 Inferior laryngeal nerve (branch of recurrent nerve)
17 Trachea
18 Arytenoid cartilage
19 **Vocal ligament**
20 **Vocalis muscle** (part of thyroarytenoid muscle)
21 Thyrohyoideus muscle
22 **Cricothyroideus muscle**
23 Root of tongue
24 Cuneiform tubercle
25 Corniculate tubercle
26 Aryepiglottic muscle

Laryngeal muscles I (lateral aspect). Thyroid cartilage (12) and thyroarytenoid muscle have been partly removed.

Laryngeal muscles II (lateral aspect). Half of the thyroid cartilage (12) has been removed. Dissection of the vocal ligament (19).

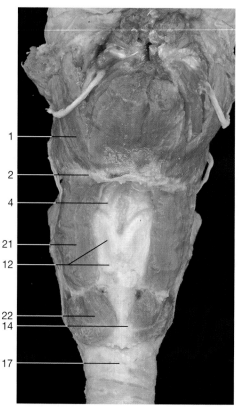

Laryngeal muscles and **larynx** (anterior aspect).

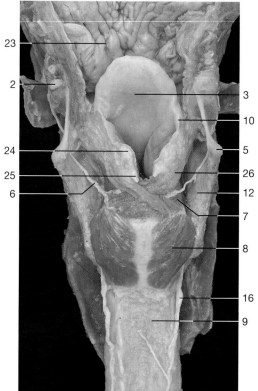

Laryngeal muscles and **larynx** (posterior aspect).

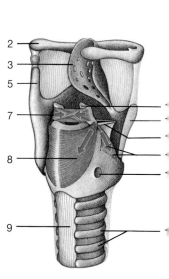

Action of internal muscles of the larynx. (Schematic drawing

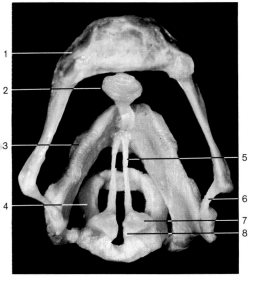

Laryngeal cartilages (superior aspect).

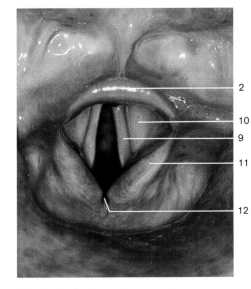

Glottis in vivo (superior aspect).

1 **Hyoid bone**
2 Epiglottis
3 **Thyroid cartilage**
4 **Cricoid cartilage**
5 **Vocal ligament**
6 Thyrohyoid ligament
7 **Arytenoid cartilage**
8 Corniculate cartilage
9 **Vocal fold**
10 **Vestibular fold**
11 Aryepiglottic fold
12 Interarytenoid notch
13 Mandible
14 Anterior belly of
   digastric muscle
15 Mylohyoid muscle
16 Pyramidal lobe of
   thyroid gland
17 Sternohyoid and
   sternothyroid muscles
18 Common carotid
   artery
19 Internal jugular vein
20 **Rima glottidis**
21 Sternocleidomastoid
   muscle
22 Transverse arytenoid
   muscle
23 Pharynx and inferior
   constrictor muscle
24 Ventricle of larynx
25 **Vocalis muscle**
26 Trachea
27 Superior cornu of
   thyroid cartilage
28 Root of tongue
   (lingual tonsil)
29 Piriform recess
30 Vocalis muscle
31 Lateral cricoarytenoid
   muscle
32 **Thyroid gland**

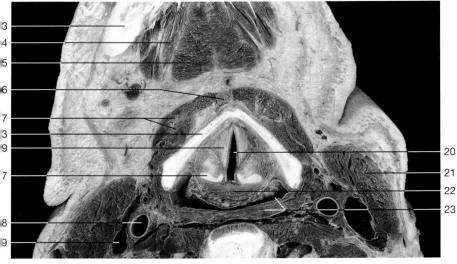

Horizontal section through the larynx at the level of the vocal folds (superior aspect).

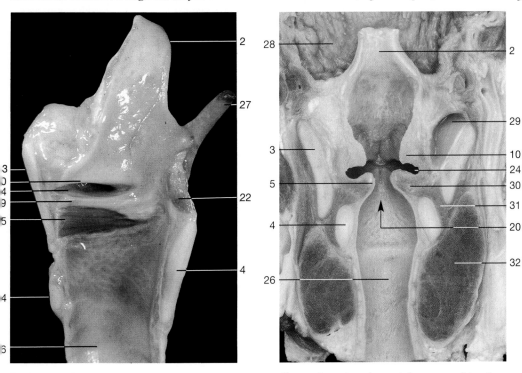

Sagittal section through the larynx.

Coronal section through larynx and trachea.

160

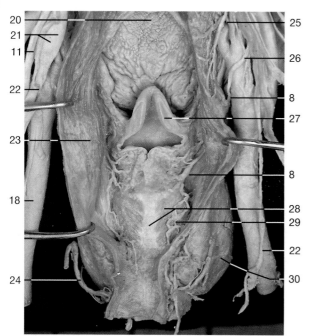

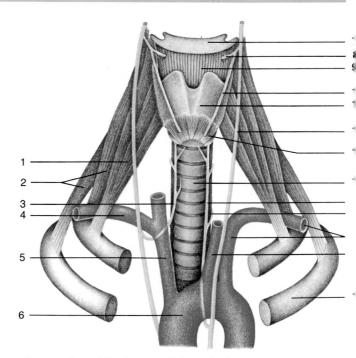

Larynx and its innervation (posterior aspect).
Dissection of superior and inferior laryngeal nerves.
Pharynx has been opened.

Innervation of the larynx. (Schematic diagram.)

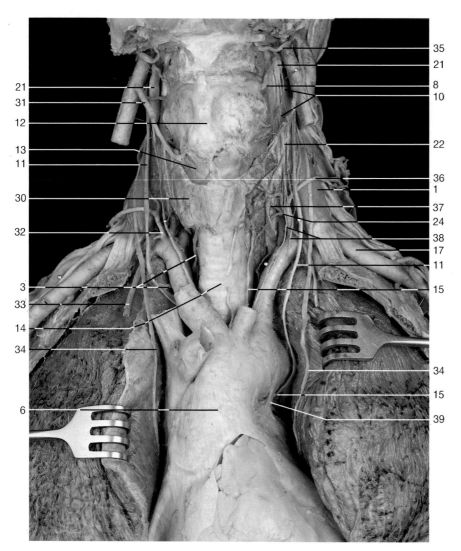

Larynx and thoracic organs (anterior aspect). Dissection of vagus and recurrent laryngeal nerves.

1   Scalenus anterior muscle
2   Scalenus medius and posterior muscles
3   Right **recurrent laryngeal nerve**
4   Right subclavian artery
5   Brachiocephalic trunk
6   Aortic arch
7   Hyoid bone
8   **Internal branch of superior laryngeal nerve**
9   Thyrohyoid membrane
10 **External branch of superior laryngeal nerve**
11 **Vagus nerve**
12 Thyroid cartilage
13 Cricothyroid muscle
14 Trachea
15 **Left recurrent laryngeal nerve**
16 Esophagus
17 Left subclavian artery
18 Left common carotid artery
19 Second rib
20 Tongue
21 Superior cervical ganglion
22 Sympathetic trunk
23 Inferior constrictor muscle of pharynx
24 **Inferior thyroid artery**
25 Glossopharyngeal nerve
26 Superior laryngeal nerve
27 Epiglottis
28 Posterior cricoarytenoid muscle and cricoid cartilage
29 Inferior laryngeal branch of recurrent laryngeal nerve
30 **Thyroid gland**
31 Superior thyroid artery
32 **Thyrocervical trunk**
33 Internal thoracic artery
34 **Phrenic nerve**
35 Hypoglossal nerve
36 Transverse cervical artery
37 Middle cervical ganglion
38 Middle cervical cardiac nerves (branches of sympathetic trunk)
39 Ligamentum arteriosum

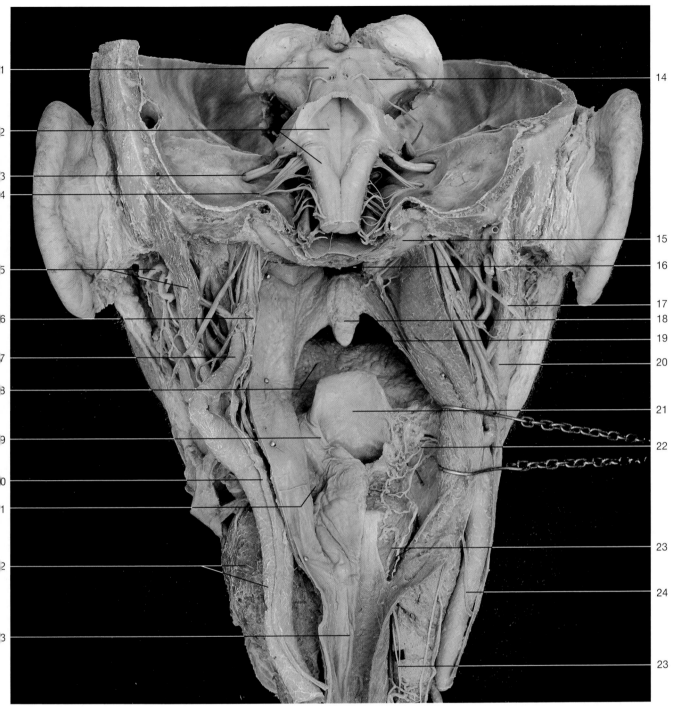

Larynx and oral cavity (posterior aspect). Mucous membrane on the right half of pharynx has been removed.

1 Midbrain (inferior colliculus)
2 Rhomboid fossa and medulla oblongata
3 Vestibulocochlear and facial nerve
4 Glossopharyngeal, vagus and accessory nerve
5 Occipital artery and posterior belly of digastric muscle
6 Superior cervical ganglion
7 **Internal carotid artery**
8 **Oral cavity** (tongue)
9 Aryepiglottic fold
10 Vagus nerve
11 **Piriform recess**
12 Thyroid gland and common carotid artery

13 Esophagus
14 Trochlear nerve
15 Occipital condyle
16 **Nasal cavity** (choana)
17 Accessory nerve
18 **Uvula** and soft palate
19 Palatopharyngeus muscle
20 External carotid artery
21 Epiglottis
22 **Internal branch of superior laryngeal nerve**
23 **Inferior laryngeal nerve**
24 Ansa cervicalis

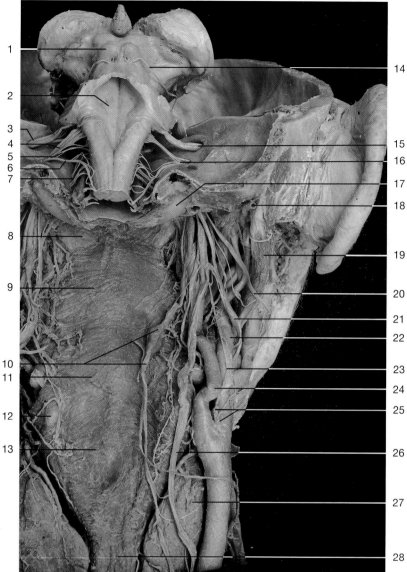

Pharynx and parapharyngeal nerves in connection with brain stem (posterior aspect).

1 Inferior colliculus of midbrain
2 Facial colliculus in **floor of rhomboid fossa**
3 Vestibulocochlear and facial nerves
4 Glossopharyngeal nerve
5 Vagus nerve
6 Accessory nerve
7 Hypoglossal nerve
8 Pharyngobasilar fascia
9 Superior constrictor muscle of pharynx
10 **Sympathetic trunk** and **superior cervical ganglion** (medially displaced)
11 Middle constrictor muscle of pharynx
12 Greater cornu of hyoid bone
13 Inferior constrictor muscle of pharynx
14 Trochlear nerve
15 **Internal acoustic meatus** with facial and vestibulocochlear nerves
16 **Jugular foramen** with glossopharyngeal, vagus and assessory nerves
17 Occipital condyle
18 Occipital artery
19 Posterior belly of digastric muscle
20 **Accessory nerve** (extracranial part)
21 **Hypoglossal nerve** (extracranial part)
22 External carotid artery
23 Carotid sinus nerve
24 **Internal carotid artery**
25 **Carotid sinus and carotid body**
26 Vagus nerve
27 Thyroid gland
28 Esophagus
29 Choanae
30 Medial pterygoid plate
31 Foramen lacerum
32 **Pharyngeal tubercle**
33 Hard palate
34 Greater and lesser palatine foramen
35 Pterygoid hamulus
36 Lateral pterygoid plate
37 Pterygoid canal
38 Foramen ovale
39 Mandibular fossa
40 Carotid canal
41 Styloid process and stylomastoid foramen

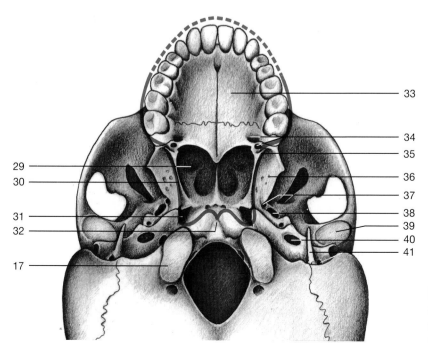

Inferior aspect of the skull. Red line = outline of superior constrictor muscle in continuation with buccinator muscle and orbicularis oris muscle. (Semischematic drawing.)

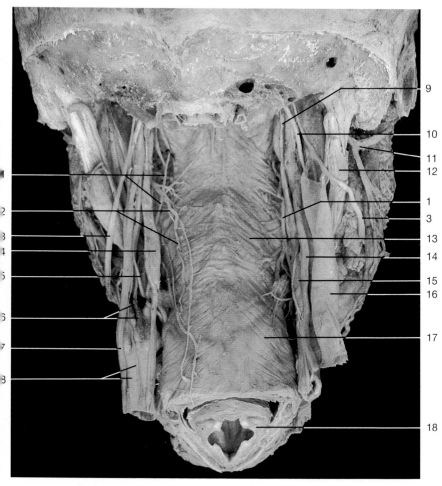

Parapharyngeal nerves and vessels. Dorsal aspect of the pharynx.

1 Ascending pharyngeal artery
2 Pharyngeal plexus
3 **Accessory nerve**
4 Superior cervical ganglion of sympathetic trunk
5 Superior laryngeal nerve
6 Carotid body and carotid sinus nerve
7 Left **vagus nerve**
8 Common carotid artery and cardiac branch of vagus nerve
9 **Glossopharyngeal nerve**
10 **Hypoglossal nerve**
11 **Facial nerve**
12 Posterior belly of digastric muscle
13 Middle constrictor muscle of pharynx
14 Right vagus nerve
15 **Sympathetic trunk**
16 **Internal jugular vein**
17 Inferior constrictor muscle of pharynx
18 Larynx
19 **Buccinator muscle**
20 Soft palate and palatine glands
21 Palatine tonsil
22 Uvula of palate
23 **Pharynx** (oral part)
24 Parotid gland
25 Longus capitis muscle
26 Medioatlantoaxial joint and anterior arch of atlas
27 **Dens of axis**
28 **Spinal cord**
29 Dura mater
30 Incisive papilla
31 **Oral vestibule**
32 Masseter muscle
33 Mandible
34 Mandibular canal with vessels and nerve
35 Medial pterygoid muscle
36 External carotid artery
37 Internal carotid artery
38 **Atlas**
39 **Vertebral artery**
40 Splenius capitis muscle
41 Semispinalis capitis muscle

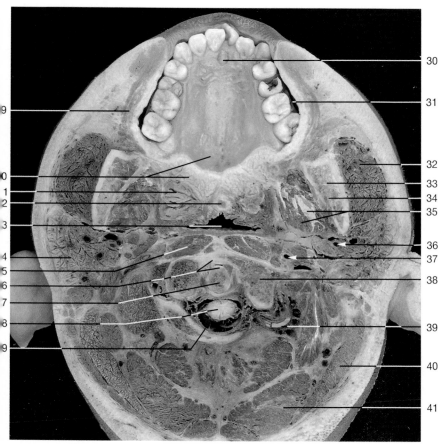

Cross section of head and neck at the level of the atlas (inferior aspect).

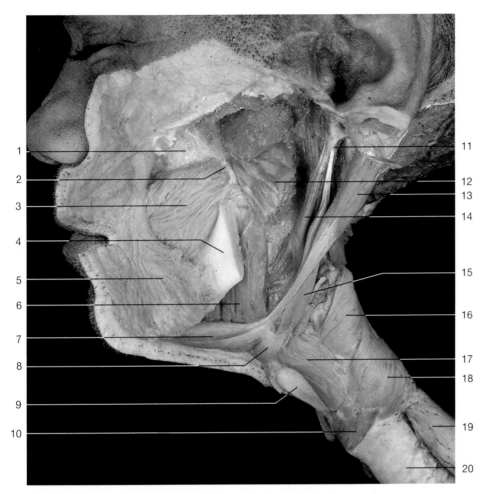

Dissection of pharynx, supra- and infrahyoid muscles I. Mandible partly removed (lateral aspect).

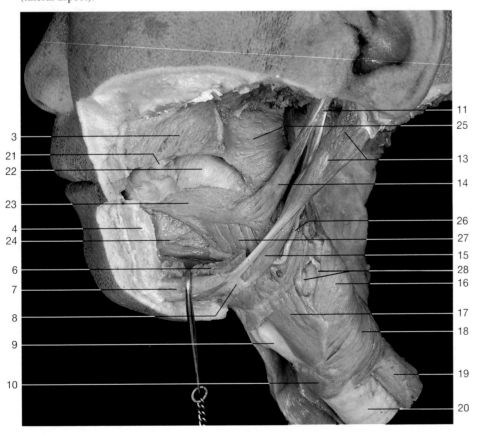

Dissection of pharynx, supra- and infrahyoid muscles II. Oral cavity opened (lateral aspect).

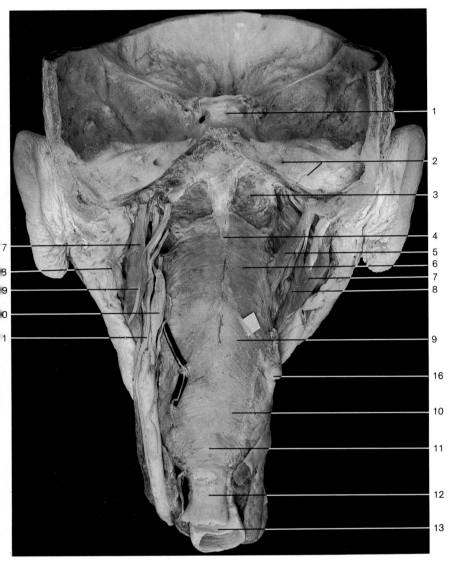

Muscles of the pharynx (posterior aspect).

1 Sella turcica
2 Internal acoustic meatus and petrous part of temporal bone
3 Pharyngobasilar fascia
4 Fibrous raphe of pharynx
5 **Stylopharyngeal muscle**
6 **Superior constrictor muscle of pharynx**
7 Posterior belly of digastric muscle
8 Stylohyoid muscle
9 **Middle constrictor muscle of pharynx**
10 **Inferior constrictor muscle of pharynx**
11 Muscle-free area (Killian's triangle)
12 Esophagus
13 Trachea
14 Thyroid and parathyroid glands
15 Medial pterygoid muscle
16 Greater horn of hyoid bone
17 Internal jugular vein
18 Parotid gland
19 Accessory nerve
20 **Superior cervical ganglion** of sympathetic trunk
21 Vagus nerve
22 Laimer's triangle (area prone to developing diverticula)
23 Orbicularis oculi muscle
24 Nasal muscle
25 Levator labii superioris and levator labii alaeque nasi muscles
26 Levator anguli oris muscle
27 Orbicularis oris muscle
28 **Buccinator muscle**
29 Depressor labii inferioris muscle
30 **Hyoglossus muscle**
31 Thyrohyoid muscle
32 Thyroid cartilage
33 Cricothyroid muscle
34 Pterygomandibular raphe
35 Tensor veli palatini muscle
36 Levator veli palatini muscle
37 Depressor anguli oris muscle
38 Mentalis muscle
39 Styloglossus muscle

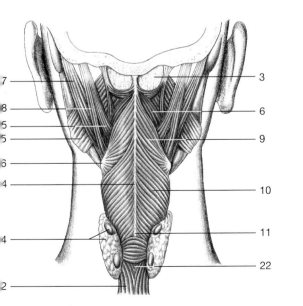

Muscles of the pharynx. (Schematic drawing.)

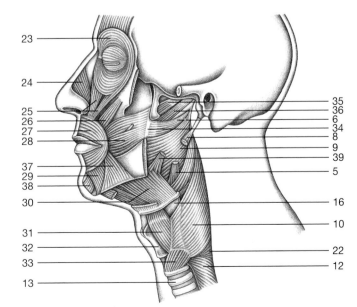

Muscles of the pharynx (lateral aspect). (Schematic drawing.)

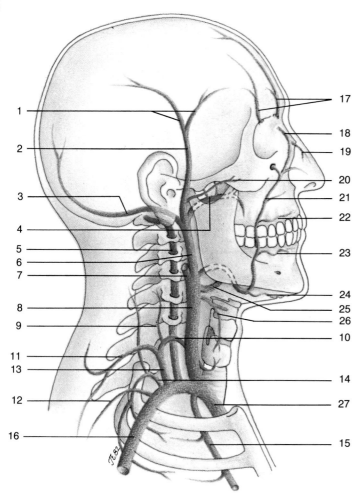

Arteries of head and neck. Diagram of the main branches
of external carotid and subclavian artery.

to page 167 ▷

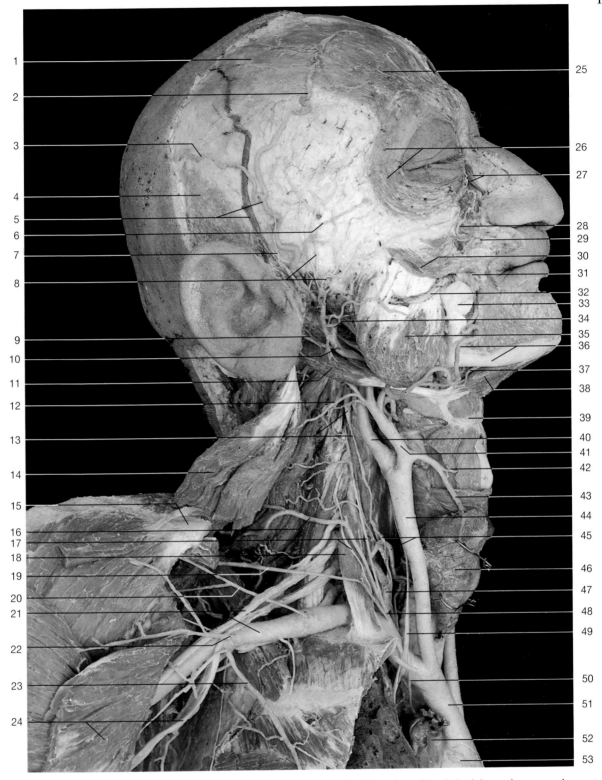

Main branches of head and neck arteries (lateral aspect). Anterior thoracic wall and clavicle partly removed; pectoralis muscles have been reflected to display the subclavian and axillary arteries.

39 Hyoid bone
40 **Internal carotid artery**
41 **External carotid artery**
42 Superior laryngeal artery
43 Superior thyroid artery
44 **Common carotid artery**
45 Thyroid ansa of sympathetic trunk and **inferior thyroid artery**

46 Thyroid gland (right lobe)
47 **Vertebral artery**
48 **Thyrocervical trunk**
49 Vagus nerve
50 Ansa subclavia of sympathetic trunk
51 **Brachiocephalic trunk**
52 Superior vena cava (divided)
53 Aortic arch

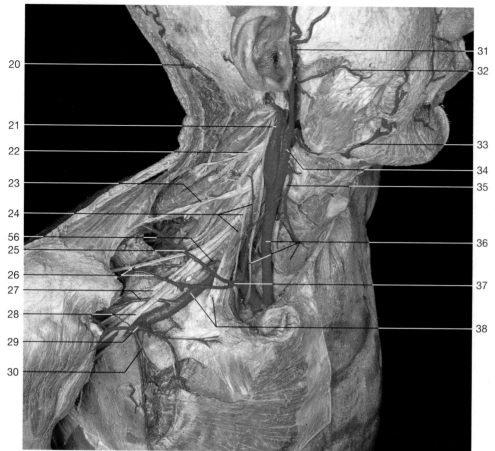

Arteries of head and neck (anterior-lateral aspect). Clavicle, sternocleidomastoid muscle and veins have been partly removed; the arteries were colored.

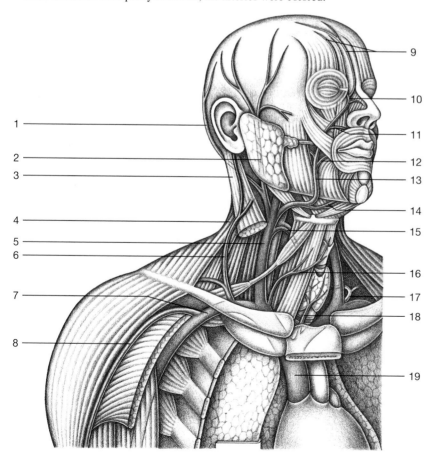

Veins of head and neck. Sternocleidomastoid muscle and anterior thoracic wall partly removed. Note the venous connection with the superior vena cava.

1 Occipital vein
2 Superficial temporal vein
3 Sternocleidomastoid muscle
4 Trapezius muscle
5 **Internal jugular vein**
6 External jugular vein
7 **Subclavian vein**
8 Cephalic vein
9 Supraorbital veins
10 Angular vein
11 Superior labial vein
12 Inferior labial vein
13 **Facial vein**
14 Submental vein
15 Superior thyroid vein
16 Anterior jugular vein
17 Thoracic duct
18 Inferior thyroid vein
19 Superior vena cava
20 Occipital artery
21 **Internal carotid artery**
22 Cervical plexus
23 Supraclavicular nerve
24 Phrenic nerve and ascending cervical artery on scalenus anterior muscle
25 Superficial cervical artery
26 Suprascapular artery and nerve
27 Brachial plexus and anterior circumflex humeral artery
28 Lateral cord of brachial plexus
29 **Thoracoacromial artery**
30 Lateral thoracic artery
31 Superficial temporal artery
32 Transverse facial artery
33 Facial artery
34 External carotid artery
35 Superior thyroid artery
36 **Common carotid artery, vagus nerve** and thyroid gland
37 **Thyrocervical trunk**
38 **Subclavian artery** and scalenus anterior muscle
39 Parotid gland and facial nerve
40 Great auricular nerve
41 External jugular vein
42 Brachial plexus
43 Cephalic vein in deltopectoral groove
44 Axillary vein and artery
45 Right brachiocephalic vein
46 **Superior vena cava**
47 Right lung (reflected)
48 Superficial temporal artery and vein
49 Facial artery and vein
50 Cervical branch of facial nerve and submandibular gland
51 **Internal jugular vein,** common carotid artery and omohyoid muscle
52 Anterior jugular vein and thyroid gland
53 Jugular venous arch
54 Left brachiocephalic vein
55 Pericardium of heart (location of right atrium)
56 Transverse cervical artery

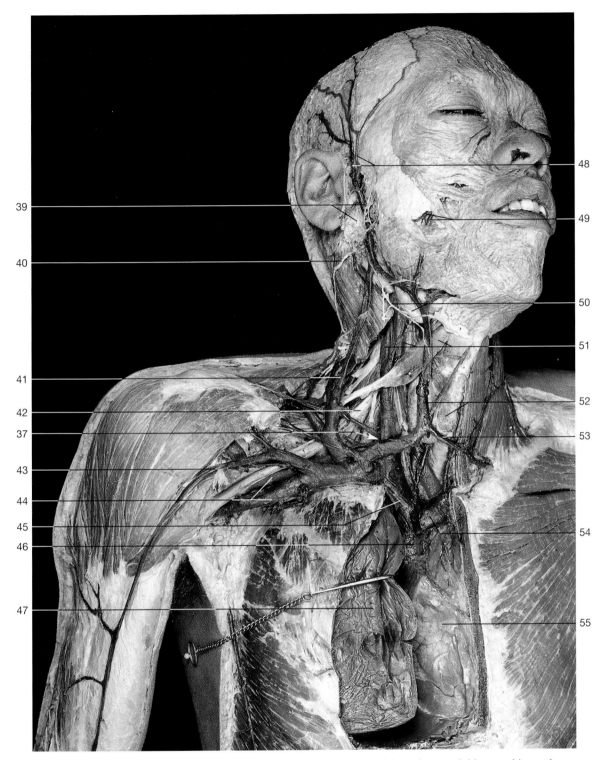

Veins of head and neck (anterior aspect). Part of the thoracic wall, clavicle and sternocleidomastoid muscle have been removed. Veins were colored blue; arteries, red.

The **internal jugular vein** is the continuation of the sigmoid sinus which drains most of the venous blood from the brain together with the external cerebrospinal fluid. By joining the subclavian vein it forms the right brachiocephalic vein, which continues on the right side directly into the superior vena cava. The common way to introduce the lead from a pacemaker device into the heart is by way of the cephalic vein. On the left side the thoracic duct joins the internal jugular vein at that point where the subclavian vein and the internal jugular vein form the

left brachiocephalic vein. Note that the subclavian vein lies in front of the scalenus anterior muscle, whereas the subclavian artery together with the plexus brachialis lies posterior to that muscle. The cephalic vein joins the axillary vein by passing into the deltopectoral triangle. The subclavian vein is strongly fixed to the first rib, so that it can be punctured with a needle at that point (underneath the sternal end of clavicle) to introduce a catheter (subclavian line).

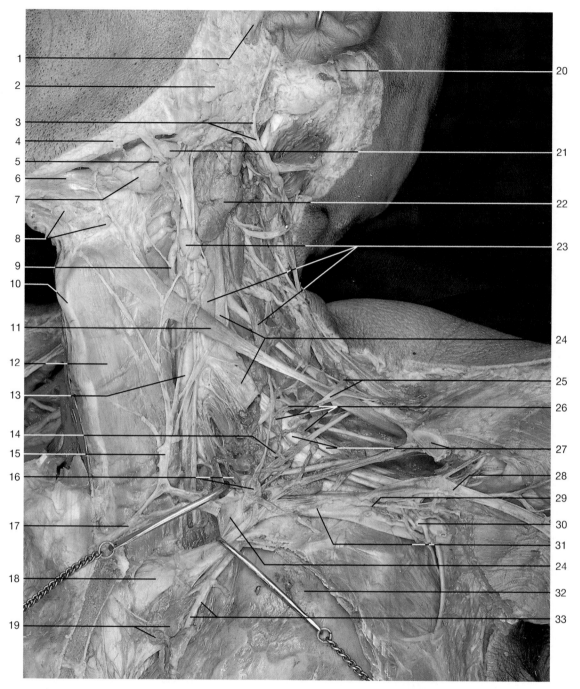

Lymph nodes and lymph vessels of the neck, left side oblique (oblique-lateral aspect). The sternocleido-mastoid muscle and the left half of the thoracic wall have been removed. Lower part of the internal jugular vein has been cut and laterally displaced to show the thoracic duct.

1	**Superficial parotid lymph node**	13	Common carotid artery	
2	Parotid gland	14	**Supraclavicular lymph nodes**	
3	Great auricular nerve	15	Anterior jugular vein	
4	Mandible	16	Thoracic duct and internal jugular vein	
5	Facial vein	17	Jugular venous arch	
6	Anterior belly of digastric muscle	18	Left brachiocephalic vein	
7	Submandibular gland	19	**Superior mediastinal lymph nodes**	
8	**Submental lymph nodes**	20	Retroauricular lymph nodes	
9	Superior thyroid artery	21	**Submandibular nodes**	
10	Thyroid cartilage	22	**Superficial cervical lymph nodes**	
11	Omohyoid muscle	23	**Jugulodigastric lymph nodes** and **jugular trunk**	
12	Sternohyoid muscle			

24	**Internal jugular vein**
25	External jugular vein
26	**Jugulo-omohyoid lymph nodes**
27	Brachial plexus
28	Cephalic vein
29	Subclavian trunk
30	**Infraclavicular lymph nodes**
31	Subclavian vein
32	Lung
33	Internal thoracic artery and vein

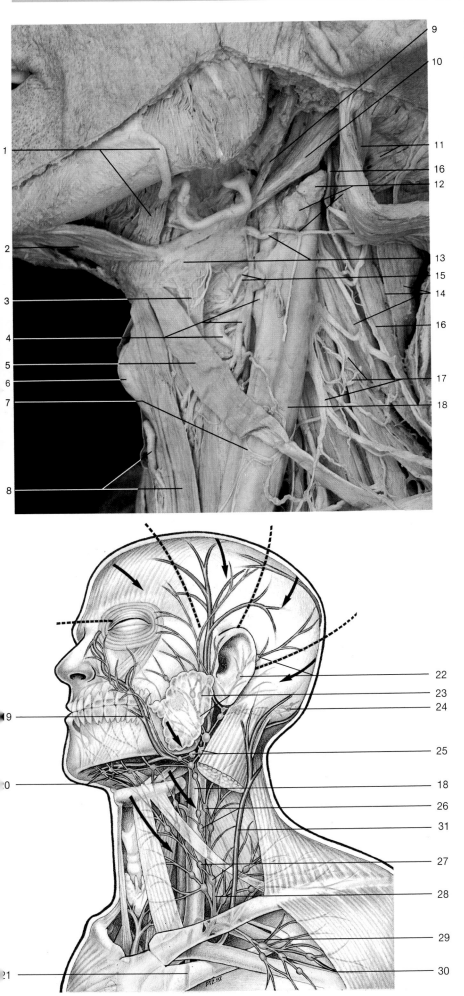

Carotid triangle, left side
(lateral aspect). Sternocleidomastoid
muscle reflected.

1   Mylohyoid muscle and facial artery
2   Anterior belly of digastric muscle
3   Thyrohyoid
4   **External carotid artery,**
    superior thyroid artery and vein
5   Omohyoid muscle
6   Thyroid cartilage
7   **Ansa cervicalis**
8   Sternohyoid muscle and superior
    thyroid artery
9   Stylohyoid muscle
10 Posterior belly of digastric muscle
11 Sternocleidomastoid muscle (reflected)
12 **Superior cervical lymph nodes** and
    sternocleidomastoid artery
13 Hyoid bone and hypoglossal nerve
    (n. XII)
14 Splenius capitis and levator
    scapulae muscles
15 Superior laryngeal artery and
    internal branch of superior
    laryngeal nerve
16 **Accessory nerve**
17 Cervical plexus
18 **Internal jugular vein**
19 Facial vein
20 Submental nodes
21 **Thoracic duct**
22 Retroauricular nodes
23 Parotid nodes
24 Occipital nodes
25 **Submandibular nodes**
26 Jugulodigastric nodes } **deep cervical
27 Jugulo-omohyoid nodes } nodes**
28 Jugular trunk
29 Subclavian trunk
30 Infraclavicular nodes
31 External jugular vein

**Lymph nodes and veins of head and
neck.** Dotted lines = border
between irrigation areas;
arrows: direction of lymph flow.

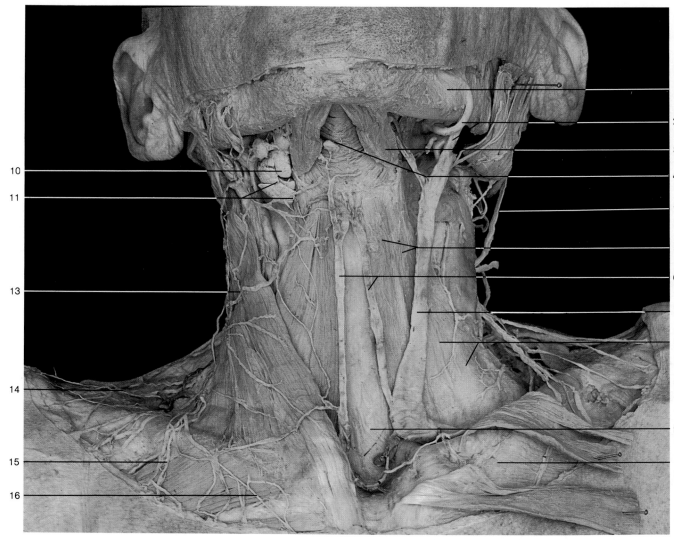

Neck (anterior aspect).
The superficial fascia has been removed.

Cross section of the neck at the level of the thyroid gland.
Notice the position of the three laminae of cervical fascia (23, 24, 25).

1 Mandible
2 **Facial artery and vein**

3 Anterior belly of digastric muscle
4 Mylohyoid muscle
5 Infrahyoid muscles (sternohyoid, sternothyroid and omohyoid)
6 **Anterior jugular veins**
7 **External jugular vein**
8 Sternocleidomastoid muscle
9 **Thyroid gland**
10 **Submandibular gland**
11 Cervical branch of facial nerve
12 Great auricular nerve ⎫ Cutaneous
13 Transverse cervical nerves ⎪ branches
14 Lateral supraclavicular nerves ⎬ of cervical
15 Middle supraclavicular nerves ⎪ plexus
16 Medial supraclavicular nerves ⎭
17 Clavicle
18 Platysma muscle
19 Prevertebral lamina of cervical fascia, covering longus colli muscle
20 Vertebral artery and vein
21 Scalenus muscles
22 Trapezius muscle
23 **Superficial lamina of cervical fascia**
24 **Pretracheal lamina of cervical fascia**
25 **Prevertebral lamina of cervical fascia** with sympathetic trunk
26 **Carotid sheath** with common carotid artery, internal jugular vein and vagus nerve
27 Cervical part of sympathetic trunk
28 Carotid sheath

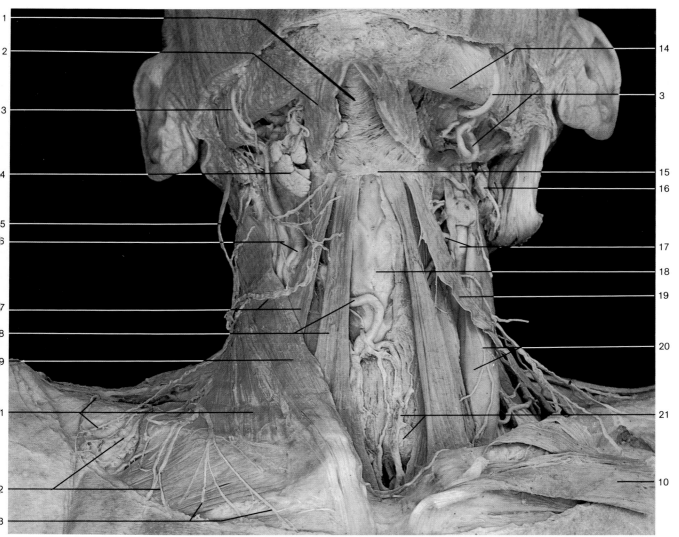

Anterior triangle (anterior aspect). The pretracheal lamina of cervical fascia and left sternocleidomastoid muscle have been removed.

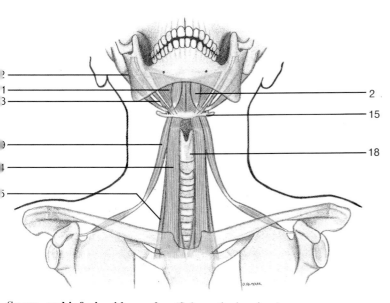

Supra- and infrahyoid muscles. (Schematic drawing.)

1 Mylohyoid muscle
2 Anterior belly of digastric muscle
3 **Facial artery**
4 **Submandibular gland**
5 Great auricular nerve
6 Internal jugular vein and common carotid artery
7 Transverse cervical nerve and omohyoid muscle
8 **Sternohyoid muscle** and **superior thyroid artery**
9 Sternocleidomastoid muscle (sternal head)
10 Left sternocleidomastoid muscle (reflected)
11 Sternocleidomastoid muscle (clavicular head)
   and lateral supraclavicular nerves
12 Middle **supraclavicular nerves**
13 Medial supraclavicular nerves
14 Mandible
15 **Hyoid bone**
16 Superficial cervical lymph nodes
17 Left superior thyroid artery and external carotid
   artery
18 **Thyroid cartilage**
19 **Omohyoid muscle** (superior belly)
20 **Internal jugular vein** and branches of ansa
   cervicalis
21 Thyroid gland and unpaired inferior thyroid vein
22 Posterior belly of digastric muscle
23 **Stylohyoid muscle**
24 **Sternohyoid muscle**
25 **Sternothyroid muscle**

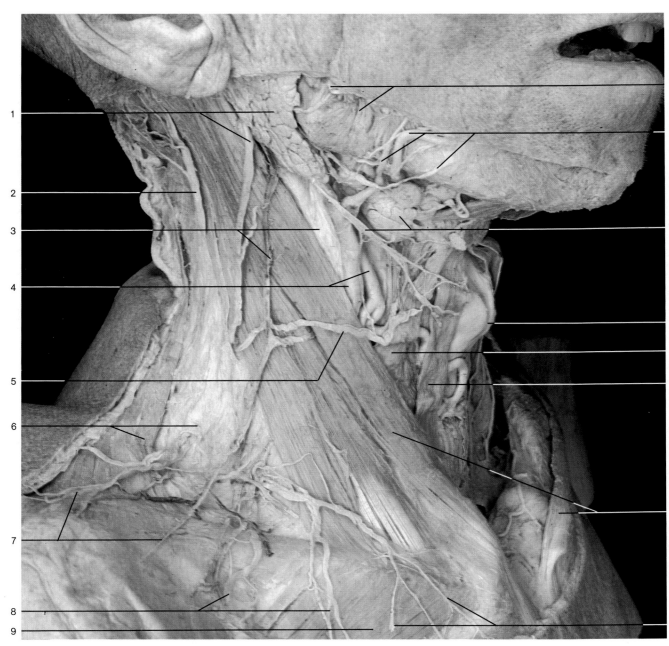

Posterior and carotid triangles (lateral aspect). Superficial dissection.

1 **Parotid gland** and **great auricular nerve**
2 **Lesser occipital nerve**
3 Internal and external jugular veins
4 Retromandibular vein and external carotid artery
5 **Transverse cervical nerve** with communicating branch to cervical branch of facial nerve
6 Trapezius muscle and superficial lamina of cervical fascia
7 Lateral supraclavicular nerves
8 Middle **supraclavicular nerves**
9 Pectoralis major muscle
10 Buccal branch of facial nerve and masseter

11 **Facial artery and vein** and mandibular branch of facial nerve
12 Cervical branch of facial nerve and submandibular gland
13 Thyroid cartilage
14 Omohyoid muscle
15 Sternohyoid muscle
16 Sternocleidomastoid muscle
17 Medial supraclavicular nerves
18 Mandibular branch of facial nerve
19 Cervical branch of facial nerve with communicating branch to transverse cervical nerve

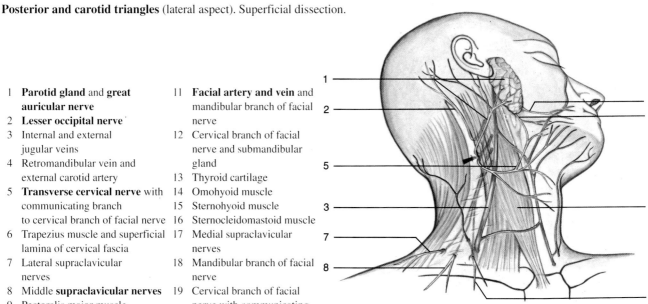

Cutaneous branches of cervical plexus. Erb's point is indicated by an arrowhead. (Schematic diagram.)

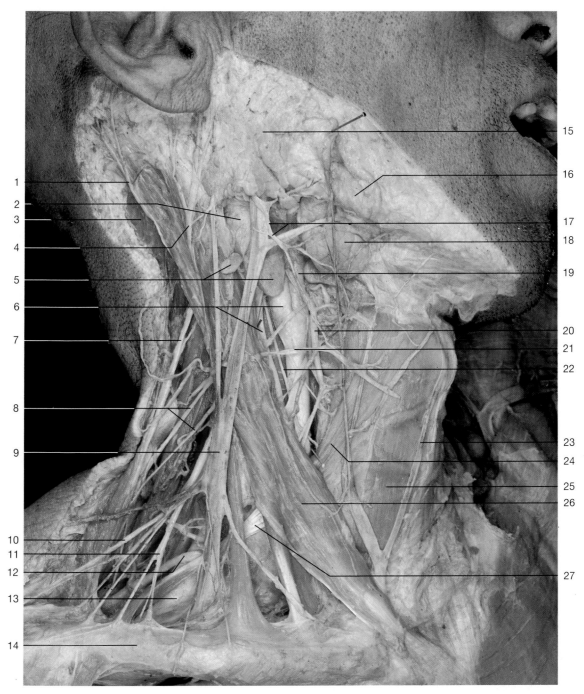

Posterior and carotid triangles (lateral aspect). Superficial dissection. The superficial lamina of cervical fascia has been removed to display the cutaneous branches of the cervical plexus and subcutaneous veins.

1	**Lesser occipital nerve**	15	Parotid gland
2	**Internal jugular vein**	16	Mandible
3	Splenius capitis muscle	17	Cervical branch of facial nerve
4	**Great auricular nerve**	18	Submandibular gland
5	Submandibular nodes	19	External carotid artery
6	Internal carotid artery and vagus nerve	20	Superior thyroid artery
7	**Accessory nerve**	21	Transverse cervical nerve
8	Muscular branches of cervical plexus	22	Superior root of ansa cervicalis
9	External jugular vein	23	Anterior jugular vein
10	**Posterior supraclavicular nerves**	24	Omohyoid muscle
11	**Middle supraclavicular nerves**	25	Sternohyoid muscle
12	Suprascapular artery	26	Sternocleidomastoid muscle
13	Pretracheal lamina of fascia of neck	27	Intermediate tendon of omohyoid muscle
14	Clavicle		

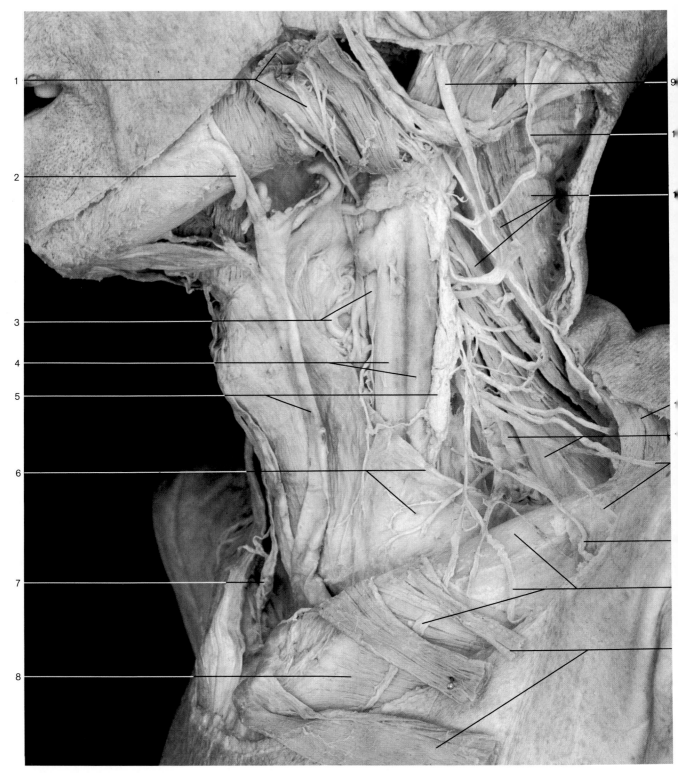

Neck, superficial dissection (lateral aspect). Sternocleidomastoid muscle has been cut and reflected to display the pretracheal lamina of the cervical fascia.

1 Sternocleidomastoid muscle (reflected) and branch of accessory nerve
2 Facial artery
3 External carotid artery and superior thyroid artery
4 **Internal jugular vein**
5 **Deep cervical lymph nodes** and external jugular vein
6 Omohyoid muscle and **pretracheal lamina of cervical fascia**
7 Anterior jugular vein
8 Pectoralis major muscle
9 **Great auricular nerve**

10 **Lesser occipital nerve**
11 Splenius capitis and levator scapulae muscles
12 Trapezius muscle
13 Scalenus medius muscle and brachial plexus
14 Posterior **supraclavicular nerves**
15 Middle supraclavicular nerve
16 Clavicle and anterior supraclavicular nerves
17 Sternocleidomastoid muscle
     (reflected)

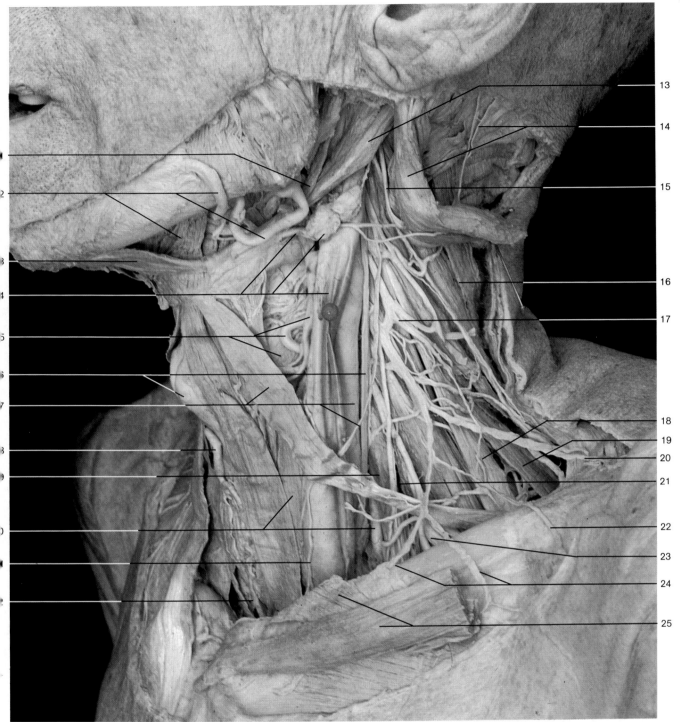

Neck, deep dissection (lateral aspect). The internal jugular vein has been reflected to expose the carotid artery and vagus nerve.

1 Stylohyoid muscle	13 Posterior belly of digastric muscle
2 Facial artery and mylohyoid muscle	14 Sternocleidomastoid muscle and lesser occipital nerve
3 Anterior belly of digastric muscle	15 **Accessory nerve**
4 **Internal jugular vein,** hypoglossal nerve, and superficial cervical lymph nodes	16 Splenius capitis muscle
5 **Superior thyroid artery and vein** and inferior pharyngeal constrictor muscle	17 **Cervical plexus**
6 Thyroid cartilage and vagus nerve	18 Scalenus posterior muscle
7 **Ansa cervicalis,** omohyoid muscle, and common carotid artery	19 Levator scapulae muscle
8 Right superior thyroid artery	20 Posterior **supraclavicular nerves**
9 Scalenus anterior muscle	21 Phrenic nerve
10 Sternothyroid muscle and inferior thyroid artery	22 Middle supraclavicular nerve
11 Muscular branches of ansa cervicalis to the infrahyoid muscles	23 **Brachial plexus**
12 Inferior thyroid vein	24 Anterior supraclavicular nerves
	25 Sternocleidomastoid muscle

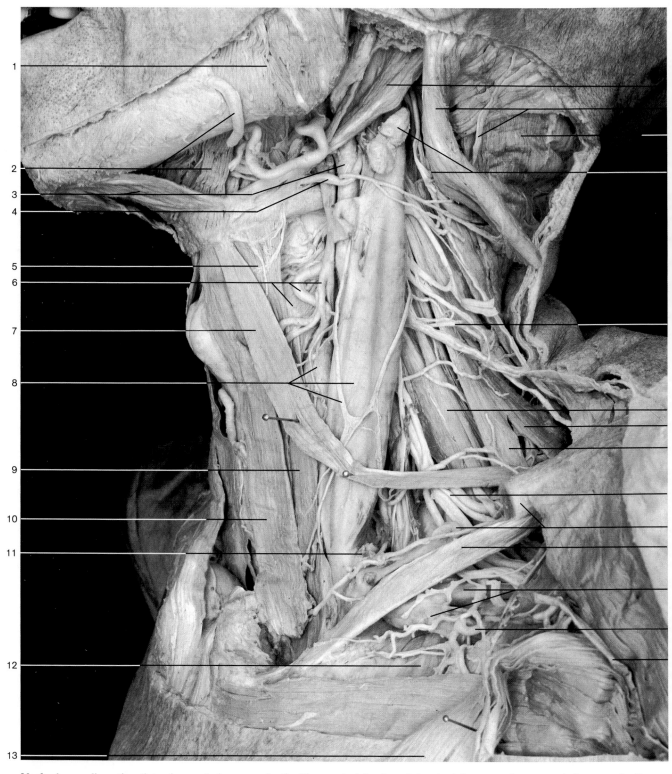

Neck, deeper dissection (lateral aspect). **Ansa cervicalis.** The cervical fascia and the clavicle are partly removed. Ansa cervicalis and infrahyoid muscles are displayed.

1 Masseter muscle	9 Sternothyroid muscle	18 **Cervical plexus**
2 Mylohyoid muscle and facial artery	10 Sternohyoid muscle	19 Scalenus medius muscle
3 **External carotid artery** and anterior belly of digastric muscle	11 **Thoracic duct**	20 Levator scapulae muscle
	12 Pectoralis minor muscle	21 Scalenus posterior muscle
4 **Hypoglossal nerve**	13 Pectoralis major muscle	22 Brachial plexus
5 Thyrohyoid muscle	14 Posterior belly of digastric muscle	23 Transverse cervical artery and clavicle
6 Superior thyroid artery and vein and inferior pharyngeal constrictor muscle	15 Sternocleidomastoid muscle and lesser occipital nerve	
		24 Subclavius muscle
7 Omohyoid muscle (superior belly)	16 Splenius capitis muscle	25 **Subclavian artery and vein**
8 **Ansa cervicalis,** thyroid gland and **internal jugular vein**	17 Superficial cervical lymph nodes and accessory nerve	26 Thoracoacromial artery
		27 Cephalic vein

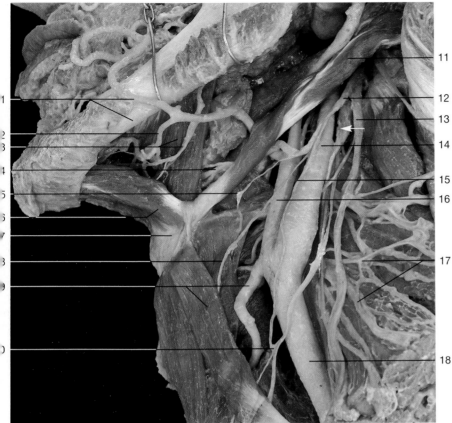

1 **Facial artery** and mandible
2 Submental artery
3 Mylohyoid muscle and nerve
4 **Hypoglossal nerve**
   (lingual branches)
5 Thyrohyoid branch of hypoglossal
   nerve (n. XII)
6 Anterior belly of digastric muscle
7 Hyoid bone
8 Omohyoid branch of hypoglossal
   nerve (n. XII)
9 Omohyoid muscle and superior
   thyroid artery
10 **Ansa cervicalis**
11 Posterior belly of digastric muscle
12 **Hypoglossal nerve** (n. XII)
13 **Vagus nerve** (n. X)
14 Internal carotid artery
15 Superior root of ansa cervicalis
16 **External carotid artery**
17 Cervical plexus
18 Common carotid artery

Neck, submandibular region (lateral aspect). **Hypoglossal nerve** (n. XII). Mandible slightly elevated. Arrow = superior cervical ganglion.

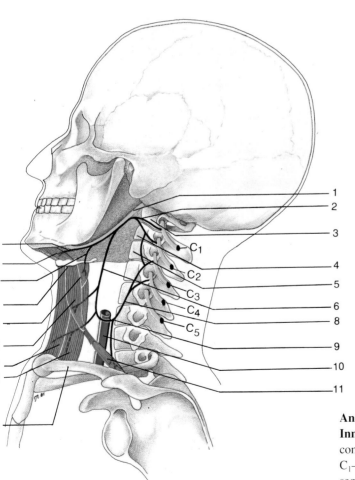

1 **Hypoglossal nerve** (n. XII)
2 Communication from the ventral ramus
   of the first cervical spinal nerve
3 Atlas
4 Axis
5 Third cervical vertebra
6 Superior root of ansa cervicalis
7 Thyrohyoid branch of hypoglossal nerve
8 Inferior root of ansa cervicalis
9 **Ansa cervicalis**
10 Internal jugular vein
11 Inferior belly of omohyoid muscle
12 Geniohyoid branch of hypoglossal nerve
13 Geniohyoid muscle
14 Hyoid bone
15 Thyrohyoid muscle
16 Superior belly of omohyoid muscle
17 Sternohyoid muscle
18 Sternothyroid muscle
19 Clavicle

Ansa cervicalis.

Innervation of infrahyoid muscles. Cervical plexus and its communication with the hypoglossal nerve.
C_1–C_4 = ventral rami of cervical spinal nerves of the first four segments.

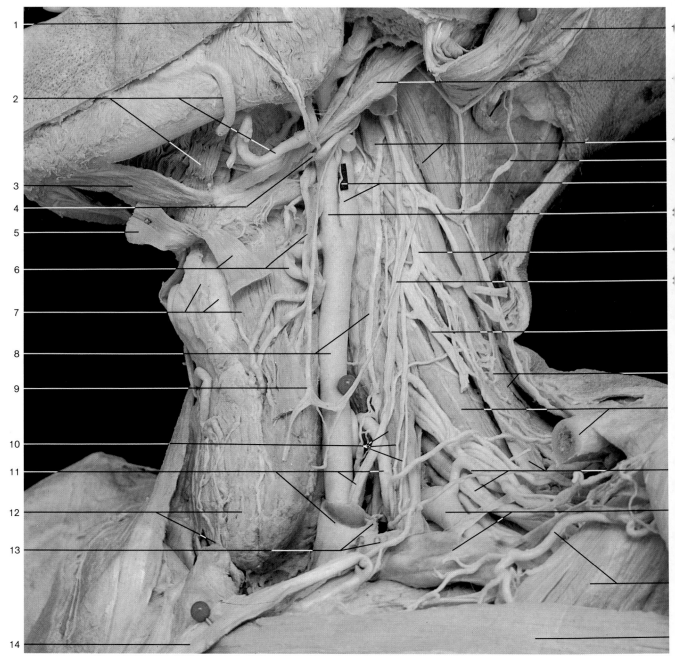

Neck, deep dissection (lateral aspect). Clavicle partly removed to show the slit between the scalenus muscles. Internal jugular vein removed.

1	Masseter muscle
2	Mylohyoid muscle and **facial artery**
3	Anterior belly of digastric muscle
4	**Hypoglossal nerve**
5	Sternohyoid muscle
6	Omohyoid muscle, superior thyroid artery and vein
7	Sternothyroid muscle, thyroid cartilage, and pyramidal lobe of thyroid gland
8	Common carotid artery and sympathetic trunk
9	**Ansa cervicalis**
10	**Phrenic nerve,** ascending cervical artery and anterior scalenus muscle
11	Inferior thyroid artery, vagus nerve and internal jugular vein (cut)
12	**Thyroid gland** and unpaired inferior thyroid venous plexus
13	Thoracic duct and left subclavian trunk
14	Subclavius muscle (reflected)
15	Sternocleidomastoid muscle (reflected)
16	Posterior belly of digastric muscle
17	**Superior cervical ganglion** and splenius muscle
18	**Lesser occipital nerve**
19	Internal carotid artery and branch of the glossopharyngeal nerve to the carotid body
20	**External carotid artery**
21	**Cervical plexus** and **accessory nerve**
22	Inferior root of ansa cervicalis
23	Supraclavicular nerve
24	Levator scapulae muscle
25	Scalenus medius muscle and clavicle
26	Transverse cervical artery, brachial plexus, and scalenus posterior muscle
27	**Subclavian artery and vein**
28	Thoracoacromial artery and pectoralis minor muscle
29	Pectoralis major muscle

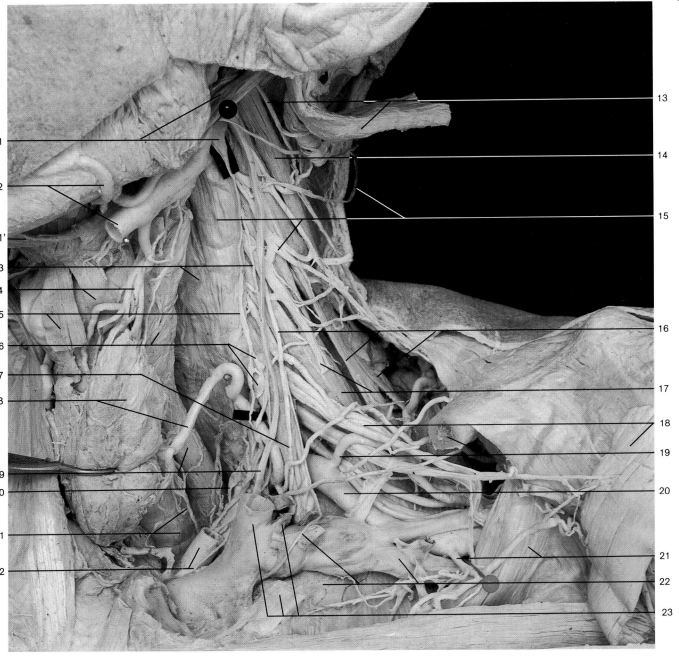

Neck, deepest dissection (anterolateral aspect). Thyroid gland reflected to expose the esophagus and the recurrent laryngeal nerve.

1 **Superior cervical ganglion** of sympathetic trunk and posterior belly of digastric muscle
1' Anterior belly of digastric muscle
2 **Facial artery** and common carotid artery (reflected anteriorly)
3 Ascending cervical artery and longus colli muscle
4 Omohyoid muscle and superior thyroid artery
5 **Sympathetic trunk** and sternohyoid muscle
6 Middle cervical ganglion and inferior pharyngeal constrictor muscle
7 Scalenus anterior muscle and phrenic nerve
8 **Thyroid gland** and **inferior thyroid artery**
9 Vagus nerve and esophagus
10 **Stellate ganglion**
11 **Recurrent laryngeal nerve** and trachea

12 Common carotid artery and cervical cardiac branch of vagus nerve
13 Sternocleidomastoid muscle and accessory nerve
14 Splenius capitis muscle
15 Lesser occipital nerve, longus capitis muscle and cervical plexus
16 **Phrenic nerve,** scalenus posterior muscle and levator scapulae muscle
17 Supraclavicular nerves and scalenus medius muscle
18 Brachial plexus and pectoralis major muscle (clavicular head)
19 Transverse cervical artery and clavicle
20 **Subclavian artery**
21 **Thoracoacromial artery** and pectoralis minor muscle
22 First rib, accessory phrenic nerve and subclavian vein
23 Internal jugular vein, thoracic duct and subclavius muscle

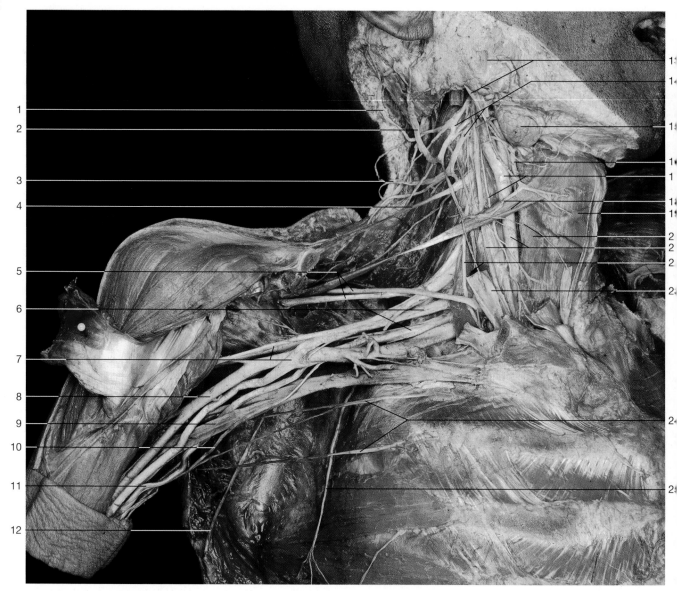

Neck and arm, deepest dissection (anterior-lateral aspect). Cervical and brachial plexus and their relation to the blood vessels are shown. Note the location and content of scalene triangle. Sternocleidomastoid muscle and clavicle have been removed; the internal jugular vein was divided to display the roots of cervical and brachial plexus.

1 Lesser occipital nerve
2 Great auricular nerve
3 Cutaneous branches of cervical plexus
4 Supraclavicular nerve
5 Suprascapular nerve and artery
6 **Brachial plexus**
7 **Median nerve** (with two roots) and musculocutaneous nerve
8 Axillary artery
9 Axillary vein
10 Medial brachial cutaneous nerve
11 **Ulnar nerve**
12 Thoracodorsal nerve
13 Parotid gland and facial nerve (cervical branch)
14 **Cervical plexus**
15 Submandibular gland
16 Superior thyroid artery

17 Common carotid artery dividing in internal and external carotid artery and superior root of ansa cervicalis
18 Omohyoid muscle and cervical branch of facial nerve joining the transverse cervical nerve (C_2, C_3)
19 Sternohyoid muscle
20 Transverse cervical nerve and sternothyroid muscle
21 **Common carotid artery** and **vagus nerve**
22 **Phrenic nerve** and scalenus anterior muscle
23 Internal jugular vein
24 Intercostobrachial nerves
25 Long thoracic nerve

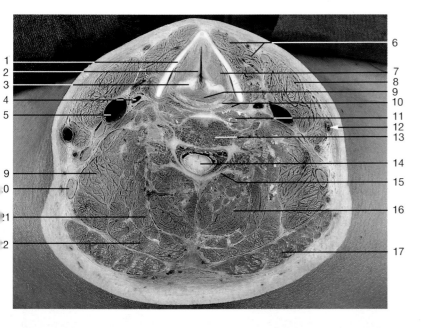

◁ **Horizontal section through the neck** at the level of the fissure of glottis, viewed from above.

1 **Thyroid cartilage**
2 **Vocal fold** and **glottis** (rima glottidis)
3 Arytenoid cartilage
4 Common carotid artery
5 **Internal jugular vein**
6 Infrahyoid muscles
7 Lateral thyroarytenoid muscle
8 Sternocleidomastoid muscle
9 Transverse arytenoid muscle
10 Laryngopharynx and inferior constrictor muscle of pharynx
11 Longus colli muscle
12 External jugular vein
13 Body of cervical vertebra (C_5)
14 **Spinal cord**
15 Vertebra arch
16 Deep muscles of neck (semispinalis cervicis muscle)
17 Trapezius muscle
18 Rima glottidis
19 Levator scapulae muscle
20 Lymph node
21 Semispinalis capitis muscle
22 Splenius capitis muscle

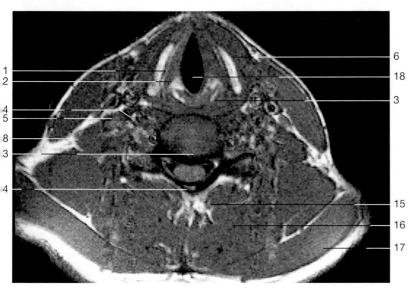

◁ **Section through the neck at the level of larynx.** (MRI scan.)

1 Hyoid bone
2 Thyroid cartilage
3 **Cervical plexus** (C_1–C_4)
4 **Phrenic nerve** (C_4)
5 Scalenus anterior muscle
6 **Brachial plexus** (C_5–T_1)
7 Scalenus medius and posterior muscles
8 Subclavian artery
9 Subclavian vein
10 Superior vena cava
11 Cricoid cartilage
12 Thyroid gland
13 **Internal jugular vein**
14 **Common carotid artery**
15 Inferior thyroid vein
16 Ascending aorta
17 Descending aorta
18 Second rib

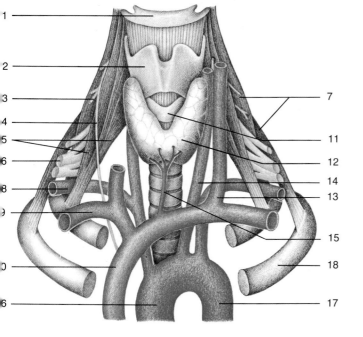

◁ **Scalene triangle, arrangements of blood vessels, and brachial plexus at the lower part of the neck.** (Schematic diagram.)

Trunk

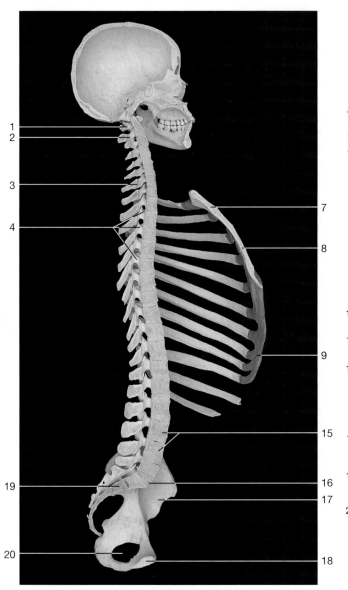

Median sagittal section through the vertebral column, head, and thorax of the adult.

Skeleton of the trunk, vertebral column, thorax, and pelvis (posterior aspect).

1	Atlas
2	Axis
3	Seventh cervical vertebra (vertebra prominens)
4	Vertebral canal
5	First rib
6	Clavicle
7	Manubrium sterni
8	Body of sternum
9	Costal arch
10	Acromion
11	Spine of scapula
12	Glenoid cavity (lateral angle of scapula)
13	Eleventh rib

14	Twelfth rib
15	Lumbar vertebrae
16	Sacral promontory
17	Hip bone
18	Symphysis pubis
19	Sacrum
20	Obturator foramen
21	Acetabulum
22	Scapula with coracoid process
23	Posterior superior iliac spine
24	Posterior inferior iliac spine
25	Ischial spine
26	Ischial tuberosity

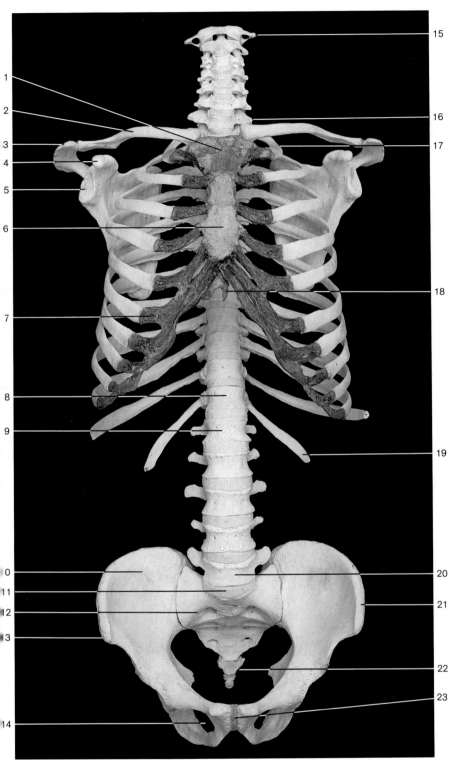

1   Manubrium sterni
2   **Clavicle**
3   Acromion
4   Coracoid process
5   Glenoid cavity
6   Body of **sternum**
7   Costal cartilage
8   Body of the twelfth **thoracic vertebra**
9   Body of the first **lumbar vertebra**
10 Hip bone
11 Sacral promontory
12 **Sacrum**
13 Anterior superior iliac spine
14 Obturator foramen
15 Atlas
16 Seventh **cervical vertebra**
17 First rib
18 Xiphoid process
19 Twelfth rib
20 Body of the fifth lumbar vertebra
21 Iliac crest
22 **Coccyx**
23 Symphysis pubis

Skeleton of the trunk, vertebral column, pelvis, thorax, and shoulder girdle (anterior aspect).

The trunk is divided into segments best visible in the thoracic region, where each segment consists of a pair of ribs connected anteriorly by the sternum and posteriorly by a thoracic vertebra. In the lumbar part of the vertebral column, only vestiges of ribs are present which form what appear to be the transverse processes. In cervical vertebrae, remnants of ribs are part of the transverse processes. Each segment also comprises muscles (e.g., intercostal muscles), nerves, and vessels. However, in the cervical and lumbar region the muscular segments fuse with each other, forming large muscle plates, for example, the oblique muscles of the abdomen, while vessels and nerves still retain their segmental pattern.

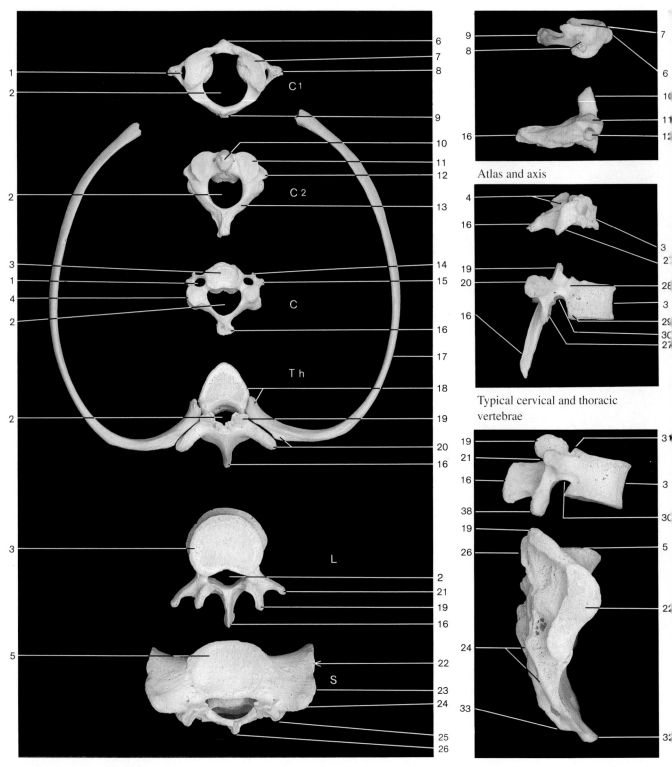

Representative vertebrae from each region of the vertebral column
(superior aspect). From top to bottom: atlas (C₁), axis (C₂), cervical vertebra (C),
thoracic vertebra (Th), lumbar vertebra (L), and sacrum (S).

Atlas and axis

Typical cervical and thoracic
vertebrae

Typical lumbar vertebra and sacrum

**Representative vertebrae from
each region of the vertebral column**
(lateral aspect, ventral surface on the
right).

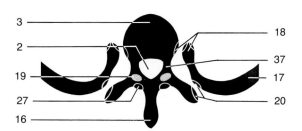

General organization of ribs and vertebrae. (Schematic diagram.)

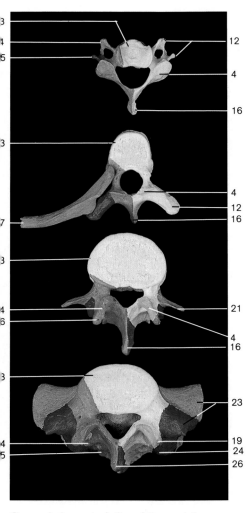

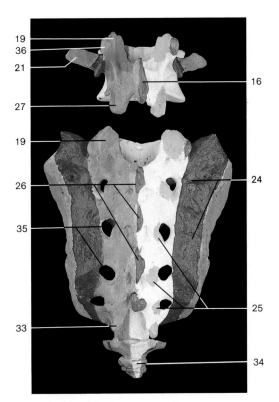

General characteristics of the vertebrae.
Typical cervical, thoracic, lumbar vertebrae
and sacrum.

**General characteristics of lumbar
vertebrae and sacrum** (posterior aspect).

Green = Ribs or homologous processes
Red = Muscular processes (transverse and spinous processes)
Orange = Laminae and articular processes
Yellow = Articular facets

1 Foramen transversarium	20 Transverse process and tubercle of rib articulating with each other (costotransverse joint)
2 Vertebral foramen	21 Transverse process
3 Body of vertebra	22 Auricular surface
4 Superior articular facet	23 Lateral part of sacrum
5 Base of sacrum	24 Lateral sacral crest
6 Anterior tubercle of atlas	25 Intermediate sacral crest
7 Superior articular facet of atlas	26 Median sacral crest
8 Transverse process	27 Inferior articular facet
9 Posterior tubercle of atlas	28 Superior demifacet for head of rib
10 Dens of axis	29 Inferior demifacet for head of rib
11 Superior articular surface	30 Inferior vertebral notch
12 Transverse process	31 Superior vertebral notch
13 Arch of vertebra	32 Apex of the sacrum
14 Anterior tubercle of transverse process	33 Sacral cornu
15 Posterior tubercle of transverse process	34 Coccyx
16 Spinous process	35 Dorsal sacral foramina
17 Shaft of rib	36 Mamillary process
18 Body of vertebra and head of rib articulating with each other (costovertebral joint)	37 Pedicle
19 Superior articular process	38 Inferior articular process

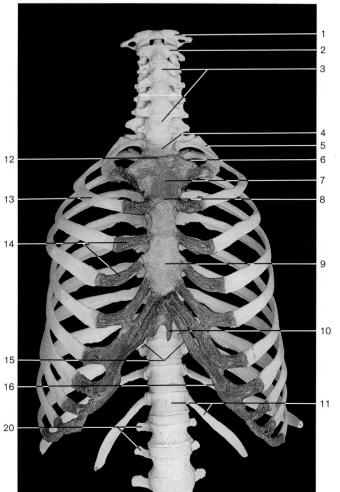

Skeleton of the thorax (anterior aspect).

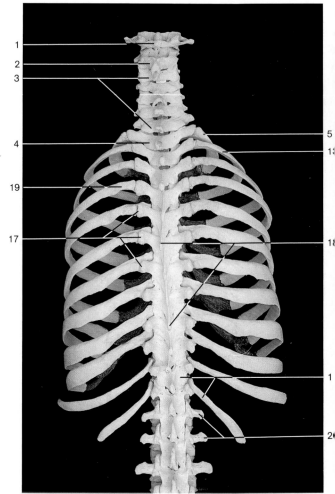

Skeleton of the thorax (posterior aspect).

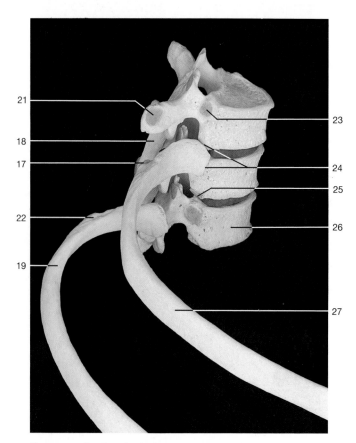

Costovertebral articulation (right lateral aspect).

1   Atlas
2   Axis
3   **Cervical vertebrae**
4   First thoracic vertebra
5   First rib
6   Facet for clavicle and clavicular notch
7   **Manubrium sterni**
8   Sternal angle
9   Body of sternum
10 Xiphoid process
11 Twelfth thoracic vertebra and rib
12 Jugular notch
13 Second rib
14 **Costal cartilages**
15 Infrasternal angle
16 **Costal arch**
17 Costotransverse joints between the transverse processes
    of thoracic vertebra and the tubercles of the ribs
18 Spinous processes
19 Costal angle
20 Transverse processes of lumbar vertebrae
21 Facet for articulation with rib
22 Tubercle of rib
23 Superior facet for articulation with head of rib
24 Articulation of head of rib with two vertebrae
25 Inferior facet for articulation with head of rib
26 Body of thoracic vertebra
27 Body or shaft of rib

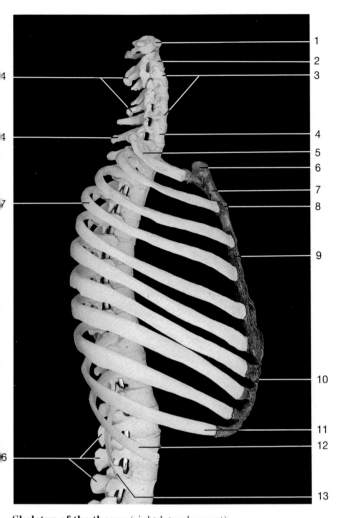

Skeleton of the thorax (right lateral aspect).

1   Atlas
2   Axis
3   **Cervical vertebrae**
4   Seventh cervical vertebra (vertebra prominens)
5   First rib
6   Facet for clavicle
7   **Manubrium sterni**
8   Sternal angle
9   Body of sternum
10 Costal arch
11 Tenth rib
12 Eleventh rib
13 Twelfth rib
14 Spinous processes of cervical vertebrae
15 Spinous processes of thoracic vertebrae
16 Spinous processes of lumbar vertebrae
17 Costal angle
18 Intervertebral foramina
19 Intervertebral discs
20 **Cervical curvature**
21 **Thoracic curvature**
22 **Lumbar curvature**
23 Sacrum
24 Coccyx

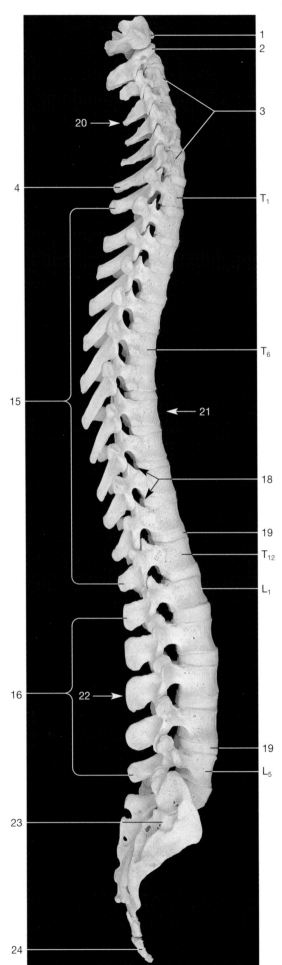

Vertebral column (right lateral aspect).

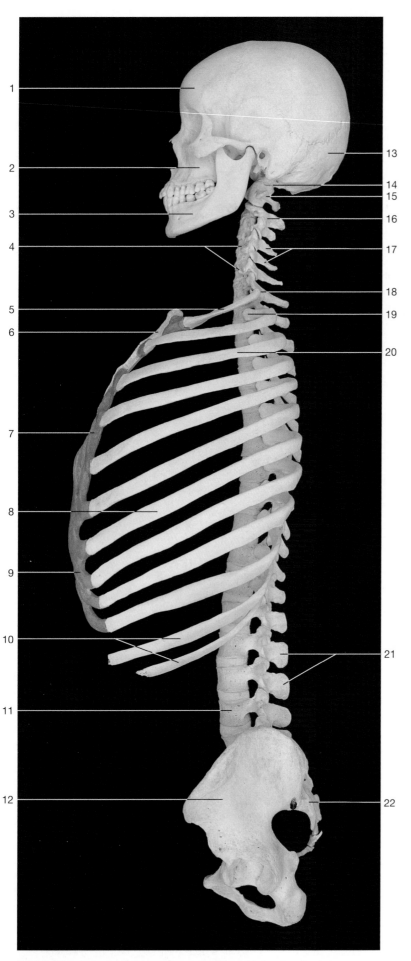

Vertebral column and thorax in connection with head and pelvis (lateral aspect).

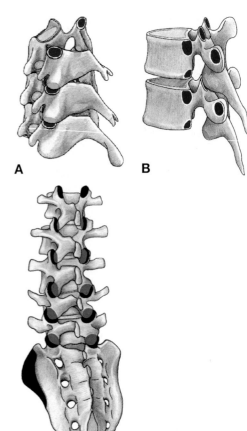

A   B

C

Articulations of the cervical (A), thoracic (B) and lumbar (C) vertebrae (lateral or oblique posterior aspect). Blue = articular facets.

 1 Frontal bone
 2 Maxilla
 3 Mandible
 4 Bodies of cervical vertebrae
 5 **First rib**
 6 Manubrium of sternum
 7 **Sternum** (corpus sterni)
 8 Seventh rib (last of the true ribs)
 9 Costal arch (arcus costalis)
10 **Floating ribs** (costae fluctuantes)
11 Body of fourth lumbar vertebra
12 **Pelvis**
13 Occipital bone
14 **Atlanto-occipital joint**
15 Atlas
16 Axis
17 Spinous processes of cervical vertebrae (C$_4$, C$_5$)
18 Costotransverse joint of first rib
19 Head of second rib
20 Third rib
21 Spinous processes of lumbar vertebrae (L$_2$, L$_3$)
22 Sacrum

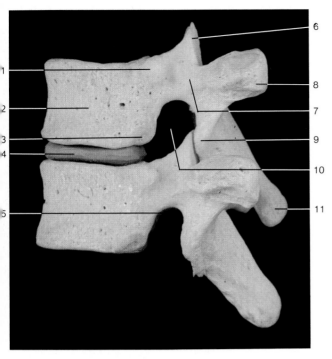

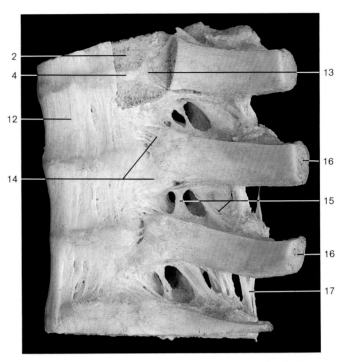

Two **thoracic vertebrae** (left lateral aspect).

Ligaments of thoracic vertebrae and costovertebral joints
(left anterolateral aspect). In the upper joint, most of the
radiate ligament and the anterior part of the head of the rib
have been removed to expose the two joint cavities and the
interposed intra articular ligament.

1 Superior demifacet for head of rib	9 Inferior articular process
2 Body of vertebra	10 Intervertebral foramen
3 Inferior demifacet for head of rib	11 Spinous process
4 Intervertebral disc	12 Anterior longitudinal ligament
5 Inferior vertebral notch	13 Intra articular ligament
6 Superior articular facet and superior articular process	14 Radiate ligament
7 Pedicle	15 Superior costotransverse ligament
8 Transverse process and facet for tubercle of rib	16 Body of rib
	17 Intertransverse ligament

Costovertebral joints. Two thoracic vertebrae with an
articulating rib (separated). Axis of movement indicated by
dotted line. Blue = articular facets. (Schematic diagram.)

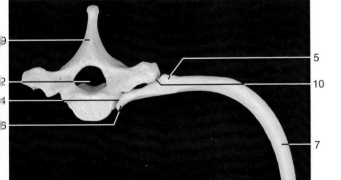

Location of costovertebral joints (superior aspect).

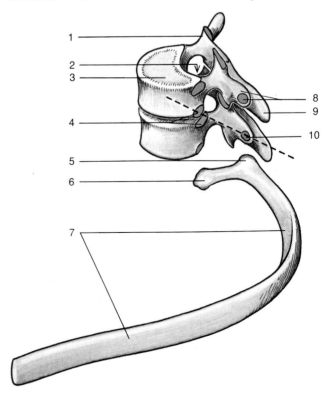

1 Superior articular process	7 Shaft or body of rib
2 Vertebral canal	8 Transverse process with articular facet
3 Body of thoracic vertebra	9 Spinous process
4 Costovertebral joint (articular facets)	10 Costotransverse joint (articular facets)
5 Tubercle of rib	
6 Head of rib	

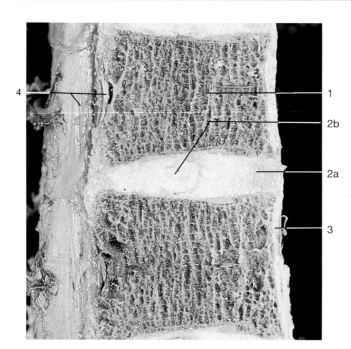

Median-sagittal section of the bodies of the vertebrae, showing the **intervertebral discs,** each of which consists of an outer laminated portion and an inner core.

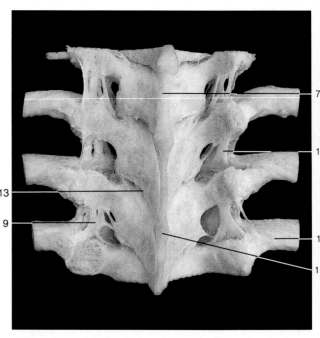

Ligaments of the vertebral column (dorsal aspect).

1 Body of vertebra	8 Interspinous ligament
2 **Intervertebral disc**	9 **Intertransverse ligament**
a Outer portion (anulus fibrosus)	10 Superior costotransverse ligament
b Inner core (**nucleus pulposus**)	11 Transverse process of thoracic
3 Anterior longitudinal ligament	vertebra
4 Posterior longitudinal ligament and spinal dura mater	12 Rib
5 Transverse process of lumbar vertebra	13 **Ligamentum flavum**
6 Sacrum	14 Spinous process
7 **Supraspinous ligament**	15 Intervertebral foramen

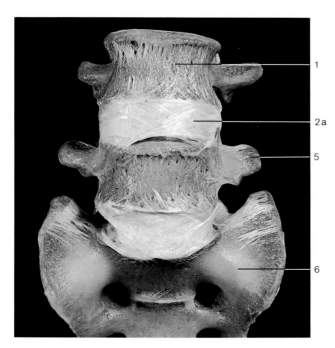

The two caudal lumbar vertebrae and the sacrum with their intervertebral discs (anterior aspect). Anterior longitudinal ligament removed.

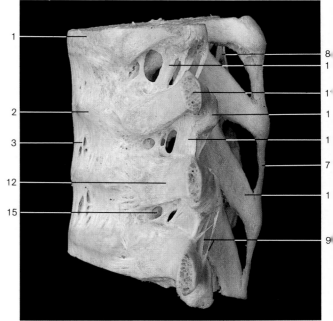

Ligaments of the vertebral column, thoracic part (left lateral aspect).

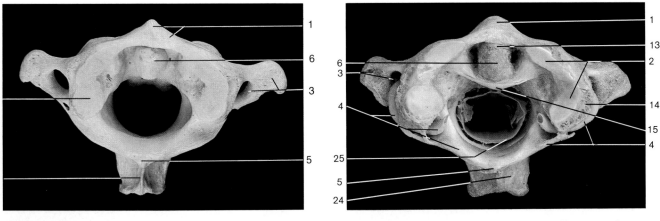

Atlas and axis (from above).

Median atlantoaxial joint and transverse ligament of atlas (from above). Dens of axis partly severed.

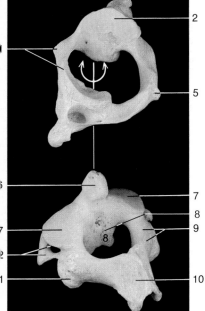

1 Anterior arch of **atlas** with anterior tubercle
2 Superior articular facet of atlas
3 **Foramen transversarium** and transverse process
4 Posterior arch of atlas and vertebral artery
5 Posterior tubercle of atlas
6 **Dens of axis**
7 Superior articular surface of axis
8 Body of axis
9 Pedicle and lamina of axis
10 Spinous process
11 Inferior articular process
12 Transverse process and foramen transversarium of axis
13 **Median atlantoaxial joint** (anterior part)

14 Articular capsule of **atlanto-occipital joint**
15 Transverse ligament of atlas
16 Occipital bone
17 **Atlanto-occipital joint**
18 **Lateral atlantoaxial joint**
19 Third cervical vertebra
20 Superior longitudinal band of cruciform ligament
21 Alar ligaments
22 Transverse ligament of atlas
23 Inferior longitudinal band of cruciform ligament
24 Spinous process of axis
25 Dura mater
26 Occipital bone

Atlas and axis. Left oblique posterolateral aspect, demonstrating the articulation of the dens of axis with atlas (cf. arrows).

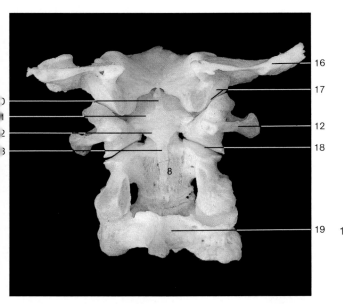

Atlanto-occipital and atlanto-axial joints (posterior aspect). Posterior part of occipital bone, posterior arch of atlas and axis have been removed to show the cruciform ligament.

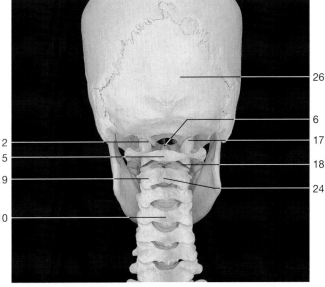

Head and cervical spine (posterior aspect). Bones of atlanto-occipital and atlantoaxial joints.

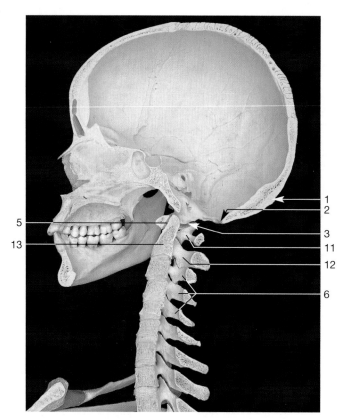

Cervical vertebral column in relation to the head
(midsagittal section) (medial aspect).

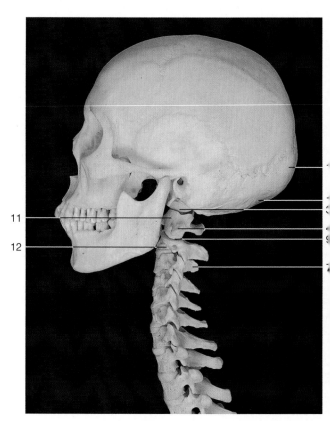

Atlas and axis in relation to the head (lateral aspect).

1 External occipital protuberance
2 Foramen magnum
3 Atlanto-occipital joint
4 Transverse process of atlas
5 Median atlantoaxial joint
6 Vertebral canal
7 Spinous process of third cervical vertebra
8 Occipital condyle

 9 Lateral atlantoaxial joint
10 Occipital bone
11 Atlas
12 Axis
13 Dens of axis
14 Hypoglossal canal
15 Spinous process of axis

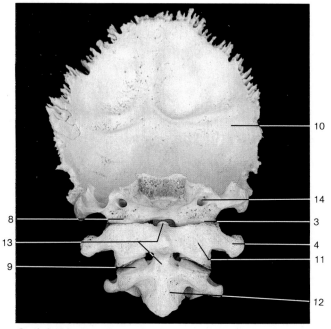

Occipital bone, atlas and axis (anterior aspect).

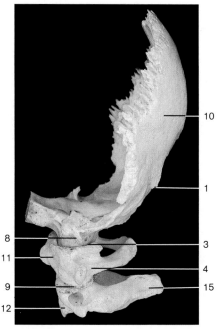

Occipital bone, atlas and axis (left lateral aspect).

1   Axillary vein
2   Intercostobrachial nerves
3   Subscapularis muscle and
    thoracodorsal nerve
4   Long thoracic nerve, lateral
    thoracic artery and vein
5   Latissimus dorsi muscle
6   **External intercostal** muscles
7   **Serratus anterior** muscle
8   Lateral cutaneous branches of
    intercostal nerves
9   External abdominal oblique muscle
10 Clavicle (divided)
11 Second rib (costochondral
    junction)
12 **Internal intercostal muscles**
13 External intercostal membrane
14 Position of xiphoid process
15 Costal arch or margin
16 Anterior layer of rectus sheath

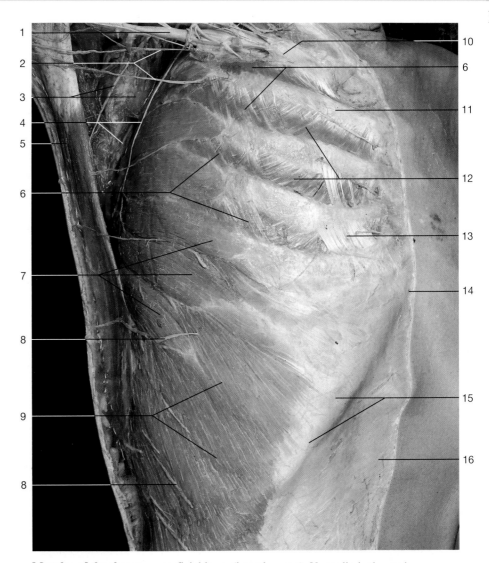

Muscles of the thorax, superficial layer (lateral aspect). Upper limb elevated.
Pectoralis major and minor muscles have been removed.

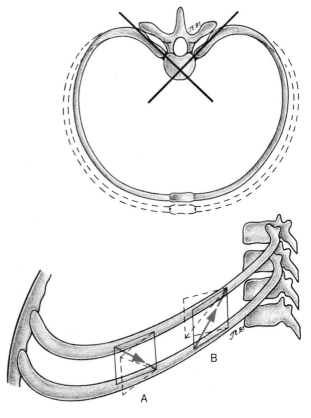

**Effect of intercostal muscles on the costovertebral and
costotransverse joints.** Axes of movement indicated by lines;
direction of movements indicated by red arrows.
A   Action of internal intercostal muscles (expiration)
B   Action of external intercostal muscles (inspiration)

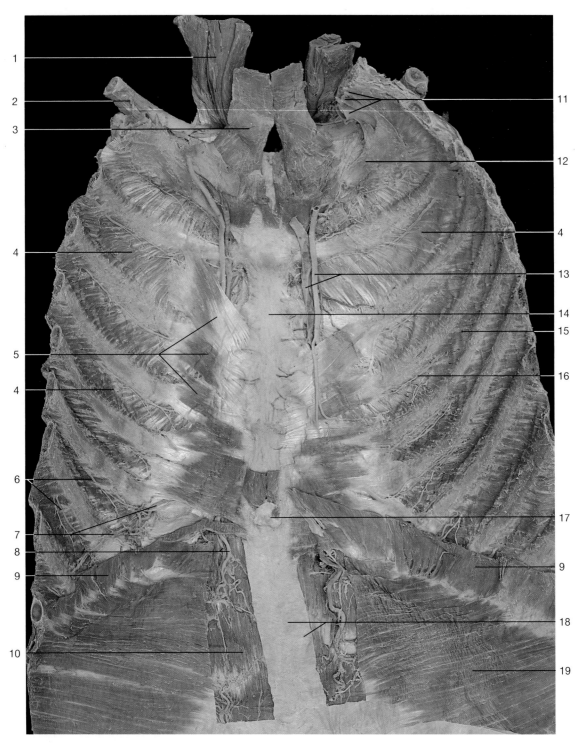

Anterior thoracic wall (posterior aspect). Diaphragm partly removed, posterior layer of rectus sheath fenestrated on both sides.

1	Sternocleidomastoid muscle (divided)	11	Subclavian artery and brachial plexus
2	Clavicle	12	First rib
3	Sternothyroid muscle	13	Internal thoracic artery and vein
4	**Internal intercostal muscle**	14	Sternum
5	**Transversus thoracic muscle**	15	Innermost intercostal muscle
6	Intercostal arteries and nerves	16	Intercostal artery and vein
7	Musculophrenic artery	17	Xiphoid process
8	Superior epigastric artery and vein	18	Linea alba and posterior layer of
9	Diaphragm (divided)		rectus sheath
10	Rectus abdominis muscle	19	**Transversus abdominis muscle**

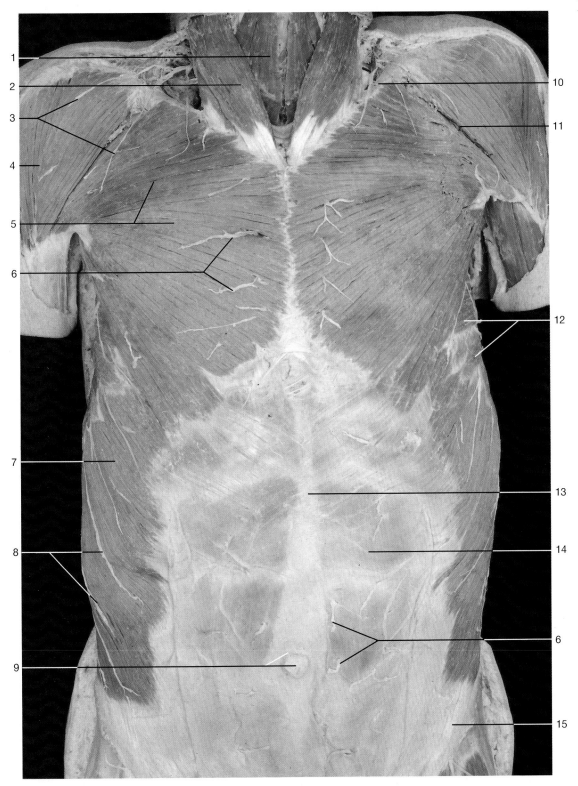

Superficial muscles of the anterior thoracic and abdominal wall. The fascia of pectoralis major muscle and the abdominal wall have been removed; the anterior layer of the sheath of the rectus abdominis muscle is displayed.

1 Sternohyoid muscle
2 Sternocleidomastoid muscle
3 Supraclavicular nerves (branches of cervical plexus)
4 Deltoid muscle
5 **Pectoralis major muscle**
6 **Anterior cutaneous branches of intercostal nerves**
7 External abdominal oblique muscle
8 **Lateral cutaneous branches of intercostal nerves**

9 Umbilicus and umbilical ring
10 Clavicle
11 Cephalic vein
12 Serratus anterior muscle
13 Linea alba
14 **Sheath of rectus abdominis** muscle (anterior layer)
15 Inguinal ligament

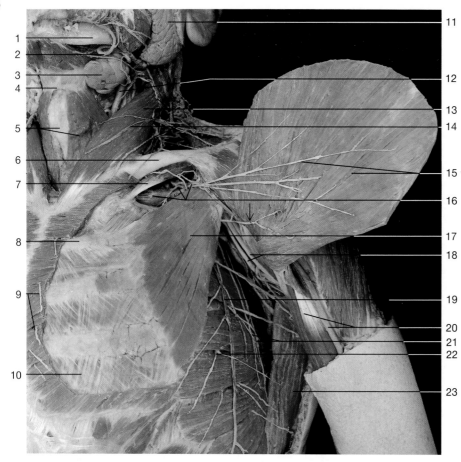

1 Mandible
2 Facial artery
3 Submandibular gland
4 Hyoid bone
5 Thyroid cartilage and
   sternohyoid muscle
6 Clavicle
7 Subclavius muscle
8 Second rib
9 Anterior cutaneous branches of
   intercostal nerves
10 External intercostal membrane
11 Parotid gland
12 External carotid artery
13 Sternocleidomastoid muscle and
   cutaneous branches of cervical plexus
14 Supraclavicular nerves
15 Pectoralis major muscle and lateral
   pectoral nerves
16 Thoracoacromial artery and
   subclavian vein
17 **Pectoralis minor muscle**
18 **Median and ulnar nerve**
19 Thoracoepigastric vein
20 Cephalic vein and long head of
   biceps brachii muscle
21 **Lateral thoracic artery and long
   thoracic nerve**
22 Lateral cutaneous branches of
   intercostal nerve
23 Latissimus dorsi muscle
24 Median nerve
25 Axillary artery
26 Intercostobrachial nerves
27 **Thoracodorsal nerve**
28 Long thoracic nerve
29 Latissimus dorsi muscle
30 **Serratus anterior muscle**
31 Thoracoacromial artery
32 Clavicle
33 External intercostal muscle
34 Third rib
35 **Internal intercostal muscle**
36 Anterior intercostal artery and vein,
   and intercostal nerve
37 Costal arch or margin

Thoracic wall I (anterior aspect). Left pectoralis major muscle has been divided and reflected. Note the connection of the cephalic vein with the subclavian vein. Arrow: medial pectoral nerve.

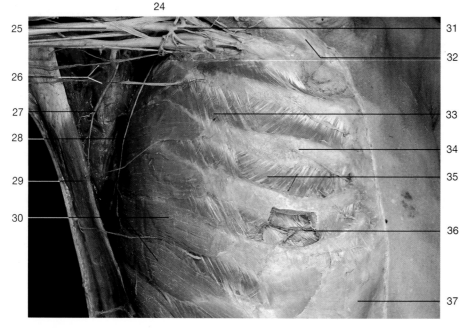

Thoracic wall (lateral aspect). Pectoralis major and minor muscles have been removed. A section of the fourth rib has been cut and removed to display the intercostal vessels and nerve.

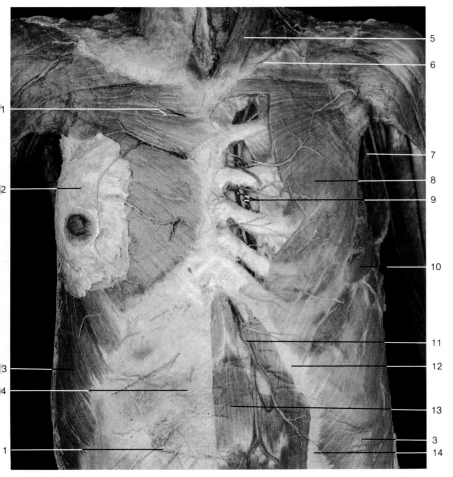

1 Anterior perforating branches
  of intercostal nerve
2 Mammary gland
3 External abdominal oblique muscle
4 Rectus sheath (anterior layer)
5 Sternocleidomastoid muscle
6 Clavicle
7 Lateral thoracic artery
  and vein
8 Pectoralis major muscle
9 **Internal thoracic artery**
  and vein
10 Serratus anterior muscle
11 **Superior epigastric artery**
   and vein
12 Costal margin
13 Rectus abdominis muscle
14 Cut edge of the anterior layer
   of the rectus sheath
15 Subclavian artery
16 Highest intercostal artery
17 Internal thoracic artery
18 Musculophrenic artery
19 Superficial epigastric artery
20 Deep circumflex iliac artery
21 Superior epigastric artery
22 Inferior epigastric artery
23 Superficial circumflex iliac artery

Thoracic wall II (anterior aspect). Dissection of the **internal thoracic artery and vein.** Left pectoralis major muscle partly removed. Anterior lamina of the rectus sheath on the left side has been removed.

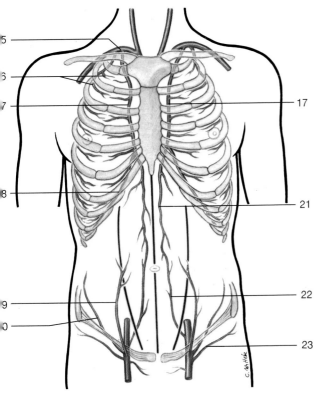

Main arteries of thoracic and abdominal wall.

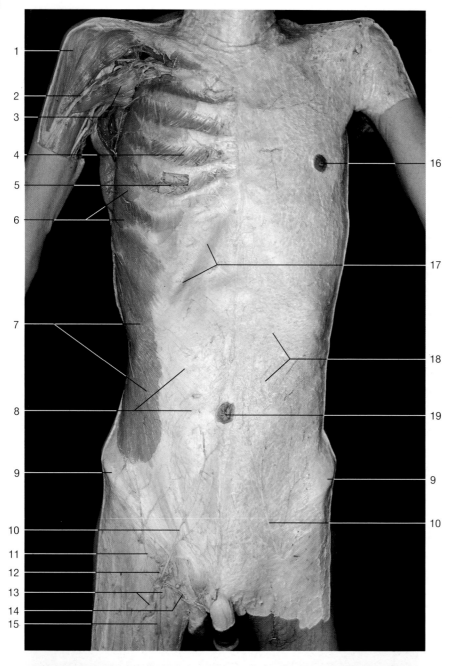

1 Deltoid muscle
2 Cephalic vein
3 Pectoralis major muscle (divided)
4 **Internal intercostal muscle**
5 **Intercostal artery and vein** (intercostal space, fenestrated)
6 Serratus anterior muscle
7 **External abdominal oblique muscle**
8 **Anterior layer of rectus sheath**
9 Iliac crest
10 Superficial epigastric vein
11 Superficial circumflex iliac vein
12 Saphenous opening
13 Superficial inguinal lymph nodes
14 Superficial external pudendal veins
15 Great saphenous vein
16 Nipple
17 Costal margin
18 Subcutaneous fatty tissue
19 Umbilicus
20 Anterior layer of rectus sheath
21 Rectus abdominis muscle
22 Posterior layer of rectus sheath
23 **Internal abdominal oblique muscle**
24 **External abdominal oblique muscle** (cut)
25 **Transversus abdominis muscle**
26 Transversal fascia and peritoneum
27 Psoas major muscle
28 Body of lumbar vertebra (L$_4$)
29 Quadratus lumborum muscle
30 Medial tract of erector spinae muscle
31 Lateral tract of erector spinae muscle (longissimus and iliocostalis muscles)
32 Small intestine
33 Left ureter
34 **Abdominal aorta**
35 **Inferior vena cava**
36 Descending colon
37 Spinous process

Thoracic and abdominal wall I. Right pectoralis major and minor muscles are divided. Muscles of thoracic and abdominal wall on right side are displayed.

Horizontal section of the trunk at the level of the umbilicus, superior to arcuate line (inferior aspect).

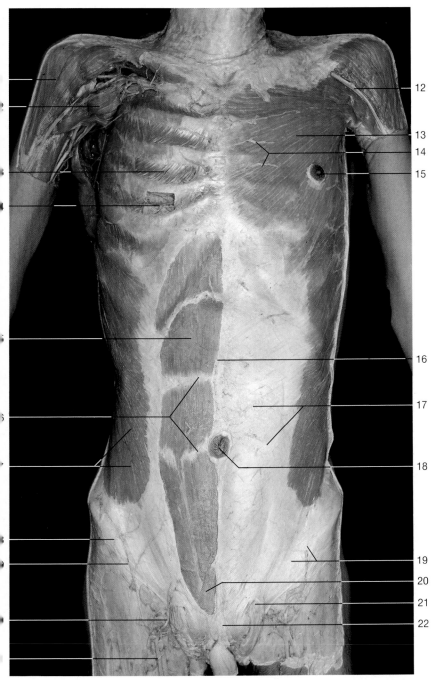

1 Deltoid muscle
2 Pectoralis major muscle (divided)
3 **Internal intercostal muscle**
4 Intercostal artery and vein
5 **Rectus abdominis muscle**
6 Tendinous intersections
7 **External abdominal oblique muscle**
8 Anterior superior iliac spine
9 Superficial circumflex iliac vein
10 Superficial epigastric vein
11 Great saphenous vein
12 Cephalic vein
13 **Pectoralis major muscle**
14 Anterior cutaneous branches of
    intercostal nerves
15 Nipple
16 Linea alba
17 **Anterior layer of rectus sheath**
18 Umbilicus
19 **Inguinal ligament**
20 Pyramidal muscle
21 Superficial inguinal ring and spermatic
    cord
22 Suspensory ligament of penis
23 Longissimus and iliocostalis muscles
24 Multifidus muscle
25 Quadratus lumborum muscle
26 Latissimus dorsi muscle
27 Psoas major muscle
28 Spinous process
29 Body of first lumbar vertebra
30 **Transversus abdominis muscle**
31 **Internal abdominal oblique muscle**

Thoracic and abdominal wall II. Right pectoralis major and minor muscles and anterior layer of rectus sheath have been removed on the right side.

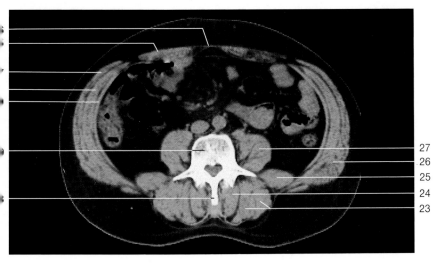

Horizontal section through the body at the level of fourth lumbar vertebra; seen from below. (CT scan.)

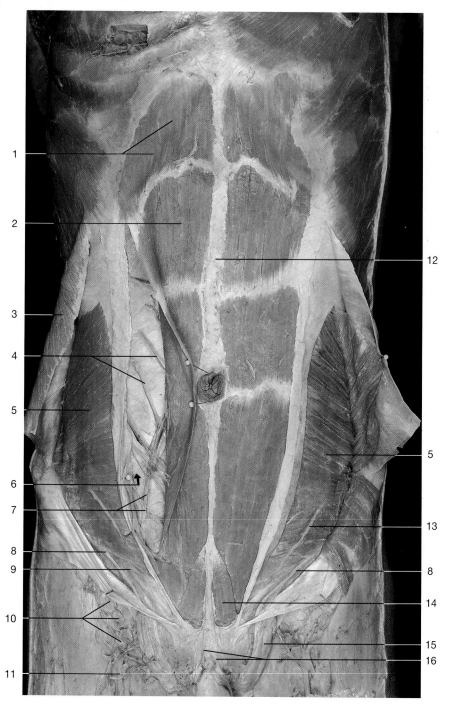

Thoracic and abdominal wall III. External abdominal oblique muscle has been divided and reflected on both sides. The right rectus muscle has been reflected medially to display the posterior layer of rectus sheath. Arrow: location of arcuate line.

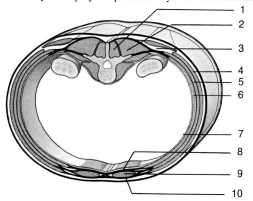

Horizontal section of the trunk superior to arcuate line. (Schematic drawing.)

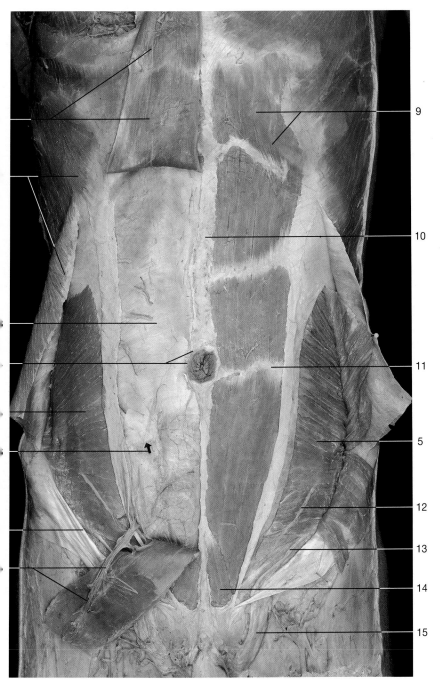

1 **Rectus abdominis muscle** (reflected)
2 External abdominal oblique muscle (divided)
3 Posterior layer of rectus sheath
4 Umbilical ring
5 **Internal abdominal oblique muscle**
6 Arcuate line (arrow)
7 Inguinal ligament
8 **Inferior epigastric artery and vein** and rectus abdominis muscle (divided and reflected)
9 Costal margin
10 Linea alba
11 Tendinous intersection
12 Iliohypogastric nerve
13 **Ilioinguinal nerve**
14 **Pyramidal muscle**
15 Spermatic cord

Thoracic and abdominal wall IV. External abdominal oblique muscle has been divided and reflected on both sides. The right rectus muscle has been cut and reflected to display the posterior layer of rectus sheath. Arrow: location of arcuate line.

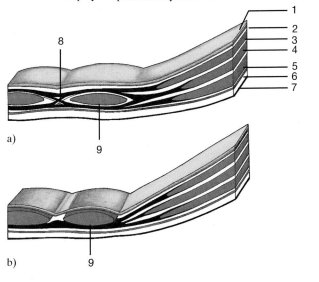

1 Peritoneum
2 Transversalis fascia (green)
3 Transversus abdominis muscle
4 Internal abdominal oblique muscle
5 External abdominal oblique muscle
6 Fascia of external abdominal oblique muscle (green)
7 Skin
8 Linea alba
9 Rectus abdominis muscle

Transverse sections through the abdominal wall superior (a) and inferior (b) to arcuate line.

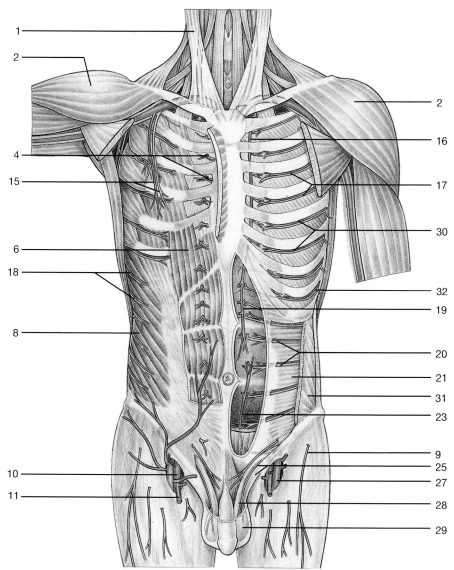

1 Sternocleidomastoid muscle
2 Deltoid muscle
3 Pectoralis major muscle
4 **Anterior cutaneous branches of
intercostal nerves**
5 Cut edge of anterior layer of rectus
sheath
6 **Rectus abdominis muscle**
7 Tendinous intersection
8 External abdominal oblique muscle
9 Lateral femoral cutaneous nerve
10 Femoral vein
11 Great saphenous vein
12 Medial supraclavicular nerves
13 Pectoralis minor muscle (reflected)
and medial pectoral nerves
14 Axillary vein
15 Long thoracic nerve and lateral
thoracic artery
16 Internal thoracic artery
17 **Intercostal nerves**
18 **Lateral cutaneous branches of
intercostal nerves**
19 Superior epigastric artery
20 Thoracoabdominal (intercostal)
nerves
21 Transversus abdominis muscle
22 Posterior layer of rectus sheath
23 **Inferior epigastric artery**
24 Lateral femoral cutaneous nerve
25 Inguinal ligament and ilioinguinal
nerve
26 Femoral nerve
27 Femoral artery
28 Spermatic cord
29 Testis
30 **Posterior intercostal arteries**
31 Internal abdominal oblique muscle
32 Lateral cutaneous branch of
intercostal nerve
33 Dorsal branch of spinal nerve
34 Latissimus dorsi muscle
35 Deep muscles of the back (medial
and lateral tract)
36 Anterior layer of rectus sheath
37 Posterior layer of rectus sheath
38 Thoracolumbar fascia
39 Spinal cord
40 Aorta
41 Ventral root ⎫ of spinal
42 Dorsal root ⎭ nerve

Thoracic and abdominal wall (schematic drawing). Note the segmental
organization of the blood vessels and nerves. Right side: superficial layers;
left side: deeper layers.

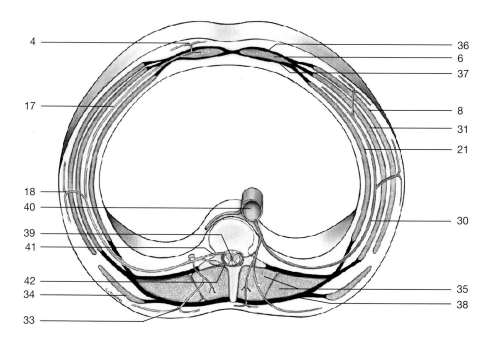

**Horizontal section of the
abdominal wall** (from below)
showing the location of the
intercostal arteries (left side)
and nerves (right side).

Thoracic wall and abdominal wall V.

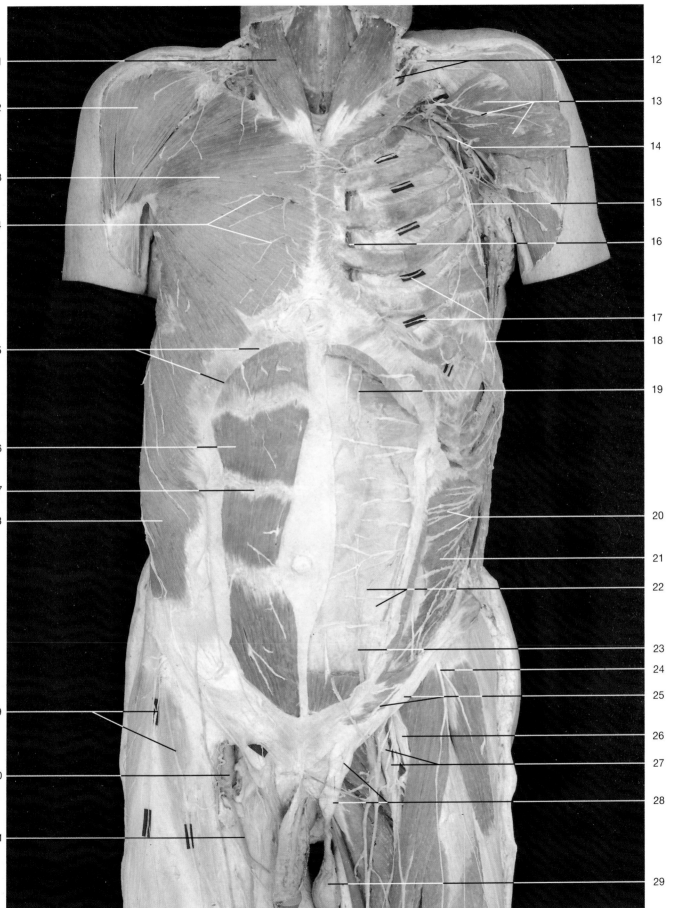

Thoracic wall and abdominal wall V. Right side: superficial layers; left side: deeper layers (anterior aspect). Pectoralis major and minor muscles, the external and internal intercostal muscles on the left side have been removed to display the intercostal nerves. The anterior layer of rectus sheath, the left rectus abdominis muscle and the external and internal abdominal oblique muscles have been removed to show the thoracoabdominal nerves within the abdominal wall.

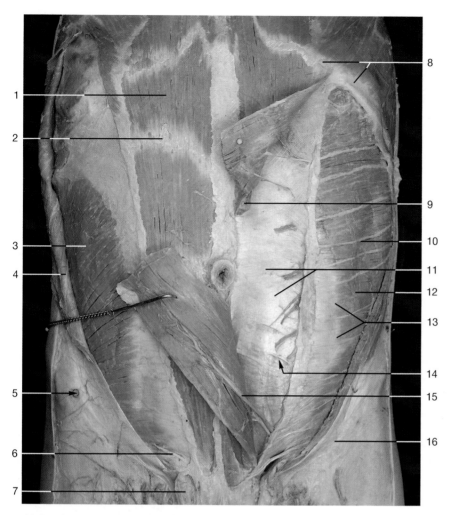

1	**Rectus abdominis muscle**
2	Tendinous intersection
3	**Internal abdominal oblique muscle**
4	External abdominal oblique muscle (reflected)
5	Anterior superior iliac spine
6	Ilioinguinal nerve
7	Spermatic cord
8	Costal margin
9	Superior epigastric artery
10	**Thoracoabdominal** (intercostal) **nerves**
11	Posterior layer of rectus sheath
12	**Transversus abdominis muscle**
13	Semilunar line
14	Arcuate line
15	**Inferior epigastric artery**
16	Inguinal ligament

Abdominal wall with vessels and nerves. The left rectus abdominis muscle has been divided and reflected to display the inferior epigastric vessels. The left internal abdominal oblique muscle has been removed to show the thoracoabdominal nerves.

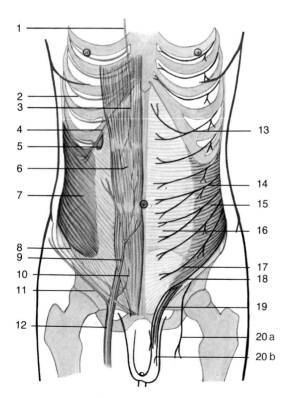

1	Internal thoracic artery
2	Intercostal artery
3	Superior epigastric artery
4	Musculophrenic artery
5	Gallbladder
6	Rectus abdominis muscle
7	External abdominal oblique muscle
8	Deep circumflex iliac artery
9	Superficial epigastric artery
10	Inferior epigastric artery
11	Superficial circumflex iliac artery
12	Femoral artery
13	Intercostal nerve
14	Thoracoabdominal nerve (T_{10})
15	Transversus abdominis muscle
16	Posterior layer of the rectus sheath
17	Iliohypogastric nerve (L_1)
18	Ilioinguinal nerve (L_1)
19	Spermatic cord
20	Genitofemoral nerve (L_1, L_2)
	a Femoral branch
	b Genital branch

Arteries and nerves which supply the thoracic and abdominal wall. Note their segmental arrangement. (Schematic drawing.)

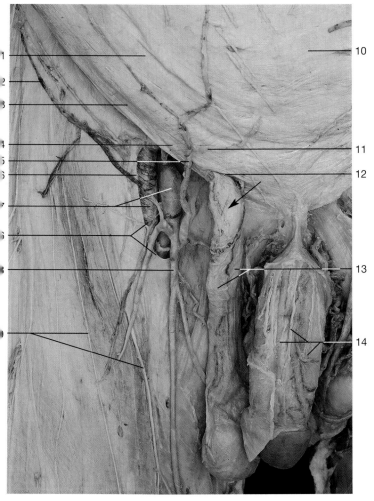

Inguinal canal in the male I (superficial layer, anterior aspect).
There is a small inguinal hernia (arrow).

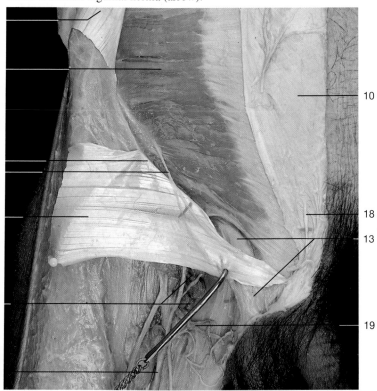

Inguinal canal in the male II, right side (anterior aspect).
The external abdominal oblique muscle has been divided to display
the inguinal canal.

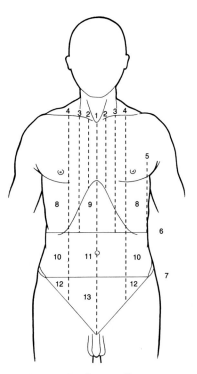

Regions and reference lines
for delineating surface projections.

Reference lines and regions
1 Median line
2 Lateral sternal line
3 Parasternal line
4 Midclavicular line
5 Axillary line
6 Transpyloric plane
7 Transtubercular plane
8 Hypochondriac region
9 Epigastric region
10 Lumbar region
11 Umbilical region
12 Iliac region
13 Hypogastric region

1 Aponeurosis of external abdominal oblique muscle
2 Superficial circumflex iliac vein
3 **Inguinal ligament**
4 Lateral crus of inguinal ring
5 Superficial epigastric vein
6 Saphenous opening
7 **Femoral artery and vein**
8 **Great saphenous vein**
9 Anterior cutaneous branches of femoral nerve
10 **Anterior layer of rectus sheath**
11 Intercrural fibers
12 **Superficial inguinal ring**
13 Spermatic cord and genital branch
    of genitofemoral nerve
14 Penis with dorsal nerves and deep dorsal vein
    of penis
15 Aponeurosis of external abdominal oblique
    muscle (divided and reflected)
16 **Internal abdominal oblique muscle**
17 Ilioinguinal nerve
18 Anterior cutaneous branches of iliohypogastric
    nerve
19 Superficial external pudendal veins

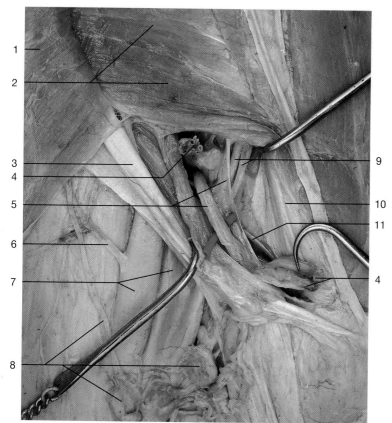

Inguinal canal in the male III. Deep dissection (anterior aspect, right side). Spermatic cord with exception of ductus deferens (probe) has been divided and reflected.

1 Internal abdominal oblique muscle (reflected)
2 Transversus abdominis muscle
3 Inguinal ligament
4 **Spermatic cord** with the exception of the ductus deferens (divided and reflected)
5 **Ductus deferens** and interfoveolar ligament
6 Superficial circumflex iliac artery
7 **Femoral artery and vein**
8 Superficial inguinal lymph nodes and inguinal lymph vessel
9 **Inferior epigastric artery and vein**
10 Falx inguinalis or conjoint tendon (cut)
11 Pubic branch of inferior epigastric artery
12 Superficial inguinal ring
13 Penis
14 External abdominal oblique muscle
15 Anterior superior iliac spine
16 Intercrural fibers
17 Fascia lata and sartorius muscle
18 Saphenous opening and great saphenous vein
19 Deep inguinal ring
20 Skin of scrotum and dartos muscle
21 Cremaster muscle
22 Internal spermatic fascia
23 Ductus deferens
24 Epididymis
25 Peritoneum (blue)
26 Remnant of processus vaginalis
27 Tunica vaginalis testis
28 Rectus abdominis muscle
29 Spermatic cord with ductus deferens covered by external spermatic fascia
30 Anterior layer of rectus sheath
31 Suspensory ligament of penis
32 **Testis and epididymis**
33 Ductus deferens
34 Pampiniform venous plexus and testicular artery
35 Inferior epigastric artery
36 Lateral femoral cutaneous nerve
37 Ilioinguinal nerve
38 **Femoral nerve**
39 Sartorius muscle
40 Deep dorsal vein of penis

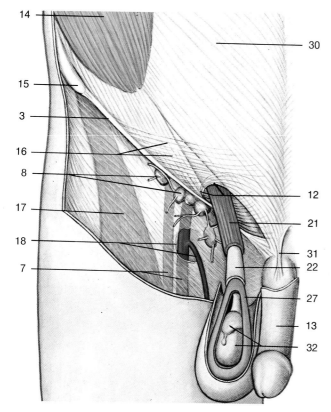

General characteristics of lower part of anterior abdominal wall and inguinal canal. (Schematic drawing.)

Inguinal hernias may either pass through the inguinal canal lateral to the inferior epigastric artery (indirect or lateral inguinal hernias, A and C) or directly penetrate the abdominal wall through the inguinal triangle located medial to the inferior epigastric artery (direct or medial inguinal hernias, B). The lateral hernias can be congenital if the vaginal process remains open (C) or acquired (A) if the hernia develops independently of a patent processus vaginalis.

Femoral hernias generally protrude through the femoral ring below the inguinal ligament. Proper assessment of the site of herniation requires the identification of both the inguinal ligament and the epigastric artery.

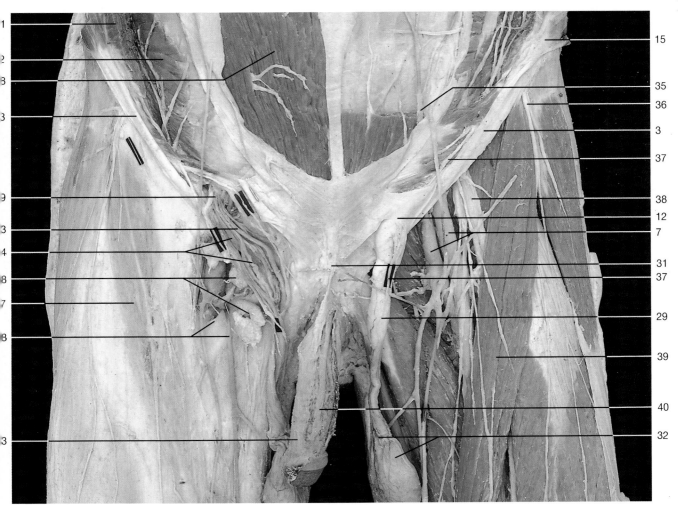

Inguinal and femoral region in the male (anterior aspect). On the right, the spermatic cord was dissected to display the ductus deferens and the accompanying vessels and nerves. The fascia lata on the left side has been removed.

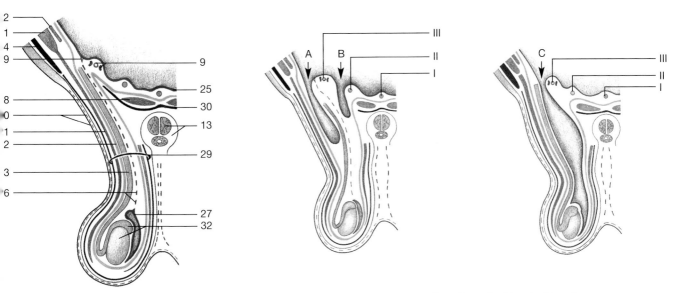

Layers of spermatic cord and types of hernias. Left: normal situation; middle: location of acquired inguinal hernias;
A = indirect; B = direct inguinal hernia. Right: congenital indirect inguinal hernia (C); the vaginal process remained open.
I   = Median umbilical fold containing urachus chord.
II   = Medial umbilical fold with remnants of umbilical artery.
III = Lateral umbilical fold with inferior epigastric artery and vein.

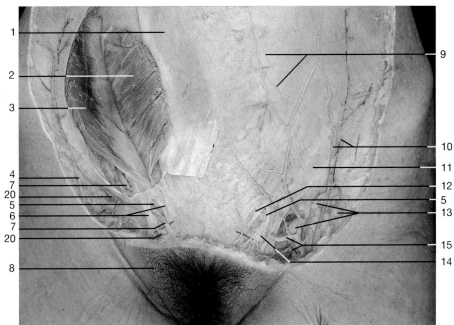

1 Aponeurosis of external abdominal
   oblique muscle
2 Internal abdominal oblique muscle
   (divided and reflected)
3 Transversus abdominis muscle
4 Superficial circumflex iliac artery and
   vein
5 Superficial inguinal ring with fat pad
6 Medial and lateral crural fibers
7 **Round ligament** (ligamentum teres uteri)
8 Labium majus pudendi
9 Anterior layer of rectus sheath
10 Superficial epigastric artery and vein
11 **Inguinal ligament**
12 Cutaneous branch of ilioinguinal nerve
13 Superficial inguinal lymph nodes
14 Entrance of round ligament into the
   labium majus
15 External pudendal artery and vein
16 Position of deep inguinal ring
17 **Ilioinguinal nerve**
18 Internal abdominal oblique muscle
19 Pubic branch of inferior epigastric
   artery
20 Genital branch of genitofemoral nerve
21 Fat pad of inguinal canal
22 Ilioinguinal nerve
23 Sheath of round ligament
   (inguinal canal)
24 Transversalis fascia

Inguinal region in the female (anterior aspect). Left side: superficial layer;
right side: external and internal abdominal oblique muscle divided and reflected.

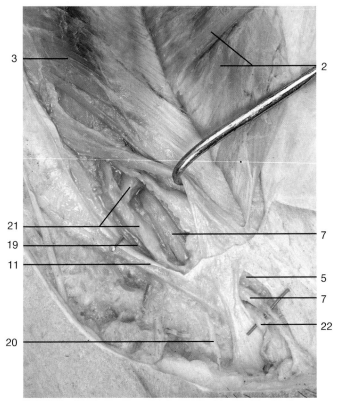

Inguinal canal of the female I (anterior aspect, right side).
The external abdominal oblique muscle has been divided and
reflected, to display the ilioinguinal nerve and the round
ligament.

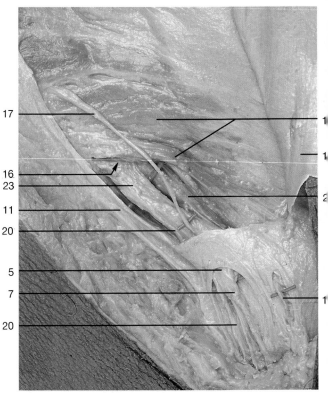

Inguinal canal of the female II (anterior aspect, right side).
The external and internal abdominal oblique muscle have
been divided and reflected to show the content of the inguinal
canal.

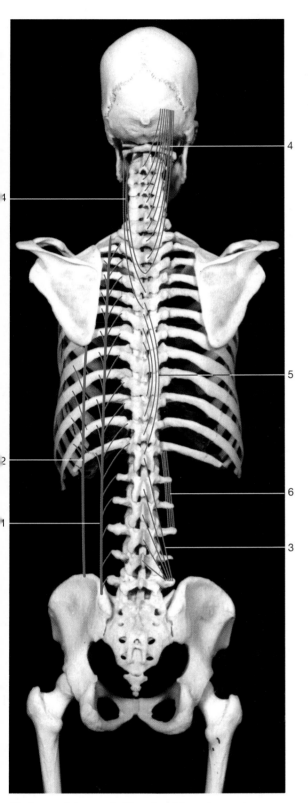

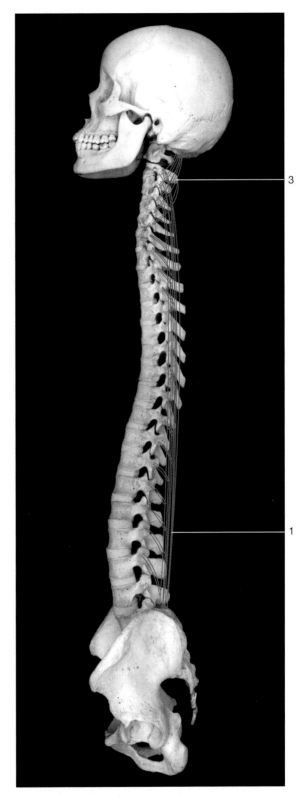

Skeleton of the trunk (dorsal and lateral aspect).
The long muscles of the back [longissimus (1) and iliocostalis (2) muscle] originate at the sacrum and pelvis and insert at the spinous or transverse processes of the vertebrae or at the ribs. There are also muscles which insert at the occipital bone. The long muscles form the lateral tract, whereas muscles of the medial tract are situated within the groove between the spinous and transverse processes of the vertebrae [transversospinal (3) and spinotransversal (4) muscles] or between the spinous processes [spinalis muscles (5)] or between the transverse processes [intertransversarii muscles (6)] of the vertebrae.

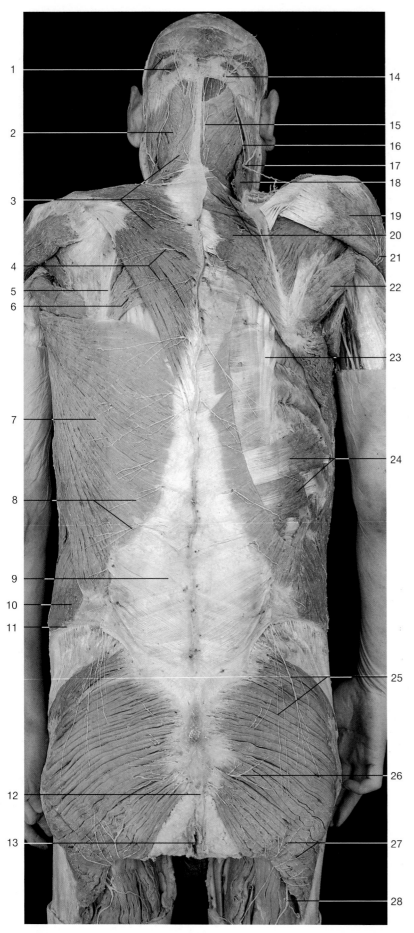

Innervation of the back I. Superficial (left) and deeper (right) layers. Right trapezius and latissimus dorsi muscles removed.

1   Occipital belly of occipitofrontalis muscle
2   Splenius capitis muscle
3   **Trapezius muscle**
4   **Medial cutaneous branches of dorsal rami of spinal nerves**
5   Medial margin of scapula
6   Rhomboid major muscle
7   **Latissimus dorsi muscle**
8   **Lateral cutaneous branches of dorsal rami of spinal nerves**
9   Thoracolumbar fascia
10 External abdominal oblique muscle
11 Iliac crest
12 Last coccygeal vertebra
13 Anus
14 Greater occipital nerve
15 Third occipital nerve
16 Lesser occipital nerve
17 Cutaneous branches of cervical plexus
18 Levator scapulae muscle
19 Deltoid muscle
20 **Rhomboid major and minor muscles**
21 Upper lateral cutaneous nerve of arm (branch of axillary nerve)
22 **Teres major muscle**
23 Iliocostalis thoracis muscle
24 Serratus posterior inferior muscle
25 Superior cluneal nerves
26 Middle cluneal nerves
27 Inferior cluneal nerves
28 Posterior femoral cutaneous nerve

▷

To page 213:
1   **Trapezius muscle**
2   Infraspinatus muscle
3   Left **latissimus dorsi muscle**
4   Thoracolumbar fascia
5   Splenius cervicis muscle
6   Serratus posterior superior muscle
7   **Medial branches of dorsal rami of thoracic spinal nerves**
8   **Lateral branches of dorsal rami of thoracic spinal nerves**
9   Iliocostalis muscle
10 Serratus posterior inferior muscle
11 Latissimus dorsi muscle (reflected)

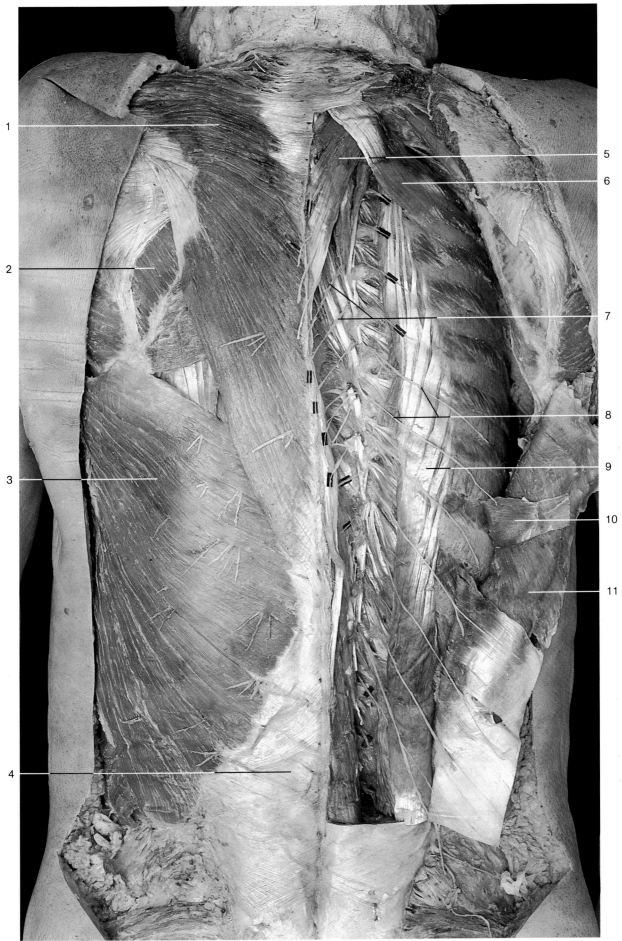

Innervation of the back II. Dissection of the dorsal branches of spinal nerves. On the right, longissimus thoracis muscle has been removed and iliocostalis muscle laterally reflected.

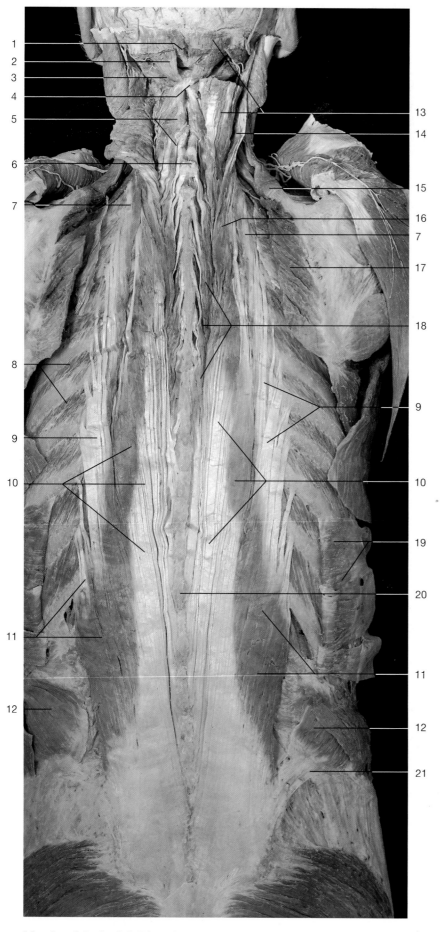

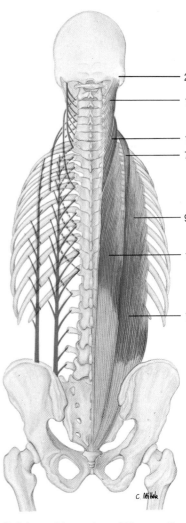

**Origin and insertion of iliocostalis
and longissimus muscles.**
(Schematic drawing.)

1   Rectus capitis posterior minor muscle
2   Rectus capitis posterior major muscle
3   Obliquus capitis inferior muscle
4   Spinous process of axis
5   Semispinalis cervicis muscle
6   Spinous process of seventh vertebra
7   **Iliocostalis cervicis muscle**
8   External intercostal muscles
9   **Iliocostalis thoracis muscle**
10 **Longissimus thoracis muscle**
11 **Iliocostalis lumborum muscle**
12 Internal abdominal oblique muscle
13 Semispinalis capitis muscle (divided)
14 **Longissimus capitis muscle**
15 Levator scapulae muscle
16 **Longissimus cervicis muscle**
17 Rhomboid major muscle
18 **Spinalis thoracis muscle**
19 Serratus posterior inferior muscle
    (reflected)
20 Spinous process of second lumbar
    vertebra
21 Iliac crest
22 Mastoid process

Muscles of the back I. Dissection of the erector spinae muscle (lateral column
of the intrinsic back muscles).

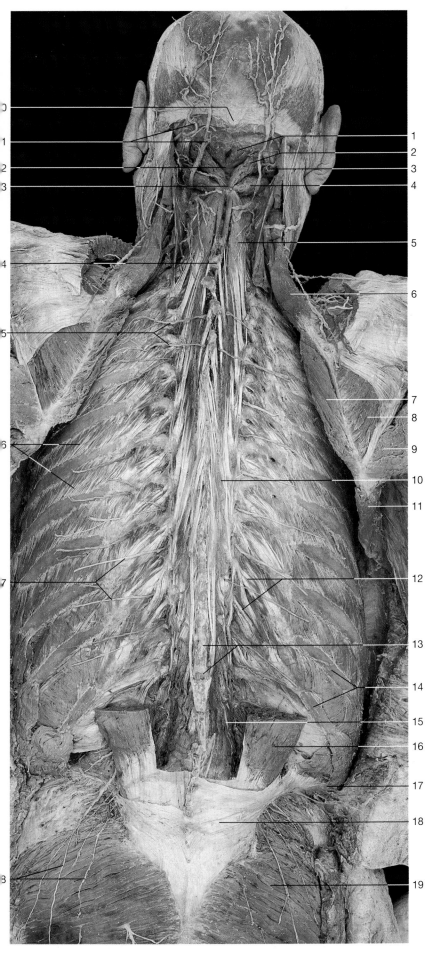

1 Rectus capitis posterior minor muscle
2 Rectus capitis posterior major muscle
3 Obliquus capitis superior muscle
4 Obliquus capitis inferior muscle
5 **Semispinalis cervicis muscle**
6 Levator scapulae muscle
7 Rhomboideus major muscle
8 Scapula with infraspinatus muscle
9 Teres major muscle
10 **Spinalis muscle**
11 Latissimus dorsi muscle
12 **Levatores costarum muscles**
13 Spinous processes of lumbar vertebrae
14 Ribs (Th_{11}, Th_{12})
15 **Multifidus muscle**
16 Longissimus and iliocostalis
   muscles (cut)
17 Iliac crest (lumbar triangle)
18 Thoracolumbar fascia
19 Gluteus maximus muscle
20 Protuberantia occipitalis externa
21 Occipital artery and greater occipital
   nerve (C_2)
22 Spinous process of atlas
23 Spinous process of axis
24 Spinous process of seventh cervical
   vertebra (vertebra prominens)
25 Medial branches of dorsal branches
   of spinal nerves
26 External intercostal muscles
27 Lateral branches of dorsal branches
   of spinal nerves
28 Superior cluneal nerves

Muscles of the back II. Dissection of the deeper layer of the intrinsic muscles of
the back (longissimus and iliocostalis muscles are cut).

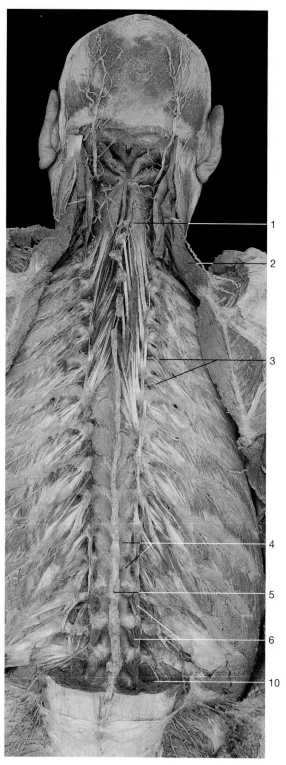

Muscles of the back III. Deepest layer.

1 **Semispinalis cervicis muscle**
2 Levator scapulae muscle
3 **Levatores costarum muscles**
4 Vertebral arches of lumbar vertebrae
5 Supraspinal ligaments
6 **Intertransverse lumbar muscles**
7 **Lumbar rotator muscles**
8 Cutaneous branches of spinal nerves
9 Lumbar interspinal muscles
10 Longissimus and iliocostalis muscle (cut)
11 Spinal muscle of the back
12 **Multifidus muscle**
13 Tenth rib (T$_{10}$)

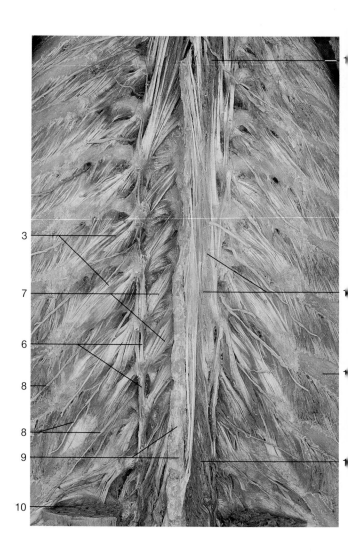

Muscles of the back III. Deepest layer. Lumbar region (higher magnification).

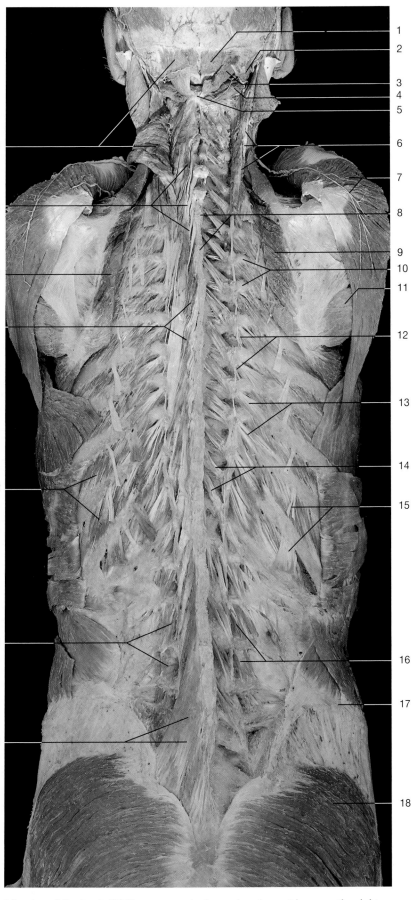

Muscles of the back IV. Transversospinal muscles, deepest layer on the right, where all parts of semispinalis and multifidus muscles have been removed.

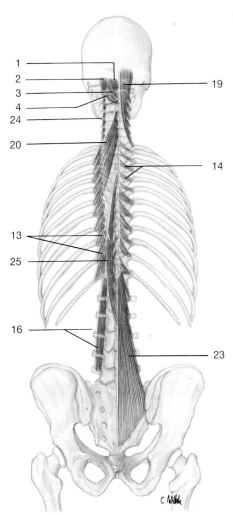

Medial column of intrinsic muscles of the back. Transversospinal and intertransversal system. (Schematic drawing.)

1 Rectus capitis posterior minor muscle
2 Obliquus capitis superior muscle
3 Rectus capitis posterior major muscle
4 Obliquus capitis inferior muscle
5 Spinous process of axis
6 **Longissimus capitis muscle**
7 Trapezius muscle (reflected) and accessory nerve (n. XI)
8 Spinous processes
9 Rhomboid major muscle
10 Transverse processes of thoracic vertebrae
11 Teres major muscle
12 Intertransverse ligaments
13 **Levatores costarum muscles**
14 **Rotatores muscles**
15 Tendons of iliocostalis muscle
16 Intertransversarii lumborum muscles (lateral)
17 Iliac crest
18 Gluteus maximus muscle
19 Semispinalis capitis muscle
20 **Semispinalis cervicis muscle**
21 Semispinalis thoracis muscle
22 **External intercostal muscles**
23 **Multifidus muscle**
24 Posterior cervical intertransversarii muscles
25 Spinalis thoracis muscle

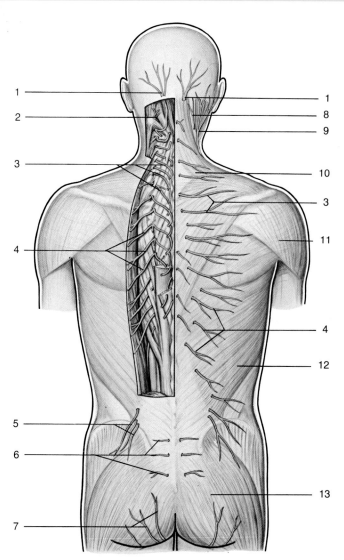

1 Greater occipital nerve (C_2)
2 Suboccipital nerve (C_1)
3 **Medial branches of dorsal rami of spinal nerves**
4 **Lateral branches of dorsal rami of spinal nerves**
5 Superior cluneal nerves ($L_1–L_3$)
6 Middle cluneal nerves ($S_1–S_3$)
7 Inferior cluneal nerves (derived from branches of the sacral plexus, ventral rami)
8 Lesser occipital nerve
9 Great auricular nerve
10 Trapezius muscle
11 Deltoid muscle
12 Latissimus dorsi muscle
13 Gluteus maximus muscle
14 External intercostal muscle
15 Internal intercostal muscle
16 Innermost intercostal muscle
17 Dorsal ramus of spinal nerve
18 **Spinal nerve** and **spinal ganglion**
19 Sympathetic trunk with ganglion
20 Intercostal nerve
21 Lateral cutaneous branch ⎫ of **intercostal nerve**
22 Anterior cutaneous branch ⎭

General characteristics of the innervation of the back.
Distribution of dorsal branches of spinal nerves. Note the segmental arrangement of the innervation of the dorsal part of the trunk. (Schematic drawing.)

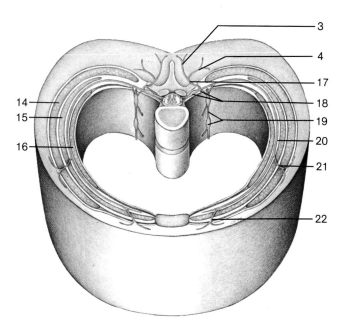

Position and branches of spinal nerves in one segment of thoracic wall. (Schematic drawing.)

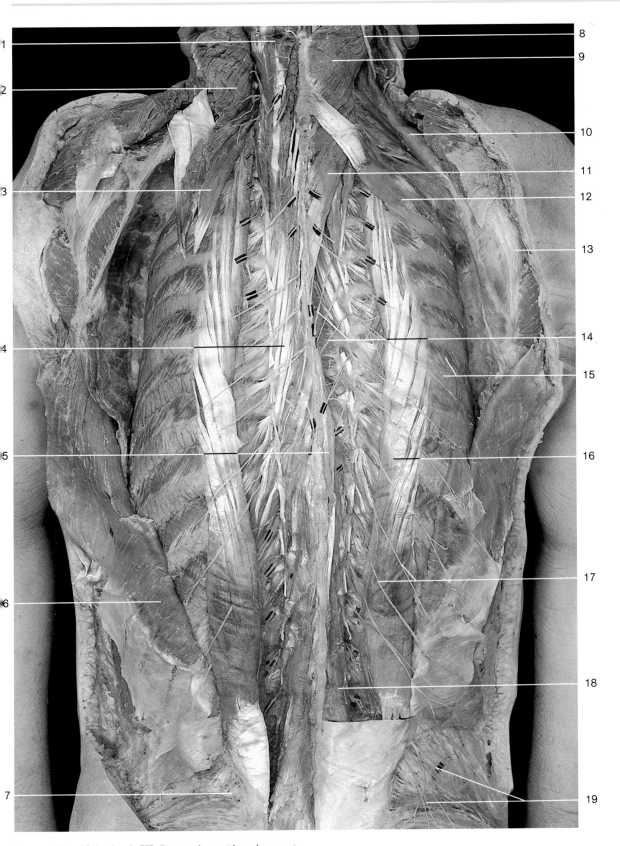

Innervation of the back III. Deeper layer (dorsal aspect).

1 Semispinalis capitis muscle
2 Left splenius capitis muscle
   (cut and reflected)
3 Left splenius cervicis muscle
   (cut and reflected)
4 Semispinalis thoracis muscle
5 **Spinalis thoracis muscle**
6 Latissimus dorsi muscle (reflected)

7 Iliac crest
8 Lesser occipital nerve
9 Splenius capitis muscle
10 Levator scapulae muscle
11 **Splenius cervicis muscle**
12 Serratus posterior superior muscle
13 Scapula

14 **Medial branches of dorsal rami**
   of spinal nerves
15 Rib and external intercostal muscle
16 Iliocostalis thoracis muscle
17 **Lateral branches of dorsal rami**
   of spinal nerves
18 Multifidus muscle
19 Superior cluneal nerves

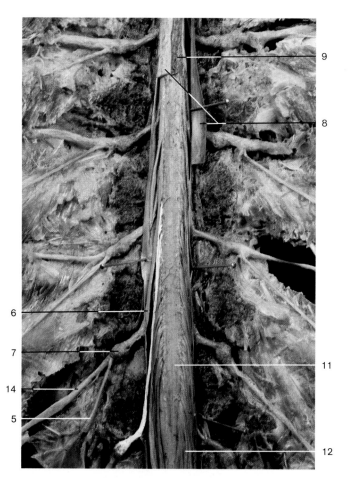

Lumbar portion of spinal cord. Note the relation between the nervous and muscular segments.

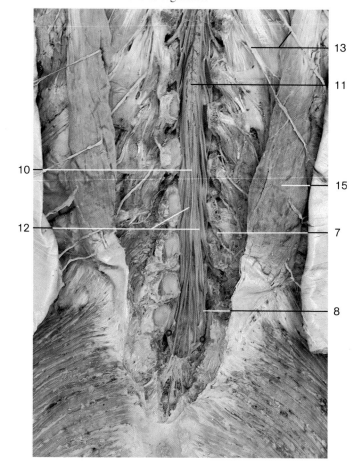

Terminal part of spinal cord. Dura removed.

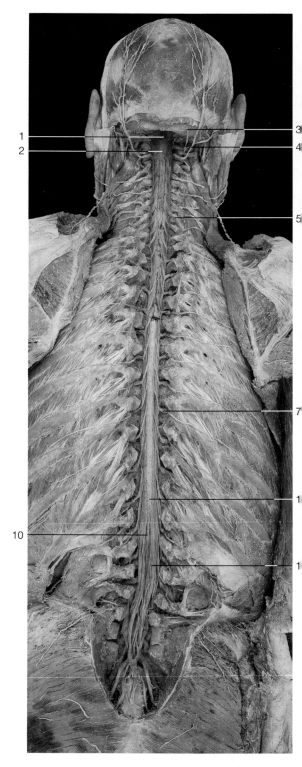

Innervation of the back IV. Spinal cord in the vertebral canal (opened). Longissimus dorsi and iliocostal muscles have been removed.

1	Cerebellomedullary cistern	9	Spinal arachnoid mater
2	Medulla oblongata	10	Filum terminale
3	Third cervical nerve (C$_3$)	11	Conus medullaris
4	Greater occipital nerve (C$_2$)	12	Cauda equina
5	Dorsal primary ramus	13	Lateral branches of dorsal rami of spinal nerves
6	Dorsal roots	14	Ventral ramus of spinal nerve (intercostal nerve)
7	Spinal ganglion		
8	Spinal dura mater	15	Iliocostalis muscle

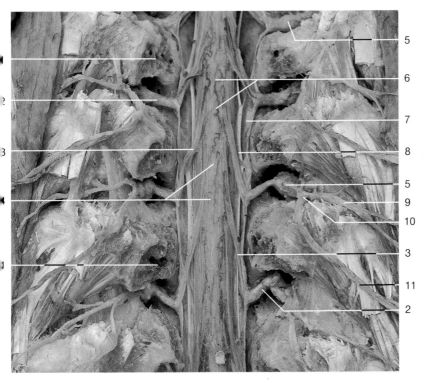

1 Arch of vertebra (divided)
2 Spinal nerve with meningeal coverings
3 Dorsal roots of thoracic spinal nerves
4 Spinal cord (thoracic portion)
5 Spinal ganglia with meningeal coverings
6 Pia mater with blood vessels
7 Dura mater (opened)
8 Denticulate ligament
9 Lateral branch of dorsal ramus
10 Dorsal ramus of spinal nerve
   (dividing into a medial and lateral branch)
11 Medial branch of dorsal ramus
   of spinal nerve
12 Spinal dura mater
13 Spinal nerves of sacral segments
14 Filum terminale

Thoracic portion of spinal cord (dorsal aspect). Vertebral canal and dura mater opened.

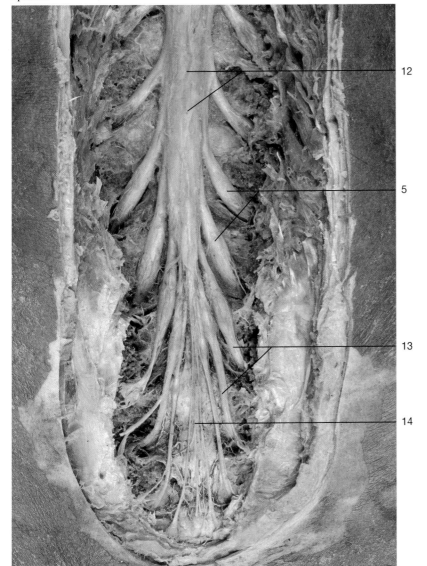

Terminal part of spinal cord with dura mater (dorsal aspect). Dorsal part of sacrum removed.

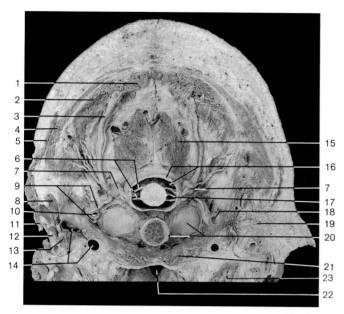

1 Trapezius muscle
2 Semispinalis capitis muscle
3 **Dorsal ramus of spinal nerve**
4 Sternocleidomastoid muscle
5 Platysma muscle
6 **Dorsal and ventral roots of spinal nerves**
7 **Spinal ganglion**
8 Posterior belly of digastric muscle
9 **Ventral ramus of spinal nerve**
10 Vertebral artery
11 Great auricular nerve
12 Superficial temporal artery
13 Styloid process
14 Internal jugular vein and internal carotid artery
15 Rectus capitis posterior major muscle
16 Dura mater and subarachnoid space
17 Denticulate ligament
18 Vertebral artery
19 Parotid gland
20 Dens of axis (divided) and inferior articular facet of atlas
21 Longus capitis muscle
22 Pharyngeal cavity
23 Medial pterygoid muscle
24 Periosteum of vertebral canal
25 Posterior spinal arteries
26 Anterior spinal artery

Meningeal coverings
27 Dura mater
28 Subdural space
29 Extradural or epidural space with venous plexus and fatty tissue
30 Arachnoid (green)
31 Subarachnoid space
32 Pia mater (pink)
33 Nucleus pulposus
34 Crus of diaphragm
35 Intervertebral disc
36 Body of first lumbar vertebra
37 Spinal cord
38 Conus medullaris
39 Cauda equina
40 Filum terminale
41 Spinous process

Horizontal section of the neck. Dissection of the second cervical spinal nerve. Posterior surface at top of figure.

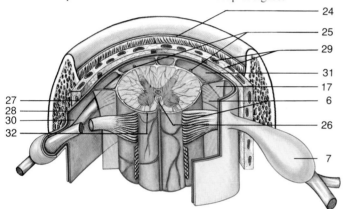

Meningeal coverings of the spinal cord (anterior aspect). (Schematic drawing.)

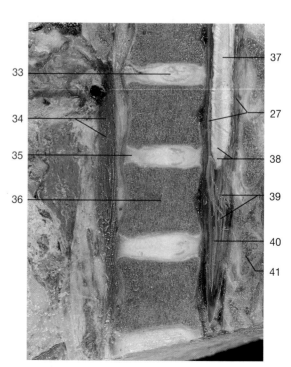

Sagittal section through the vertebral canal, T_9–L_2. (MRI scan.)

Sagittal section through vertebral canal, T_{12}–L_2. Notice red bone marrow (unfixed).

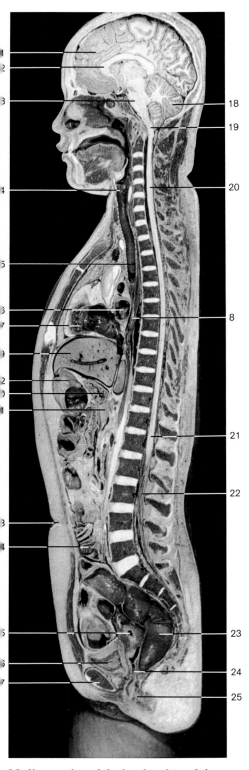

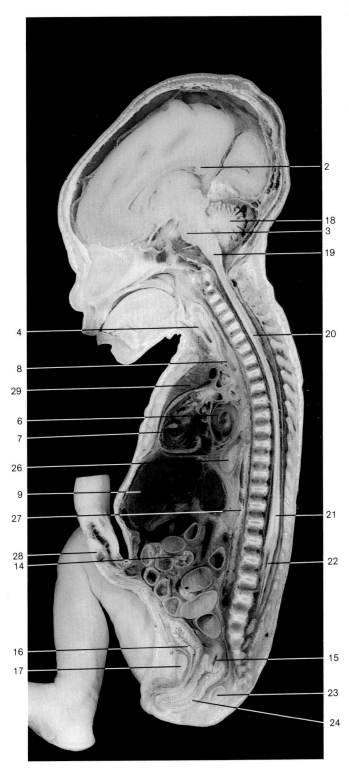

Median section of the head and trunk in the adult (female). The conus medullaris of the spinal cord is located at the level of L₁.

Median section of the head and trunk in the neonate. Note that in the neonate the conus medullaris of the spinal cord extends far more caudally than in the adult.

1	Cerebrum	11	Pancreas
2	Corpus callosum	12	Transverse colon
3	Pons	13	Umbilicus
4	Larynx	14	Small intestine
5	Trachea	15	Uterus
6	Left atrium	16	Urinary bladder
7	**Right ventricle**	17	Pubic symphysis
8	Esophagus	18	Cerebellum
9	**Liver**	19	Medulla oblongata
10	Stomach	20	**Spinal cord**

21	**Conus medullaris**
22	**Cauda equina**
23	Rectum
24	Vagina
25	Anus
26	Inferior vena cava
27	Aorta
28	Umbilical cord
29	Thymus

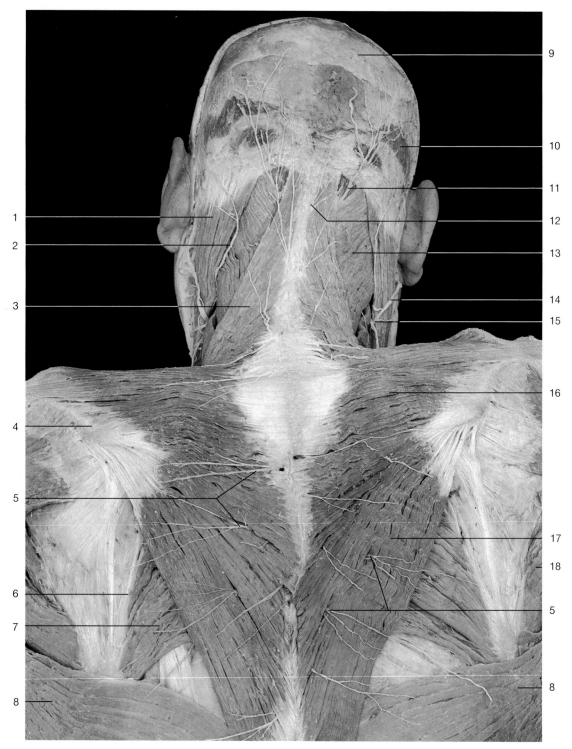

Dorsal aspect of the neck I. Superficial layer. Nuchal region and shoulder.

1 Sternocleidomastoid muscle
2 **Lesser occipital nerve**
3 Descending fibers of trapezius muscle
4 Spine of scapula
5 **Medial cutaneous branches of dorsal rami of spinal nerves**
6 Medial margin of scapula
7 Rhomboid major muscle
8 Latissimus dorsi muscle
9 Galea aponeurotica

10 Occipital belly of occipitofrontalis muscle
11 **Greater occipital nerve**
12 Third occipital nerve
13 Splenius capitis muscle
14 **Great auricular nerve**
15 Cutaneous nerves of cervical plexus
16 Transverse fibers of trapezius muscle
17 Ascending fibers of trapezius muscle
18 Teres major muscle

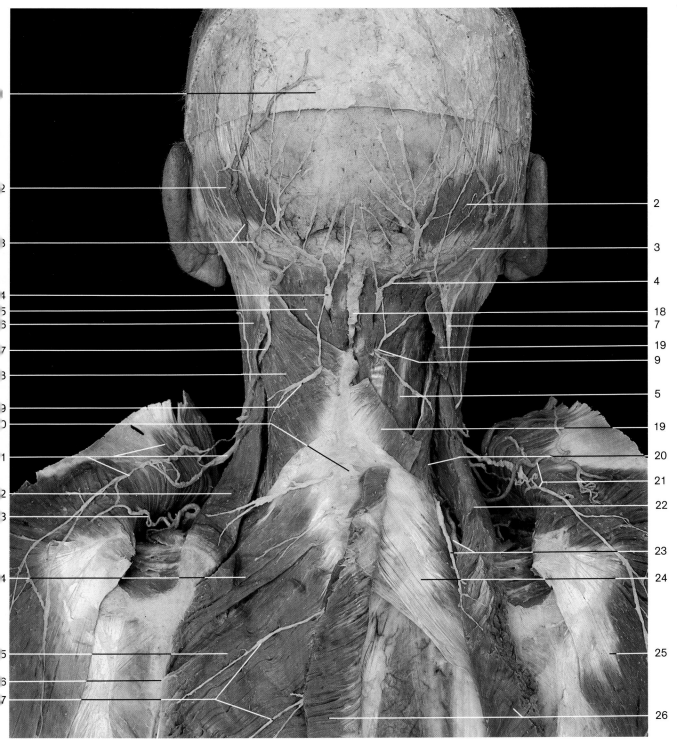

Dorsal aspect of neck II. Deeper layer. The left trapezius muscle has been divided and reflected. On the right, trapezius, rhomboid and splenius muscles have been divided. Right levator scapulae muscle has been slightly reflected.

1 Galea aponeurotica
2 Occipital belly of occipitofrontalis muscle
3 Occipital artery
4 **Greater occipital nerve** (C_2)
5 Semispinalis capitis muscle
6 Sternocleidomastoid muscle
7 Lesser occipital nerve
8 Left splenius capitis muscle
9 Third occipital nerve (C_3)
10 Spinous process of vertebra prominens (C_7)

11 Left trapezius muscle and **accessory nerve**
12 Levator scapulae muscle
13 Superficial branch of transverse cervical artery
14 Rhomboid minor muscle
15 Rhomboid major muscle
16 Medial margin of scapula
17 **Medial branches of dorsal rami of spinal nerves**
18 Ligamentum nuchae
19 Splenius capitis muscle (divided)

20 Splenius cervicis muscle
21 Right **accessory nerve** and superficial branch of transverse cervical artery
22 Right levator scapulae muscle
23 Dorsal scapular nerve and deep branch of transverse cervical artery
24 Serratus posterior superior muscle
25 Right trapezius muscle (divided and reflected)
26 Right rhomboid major muscle (divided and reflected)

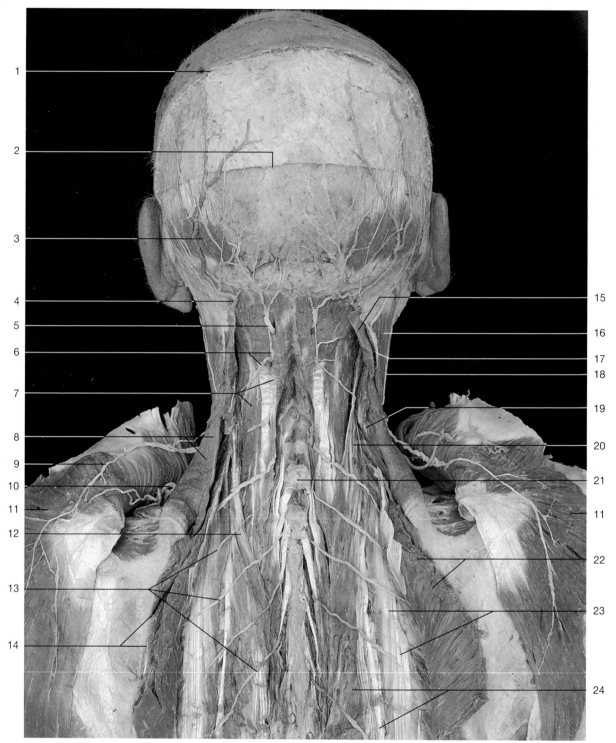

Dorsal aspect of neck III. Deepest layer. Nuchal region. Trapezius muscle and splenius capitis and cervicis muscles have been divided and partly removed or reflected.

1	Skin of scalp
2	Galea aponeurotica
3	Occipital belly of occipitofrontalis muscle
4	**Occipital artery**
5	**Greater occipital nerve**
6	Third occipital nerve
7	Semispinalis capitis muscle
8	Levator scapulae muscle
9	**Accessory nerve** (n. XI)
10	Superficial cervical artery
11	Trapezius muscle (reflected)
12	Longissimus cervicis muscle
13	**Medial cutaneous branches of dorsal rami of spinal nerves**
14	Medial margin of scapula
15	Splenius capitis muscle (divided)
16	Sternocleidomastoid muscle
17	**Lesser occipital nerve**
18	Great auricular nerve
19	Splenius cervicis muscle
20	Longissimus cervicis muscle
21	Spinous process of seventh cervical vertebra (vertebra prominens)
22	Rhomboid muscles (divided)
23	Iliocostalis thoracis muscle
24	Longissimus thoracis muscle

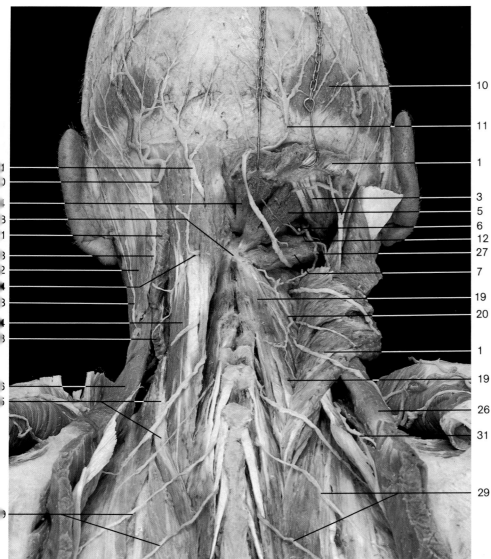

1 Semispinalis capitis muscle
   (divided)
2 External occipital protuberance
3 Obliquus capitis superior
   muscle
4 Rectus capitis posterior minor
   muscle
5 Rectus capitis posterior major
   muscle
6 Vertebral artery
7 Obliquus capitis inferior muscle
8 **Spinous process of axis**
9 Third cervical vertebra
10 Occipital belly of
   occipitofrontalis muscle
11 **Greater occipital nerve**
12 Suboccipital nerve (C_1)
13 Lesser occipital nerve
14 Third occipital nerve (C_3)
15 Mastoid process and
   splenius capitis muscle
16 Atlas
17 Axis
18 Spinous process of third
   cervical vertebra
19 Right semispinalis cervicis
   muscle
20 Deep cervical artery
21 Left splenius capitis muscle
   (divided)
22 Left sternocleidomastoid
   muscle
23 Great auricular nerve
24 Left **semispinalis capitis muscle**
25 Left longissimus cervicis muscle
26 Levator scapulae muscle
27 Muscular branch of
   vertebral artery
28 Left semispinalis cervicis
   muscle (divided)
29 **Medial branches of dorsal
   rami of spinal nerves**
30 **Occipital artery**
31 Dorsal scapular nerve

Dorsal aspect of neck IV. Deepest layer, suboccipital triangle; right semispinalis capitis muscle divided and reflected.

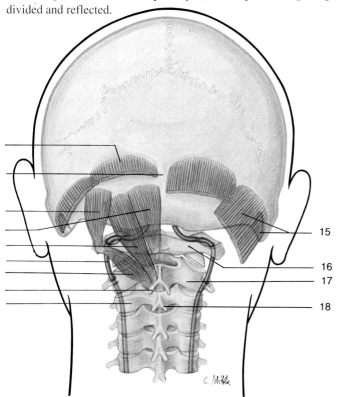

Suboccipital triangle and position of the vertebral artery.
(Schematic drawing.)

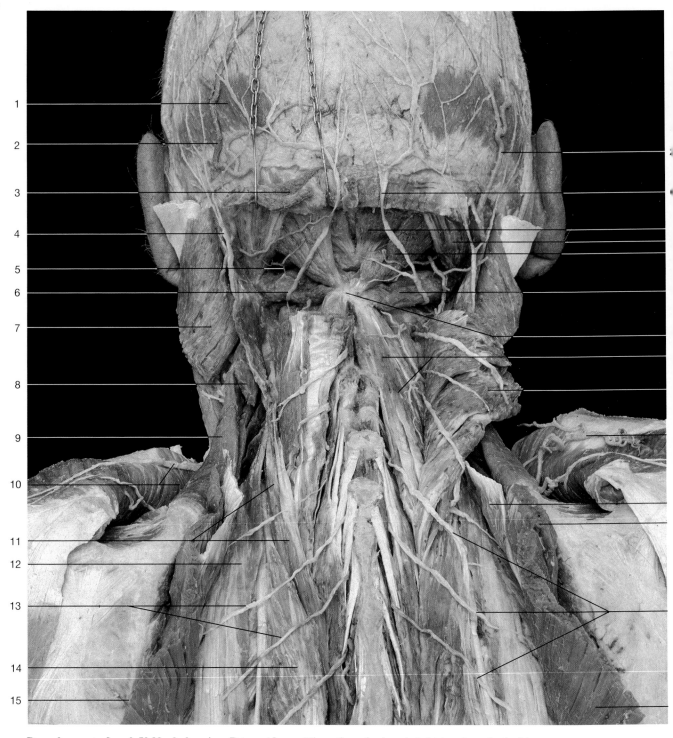

Dorsal aspect of neck V. Nuchal region. Deepest layer. Dissection of suboccipital triangle on both sides.

1 Occipital belly of occipitofrontalis muscle	11 Longissimus cervicis muscle	21 Semispinalis cervicis muscle
2 **Occipital artery**	12 Iliocostalis cervicis muscle	22 Semispinalis capitis muscle
3 Insertion of semispinalis capitis muscle (divided)	13 **Medial cutaneus branches of dorsal rami**	(divided and reflected)
4 Lesser occipital nerve (from cervical	**of spinal nerves** (C_7, C_8)	23 Transverse cervical artery
plexus)	14 Longissimus thoracis muscle	(superficial branch)
5 Suboccipital nerve (C_1)	15 Medial margin of scapula	24 Serratus posterior superior muscle
6 **Greater occipital nerve** (C_2)	16 **Rectus capitis posterior minor muscle**	(divided and reflected)
7 Splenius capitis muscle (reflected)	17 **Obliquus capitis superior muscle**	25 Rhomboid minor muscle
8 Splenius cervicis muscle	18 **Rectus capitis posterior major muscle**	(divided and reflected)
9 Levator scapulae muscle	19 **Obliquus capitis inferior muscle**	26 Rhomboid major muscle
10 Accessory nerve (n. XI), trapezius muscle	20 Spinous process of axis	(divided and reflected)

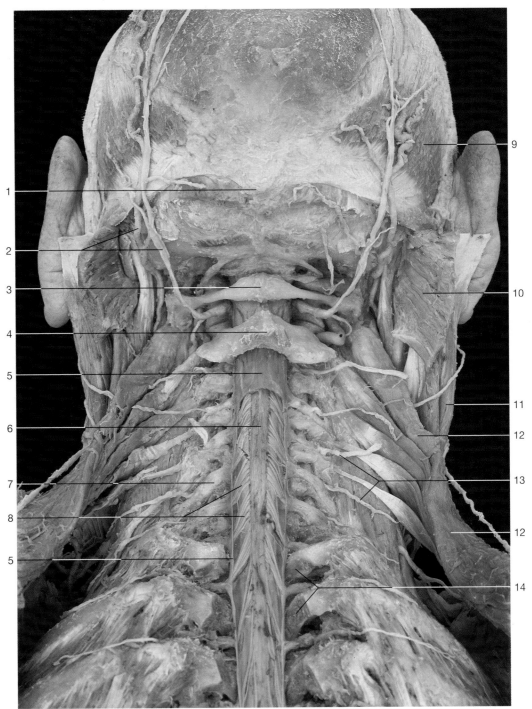

Dorsal aspect of the neck VI. Nuchal region (deepest layer). The vertebral canal caudally of the atlas and axis has been opened to show the spinal cord (dura mater has been partly removed).

1　Protuberantia occipitalis externa
2　Greater occipital nerve (C₂) and occipital artery
3　**Atlas** (posterior arch)
4　**Axis** (posterior arch)
5　Dura mater
6　**Spinal cord**
7　Spinal ganglion

8　Posterior root filaments (fila radicularia posterior)
9　Occipital belly of occipitofrontalis muscle
10　Splenius capitis muscle (cut and reflected)
11　Sternocleidomastoid muscle
12　Levator scapulae muscle
13　Posterior branches of spinal nerves
14　Arches of cervical vertebrae (cut)

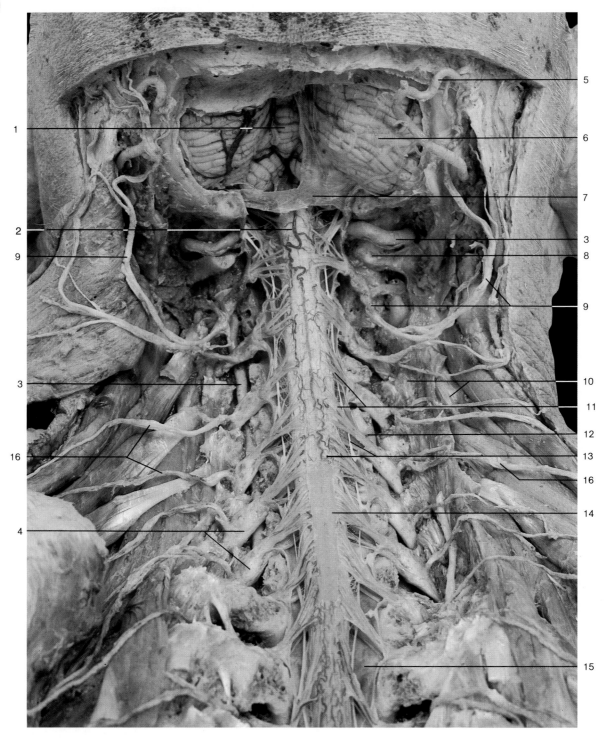

Neck, deepest layer. Spinal cord and medulla oblongata (dorsal aspect). Cranial cavity opened.

1 Vermis of the cerebellum
2 Medulla oblongata and posterior spinal artery
3 Vertebral artery
4 **Spinal ganglion**
5 Occipital artery
6 Cerebellum
7 **Cerebellomedullary cistern**
8 Atlas

9 Greater occipital nerve (C$_2$)
10 Levator scapulae muscle and intertransverse ligament
11 **Dorsal roots of spinal nerves**
12 Vertebral arch
13 **Denticulate ligament and arachnoid mater**
14 Area where pia mater has been removed
15 Dura mater
16 **Dorsal rami of spinal nerves**

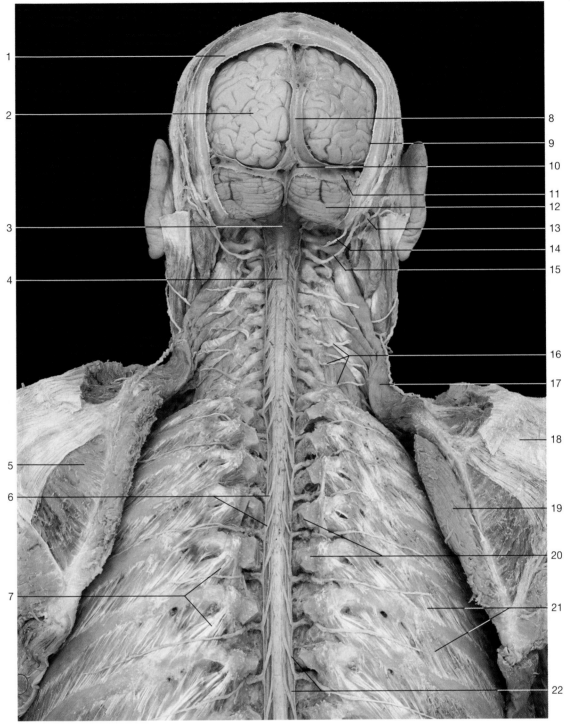

Neck (deepest layer). **Dissection of medulla oblongata and spinal cord** in relation to the brain (dorsal aspect).

1 Calvaria
2 Left hemisphere of the brain
3 Cerebellomedullary cistern
4 **Spinal cord**
5 Scapula with infraspinous muscle
6 Root filaments (fila radicularia posterior)
7 Levatores costarum muscles
8 Falx cerebri with sinus sagittalis superior
9 Subarachnoidal space
10 Confluens sinuum
11 Transverse sinus
12 Cerebellum
13 Occipital artery
14 Suboccipital nerve (C$_1$)
15 **Greater occipital nerve** (C$_2$)
16 Posterior branches of spinal nerves
17 Levator scapulae muscle
18 Deltoid muscle
19 Rhomboid muscles
20 Vertebral arches (cut)
21 External intercostal muscle
22 Dura mater

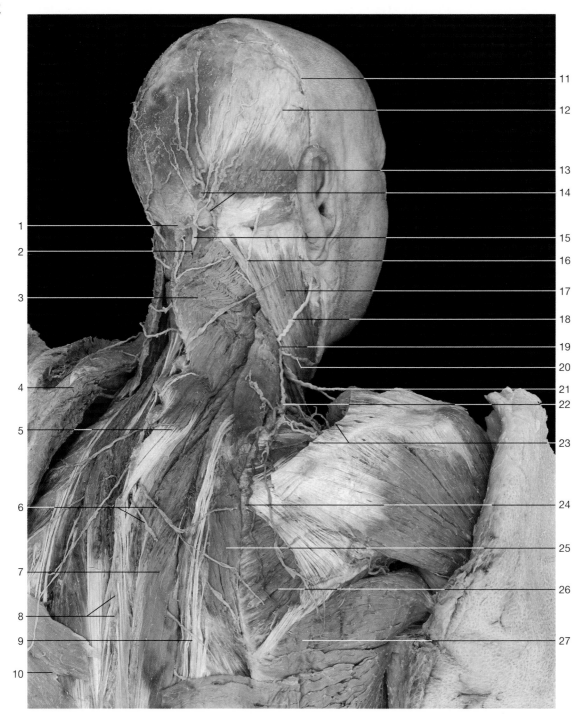

Dissection of neck and back, deeper layer (oblique lateral aspect after removal of trapezius muscle).

1	Protuberantia occipitalis externa	15	**Greater occipital nerve** (C_2)
2	Semispinalis capitis muscle	16	Lesser occipital nerve
3	**Splenius capitis muscle**	17	**Sternocleidomastoid muscle**
4	Scapula	18	Great auricular nerve
5	**Splenius cervicis muscle**	19	**Punctum nervosum**
6	Posterior branches of spinal nerves	20	Transverse cervical nerve
7	**Longissimus muscle**	21	Supraclavicular nerves
8	Spinous processes of thoracic vertebrae	22	**Accessory nerve (n. XI)**
9	Iliocostalis muscle	23	Trapezius muscle (cut edge)
10	Latissimus dorsi muscle	24	Medial margin of scapula
11	Epidermis of the head (scalp)	25	Rhomboid muscle
12	Galea aponeurotica	26	Infraspinous muscle
13	Occipital belly of occipitofrontalis muscle	27	Teres major muscle
14	Occipital artery		

Thoracic Organs

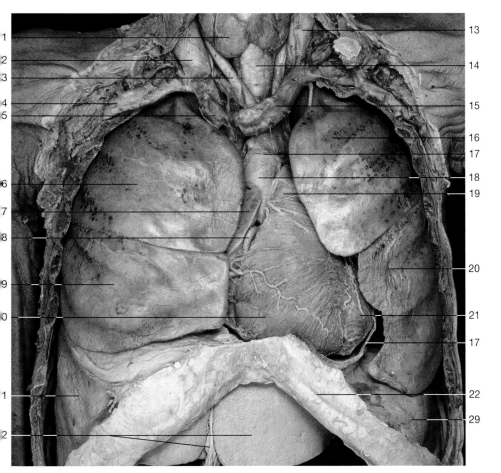

1	Thyroid gland
2	Internal jugular vein
3	Right common carotid artery
4	Right axillary vein
5	Right brachiocephalic vein
6	Superior lobe of right lung
7	Right atrium
8	Right coronary artery
9	Middle lobe of right lung
10	**Right ventricle**
11	Diaphragm
12	Liver (left lobe) and falciform ligament
13	Left internal jugular vein
14	**Trachea**
15	Left brachiocephalic vein
16	Superior lobe of left lung
17	Cut edge of pericardium
18	**Ascending aorta**
19	**Pulmonary trunk**
20	Inferior lobe of left lung
21	**Left ventricle**
22	Costal margin
23	Right pulmonary artery
24	Esophagus
25	Descending aorta
26	Pericardium
27	Aortic valve
28	Thymus
29	Diaphragm

Thoracic organs, heart and lungs in situ (ventral aspect). Anterior thoracic wall, parietal pleura and pericardium had been removed.

Divisions of mediastinum	Main content
Superior mediastinum (yellow)	Trachea, brachiocephalic veins, thymus, aortic arch, esophagus, thoracic duct
Middle mediastinum (light blue)	Heart, ascending aorta, pulmonary trunk, pulmonary veins, phrenic nerves
Posterior mediastinum (red)	Esophagus with vagus nerves, descending aorta, thoracic duct, sympathetic trunks
Anterior mediastinum (pink)	Small vessels, connective and fatty tissue, and thymus in the child

Sagittal section through thoracic cavity. The divisions of the mediastinum are indicated by colors.

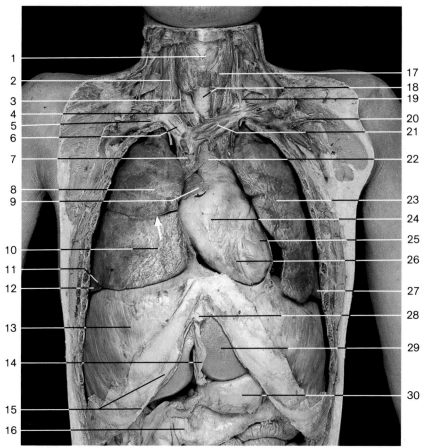

1 Cricothyroid muscle
2 Right internal jugular vein
3 Vagus nerve
4 Right common carotid artery
5 Right subclavian vein
6 Right brachiocephalic vein
7 Superior vena cava
8 Upper lobe of right lung
9 Right auricle
10 Middle lobe of right **lung**
11 Oblique fissure of right lung
12 Lower lobe of right lung
13 **Diaphragm**
14 Falciform ligament
15 Costal margin
16 Transverse colon
17 Thyroid gland
18 Trachea
19 Left internal jugular vein
20 Left cephalic vein
21 Left brachiocephalic vein
22 Pericardium (cut edge)
23 Upper lobe of left **lung**
24 **Right ventricle**
25 **Left ventricle**
26 Anterior interventricular sulcus
27 Lower lobe of left lung
28 Xiphoid process
29 **Liver**
30 **Stomach**
31 Pectoralis major muscle

Positions of thoracic organs. The anterior thoracic wall has been removed.
Arrow: horizontal fissure of right lung.

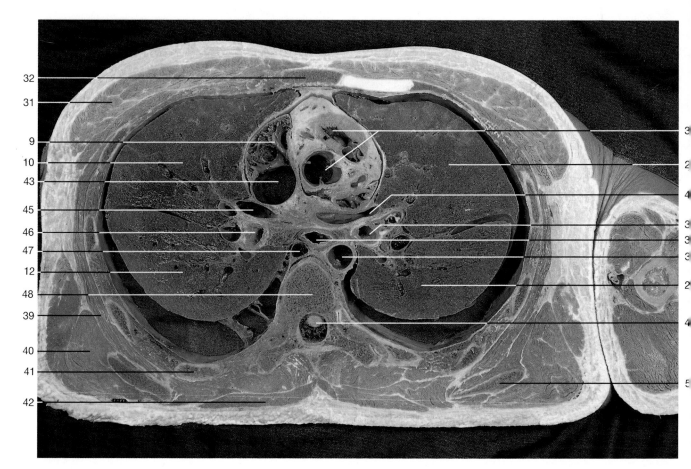

Horizontal section through the thorax at the level of the seventh thoracic vertebra (from below).

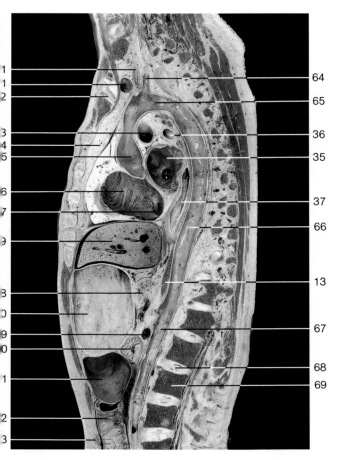

1	64
1	65
2	
3	36
4	35
5	
6	37
7	66
9	
3	13
0	
9	67
0	
1	68
	69
2	
3	

Sagittal section through the left thorax, 2 cm lateral to the median plane.

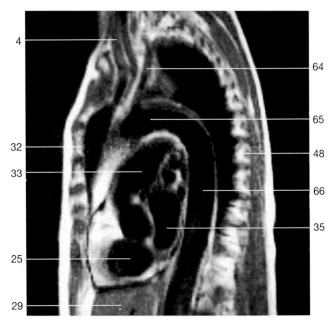

4	64
32	65
33	48
25	66
29	35

Sagittal section through the thorax. MRI scan.

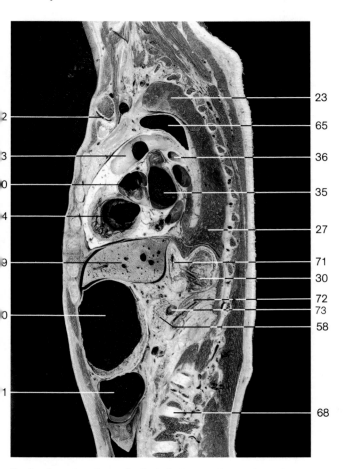

2	23
	65
3	36
0	35
4	27
9	71
	30
0	72
	73
	58
1	
	68

Sagittal section through the left thorax, 3.5 cm lateral to the median plane.

32 Sternum
33 Pulmonary trunk
34 Left ventricle and bulb of aorta
35 Left atrium
36 Left main bronchus
37 **Esophagus**
38 Descending aorta
39 Serratus anterior muscle
40 Teres major muscle
41 Rib
42 Trapezius muscle
43 Right atrium
44 Left pulmonary vein
45 Right pulmonary vein
46 Right main bronchus
47 Azygos vein
48 Body of vertebra
49 Spinal cord
50 Scapula
51 Left common carotid artery
52 Sternoclavicular articulation with disc
53 Right pulmonary artery
54 Remnants of thymus
55 Aortic bulb
56 Right atrium
57 Entrance of inferior vena cava in right atrium
58 **Pancreas**
59 Left renal vein
60 **Duodenum**
61 Transverse colon (dilated)
62 Small intestine
63 Umbilicus
64 Left subclavian artery
65 Aortic arch
66 **Thoracic aorta**
67 Abdominal aorta
68 Intervertebral disc
69 Body of lumbar vertebra
70 Aortic valve
71 Cardia of stomach
72 Suprarenal gland
73 Splenic vein

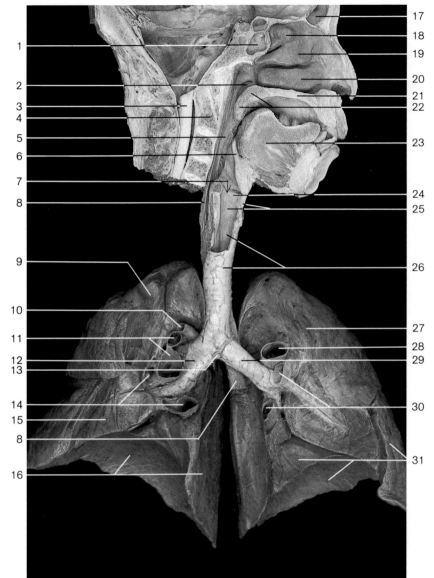

1 Sphenoid sinus
2 Pharyngeal opening of auditory tube
3 Spinal cord
4 Dens of axis
5 **Oropharynx** (oropharyngeal isthmus)
6 Epiglottis
7 Entrance of larynx
8 Esophagus
9 Upper lobe of right lung
10 Azygos vein
11 Branches of pulmonary artery
12 **Right main bronchus**
13 **Bifurcation of trachea**
14 Tributaries of right pulmonary veins
15 Middle lobe of right lung
16 Lower lobe of right lung
17 Frontal sinus
18 Superior nasal concha
19 Middle nasal concha
20 Inferior nasal concha
21 Hard palate
22 Soft palate with uvula
23 Tongue
24 Vocal fold
25 Larynx
26 Trachea
27 Upper lobe of left lung
28 Left pulmonary artery
29 **Left main bronchus**
30 Left pulmonary veins
31 Lower lobe of left lung

Respiratory system. The lungs have been fixed in expiration and turned laterally. Head bisected and turned laterally.

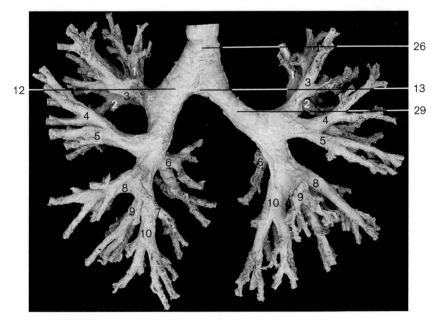

Bronchial tree (ventral aspect). The lung tissue has been removed. The bronchopulmonary segments are numbered 1–10.

▷
To page 237:

1 Nasal cavity
2 Pharynx
3 Larynx (thyroid cartilage)
4 Trachea
5 Upper lobe of right lung
6 Bifurcation of trachea
7 Right main bronchus
8 Horizontal fissure of right lung
9 Middle lobe of right lung
10 Oblique fissures of lungs
11 Lower lobe of right lung
12 Clavicle
13 Upper lobe of left lung
14 Left main bronchus
15 Bronchi supplying bronchopulmonary segments
16 Lower lobe of left lung
17 Costal margin
18 Hyoid bone
19 Right superior lobe bronchus
20 Right middle lobe bronchus
21 Right inferior lobe bronchus
22 Left superior lobe bronchus
23 Left inferior lobe bronchus
24 Segmental bronchi
25 Branches of pulmonary arteries
26 Branches of pulmonary veins

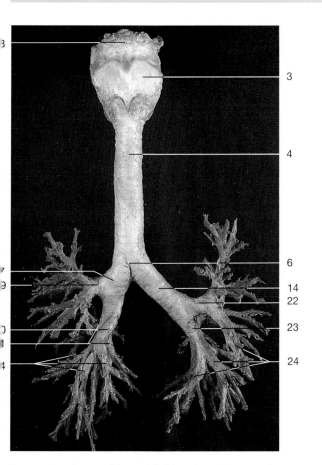

Larynx, trachea and bronchial tree (anterior aspect).

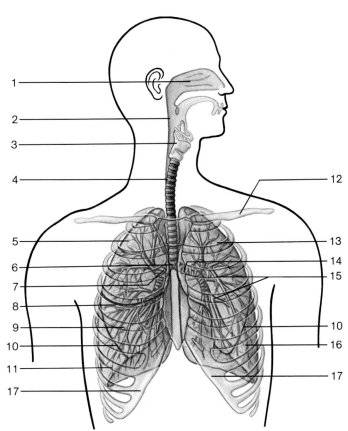

Organization and positions of respiratory organs.
(Schematic drawing.)

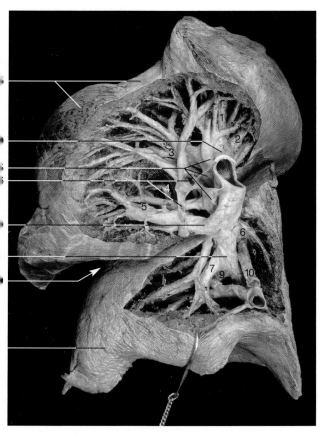

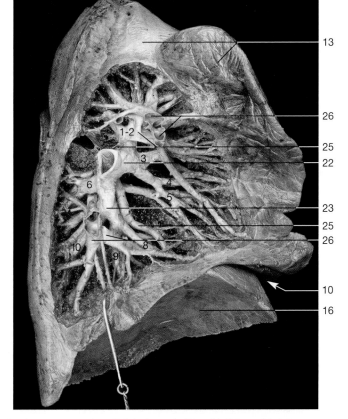

Mediastinal dissection of the bronchial tree, pulmonary veins, and pulmonary arteries of right lung (left) and left lung (right) (medial aspect). Segmental bronchi are numbered 1–10.

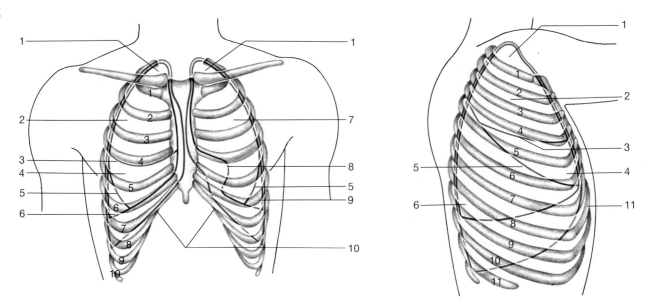

Surface projections of lungs and pleura on the thoracic wall. Left: anterior aspect; right: right-lateral aspect.
Red = margins of the lung; blue = margins of pleura. The numbers indicate ribs.

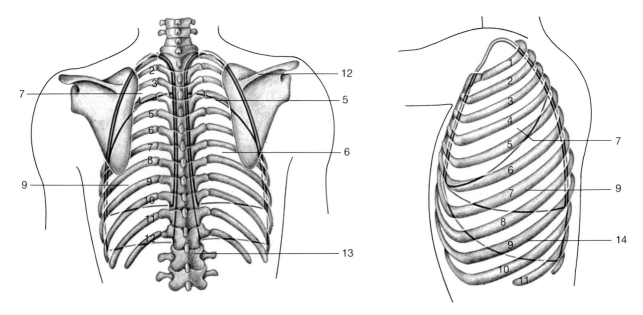

Surface projections of lungs and pleura on thoracic wall. Left: posterior aspect; right: left-lateral aspect.
Red = margins of lung; blue = margins of pleura. The numbers indicate ribs.

1 Apex of lung	6 Lower lobe of right lung	11 Costal margin
2 Upper lobe of right lung	7 Upper lobe of left lung	12 Spine of scapula
3 Horizontal fissure of right lung	8 Cardiac notch of left lung	13 First lumbar vertebra
4 Middle lobe of right lung	9 Lower lobe of left lung	14 Space between border of lung and pleura
5 Oblique fissures of lungs	10 Infrasternal angle	(costodiaphragmatic recess)

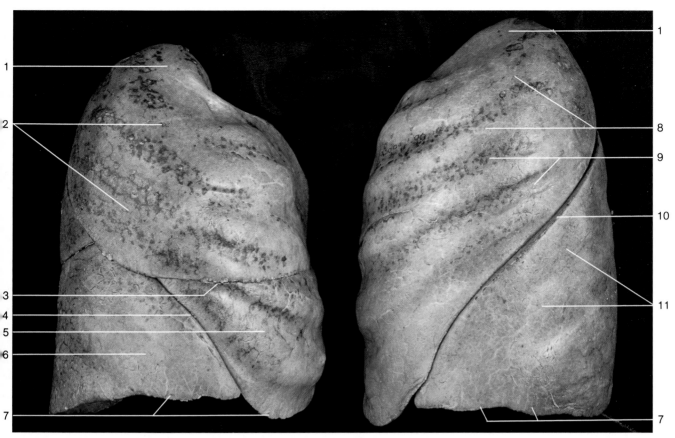

Right lung (lateral aspect).

Left lung (lateral aspect) .

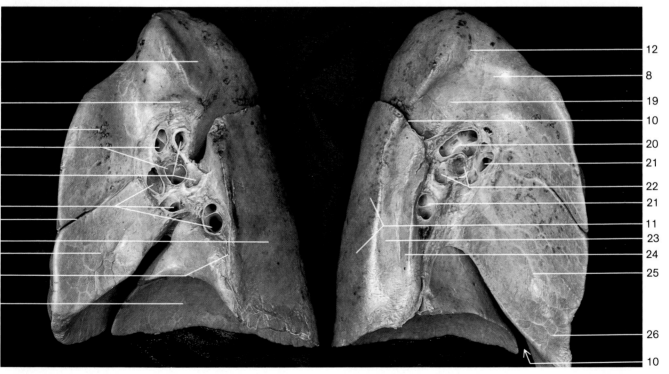

Right lung (medial aspect).

Left lung (medial aspect).

1	Apex of lung	8	Upper lobe of left lung
2	Upper lobe of right lung	9	Impressions of ribs
3	Horizontal fissure of right lung	10	Oblique fissure of left lung
4	Oblique fissure of right lung	11	Lower lobe of left lung
5	Middle lobe of right lung	12	Groove of subclavian artery
6	Lower lobe of right lung	13	Groove of azygos arch
7	Inferior border	14	Branches of right pulmonary artery

15	Bronchi	22	Left secondary bronchi
16	Right pulmonary veins	23	Groove of thoracic aorta
17	Pulmonary ligament	24	Groove of esophagus
18	Diaphragmatic surface	25	Cardiac impression
19	Groove of aortic arch	26	Lingula
20	Left pulmonary artery		
21	Branches of left pulmonary veins		

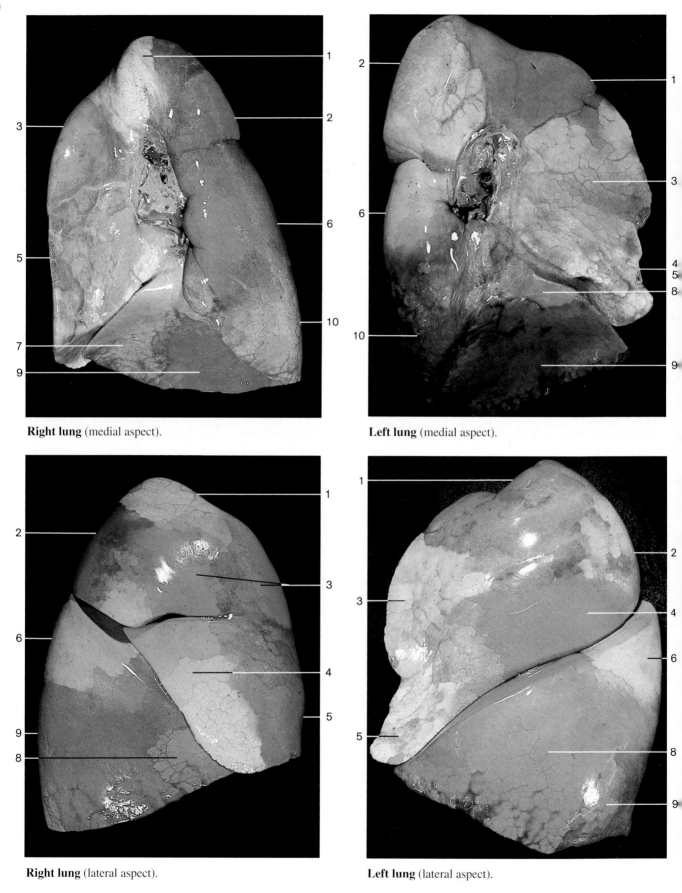

Right lung (medial aspect).

Left lung (medial aspect).

Right lung (lateral aspect).

Left lung (lateral aspect).

The bronchopulmonary segments of the lungs are differentiated by the various colors. Notice that there is no segment in the left lung that corresponds to the seventh segment of the right lung. Compare with the schematic drawing on the facing page.

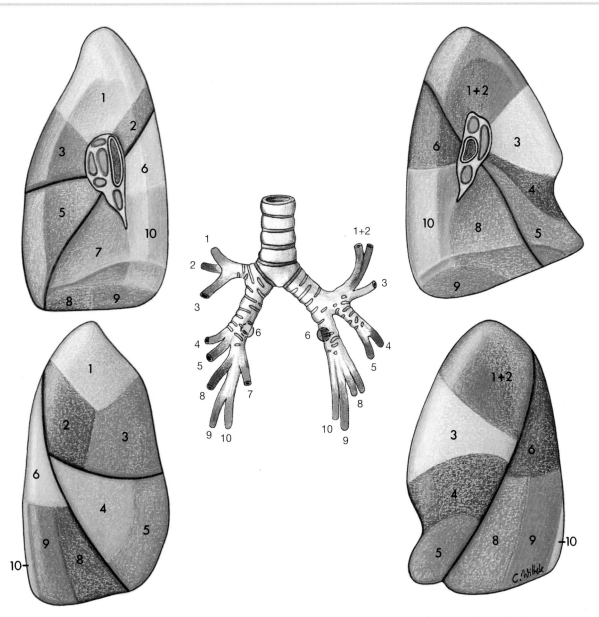

Distribution of bronchopulmonary segments of the lungs and their relation to the bronchial tree (after J. F. Huber).

The bronchopulmonary segments are morphologically and functionally separate independent respiratory units of the lung tissue. Each segment is surrounded by connective tissue which is continuous with the visceral pleura. The segmental bronchi in a segment are central, closely accompanied by branches of the pulmonary arteries, whereas the tributaries of the pulmonary veins run **between** the segments. Thus, the veins serve two adjacent segments which drain for the most part into more than one vein. A bronchopulmonary segment is therefore not a complete vascular unit, but segmentation is the result of a specific architecture of the lung vasculature.

Right lung				**Left lung**			
1 Apical segment	} Upper lobe bronchus			1+2 Apico-posterior segment	} Superior division		} Upper lobe bronchus
2 Posterior segment							
3 Anterior segment				3 Anterior segment			
4 Lateral segment	} Middle lobe bronchus			4 Superior lingular segment	} Inferior division		
5 Medial segment				5 Inferior lingular segment			
6 Superior (apical) segment	} Lower lobe bronchus			6 Superior (apical) segment	} Lower lobe bronchus		
7 Medial basal segment				7 Absent			
8 Anterior basal segment				8 Anteromedial basal segment			
9 Lateral basal segment				9 Lateral basal segment			
10 Posterior basal segment				10 Posterior basal segment			

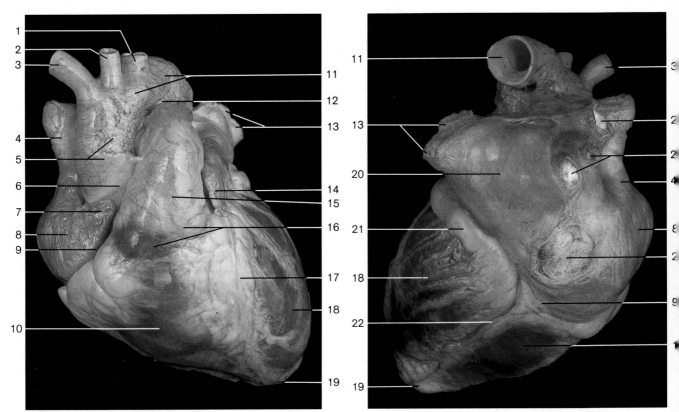

Heart of 30-year-old woman (anterior aspect).

Heart of 30-year-old woman (oblique posterior view).

1 Left subclavian artery	9 Coronary sulcus
2 Left common carotid artery	10 **Right ventricle**
3 Brachiocephalic trunk	11 Aortic arch
4 Superior vena cava	12 Ligamentum arteriosum
5 Ascending aorta	13 Left pulmonary veins
6 Bulb of the aorta	14 Left auricle
7 Right auricle	15 **Pulmonary trunk**
8 **Right atrium**	16 Sinus of pulmonary trunk
	17 Anterior interventricular sulcus

18 **Left ventricle**
19 Apex of the heart
20 **Left atrium**
21 Epicardial fat overlying coronary sinus
22 Posterior interventricular sulcus
23 Right pulmonary artery
24 Right pulmonary veins
25 Inferior vena cava

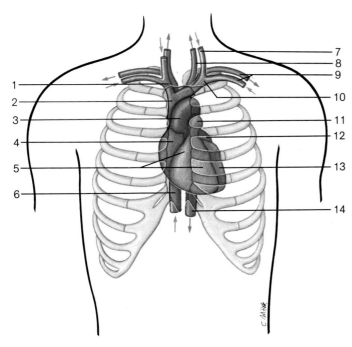

Position of heart and its vessels within the thorax.
(Schematic drawing.)

1 Right brachiocephalic vein
2 Superior vena cava
3 Ascending aorta
4 Right atrium
5 Right ventricle
6 Inferior vena cava
7 Left internal jugular vein
8 Left common carotid artery
9 Left axillary artery and vein
10 Left brachiocephalic vein
11 Pulmonary trunk
12 Left auricle
13 Left ventricle
14 Descending aorta

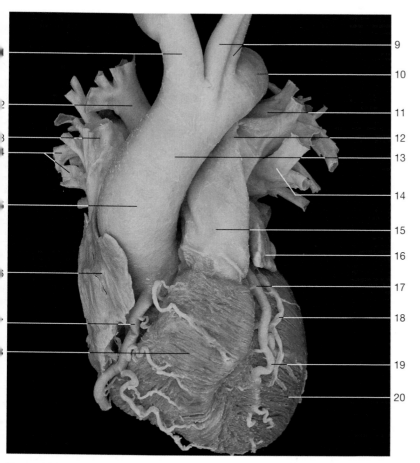

1 Brachiocephalic trunk
2 Right pulmonary artery
3 Superior vena cava
4 Right pulmonary veins
5 **Ascending aorta**
6 Right atrium
7 **Right coronary artery**
8 **Right ventricle**
9 Left common carotid artery and left
   subclavian artery
10 Descending aorta (thoracic part)
11 Ligamentum arteriosum (remnant of
    ductus arteriosus Botalli)
12 Left pulmonary artery
13 **Aortic arch**
14 Left pulmonary veins
15 **Pulmonary trunk**
16 Left atrium
17 **Left coronary artery**
18 Diagonal branch of left coronary artery
19 Interventricular branch of left coronary
    artery
20 **Left ventricle**
21 Right brachiocephalic vein
22 Thoracic wall
23 Liver
24 Aortic valve
25 Chordae tendineae
26 Papillary muscles
27 Stomach

Heart with related vessels. Dissection of coronary arteries (anterior aspect, systolic phase of heart action).

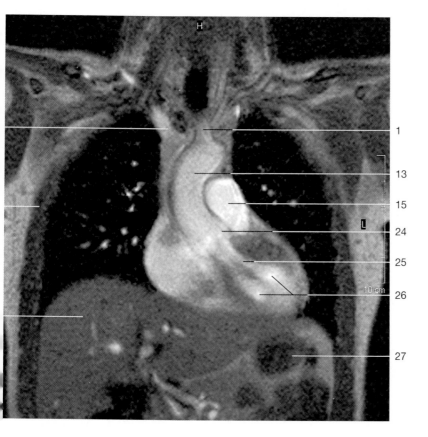

Coronal section through the thorax at the level of the ascending aorta (MRI scan, courtesy of Prof. W. Bautz, University of Erlangen, Germany).

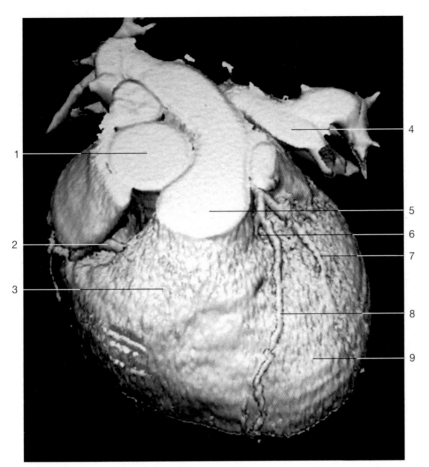

1   Ascending aorta
2   **Right coronary artery**
3   Right ventricle
4   Left atrium
5   **Pulmonary trunk**
6   Septal branch of left coronary artery
7   Diagonal branch
8   **Anterior interventricular branch** of left
    coronary artery
9   Left ventricle
10 Aortic root
11 Superior vena cava
12 Circumflex branch of left coronary artery
13 Sternum

Human heart (3-D reconstruction of electron beam CT scans as "Shaded Surface Display"[1]).

Electron beam tomographic image of the human heart (axial section after injection of contrast medium[1]).

[1] Courtesy of Drs. W. Moshage, S. Achenbach
     and D. Ropers, Dept. of Internal Medicine II
     (Chairman: Prof. W. G. Daniel), University of
     Erlangen-Nürnberg, Germany.

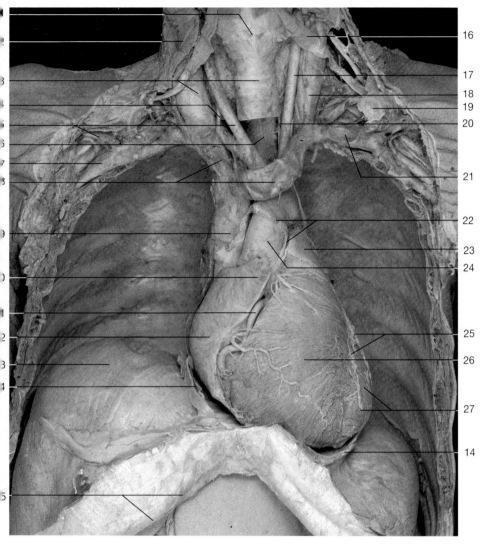

1 Larynx (thyroid cartilage)
2 Sternocleidomastoid muscle (divided)
3 Trachea (divided) and right internal jugular vein
4 Vagus nerve
5 Right common carotid artery and cephalic vein
6 Esophagus
7 Right axillary vein
8 Right and left brachiocephalic veins
9 **Superior vena cava**
10 Right auricle
11 Right **coronary artery**
12 **Right atrium**
13 Diaphragm
14 Pericardium (cut edges)
15 Costal margin
16 Omohyoid muscle
17 Left **common carotid artery**
18 Left internal jugular vein
19 Clavicle (divided)
20 Left recurrent laryngeal nerve
21 **Subclavian vein**
22 Pericardial reflection
23 **Pulmonary trunk**
24 **Ascending aorta**
25 Anterior interventricular sulcus and anterior interventricular branch of left coronary artery
26 **Right ventricle**
27 **Left ventricle**
28 Aortic valve
29 Tricuspid or right atrioventricular valve
30 Inferior vena cava
31 Pulmonary veins
32 Pulmonary valve
33 Left atrioventricular (bicuspid or mitral) valve

Heart and related vessels in situ (anterior aspect). Anterior thoracic wall, pericardium and epicardium have been removed; trachea divided.

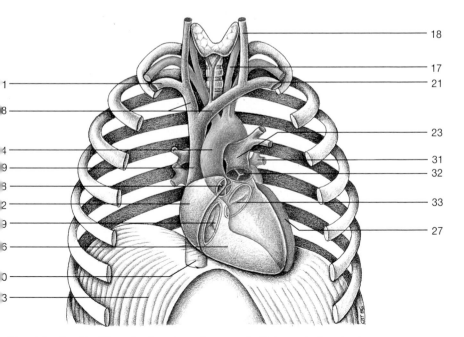

Heart in situ. Position of valves (anterior aspect). (Schematic drawing.)

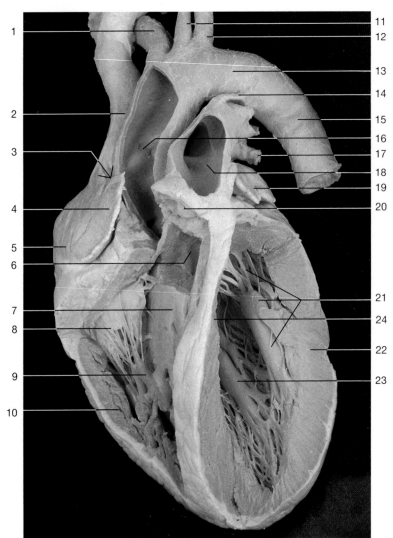

1
2
3
4
5
6
7
8
9
10

11
12
13
14
15
16
17
18
19
20
21
24
22
23

1 Brachiocephalic trunk
2 Superior vena cava
3 Sulcus terminalis
4 Right auricle
5 Right atrium
6 **Aortic valve**
7 Conus arteriosus (interventricular septum)
8 **Right atrioventricular (tricuspid) valve**
9 **Anterior papillary muscle**
10 Myocardium of right ventricle
11 Left common carotid artery
12 Left subclavian artery
13 **Aortic arch**
14 Ligamentum arteriosum (remnant of ductus arteriosus)
15 Thoracic aorta (descending aorta)
16 **Ascending aorta**
17 Left pulmonary vein
18 **Pulmonary trunk**
19 Left auricle
20 Pulmonic valve
21 **Anterior papillary muscle** with chordae tendineae
22 Myocardium of left ventricle
23 Posterior papillary muscle
24 Interventricular septum
25 Right and left brachiocephalic veins
26 **Chordae tendineae**
27 Papillary muscles of right ventricle
28 Left atrium
29 Infundibulum
30 Anterior papillary muscle of left ventricle
31 Left atrioventricular (bicuspid or mitral) valve and chordae tendineae
32 Apex of heart
33 Inferior vena cava
34 Liver
35 Aorta (pars abdominalis)

Anterior aspect of the heart. Dissection of the four valves.

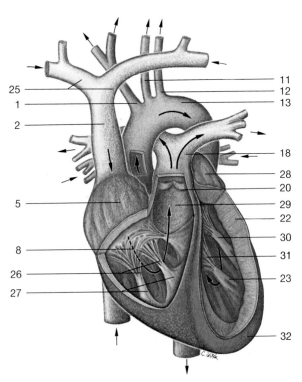

Circulation within the heart (anterior aspect; arrows = direction of blood flow).

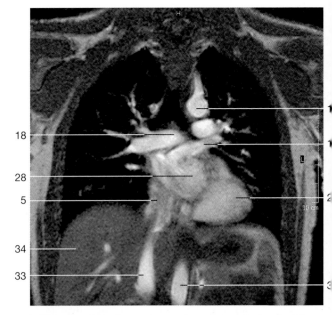

MRI scan of the heart (coronal section at the level of the left atrium).

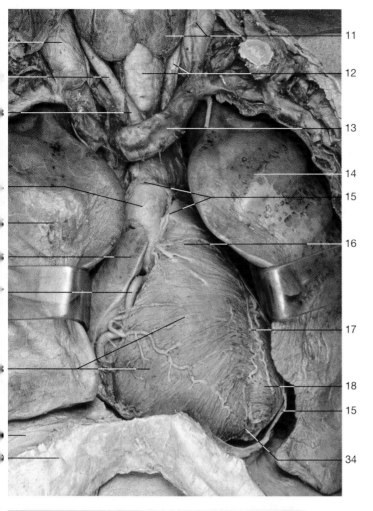

Heart in situ. Myocardium and coronary arteries (anterior aspect).

1   Internal jugular vein
2   Common carotid artery
3   Brachiocephalic trunk
4   **Ascending aorta**
5   Right lung
6   Right auricle
7   **Right coronary artery**
8   **Myocardium of right ventricle**
9   Diaphragm
10 Costal margin
11 Thyroid gland and internal jugular vein
12 Trachea and left common carotid artery
13 Left brachiocephalic vein
14 Left lung
15 **Pericardium** (cut edge)
16 Pulmonary trunk
17 Anterior interventricular artery
18 **Myocardium of left ventricle**
19 **Muscular vortex** (right ventricle)
20 Posterior interventricular sulcus
21 Anterior interventricular sulcus
22 **Muscular vortex** (left ventricle)
23 Aortic arch
24 Left atrium
25 Coronary sinus
26 Superior vena cava
27 Right pulmonary vein
28 Right atrium
29 Inferior vena cava
30 Coronary sulcus
31 Myocardium of left ventricle
32 Left pulmonary artery
33 Left pulmonary vein
34 Apex of heart

Heart (posterior aspect). The myocardium of the left ventricle has been fenestrated to show the muscle fiber bundles of the deeper layer with their more circular course.

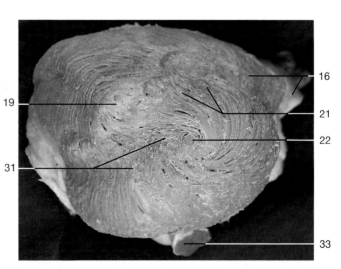

Vortex of cardiac muscle fibers (from below).

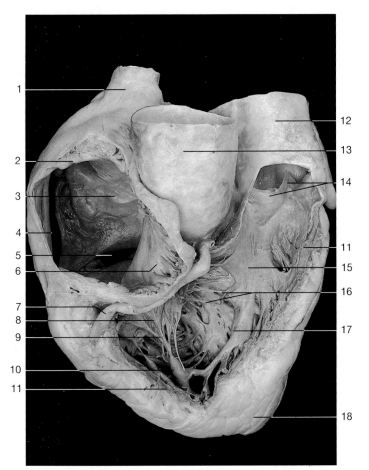

1   Superior vena cava
2   Crista terminalis
3   Fossa ovalis
4   Opening of inferior vena cava
5   Opening of coronary sinus
6   Right auricle
7   Right coronary artery and coronary sulcus
8   **Anterior cusp** of **tricuspid valve**
9   Chordae tendineae
10 **Anterior papillary muscle**
11 Myocardium
12 Pulmonary trunk
13 Ascending aorta
14 **Pulmonic valve**
15 Conus arteriosus (interventricular septum)
16 Septal papillary muscles
17 Septomarginal or moderator band
18 Apex of heart
19 Left auricle
20 **Aortic valve**
21 **Left ventricle**
22 Pulmonary veins
23 Position of fossa ovalis
24 **Left atrium**
25 **Left atrioventricular** (bicuspid or **mitral) valve**
26 Right atrium
27 Pericardium
28 Posterior papillary muscle
29 **Right ventricle**
30 Interventricular septum

Right heart (anterior aspect). Anterior wall of right atrium and ventricle removed.

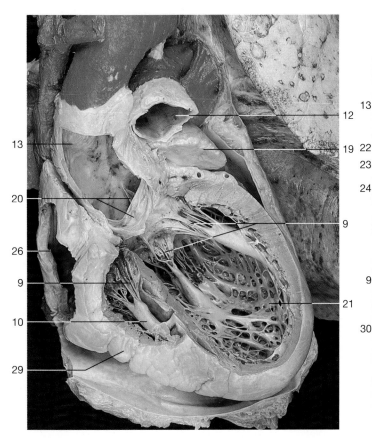

Heart, left ventricle with mitral valve, papillary muscles and aortic valve (anterior portion of the heart removed).

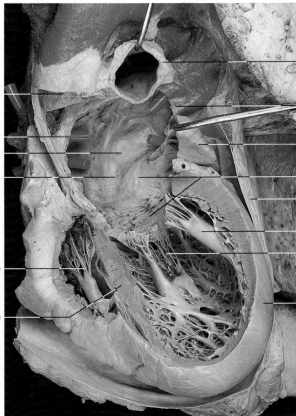

Heart, left ventricle and atrium (opened) showing the posterior part of the mitral valve with papillary muscles.

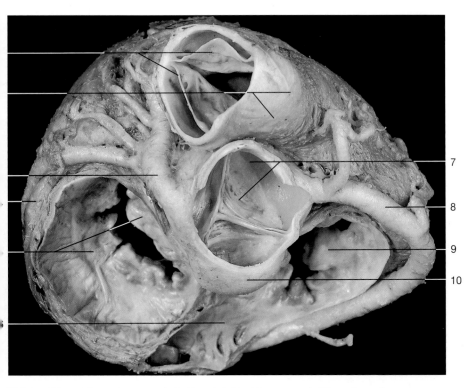

1   Pulmonic valve
2   Sinus of pulmonary trunk
3   Left coronary artery
4   Great cardiac vein
5   Left atrioventricular (mitral) valve
6   Coronary sinus
7   Aortic valve
8   Right coronary artery
9   Right atrioventricular (tricuspid) valve
10 Bulb of aorta
11 Anterior semilunar cusp of pulmonic valve
12 Left semilunar cusp of pulmonic valve
13 Right semilunar cusp of pulmonic valve
14 Left semilunar cusp of aortic valve
15 Right semilunar cusp of aortic valve
16 Posterior semilunar cusp of aortic valve
17 Right atrium
18 Anterior cusp of tricuspid valve
19 Chordae tendineae
20 Trabeculae carneae
21 Interventricular septum
22 Septal cusp of tricuspid valve
23 Anterior papillary muscle
24 Myocardium of right ventricle

Valves of heart (superior aspect). Left and right atria removed. Dissection of coronary arteries. Above: anterior wall of the heart.

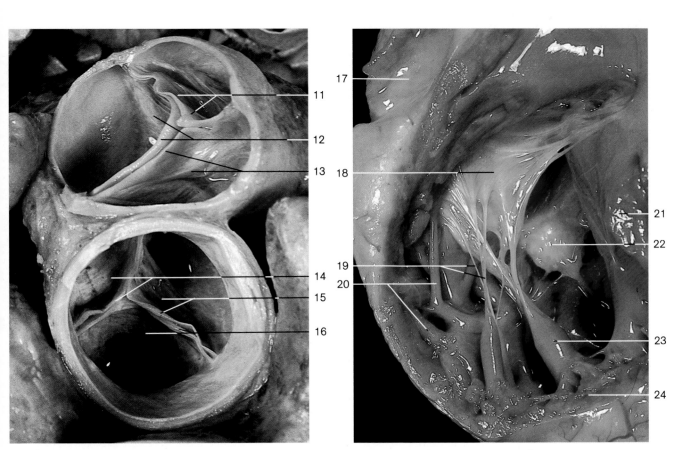

Pulmonic and aortic valves (from above). Anterior wall of the heart at the top. Both valves are closed.

Right atrioventricular (tricuspid) valve (anterior aspect after removal of the anterior wall of the right ventricle).

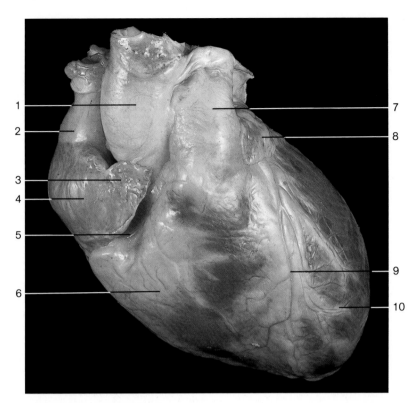

Heart, fixed in **diastole** (anterior aspect). The ventricles are relaxed, atria contracted.

1 Ascending aorta
2 Superior vena cava
3 Right auricle
4 **Right atrium**
5 Coronary sulcus
6 Right ventricle
7 Pulmonary trunk
8 Left auricle
9 Anterior interventricular sulcus
10 **Left ventricle**
11 Right pulmonary artery
12 Sulcus terminalis with sinoatrial node
13 Line indicating plane of position of valves
14 Myocardium of right atrium
15 Inferior vena cava
16 Valve of pulmonary trunk
17 Tricuspid valve
18 Myocardium of right ventricle

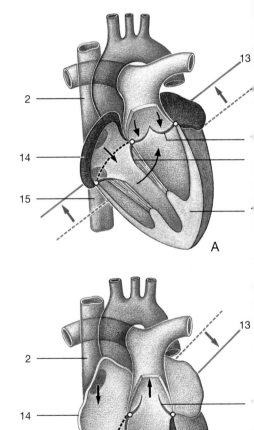

Morphological changes during heart movements. Note the changes in position of the valves (red arrows). Contracted portions of heart are indicated in black.
A. **Diastole:** muscles of the ventricles relaxed, atrioventricular valves open, semilunar valves closed.
B. **Systole:** muscles of ventricles contracted, atrioventricular valves closed, semilunar valves open.

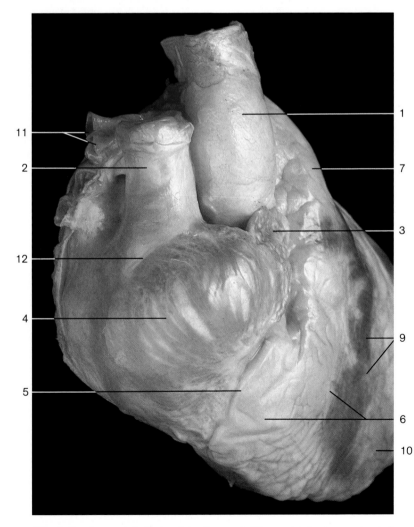

Heart, fixed in **systole** (anterolateral aspect). The ventricles are contracted, atria dilated.

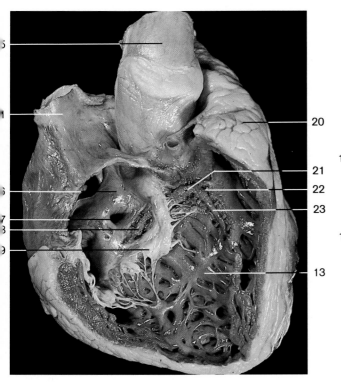

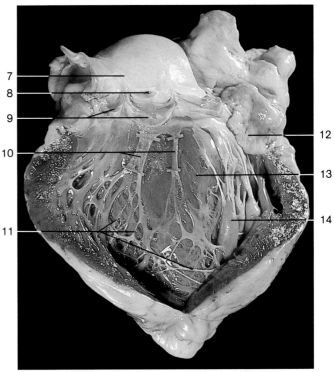

Right ventricle, dissection of **atrioventricular node, atrioventricular bundle (bundle of His)** and right limb or bundle branch (probes).

Left ventricle, dissection of the left limb or bundle branch of conducting system (probes).

1	Superior vena cava	5	Muscle fiber bundles of right atrium
2	Sulcus terminalis	6	Coronary sulcus (with right coronary artery)
3	Bulb of aorta	7	Aortic sinus
4	Sinoatrial node (arrows)	8	Entrance to left coronary artery

9   Aortic valve
10   Branches of **left bundle branch**
11   Purkinje fibers
12   Left auricle
13   Interventricular septum
14   Papillary muscles
15   Ascending aorta
16   Right atrium
17   Opening of coronary sinus
18   **Atrioventricular node**
19   Septal cusp of tricuspid valve
20   Pulmonary trunk
21   **Atrioventricular bundle** (bundle of His)
22   Bifurcation of atrioventricular bundle
23   **Right bundle branch**
24   Inferior vena cava
25   Left atrium
26   Left bundle branch
27   Papillary muscles with Purkinje fibers

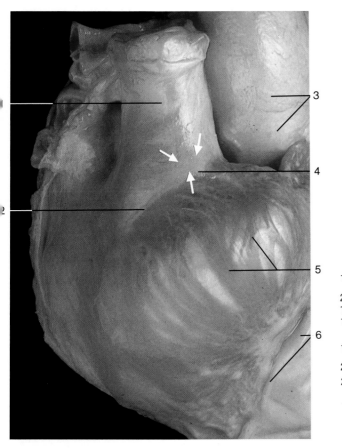

Right atrium, anterior wall, showing the location of the **sinoatrial node** (arrows).

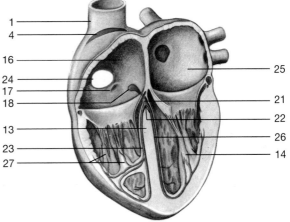

Conducting system of the heart.
(Schematic drawing.)

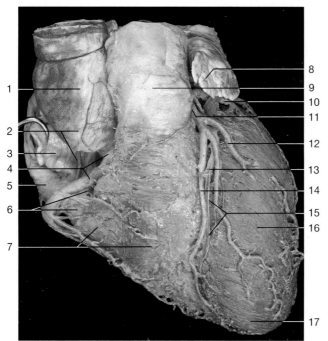

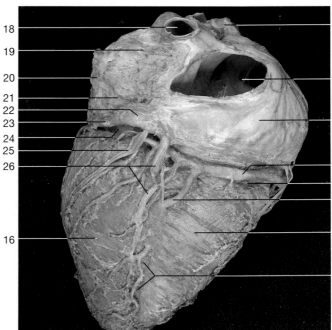

Coronary arteries (anterior aspect). The epicardium and subepicardial fatty tissue have been removed. The arteries have been injected with red resin from the aorta.

Right coronary artery and veins of the heart (dorsal aspect). The epicardium and subepicardial fatty tissue have been removed.

1   Ascending aorta
2   Aortic bulb and (in the above specimen) sinoatrial branch of right coronary artery
3   Right auricle
4   **Right coronary artery**
5   Right atrium
6   Coronary sulcus
7   Right ventricle
8   Left auricle
9   Pulmonary trunk

10   Circumflex branch of left coronary artery
11   **Left coronary artery**
12   Diagonal branch of left artery
13   Great cardiac vein
14   Anterior interventricular artery
15   Anterior interventricular sulcus
16   Left ventricle
17   Apex of heart
18   Right pulmonary vein
19   Left atrium
20   Left pulmonary veins
21   Oblique vein of left atrium (Marshall's vein)
22   **Coronary sinus**
23   **Great cardiac vein**
24   Coronary sulcus (posterior portion)
25   Posterior vein of left ventricle
26   **Middle cardiac vein**
27   Left pulmonary artery
28   Inferior vena cava
29   Right atrium
30   Posterior interventricular branch of right coronary artery
31   Posterior interventricular sulcus
32   Superior vena cava
33   Right marginal branch
34   Branch of sinoatrial node
35   Minimal cardiac veins
36   **Small cardiac vein**

Vessels of the heart. Coronary arteries (red) and veins (blue) of the heart (anterior aspect).

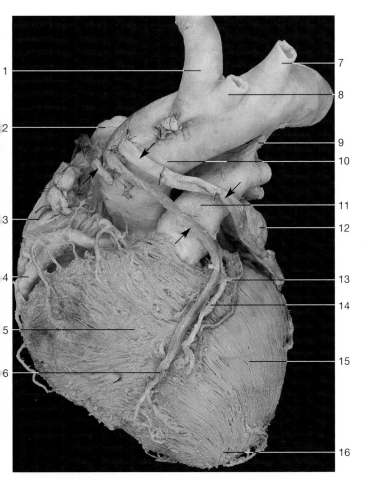

1 Brachiocephalic trunk
2 Superior vena cava
3 Right atrium
4 **Right coronary artery**
5 **Right ventricle**
6 Connection of one of the bypass vessels with the anterior interventricular artery
7 Left subclavian artery
8 Left common carotid artery
9 **Ductus arteriosus** (Botalli) (still open)
10 **Ascending aorta** with three bypass vessels implanted
11 Pulmonary trunk
12 Left atrium
13 Circumflex branch of left coronary artery
14 **Anterior interventricular branch** of left coronary artery
15 **Left ventricle**
16 Apex of heart
17 Sternum
18 Right ventricle
19 Liver
20 Spinal cord
21 **Trachea**
22 Aorta
23 Body of thoracic vertebrae
24 Pulmonary artery
25 Inferior vena cava
26 Hepatic vein

Heart, coronary vessels after implantation of three bypass vessels (anterior aspect). The ductus arteriosus (9) is still open.

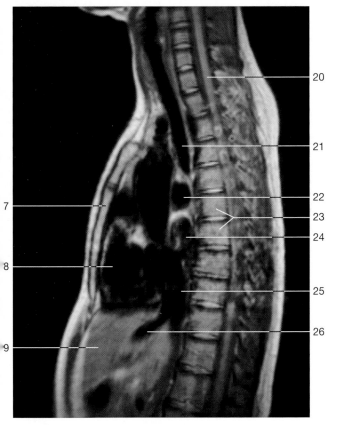

Sagittal section through the thoracic cavity (MRI scan at the level of the trachea) (21).

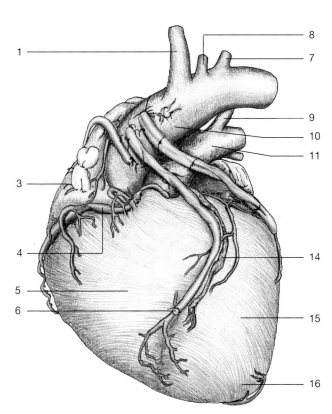

Heart, coronary vessels after implantation of three bypass vessels (yellow) (schematic drawing of the specimen above).

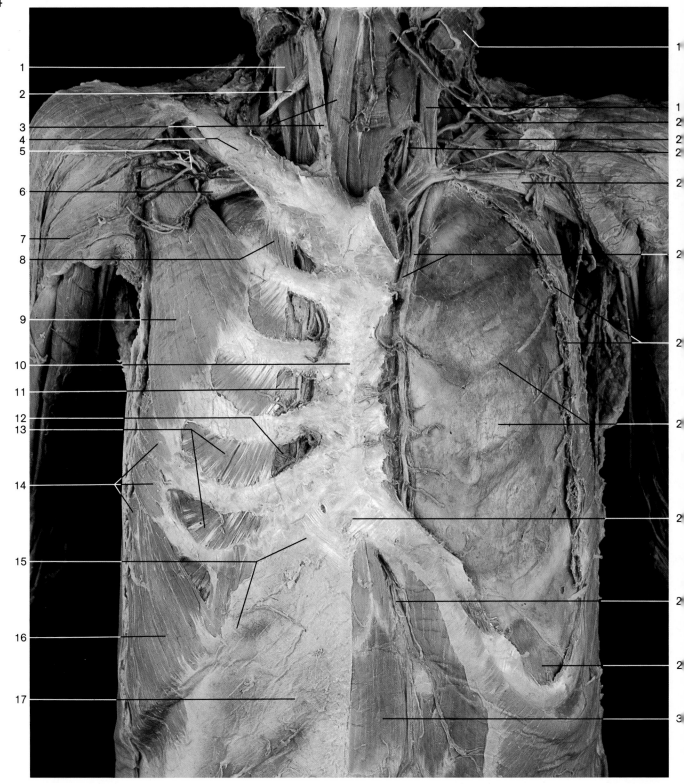

Thoracic wall and organs (ventral aspect). The left clavicle and ribs have been partially removed, and the right intercostal spaces have been opened to show the internal thoracic vein and artery.

1 Right internal jugular vein	11 Right internal thoracic artery and vein	21 Brachial plexus
2 Omohyoid muscle	12 Fascicles of transversus thoracis muscle	22 Vagus nerve
3 Sternohyoid muscle and external jugular vein	13 **Internal intercostal muscles**	23 Left axillary vein
4 Clavicle	14 Serratus anterior muscle	24 Left **internal thoracic artery and vein**
5 Thoracoacromial artery	15 Costal margin	25 Ribs and thoracic wall (cut)
6 Right **subclavian vein**	16 External abdominal oblique muscle	26 Costal pleura
7 Pectoralis major muscle	17 Anterior sheath of rectus abdominis muscle	27 Xiphoid process
8 External intercostal muscle	18 Sternocleidomastoid muscle	28 **Superior epigastric artery**
9 Pectoralis minor muscle	19 Left internal jugular vein	29 Diaphragm
10 Body of sternum	20 Transverse cervical artery	30 Rectus abdominis muscle

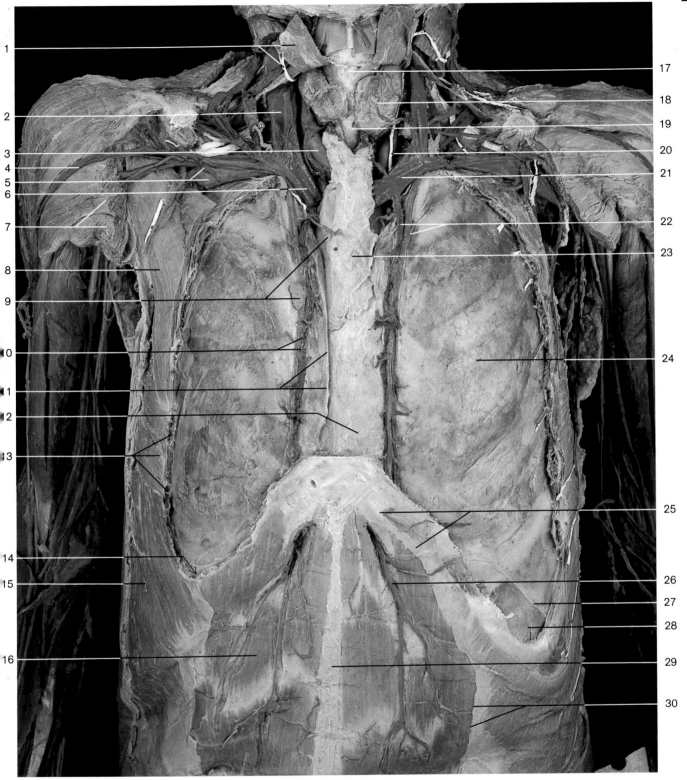

Thoracic organs, anterior mediastinum and pleura. Ribs, clavicle and sternum have been partly removed.
Red = arteries; blue = veins; green = lymph vessels and nodes.

1	Sternothyroid muscle and its nerve (a branch of the ansa cervicalis)	11 Anterior margin of costal pleura
2	Right **internal jugular vein**	12 **Pericardium**
3	Right common carotid artery	13 Fifth and sixth ribs (divided) and serratus anterior muscle
4	Cephalic vein	14 **Costodiaphragmatic recess**
5	Right **subclavian vein**	15 External abdominal oblique muscle
6	**Right brachiocephalic vein**	16 Rectus abdominis muscle
7	Pectoralis major muscle (divided)	17 Larynx (thyroid cartilage)
8	Pectoralis minor muscle (divided)	18 Thyroid gland
9	Parasternal lymph nodes	19 Trachea
10	Internal thoracic artery and vein	20 Left vagus nerve

21 Left brachiocephalic vein
22 Left **internal thoracic artery and vein**
23 Thymus
24 **Costal pleura**
25 Costal margin
26 **Superior epigastric artery**
27 Margin of costal pleura
28 **Diaphragm**
29 **Linea alba**
30 Cut edge of anterior sheath of rectus abdominis muscle

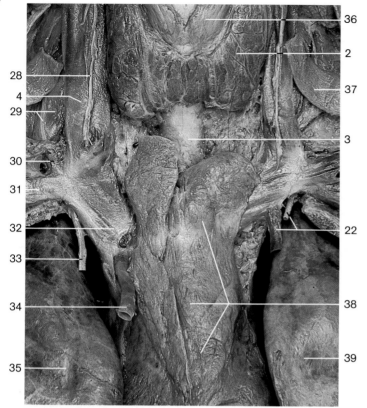

The **thymus** above the heart, showing its position and size.

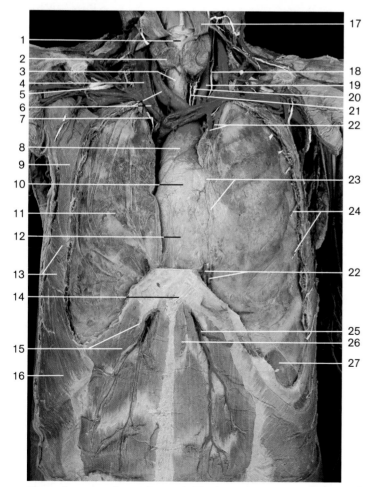

Thoracic organs (ventral aspect). The internal thoracic vessels have been removed, and the anterior margins of the pleura and lungs have been slightly reflected to display the **anterior** and **middle mediastinum,** including the **heart** and **great vessels.**

1 Larynx (thyroid cartilage)
2 Thyroid gland
3 **Trachea**
4 Internal jugular vein
5 Brachial plexus
6 Right brachiocephalic vein and common carotid artery
7 Right phrenic nerve
8 **Ascending aorta**
9 Pectoralis minor muscle (divided)
10 Pulmonary trunk (covered by pericardium)
11 **Costal pleura**
12 Pericardium and **heart**
13 Serratus anterior muscle
14 Xiphoid process
15 Costal margin
16 External abdominal oblique muscle
17 Sternothyroid muscle (divided and reflected)
18 Vagus nerve
19 Left common carotid artery
20 Left sympathetic trunk
21 Left recurrent laryngeal nerve
22 Left internal thoracic artery and vein (divided)
23 Margin of costal pleura
24 Intercostal nerves and vessels
25 Superior epigastric artery
26 Rectus abdominis muscle
27 **Diaphragm**
28 Ansa cervicalis
29 Phrenic nerve and scalenus anterior muscle
30 External jugular vein (divided)
31 Right subclavian vein
32 Right brachiocephalic vein
33 Internal thoracic artery (divided)
34 Internal thoracic vein (divided)
35 Right lung
36 Cricothyroid muscle
37 Omohyoid muscle
38 **Thymus**
39 Left lung

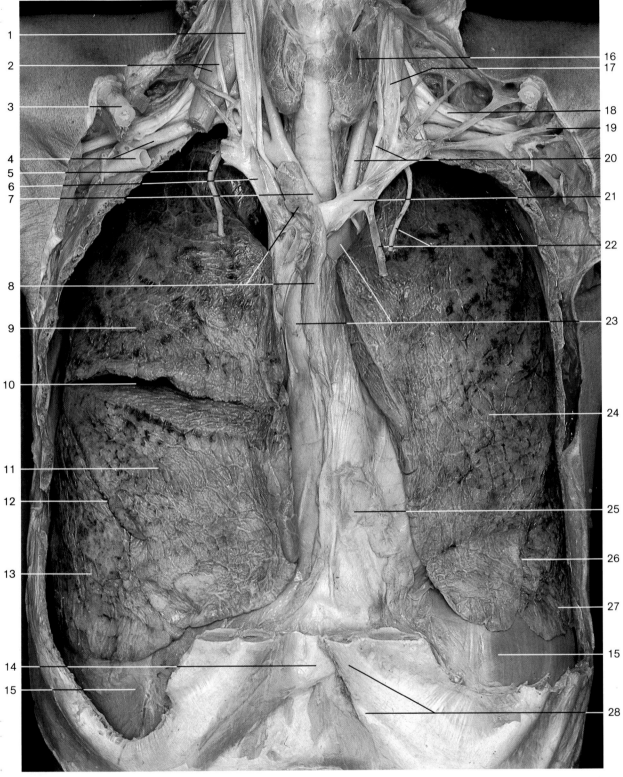

Thoracic organs (ventral aspect). The pleura has been opened and the lungs exposed. Remnants of the thymus and pericardium are seen.

1   Right internal jugular vein
2   Phrenic nerve and scalenus anterior muscle
3   Clavicle (divided)
4   Right subclavian artery and vein
5   Internal thoracic artery
6   **Right brachiocephalic vein**
7   Brachiocephalic trunk
8   Thymus (atrophic)
9   Upper lobe of right **lung**
10 Horizontal fissure of right lung (incomplete)

11 Middle lobe of right lung
12 Oblique fissure of right **lung**
13 Lower lobe of right lung
14 Xiphoid process
15 **Diaphragm**
16 **Thyroid gland**
17 Left internal jugular vein
18 Brachial plexus
19 Left cephalic vein

20 Left common carotid artery and vagus nerve
21 **Left brachiocephalic vein**
22 Internal thoracic artery and vein (divided)
23 **Ascending aorta** and aortic arch
24 Upper lobe of left **lung**
25 **Pericardium**
26 Oblique fissure of left lung
27 Lower lobe of left lung
28 Costal margin

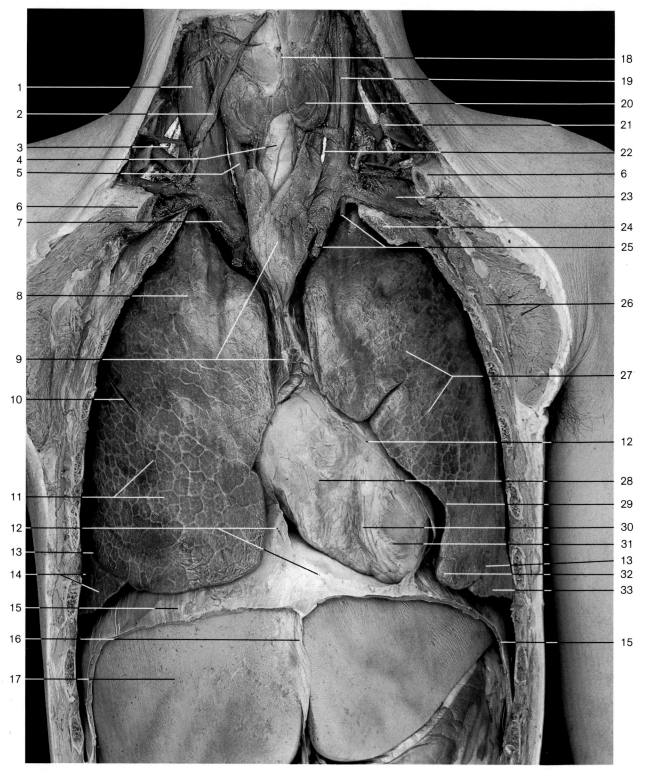

Thoracic organs (ventral aspect). The thoracic wall, costal pleura, pericardium and diaphragm have been partly removed.

1 Internal jugular vein	13 Oblique fissure of lung	25 Internal thoracic artery and vein
2 External jugular vein (displaced medially)	14 Lower lobe of right lung	26 Pectoralis major and pectoralis minor muscles
3 Brachial plexus	15 **Diaphragm**	(cut edges)
4 Trachea	16 Falciform ligament	27 **Upper lobe of left lung**
5 Right common carotid artery	17 **Liver**	28 **Right ventricle**
6 Clavicle (divided)	18 Location of larynx	29 Cardiac notch of left lung
7 Right brachiocephalic vein	19 Left internal jugular vein	30 Interventricular sulcus of heart
8 Upper lobe of right lung	20 Thyroid gland	31 **Left ventricle**
9 **Thymus** (atrophic)	21 Omohyoid muscle (divided)	32 Lingula
10 Horizontal fissure of right lung	22 Vagus nerve	33 Lower lobe of left lung
11 Middle lobe of right lung	23 Left subclavian vein	
12 Pericardium (cut edges)	24 First rib (divided)	

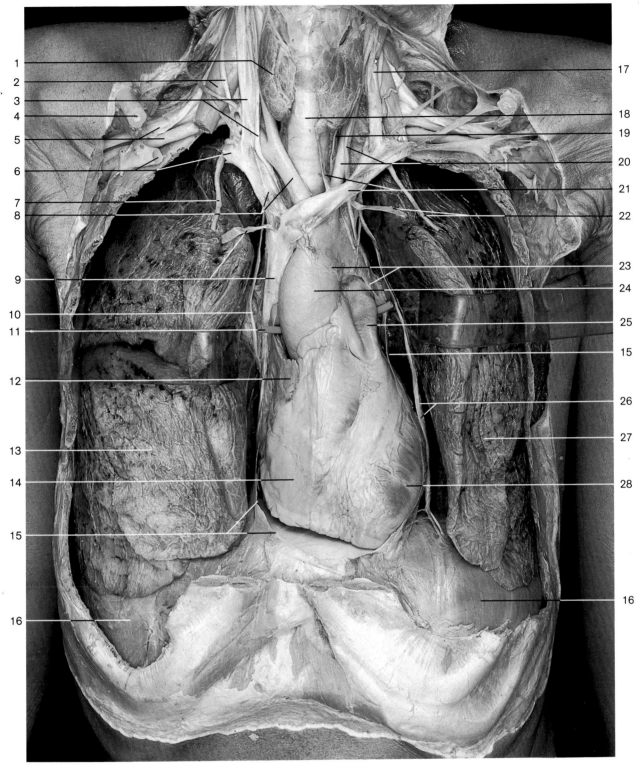

Thoracic organs, position of the heart, middle mediastinum (ventral aspect). The anterior wall of the thorax, the costal pleura and the pericardium have been removed and the lungs slightly reflected.

1 Thyroid gland	11 Transverse pericardial sinus (probe)	21 Left brachiocephalic vein and inferior thyroid vein
2 Phrenic nerve and scalenus anterior muscle	12 Right auricle	22 Left internal thoracic artery and vein (divided)
3 Vagus nerve and internal jugular vein	13 Middle lobe of right lung	23 Upper margin of pericardial sac
4 Clavicle (divided)	14 **Right ventricle**	24 **Ascending aorta**
5 Brachial plexus and subclavian artery	15 Cut edge of pericardium	25 Pulmonary trunk
6 Subclavian vein	16 Diaphragm	26 **Left phrenic nerve** and left pericardiacophrenic artery and vein
7 Internal thoracic artery	17 Internal jugular vein	27 Upper lobe of left lung
8 Brachiocephalic trunk and right brachiocephalic vein	18 Trachea	28 Left ventricle
9 **Superior vena cava** and thymic vein	19 Left recurrent laryngeal nerve	
10 **Right phrenic nerve**	20 Left common carotid artery and vagus nerve	

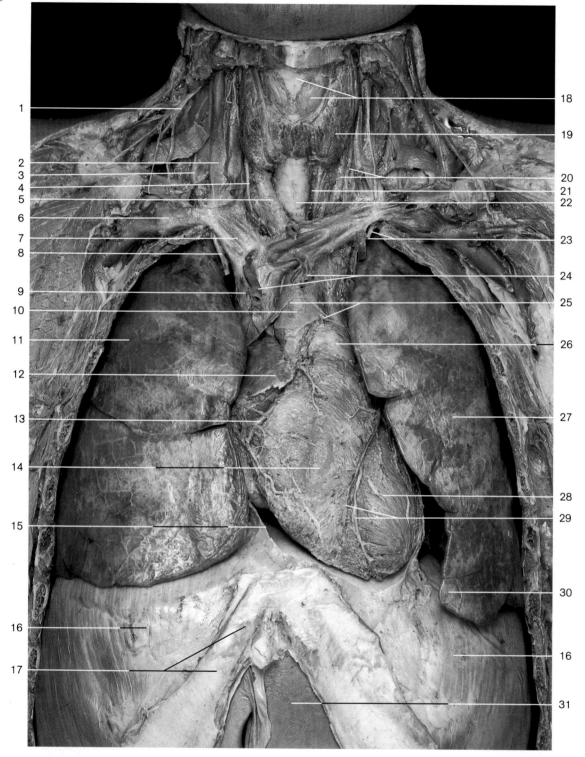

Thoracic organs, position of heart, dissection of coronary vessels in situ (ventral aspect). The anterior wall of thorax, costal pleura and pericardium have been removed.

1 Intermediate supraclavicular nerve	12 Right atrium	21 Left recurrent laryngeal nerve
2 Internal jugular vein	13 **Right coronary artery** and	22 Trachea
3 Right phrenic nerve	small cardiac vein	23 Left internal thoracic artery and vein (divided)
4 Right vagus nerve	14 **Right ventricle**	24 Thymic veins
5 Right common carotid artery	15 Cut edge of pericardium	25 Margin of pericardial sac
6 Right subclavian vein	17 Costal margin	26 Pulmonary trunk
7 Right brachiocephalic vein	18 Larynx (cricothyroid muscle and thyroid	27 Left lung
8 Right internal thoracic artery	cartilage)	28 Left ventricle
9 **Superior vena cava**	19 Thyroid gland	29 Anterior interventricular artery and vein
10 Ascending aorta	20 Left common carotid artery and	30 Lingula
11 Right lung	left vagus nerve	31 Liver

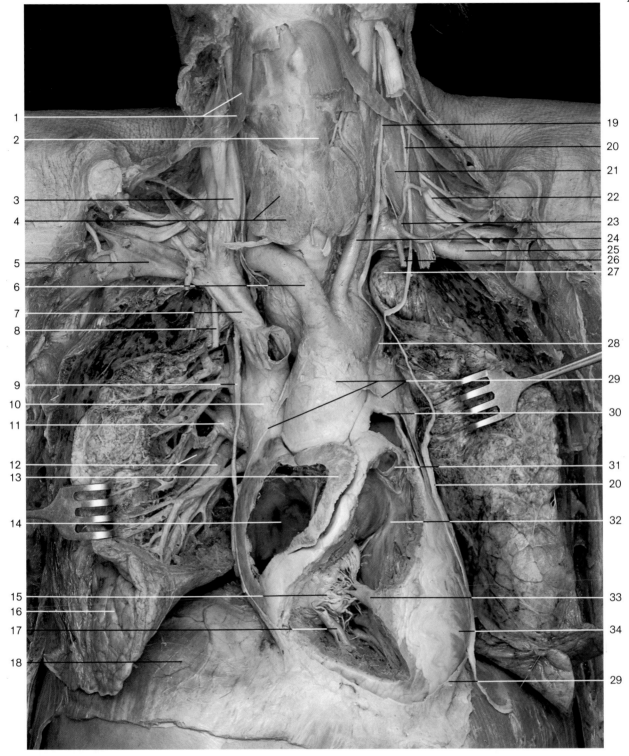

Thoracic organs, heart with valves in situ (ventral aspect). Anterior wall of thorax, pleura and anterior portion of pericardium have been removed. The right atrium and ventricle have been opened to show the right atrioventricular and pulmonary valves.

1 Omohyoid muscle	13 Right auricle	24 Left common carotid artery
2 Pyramidal lobe of thyroid gland	14 **Right atrium**	25 Left subclavian artery
3 Internal jugular vein	15 **Right atrioventricular (tricuspid) valve**	26 Left internal thoracic artery
4 Thyroid gland	16 Right lung	27 Apex of left lung
5 Right subclavian vein	17 Posterior papillary muscle	28 Left recurrent laryngeal nerve
6 Brachiocephalic trunk	18 Diaphragm	29 Cut edge of **pericardium**
7 **Right brachiocephalic vein**	19 Left **vagus nerve**	30 Pulmonary trunk (fenestrated)
8 Right internal thoracic artery	20 Left **phrenic nerve**	31 Pulmonic valve
9 Right phrenic nerve	21 Scalenus anterior muscle	32 Supraventricular crest
10 **Superior vena cava**	22 Brachial plexus	33 **Anterior papillary muscle**
11 Pulmonary vein	23 Thyrocervical trunk	34 **Left ventricle**
12 Branches of pulmonary artery		

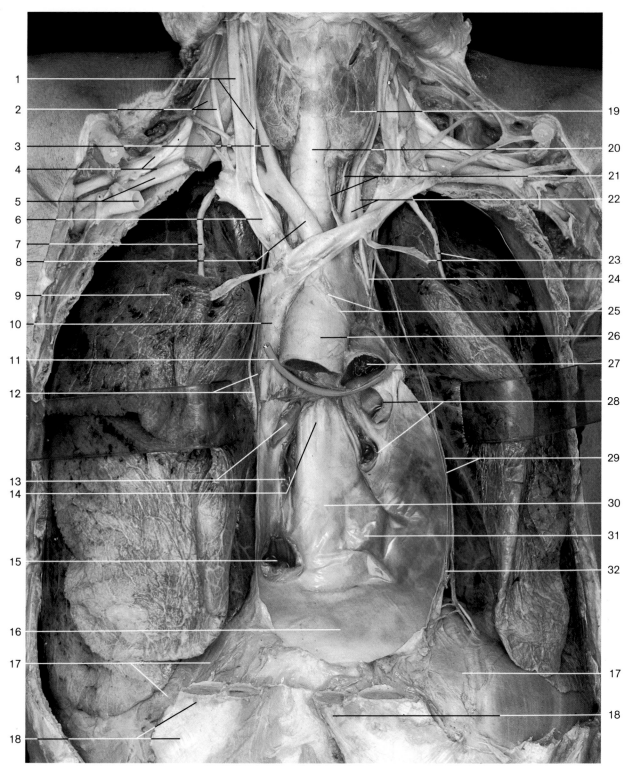

Thoracic organs, pericardium and **mediastinum** (ventral aspect). Anterior wall of thorax and heart have been removed and the lungs slightly reflected. Note probe within transverse pericardial sinus.

1 Right internal jugular vein and
   right vagus nerve
2 Right phrenic nerve and scalenus anterior muscle
3 Right common carotid artery
4 Brachial plexus
5 Right subclavian artery and vein
6 Right brachiocephalic vein
7 Right internal thoracic artery (divided)
8 **Brachiocephalic trunk**
9 Upper lobe of right lung
10 **Superior vena cava**
11 Transverse pericardial sinus (probe)

12 Right **phrenic nerve** and right
   pericardiacophrenic artery and vein
13 Right pulmonary veins
14 Oblique sinus of pericardium
15 **Inferior vena cava**
16 Diaphragmatic part of pericardium
17 Diaphragm
18 Costal margin
19 Thyroid gland
20 **Trachea**
21 Left recurrent laryngeal nerve and
   inferior thyroid vein

22 Left common carotid artery and left vagus nerve
23 Left internal thoracic artery and vein (divided)
24 **Vagus nerve** at aortic arch
25 Cut edge of pericardium
26 **Ascending aorta**
27 Pulmonary trunk (divided)
28 Left pulmonary veins
29 Left phrenic nerve and left pericardiacophrenic
   artery and vein
30 Contour of esophagus beneath pericardium
31 Contour of aorta beneath pericardium
32 **Pericardium** (cut edge)

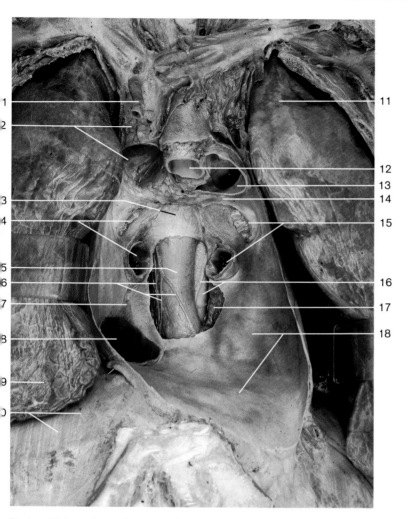

1 Internal thoracic vein
2 Superior vena cava
3 Oblique sinus of pericardium
4 Right pulmonary veins
5 Esophagus
6 Branches of right vagus nerve
7 Mesocardium
8 Inferior vena cava
9 Middle lobe of right lung
10 Diaphragm
11 Upper lobe of left lung
12 Ascending aorta
13 **Pulmonary trunk**
14 Transverse pericardial sinus
15 Left pulmonary veins
16 Descending aorta and left vagus nerve
17 Left lung (adjacent to pericardium)
18 **Pericardium**
19 Left subclavian artery
20 Vagus nerve
21 Left recurrent laryngeal nerve
22 Descending aorta
23 Pulmonary artery
24 **Left atrium**
25 **Left ventricle**
26 Coronary sinus
27 Left common carotid artery
28 Brachiocephalic trunk
29 Azygos arch
30 **Right atrium**
31 **Right ventricle**
32 Aortic arch

Pericardial sac (ventral aspect). The heart has been removed, and the posterior wall of the pericardium has been opened to show the adjacent esophagus and aorta.

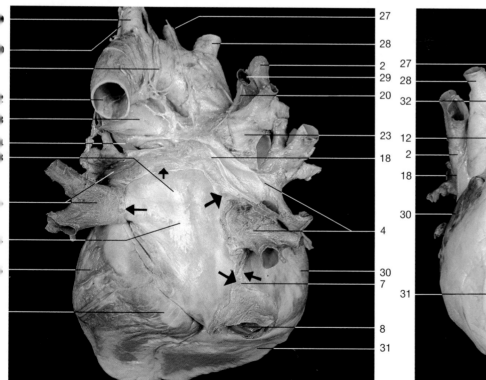

Heart with epicardium (posterior aspect). Arrows: oblique sinus.

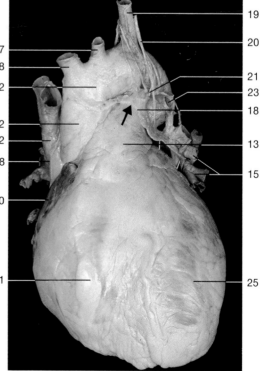

Heart with epicardium (anterior aspect).
Arrow: pericardial reflection.

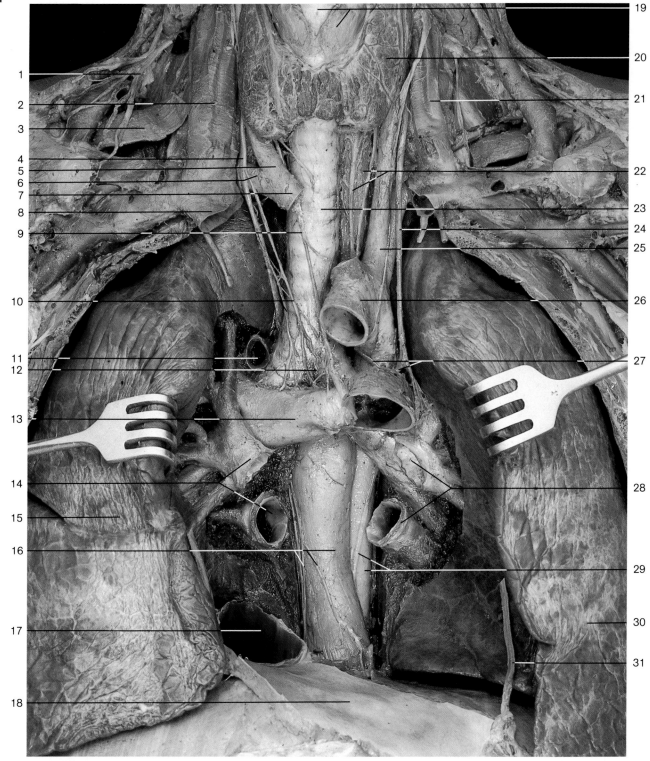

Mediastinal organs after removal of heart and pericardium (ventral aspect). Both lungs have been slightly reflected.

1 Supraclavicular nerves
2 Internal jugular vein
3 Omohyoid muscle
4 **Right vagus nerve**
5 Right common carotid artery
6 Right subclavian artery
7 Brachiocephalic trunk
8 Right brachiocephalic vein
9 Superior cervical cardiac branch
   of vagus nerve
10 Inferior cervical cardiac branches
   of vagus nerve

11 Azygos arch (divided)
12 Bifurcation of trachea
13 Right **pulmonary artery**
14 Right **pulmonary veins**
15 Right lung
16 **Esophagus** and branches
   of right vagus nerve
17 Inferior vena cava
18 Pericardium
19 Larynx (thyroid cartilage, cricothyroid muscle)
20 Thyroid gland
21 Internal jugular vein

22 Esophagus and left recurrent
   laryngeal nerve
23 **Trachea**
24 **Left vagus nerve**
25 Left common carotid artery
26 Aortic arch
27 Left recurrent laryngeal nerve
   branching off from vagus nerve
28 Left pulmonary veins
29 **Thoracic aorta** and left vagus nerve
30 Left lung
31 Left phrenic nerve (divided)

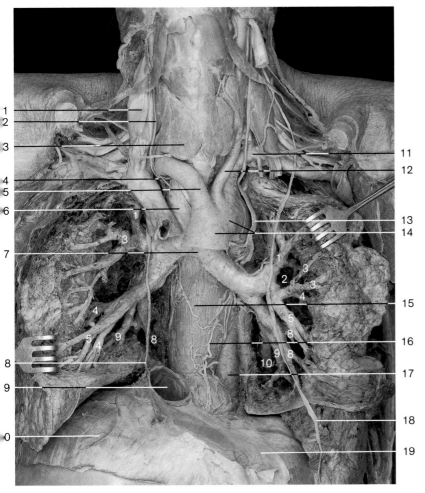

1 Internal jugular vein
2 Right vagus nerve
3 **Thyroid gland**
4 Right recurrent laryngeal nerve
5 Brachiocephalic trunk
6 Trachea
7 **Bifurcation of trachea**
8 **Right phrenic nerve**
9 Inferior vena cava
10 Diaphragm
11 Left subclavian artery
12 Left common carotid artery
13 Left **vagus nerve**
14 Aortic arch
15 **Esophagus**
16 Esophageal plexus
17 Thoracic aorta
18 **Left phrenic nerve**
19 Pericardium at the central tendon of diaphragm
20 Right pulmonary artery
21 Left pulmonary artery
22 Tracheal lymph nodes
23 Superior tracheobronchial lymph nodes
24 Bronchopulmonary lymph nodes

Bronchial tree in situ (ventral aspect). Heart and pericardium have been removed; the bronchi of the bronchopulmonary segments are dissected.
1–10 = numbers of segments (cf. p. 236 and 241).

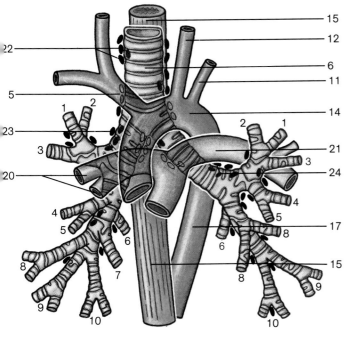

Relation of aorta, pulmonary trunk and esophagus to trachea and bronchial tree. (Schematic drawing.)
1–10 = number of segments (cf. p. 236 and 241).

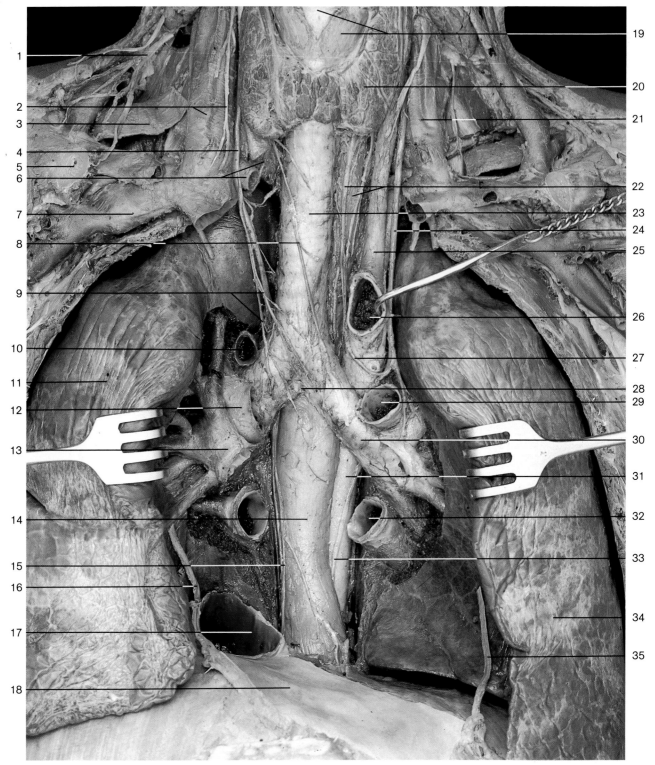

Organs of posterior mediastinum (ventral aspect). The heart with the pericardium has been removed, and the lungs and aortic arch have been slightly reflected to show the vagus nerves and their branches.

1 Supraclavicular nerves	12 **Right pulmonary artery**	24 **Left vagus nerve**
2 Right internal jugular vein with ansa cervicalis	13 **Right pulmonary veins**	25 Left common carotid artery
3 Omohyoid muscle	14 **Esophagus**	26 Aortic arch
4 **Right vagus nerve**	15 Esophageal plexus	27 Left recurrent laryngeal nerve
5 Clavicle	16 Right phrenic nerve (divided)	28 **Bifurcation of trachea**
6 Right subclavian artery and recurrent laryngeal nerve	17 Inferior vena cava	29 **Left pulmonary artery**
7 Right subclavian vein	18 Pericardium covering the diaphragm	30 Left primary bronchus
8 Superior cervical cardiac branch of vagus nerve	19 Larynx (thyroid cartilage and cricothyroid muscle)	31 Descending aorta
9 Inferior cervical cardiac branch of vagus nerve	20 Thyroid gland	32 Left pulmonary veins
10 Azygos arch (divided)	21 Left internal jugular vein	33 Branch of left vagus nerve
11 **Right lung**	22 Esophagus and left recurrent laryngeal nerve	34 **Left lung**
	23 Trachea	35 Left phrenic nerve (divided)

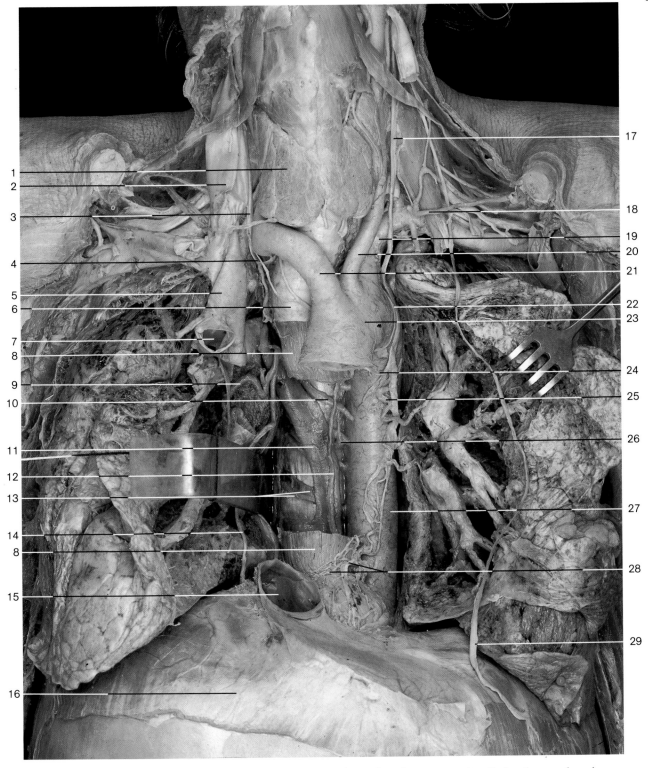

Mediastinal organs (ventral aspect). Heart and distal part of esophagus have been removed to display the vessels and nerves of the posterior mediastinum.

1	Thyroid gland	11	**Azygos vein**	21	Brachiocephalic trunk
2	Right internal jugular vein	12	**Thoracic duct**	22	Left vagus nerve
3	Right vagus nerve	13	Posterior intercostal artery and vein	23	**Aortic arch**
4	Point, where right recurrent laryngeal nerve		(in front of the vertebral column)	24	Left recurrent laryngeal nerve
	is branching off the vagus nerve	14	Right phrenic nerve	25	Left bronchial artery
5	Right brachiocephalic vein	15	Inferior vena cava	26	Lymph node
6	Trachea	16	Diaphragm	27	Thoracic aorta
7	Left brachiocephalic vein (reflected)	17	**Left vagus nerve**	28	Esophageal plexus
8	Esophagus	18	Thyrocervical trunk	29	Left phrenic nerve
9	Right bronchial artery	19	Left subclavian artery		
10	Posterior intercostal artery	20	Left common carotid artery		

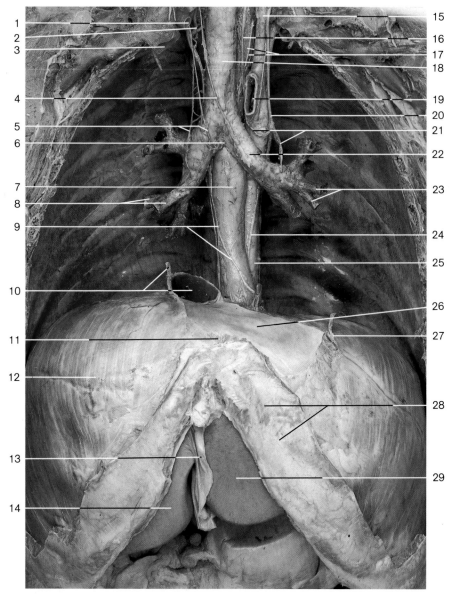

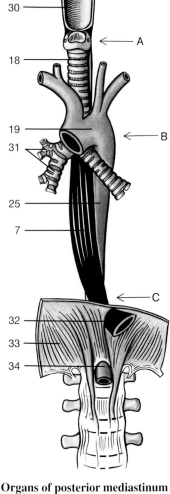

Diaphragm and organs of mediastinum (anterior aspect). Heart and lungs have been removed; the costal margin remains in place. Note the different courses of left and right vagus.

Organs of posterior mediastinum (ventral aspect). (Schematic drawing.) Three regions in which the esophagus is narrowed are shown:
A   at the level of the cricoid cartilage;
B   at the level of the aortic arch;
C   at the level of the diaphragm.

1	Right subclavian artery	14	Liver (quadrate lobe)
2	Right recurrent laryngeal nerve	15	Left common carotid artery
3	Right brachiocephalic vein	16	Left recurrent laryngeal nerve
4	Superior cervical cardiac nerve	17	Esophageal branches of left vagus nerve and esophagus
5	Inferior cervical cardiac nerves and pulmonary branches	18	**Trachea**
6	**Bifurcation of trachea**	19	Aortic arch
7	**Esophagus** (thoracic part)	20	Left vagus nerve
8	Bronchi of lateral and medial segments of middle lobe	21	Left recurrent laryngeal nerve with inferior cardiac nerve
9	Esophageal plexus and branches of right vagus nerve	22	Left primary bronchus
10	Inferior vena cava and right phrenic nerve (cut)	23	Superior and inferior lingular bronchi
11	Sternal part of diaphragm	24	Esophageal plexus of left vagus nerve
12	Costal part of **diaphragm**	25	**Descending aorta**
13	Falciform ligament of liver	26	Central tendon of diaphragm covered with pericardium
		27	Left phrenic nerve (divided)

28	Costal margin
29	**Liver,** left lobe
30	Pharynx
31	Secondary bronchi
32	Esophagus (abdominal part)
33	Diaphragm
34	Abdominal aorta

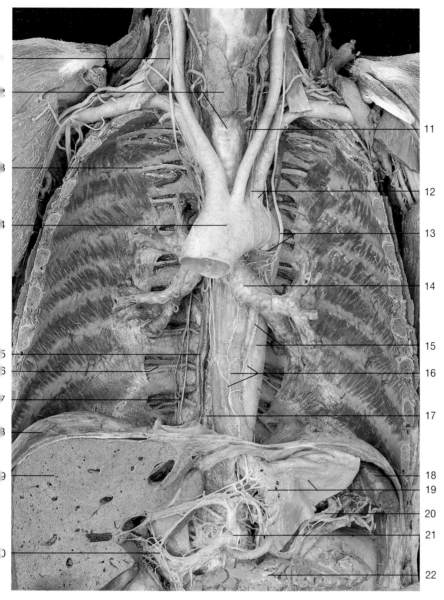

Organs of posterior mediastinum (anterior aspect).

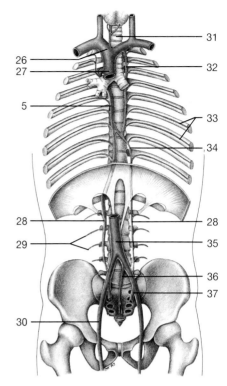

Veins of the posterior wall of thoracic and abdominal cavity. (Schematic drawing.)

1   Right vagus nerve
2   Thyroid gland and trachea
3   Intercostal nerve
4   Aortic arch
5   **Azygos vein**
6   Posterior intercostal artery
7   **Greater splanchnic nerve**
8   Diaphragm
9   Liver
10 Proper hepatic artery and hepatic plexus
11 Left recurrent laryngeal nerve
12 Inferior cervical cardiac nerves
13 Left vagus nerve and left recurrent laryngeal nerve
14 Left primary bronchus
15 Thoracic aorta and left vagus nerve
16 Esophagus and esophageal plexus
17 **Thoracic duct**
18 Spleen
19 Anterior gastric plexus and stomach (divided)
20 Splenic artery and splenic plexus
21 **Celiac trunk** and **celiac plexus**
22 Pancreas
23 Ramus communicans
24 **Sympathetic trunk** and **sympathetic ganglion**
25 **Posterior intercostal vein** and **artery** and **intercostal nerve**
26 Right brachiocephalic vein
27 Superior vena cava
28 Ascending lumbar vein
29 Lumbar veins
30 Right external iliac vein
31 Trachea
32 Accessory hemiazygos vein
33 Posterior intercostal veins
34 Hemiazygos vein
35 Inferior vena cava
36 Median sacral vein
37 Internal iliac vein

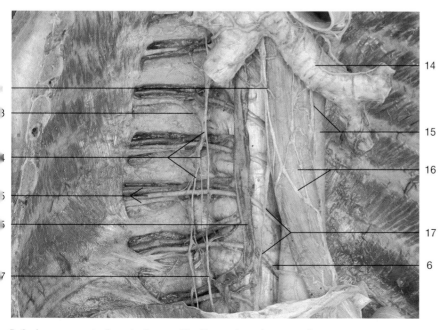

Inferior segment of posterior mediastinum (anterior aspect).

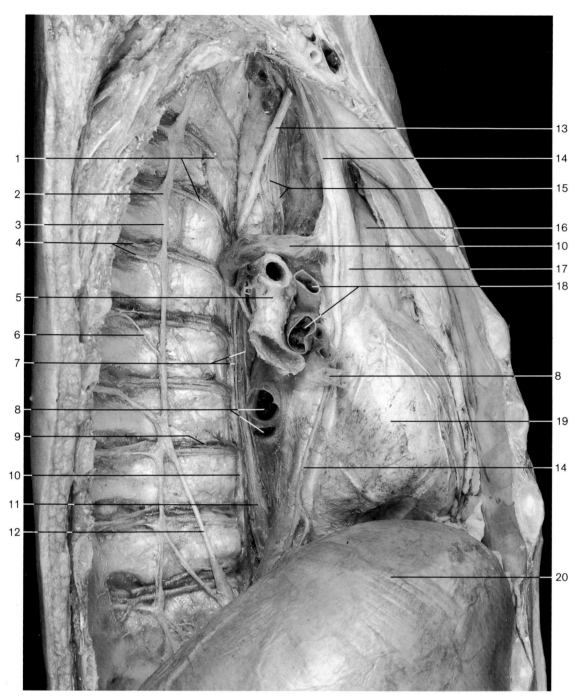

Mediastinal organs (right lateral aspect). Right lung and pleura of right half of the thorax have been removed.

1 Posterior intercostal arteries
2 Ganglion of sympathetic trunk
3 **Sympathetic trunk**
4 Vessels and nerves of the intercostal space (from above: posterior intercostal vein and artery and intercostal nerve)
5 Right primary bronchus
6 Ramus communicans of sympathetic trunk

7 Esophageal plexus (branches of right vagus nerve)
8 Pulmonary veins
9 Posterior intercostal vein
10 **Azygos vein**
11 Esophagus
12 Greater splanchnic nerve
13 **Right vagus nerve**

14 **Right phrenic nerve**
15 Inferior cervical cardiac branches of vagus nerve
16 **Aortic arch**
17 Superior vena cava
18 Right pulmonary artery
19 **Heart with pericardium**
20 Diaphragm

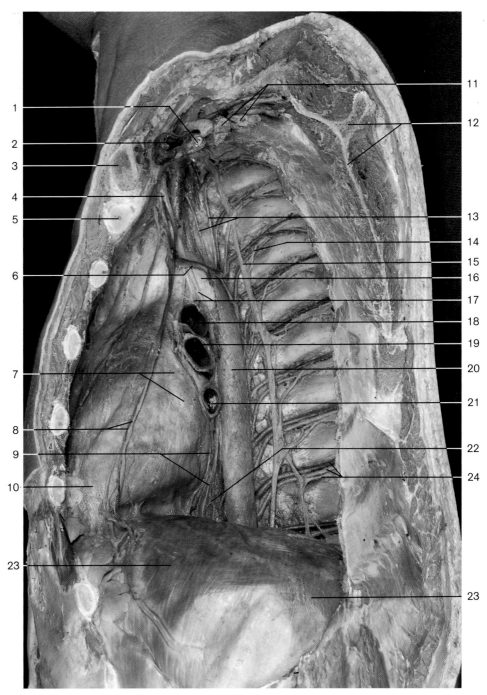

Organs of posterior and superior mediastinum (left lateral aspect).

1   Subclavian artery
2   Subclavian vein
3   Clavicle (divided)
4   **Left vagus nerve**
5   First rib (divided)
6   Left superior intercostal vein
7   **Left atrium with pericardium**
8   **Left phrenic nerve** and pericardiacophrenic
    artery and vein
9   Esophageal plexus (branches derived
    from left vagus nerve)

10 **Apex of heart with pericardium**
11 Brachial plexus
12 Scapula (divided)
13 Posterior intercostal arteries
14 Ramus communicans of sympathetic
    trunk
15 **Sympathetic trunk**
16 Aortic arch
17 Left vagus nerve and left recurrent
    laryngeal nerve
18 Left pulmonary artery

19 Left primary bronchus
20 **Thoracic aorta**
21 Pulmonary vein
22 Esophagus (thoracic part)
23 **Diaphragm**
24 Posterior intercostal artery and
    vein and intercostal nerve

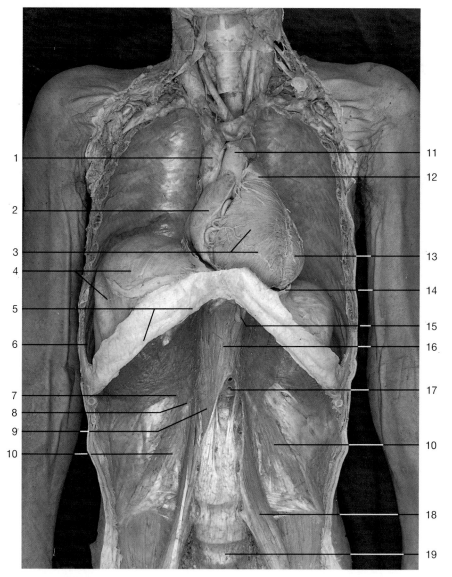

1 Superior vena cava
2 Right atrium
3 Right ventricle
4 **Costal part of diaphragm**
5 Costal margin
6 Position of costodiaphragmatic recess
7 **Lateral arcuate ligament**
8 **Medial arcuate ligament**
9 Right crus of lumbar part of diaphragm
10 Quadratus lumborum muscle
11 Ascending aorta
12 Pulmonary trunk
13 Left ventricle
14 Pericardium, diaphragm
15 Esophageal hiatus and abdominal
   part of esophagus (cut)
16 **Lumbar part of diaphragm**
17 Aortic hiatus
18 Psoas major muscle
19 Lumbar vertebra

Diaphragm in situ (anterior aspect). Anterior walls of thoracic and abdominal cavities have been removed. Natural position of the heart above the central tendon on the diaphragm is shown.

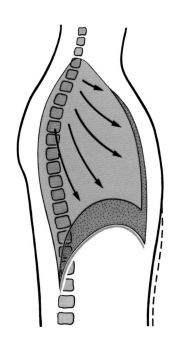

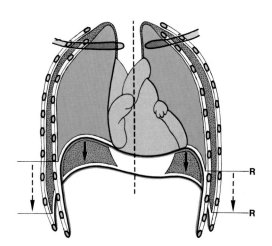

Changes in the position of the diaphragm and thoracic cage during respiration. Left: lateral aspect; right: anterior aspect. During inspiration the diaphragm moves downwards and the lower part of the thoracic cage expands forward and laterally, causing the costodiaphragmatic recess (R) to enlarge (cf. dotted arrows).

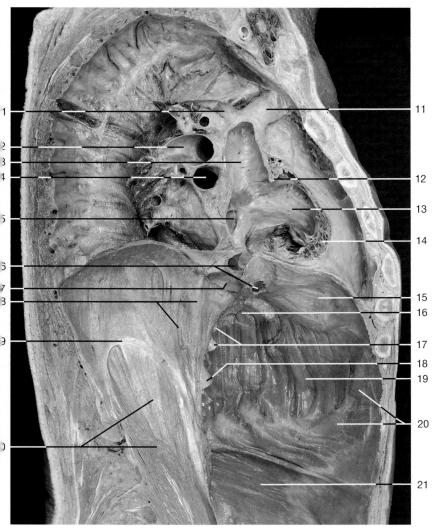

1 Azygos venous arch
2 Right pulmonary artery
3 **Superior vena cava**
4 Right pulmonary vein
5 Fossa ovalis
6 Hepatic veins
7 Inferior vena cava
8 Right crus of lumbar part of **diaphragm**
9 Medial arcuate ligament
10 Psoas major muscle
11 Left brachiocephalic vein
12 Terminal crista
13 **Right atrium**
14 Right auricle
15 Central tendon of diaphragm
16 Esophagus
17 Celiac trunk and superior mesenteric artery
18 Aorta
19 Costal part of diaphragm
20 Costal margin
21 Transversus abdominis muscle

Diaphragm. Paramedian section to the right of the median plane through thoracic and upper abdominal cavity. The plane passes through the superior and inferior vena cava just to the right of the vertebral bodies. Most of the heart remains in situ to the left of this plane (specimen is viewed from the right side).

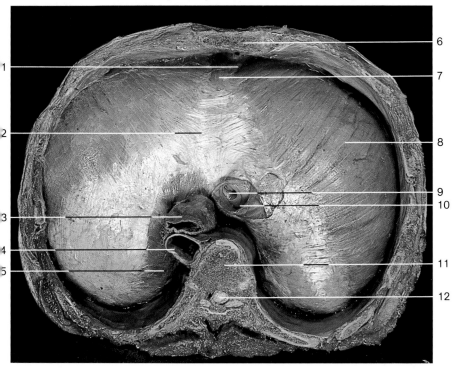

1 Sternocostal triangle
2 Central tendon (from above)
3 Esophagus
4 Aorta
5 Lumbar part of diaphragm
6 Sternum
7 Sternal part of diaphragm
8 Costal part of diaphragm
9 Entrance of hepatic veins
10 Inferior vena cava
11 Body of 9th thoracic vertebra
12 Spinal cord

Diaphragm (superior aspect). The pleura and pericardium have been removed.

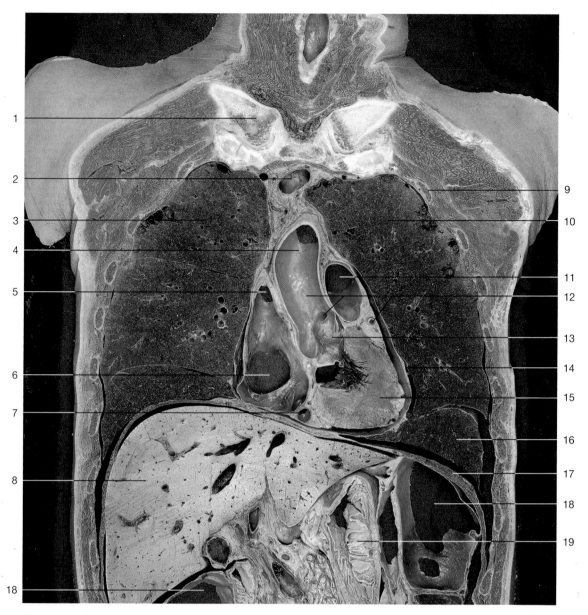

Coronal section through the thorax at the level of ascending aorta (anterior aspect).

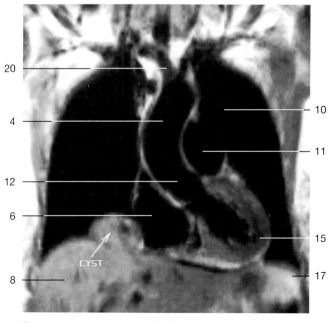

Coronal section through the thorax at the level of ascending aorta. (MRI scan.)

1 Clavicle
2 Left brachiocephalic vein
3 Superior lobe of right lung
4 Aortic arch
5 Superior vena cava
6 Right atrium (entrance of inferior vena cava)
7 Coronary sinus
8 Liver
9 Second rib
10 Superior lobe of left lung
11 Pulmonary trunk
12 Ascending aorta and left coronary artery
13 Aortic valve
14 Pericardium
15 Myocardium of left ventricle
16 Lower lobe of left lung
17 Diaphragm
18 Colic flexures
19 Stomach
20 Brachiocephalic trunk

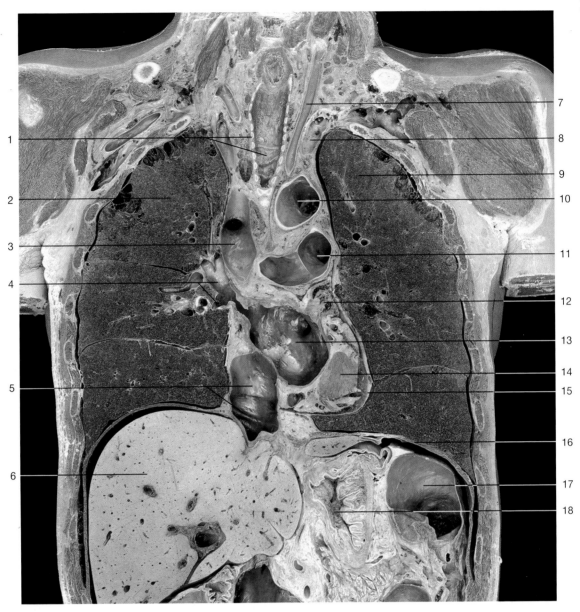

Coronal section through the thorax at the level of superior and inferior vena cava (anterior aspect).

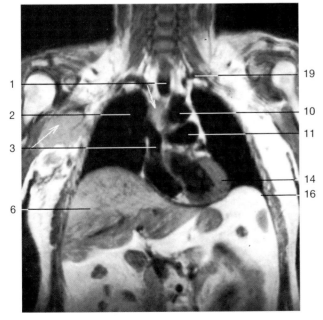

Coronal section through the thorax at the level of superior vena cava. (MRI scan.)

1 Trachea
2 Upper lobe of right lung
3 **Superior vena cava**
4 Right pulmonary veins
5 Inferior vena cava and right atrium
6 Liver
7 Left common carotid artery
8 Left subclavian vein
9 Upper lobe of left lung
10 Aortic arch
11 Left pulmonary artery
12 Left auricle
13 **Left atrium** with orifices
    of pulmonary veins
14 Left ventricle (myocardium)
15 Pericardium
16 Diaphragm
17 Left colic flexure
18 Stomach
19 Left subclavian artery

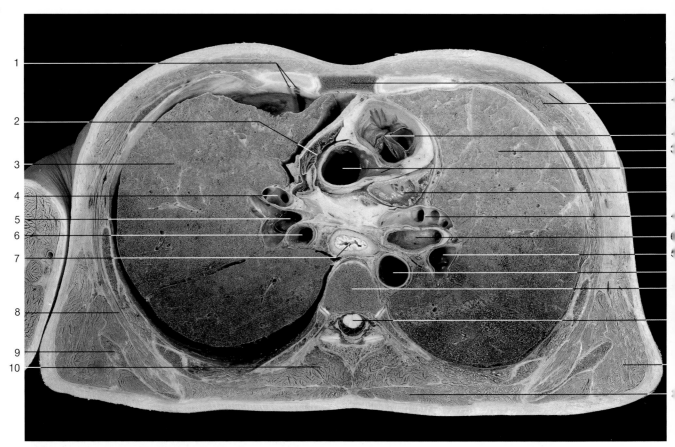

Horizontal section through the thorax at level 1 (from below).

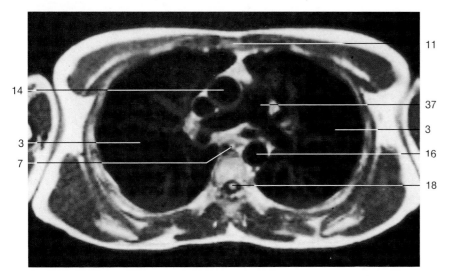

Horizontal section through the thorax at level 1 (from below). (MRI scan.)

1	Internal thoracic artery and vein	12	Pectoralis major and minor muscles
2	Right atrium	13	Conus arteriosus (right ventricle),
3	Lung		pulmonic valve
4	Pulmonary artery	14	Ascending aorta and left coronary artery
5	Pulmonary vein		(only in upper figure)
6	Primary bronchus	15	**Left atrium**
7	Esophagus	16	**Descending aorta**
8	Serratus anterior muscle	17	Thoracic vertebra
9	Scapula	18	Spinal cord
10	Longissimus thoracis muscle	19	Latissimus dorsi muscle
11	Sternum	20	Trapezius muscle

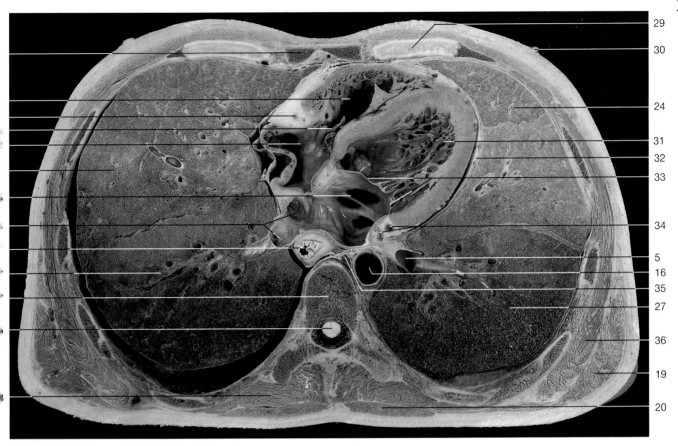

Horizontal section through the thorax at level 2 (from below).

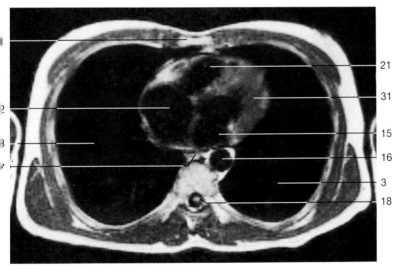

Horizontal section through the thorax at level 2 (from below).
(MRI scan.)

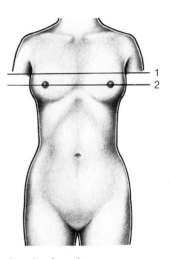

Levels of sections.

21	**Right ventricle**	31	**Left ventricle**
22	Right coronary artery	32	Pericardium
23	Right atrioventricular valve	33	Left atrioventricular valve
24	Lung (upper lobe)	34	Left coronary artery and coronary sinus
25	**Left atrium**	35	Accessory hemiazygos vein
26	Pulmonary veins	36	Serratus anterior muscle
27	Lung (lower lobe)	37	Pulmonary trunk
28	Erector muscle of spine		
29	Third costal cartilage		
30	Nipple		

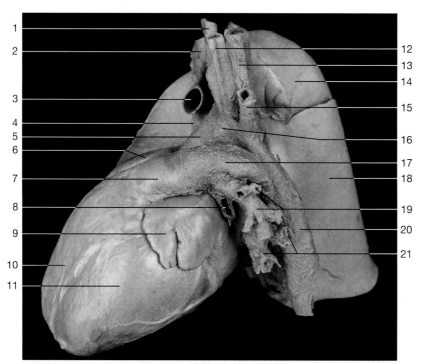

Heart and right lung of the fetus (viewed from left side). The left lung has been removed. Note the ductus arteriosus (Botalli).

Shunts in the fetal circulation system		
1. Ductus venosus (of Arantius)	between umbilical vein and inferior vena cava	bypass of liver circulation
2. Foramen ovale	between right and left atrium	bypass of pulmonary circulation
3. Ductus arteriosus (Botalli)	between pulmonary trunk and aorta	

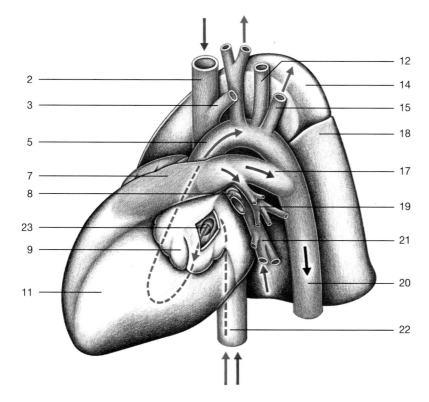

Heart of the fetus (anterior aspect). Right atrium and ventricle opened.

1 Right common carotid artery
2 Right brachiocephalic vein
3 Left brachiocephalic vein
4 Superior vena cava
5 **Ascending aorta**
6 Right auricle
7 **Pulmonary trunk**
8 Left primary bronchus
9 Left auricle
10 Right ventricle
11 Left ventricle
12 Left common carotid artery
13 Trachea
14 Superior lobe of right lung
15 Left subclavian artery
16 Aortic arch
17 **Ductus arteriosus (Botalli)**
18 Inferior lobe of right lung
19 Left pulmonary artery with branches to the left lung
20 **Descending aorta**
21 Left pulmonary veins
22 Inferior vena cava
23 **Foramen ovale**
24 Right atrium
25 Opening of inferior vena cava
26 Valve of inferior vena cava (Eustachian valve)
27 Opening of coronary sinus
28 Anterior papillary muscle of right ventricle

◁ **Heart of the fetus** (schematic drawing). Direction of blood flow indicated by arrows. Note the change in oxygenation of blood after ductus arteriosus entry into aorta.

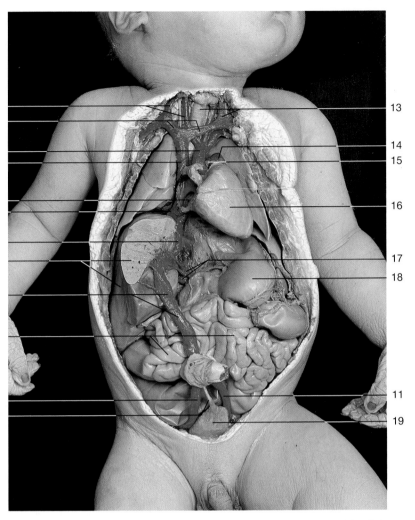

1   Internal jugular vein and right common carotid artery
2   Right and left brachiocephalic vein
3   Aortic arch
4   Superior vena cava
5   **Foramen ovale**
6   Inferior vena cava
7   **Ductus venosus**
8   Liver
9   **Umbilical vein**
10 Small intestine
11 **Umbilical artery**
12 Urachus
13 Trachea and left internal jugular vein
14 Left pulmonary artery
15 **Ductus arteriosus** (Botalli)
16 Right ventricle
17 Hepatic arteries (red) and portal vein (blue)
18 Stomach
19 Urinary bladder
20 Portal vein
21 Pulmonary veins
22 Descending aorta
23 Placenta

Thoracic and abdominal organs in the newborn (anterior aspect). The right atrium has been opened to show the foramen ovale. The left lobe of the liver has been removed.

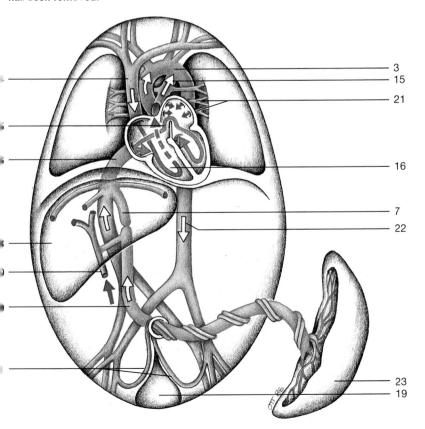

◁ **Fetal circulatory system.** (Schematic drawing.) The oxygen gradient is indicated by color.

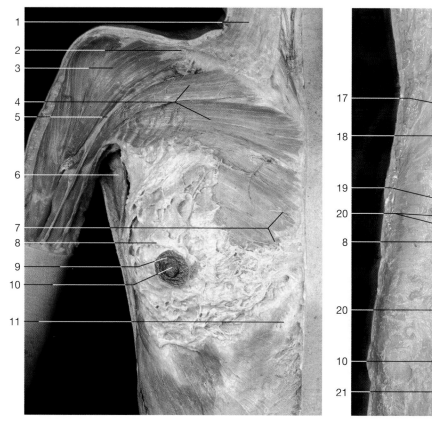

Dissection of mammary gland (anterior aspect).

Dissection of mammary gland and axillary lymph nodes.

1	Platysma muscle	8	Breast tissue
2	Clavicle	9	Areola
3	Deltoid muscle	10	Nipple (papilla)
4	Pectoralis major muscle	11	Costal margin
5	Deltopectoral groove	12	Pectoral fascia
	and cephalic vein	**13**	**Mammary gland**
6	Latissimus dorsi muscle	14	Serratus anterior muscle
7	Medial mammarian branches		(insertion)
	of intercostal nerves	15	Lactiferous sinus

16	Apical lymph nodes
17	**Axillary lymph nodes**
18	Intercostobrachial nerve
19	Lateral thoracic vein
20	Lymph vessels
21	Serratus anterior muscle
22	Medial branches of intercostal
	arteries
23	Pectoralis minor muscle

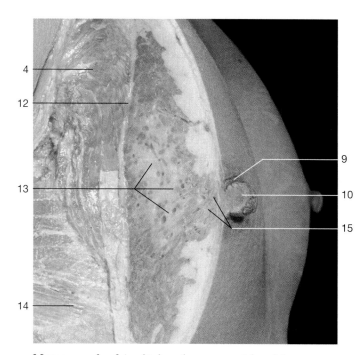

Mammary gland (sagittal section; pregnant female).

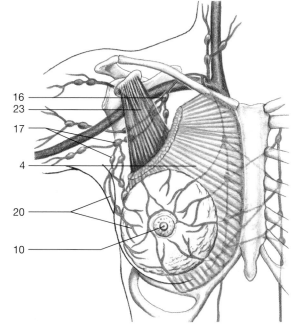

Lymphatics of the breast and axilla. Most lymph vessels drain into the axillary lymph nodes.

Abdominal Organs

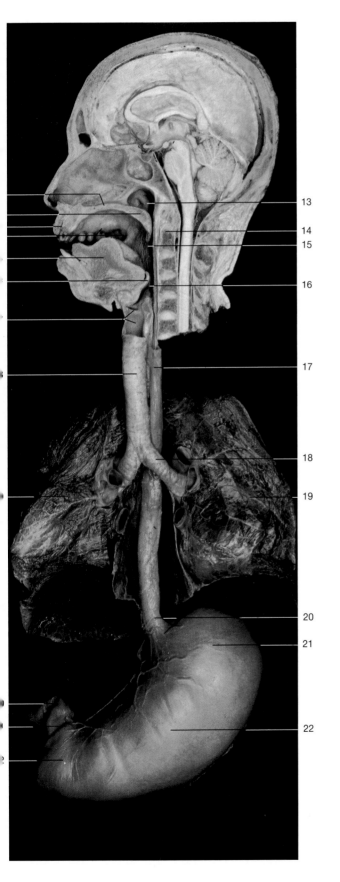

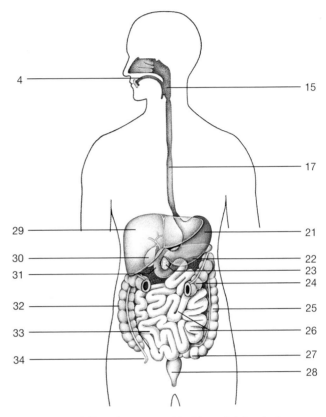

Organization of digestive system. Position of abdominal organs.

1	Hard palate	19	Left lung
2	Soft palate with uvula	20	Abdominal part of esophagus
3	Vestibule of the mouth		and cardia
4	Oral cavity proper	21	Fundus of stomach
5	Tongue	22	Body of stomach
6	Epiglottis	23	Pancreas
7	Vocal ligament and larynx	24	Transverse colon (divided)
8	Trachea	25	Descending colon
9	Right lung	26	Jejunum
10	Superior part of duodenum	27	Sigmoid colon
11	Pylorus	28	Rectum
12	Pyloric antrum	29	Liver
13	Nasopharynx	30	Gall bladder
14	Dens of axis	31	Duodenum
15	Oropharynx	32	Ascending colon
16	Laryngopharynx	33	Ileum
17	Esophagus (thoracic part)	34	Vermiform appendix
18	Left primary bronchus		

Survey of upper portion of digestive system.
Oral cavity, pharynx, esophagus, and stomach.

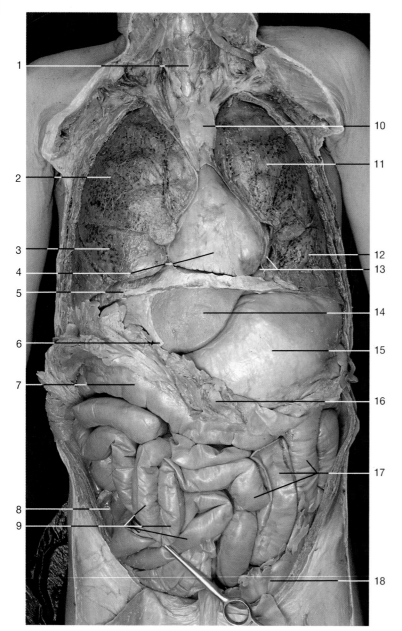

<table>
<tr><td>1</td><td>Thyroid gland</td></tr>
<tr><td>2</td><td>Upper lobe of right lung</td></tr>
<tr><td>3</td><td>Middle lobe of right lung</td></tr>
<tr><td>4</td><td>Heart</td></tr>
<tr><td>5</td><td>Diaphragm</td></tr>
<tr><td>6</td><td>Round ligament of liver (ligamentum teres)</td></tr>
<tr><td>7</td><td>Transverse colon</td></tr>
<tr><td>8</td><td>Cecum</td></tr>
<tr><td>9</td><td>Small intestine (ileum)</td></tr>
<tr><td>10</td><td>Thymus</td></tr>
<tr><td>11</td><td>Upper lobe of left lung</td></tr>
<tr><td>12</td><td>Lower lobe of left lung</td></tr>
<tr><td>13</td><td>Pericardium (cut edge)</td></tr>
<tr><td>14</td><td>Liver (left lobe)</td></tr>
<tr><td>15</td><td>Stomach</td></tr>
<tr><td>16</td><td>Greater omentum</td></tr>
<tr><td>17</td><td>Small intestine (jejunum)</td></tr>
<tr><td>18</td><td>Sigmoid colon</td></tr>
<tr><td>19</td><td>Rectus abdominis muscle</td></tr>
<tr><td>20</td><td>Small intestine (section)</td></tr>
<tr><td>21</td><td>Rib</td></tr>
<tr><td>22</td><td>Common bile duct, duodenum and pancreas</td></tr>
<tr><td>23</td><td>Inferior vena cava</td></tr>
<tr><td>24</td><td>Liver</td></tr>
<tr><td>25</td><td>Body of second lumbar vertebra</td></tr>
<tr><td>26</td><td>Right kidney</td></tr>
<tr><td>27</td><td>Cauda equina and dura mater</td></tr>
<tr><td>28</td><td>Linea alba</td></tr>
<tr><td>29</td><td>Stomach and pylorus</td></tr>
<tr><td>30</td><td>Superior mesenteric artery and vein</td></tr>
<tr><td>31</td><td>Abdominal aorta</td></tr>
<tr><td>32</td><td>Left renal artery and vein</td></tr>
<tr><td>33</td><td>Left kidney</td></tr>
<tr><td>34</td><td>Psoas major muscle</td></tr>
<tr><td>35</td><td>Deep muscles of the back</td></tr>
<tr><td>36</td><td>Pancreas adjacent to lesser sac (bursa omentalis)</td></tr>
<tr><td>37</td><td>Falciform ligament with ligamentum teres</td></tr>
</table>

Abdominal organs in situ. The greater omentum has been partly removed or reflected.

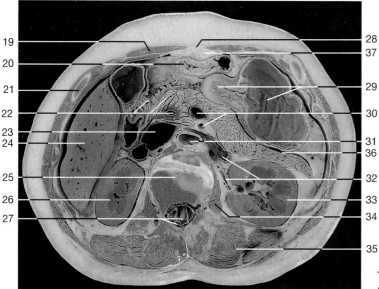

Transverse section through the abdominal cavity at the level of the second lumbar vertebra (from below).

1 Left ventricle with pericardium
2 Diaphragm
3 Remnant of liver
4 Ligamentum teres
   (free margin of falciform ligament)
5 Site of umbilicus
6 **Medial umbilical fold**
   (containing the obliterated umbilical artery)
7 **Lateral umbilical fold** (containing inferior
   epigastric artery and vein)
8 **Median umbilical fold**
   (containing remnant of urachus)
9 Head of femur and pelvic bone
10 Urinary bladder
11 Root of penis
12 Falciform ligament of liver
13 Rib (divided)
14 Iliac crest (divided)
15 Site of **deep inguinal ring** and
   lateral inguinal fossa
16 Iliopsoas muscle (divided)
17 Medial inguinal fossa
18 Supravesical fossa
19 Posterior layer of rectus sheath
20 Transversus abdominis muscle
21 Umbilicus and arcuate line
22 **Inferior epigastric artery**
23 Femoral nerve
24 Iliopsoas muscle
25 Remnant of umbilical artery
26 Femoral artery and vein
27 Tendinous intersection of rectus abdominis
   muscle
28 Rectus abdominis muscle
29 Interfoveolar ligament
30 Pubic symphysis (divided)
31 External iliac artery and vein

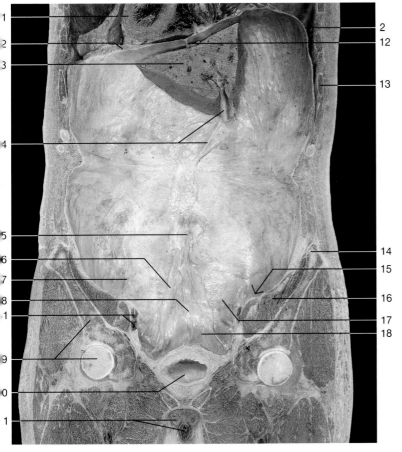

Anterior abdominal wall with pelvic cavity and thigh (frontal section, male) (internal aspect).

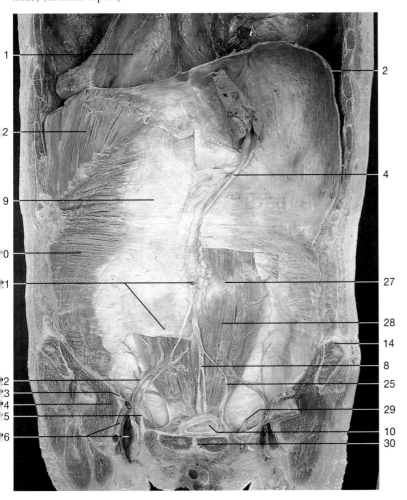

Anterior abdominal wall (male) (internal aspect). The peritoneum and parts of the posterior layer of rectus sheath have been removed. Dissection of inferior epigastric arteries and veins.

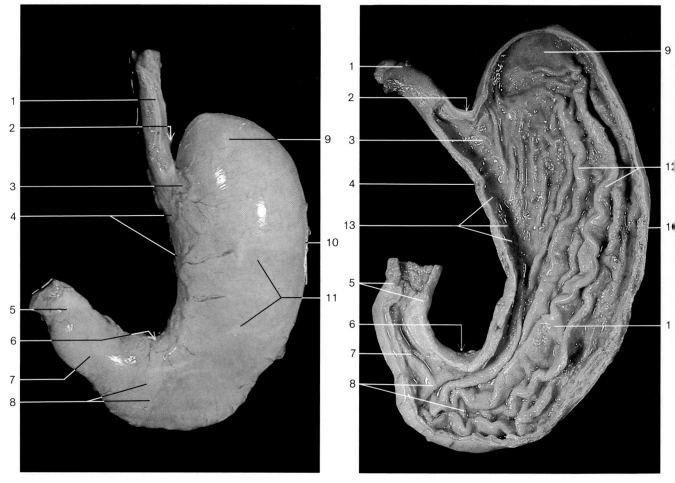

Stomach (ventral aspect).

Mucosa of posterior wall of stomach (ventral aspect).

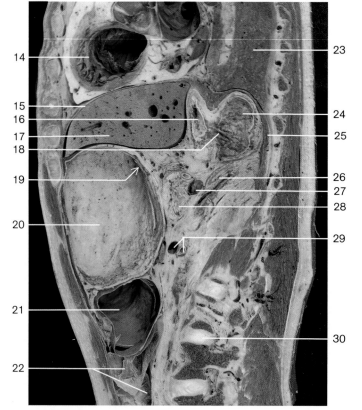

Parasagittal section through upper part of left abdominal cavity 3.5 cm lateral to median plane.

 1 Esophagus
 2 Cardiac notch
 3 **Cardiac part of stomach**
 4 Lesser curvature of stomach
 5 **Pyloric sphincter**
 6 Angular notch (incisura angularis)
 7 **Pyloric canal**
 8 Pyloric antrum
 9 Fundus of stomach
10 Greater curvature of stomach
11 Body of stomach
12 Folds of mucous membrane (gastric rugae)
13 **Gastric canal**
14 Right ventricle of heart
15 Diaphragm (cut edge)
16 Abdominal portion of esophagus
17 **Liver**
18 Cardiac part of stomach (cut edge)
19 Position of pyloric canal
20 Body of stomach
21 Transverse colon
22 Small intestine
23 Lung (cut edge)
24 Fundus of stomach (section)
25 Lumbar portion of diaphragm (cut edge)
26 Suprarenal gland
27 Splenic vein
28 Pancreas
29 Superior mesenteric artery and vein
30 Intervertebral disc

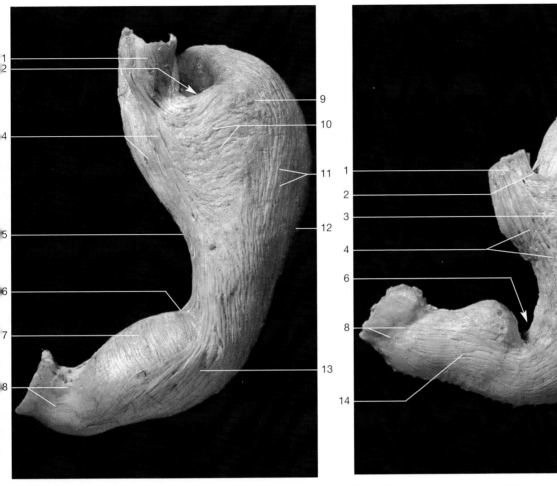

Muscular coat of stomach, outer layer (ventral aspect).

Muscular coat of stomach, middle layer (ventral aspect).

1 Esophagus (abdominal part)
2 Cardiac notch
3 Cardiac part of stomach
4 Longitudinal muscle layer at lesser curvature of stomach
5 Lesser curvature
6 Incisura angularis
7 Circular muscle layer of pyloric part of stomach
8 Pyloric sphincter muscle
9 Fundus of stomach
10 Circular muscle layer of fundus of stomach
11 Longitudinal muscle layer of greater curvature of stomach
12 Greater curvature of stomach
13 Longitudinal muscle layer (transition from body to pyloric part of stomach)
14 Pyloric part of stomach
15 Oblique muscle fibers

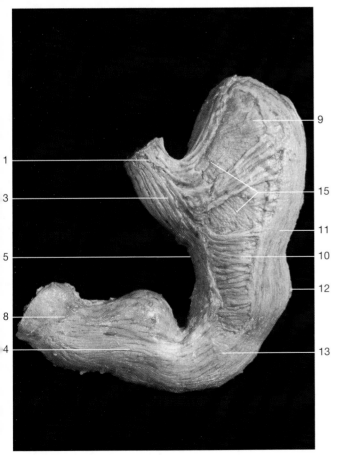

Muscular coat of stomach, inner layer (ventral aspect).

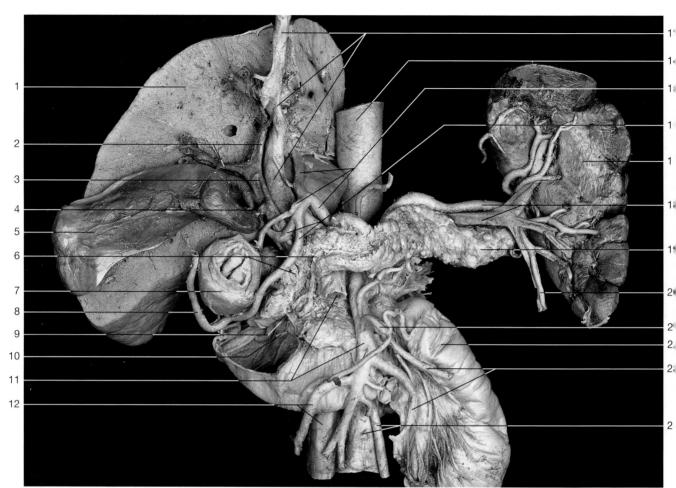

Pancreas with adjacent duodenum, spleen, liver and related arteries. The pancreatic ducts have been partly dissected. The duodenal papillae are indicated by probes. Left half of liver has been removed.

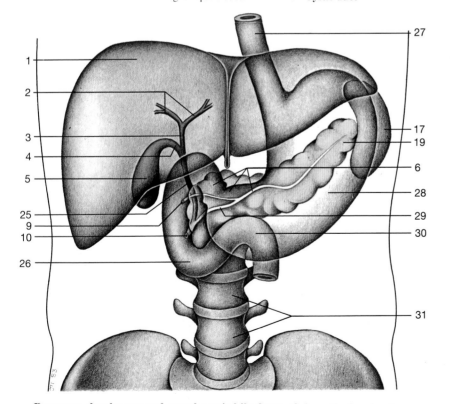

Pancreas, duodenum and extrahepatic bile ducts. (Schematic drawing.)

1 Liver
2 Left and right hepatic ducts
3 Common hepatic duct
4 **Cystic duct**
5 **Gallbladder**
6 **Pancreatic duct** and **head of pancreas**
7 Pylorus (cut)
8 Right gastro-omental (gastroepiploic) artery
9 Lesser duodenal papilla (probe)
10 Greater duodenal papilla (probe)
11 **Superior mesenteric artery and vein**
12 Inferior vena cava and ileocolic artery
13 **Portal vein,** ligamentum teres of liver and ligamentum venosum
14 Aorta
15 Common hepatic artery, left branch of hepatic artery proper, and right gastric artery
16 **Gastroduodenal artery** and right branch of hepatic artery proper
17 Spleen
18 Splenic artery and vein
19 **Tail of pancreas**
20 Left gastro-omental artery
21 Middle colic artery
22 Jejunum
23 Jejunal arteries
24 Aorta and inferior mesenteric artery
25 **Common bile duct**
26 Horizontal part of duodenum
27 Esophagus
28 Stomach
29 **Pancreatic duct**
30 Duodenojejunal flexure
31 Lumbar vertebrae

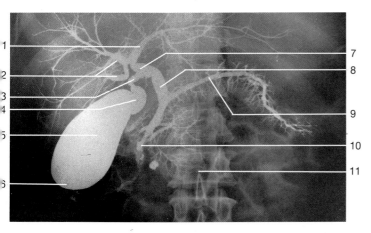

1   Left hepatic duct
2   Right hepatic duct
3   Cystic duct
4   Neck of gallbladder
5   Body of gallbladder
6   Fundus of gallbladder
7   Common hepatic duct
8   **Common bile duct**
9   **Pancreatic duct**
10   **Greater duodenal papilla**
11   Second lumbar vertebra
12   Folds of mucous membrane of gallbladder
13   Muscular coat of gallbladder
14   Neck of gallbladder (opened)
15   Cystic duct with spiral fold
16   **Lesser duodenal papilla**
17   **Accessory pancreatic duct**
18   Uncinate process
19   Plica circularis of duodenum (Kerckring's fold)
20   Head of pancreas
21   Body of pancreas
22   Tail of pancreas
23   Descending part of duodenum
24   Incisure of pancreas

Radiograph of biliary ducts, gallbladder and pancreatic duct (anterior-posterior view).

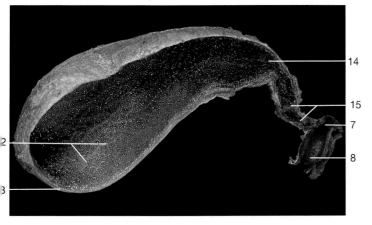

Isolated gallbladder and cystic duct (anterior aspect).
The gallbladder has been opened to display the mucous membrane.

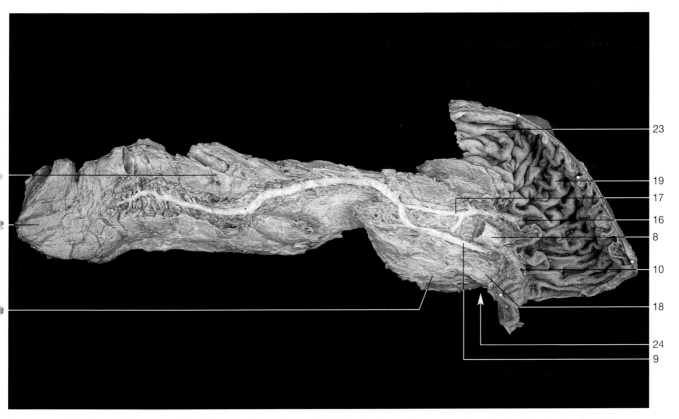

Pancreas with descending part of duodenum (posterior aspect). The duodenum was opened to display the duodenal papillae. Pancreatic duct has been dissected, the common bile duct has been divided. The sphincter of Oddi is shown.

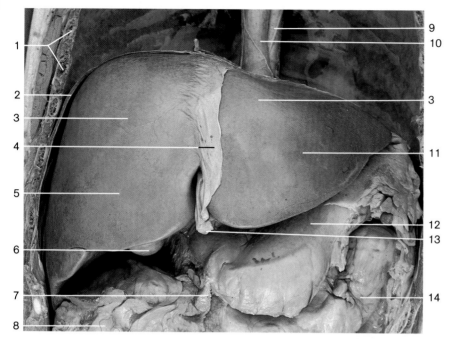

1	Ribs (cut edges)
2	Diaphragm
3	Diaphragmatic surface of liver
4	**Falciform ligament of liver**
5	Right lobe of liver
6	Fundus of gallbladder
7	Gastrocolic ligament
8	Greater omentum
9	Aorta
10	Esophagus
11	Left lobe of liver
12	Stomach
13	**Ligamentum teres**
14	Transverse colon
15	Right atrium of heart
16	Central tendon and sternal portion of diaphragm
17	Liver (cut edge)
18	Entrance to duodenum (pylorus)
19	Stomach
20	Duodenum
21	Transverse colon (divided, dilated)
22	Small intestine
23	Thoracic aorta (longitudinally divided)
24	Esophagus (longitudinally divided)
25	Esophageal hiatus of diaphragm
26	**Omental bursa** (lesser sac)
27	Splenic artery
28	Pancreas
29	Left renal vein
30	Intervertebral disc
31	Abdominal aorta (longitudinally divided)

Liver in situ (ventral aspect). Part of the diaphragm has been removed.

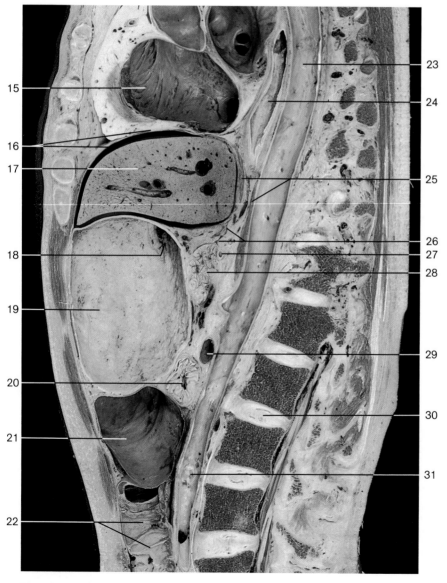

Liver in situ. Parasagittal section through the left side of the abdomen 2 cm lateral to median plane.

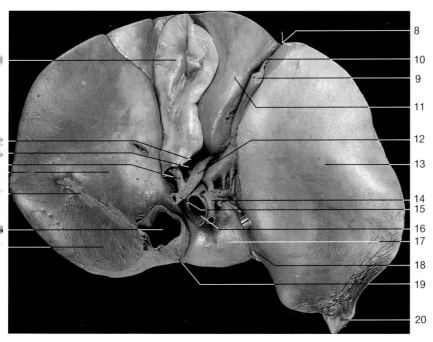

Liver (inferior aspect). Dissection of porta hepatis. Gallbladder partly collapsed. Ventral margin of liver above.

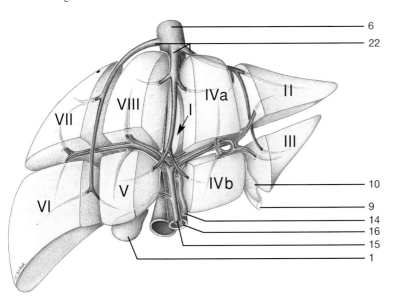

Segmentation of the liver (anterior aspect). Liver segments indicated by roman numerals.

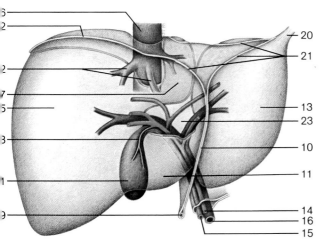

Liver (ventral aspect) (transparent drawing illustrating margins of peritoneal folds).

It should be noted that the anatomical left and right lobes of the liver do not reflect the internal distribution of the hepatic artery, portal vein, and biliary ducts. With these structures, used as criteria, the left lobe includes both the caudate and quadrate lobes, and thus the line dividing the liver into left and right functional lobes passes through the gallbladder and inferior vena cava. The three main hepatic veins drain segments of the liver which have no visible external markings.

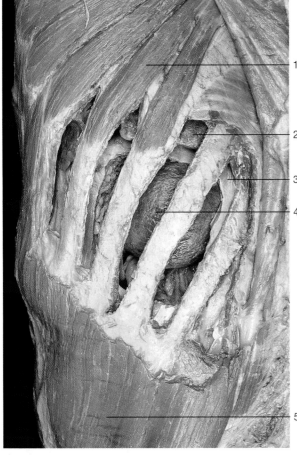

1 Serratus anterior muscle
2 Left lung
3 Diaphragm
4 Spleen
5 External abdominal oblique muscle
6 Gastrosplenic ligament
7 **Splenic artery**
8 Pancreas tail
9 Superior margin of spleen
10 Anterior border of spleen
11 Inferior vena cava
12 **Hepatic veins**
13 Liver
14 **Portal vein**
15 Paraumbilical veins within falciform ligament
16 **Superior mesenteric vein**
17 Middle colic vein
18 Right colic vein
19 Ascending colon
20 Ileocolic vein
21 Vermiform appendix and appendicular vein
22 Spleen
23 Gastric and esophageal veins
24 **Splenic vein**
25 **Inferior mesenteric vein**
26 Right gastroepiploic vein
27 Ileal veins
28 Descending colon
29 Ileum
30 Sigmoid veins
31 Superior rectal veins

Location of the spleen in situ (left-lateral aspect). Intercostal spaces and diaphragm have been fenestrated.

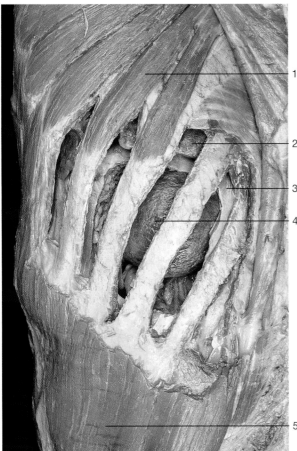

Spleen (visceral surface), hilum of spleen with vessels, nerves and ligaments.

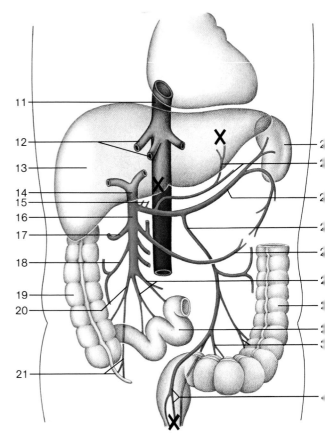

Main tributaries of portal vein. (Schematic drawing of portal circulation.) X = sites of portocaval anastomoses.

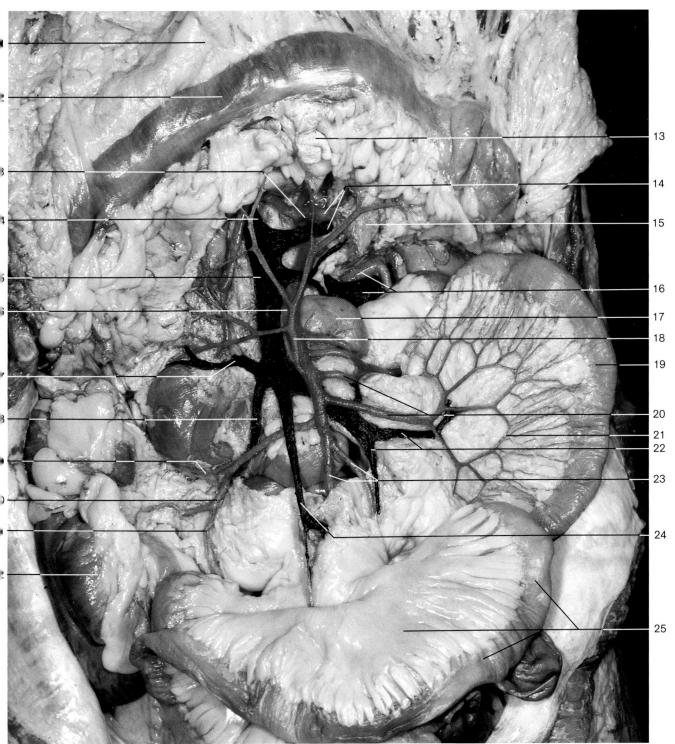

Tributaries of portal vein and branches of superior mesenteric artery (injected with colored solutions).
Blue = veins; red = arteries. One layer of peritoneum has been removed to display the vascular arcades of the intestine.
Part of the head of the pancreas and the mesocolon have also been removed to show the deeper vessels.

1	Greater omentum (reflected)	10	Ileocolic artery	19	Jejunum
2	Transverse colon (raised cranially)	11	Appendicular artery	20	Jejunal arteries
3	Celiac trunk	12	Cecum	21	Arterial arcades to intestine
4	**Portal vein**	13	Transverse mesocolon	22	Jejunal veins
5	Superior mesenteric vein	14	**Splenic artery and vein**	23	Ileal arteries
6	**Superior mesenteric artery**	15	Pancreas (divided)	24	Ileal vein
7	Right colic vein	16	Renal artery and vein	25	Ileum with mesentery
8	Ileocolic vein	17	Duodenojejunal flexure		
9	Right colic artery	18	Middle colic artery		

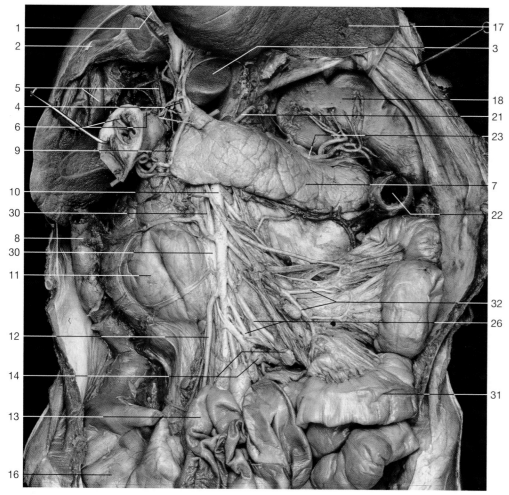

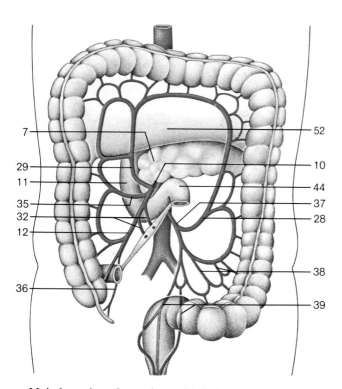

1 Ligamentum teres
2 Liver
3 Caudate lobe of liver
4 Proper hepatic artery and portal vein
5 Gallbladder and common bile duct
6 Right gastric artery and pylorus
7 **Pancreas**
8 Ascending colon
9 Gastroduodenal artery
10 **Superior mesenteric artery**
11 Duodenum
12 **Ileocolic artery**
13 Ileum
14 Mesenteric lymph nodes
15 Right common iliac artery
16 Cecum
17 Left lobe of liver
18 **Spleen**
19 Left gastro-omental (gastroepiploic) artery
20 Stomach
21 Left gastric artery
22 Left colic flexure (cut)
23 **Splenic artery**
24 Right gastro-omental (gastroepiploic) artery
25 Renal artery
26 **Ileal arteries**
27 Left kidney
28 Left colic artery
29 Middle colic artery
30 **Superior mesenteric vein**
31 Jejunum
32 **Jejunal arteries**
33 Inferior vena cava
34 Sigmoid colon
35 Right colic artery
36 Appendicular artery
37 **Inferior mesenteric artery**
38 Sigmoid arteries
39 Superior rectal artery
40 Fundus of gallbladder
41 Common bile duct
42 Portal vein
43 Beginning of jejunum
44 Duodenojejunal flexure
45 Ureter
46 Splenic artery
47 **Celiac trunk**
48 Renal vein
49 Abdominal aorta
50 Descending colon
51 Left common iliac artery
52 Transverse mesocolon

Superior mesenteric artery in relation to pancreas and duodenum. Stomach and transverse colon have been removed and the liver elevated. Note the location of the spleen. A yellow probe is inserted through the omental foramen.

Main branches of superior and inferior mesenteric arteries. (Schematic drawing.)

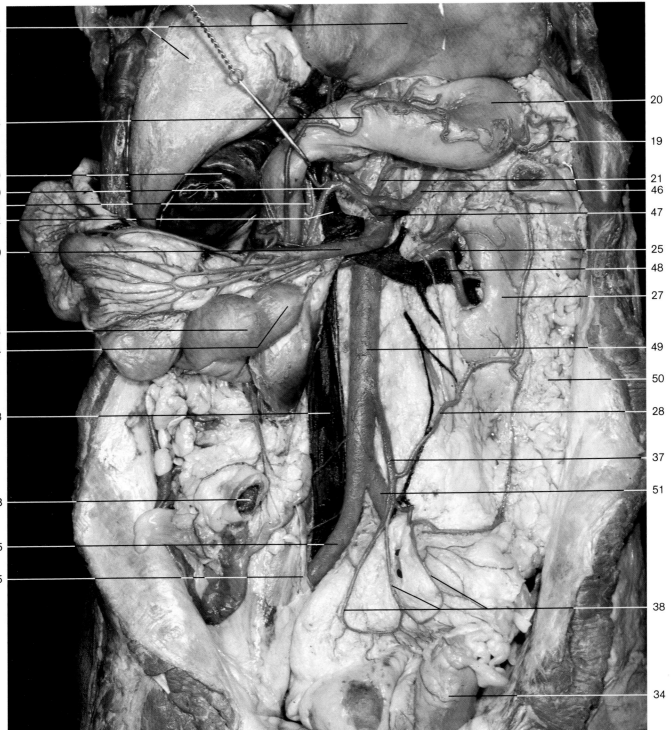

Vessels of abdominal organs; dissection of inferior mesenteric artery and celiac trunk (injected with colored solutions). Blue = veins; red = arteries. The small intestine including the duodenojejunal flexure has been reflected laterally and the stomach and liver have been raised. The peritoneum of the posterior abdominal wall has been removed to display the inferior mesenteric artery and its branches to the colon.

The **superior mesenteric artery** arises at the level of L_1 vertebra branching of the abdominal aorta. It supplies jejunum and ileum as the ascending and transverse colon. At the left colic flexure, branches of the middle colic artery (from the superior mesenteric artery) and of the left colic artery (from the inferior mesenteric artery) anastomose (so-called **Riolan's anastomosis**). The arteries unite to form loops or arches called arterial arcades from which straight vessels (vasa recta) arise. The vasa recta do not anastomose within the mesentery. Thus occlusion of these vessels may lead to necrosis of the segment of bowel concerned and ileus. Within the wall of the intestine there are many anastomoses of blood vessels, so that blockage of a single vessel is usually not dangerous. The arteries are paralleled by veins which convey blood to the portal vein. Closely related to the venous drainage are the lymph vessels which pass the mesenteric lymph nodes and finally enter the cisterna chyli.

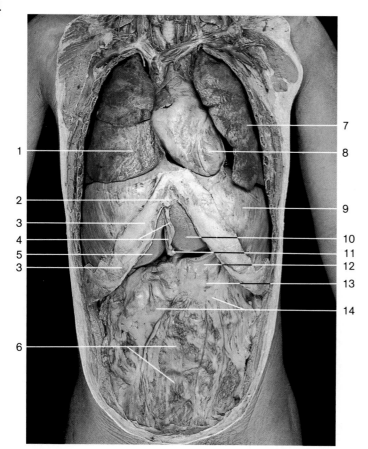

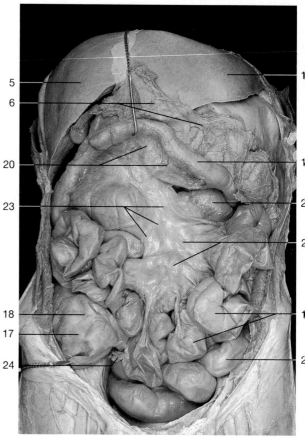

1	Middle lobe of right lung
2	Xiphoid process
3	Costal margin
4	Falciform ligament of liver
5	Quadrate lobe of liver
6	Greater omentum
7	Upper lobe of left lung
8	Heart
9	Diaphragm
10	Left lobe of liver
11	Ligamentum teres
12	Stomach
13	Gastrocolic ligament
14	Transverse colon
15	Taenia coli
16	Appendices epiploicae
17	Cecum
18	Taenia coli
19	Ileum
20	Transverse mesocolon
21	Jejunum
22	Sigmoid colon
23	Position of root of mesentery
24	Vermiform appendix
25	Duodenojejunal flexure
26	Mesentery

Abdominal organs. The anterior thoracic and abdominal walls have been removed.

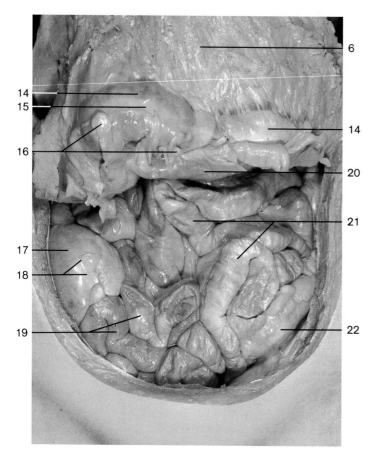

Abdominal organs. The greater omentum which is fixed to the transverse colon has been raised.

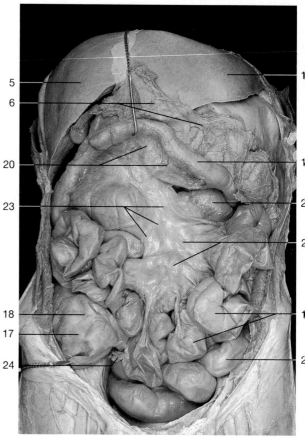

Abdominal organs (anterior aspect). The transverse colon has been reflected.

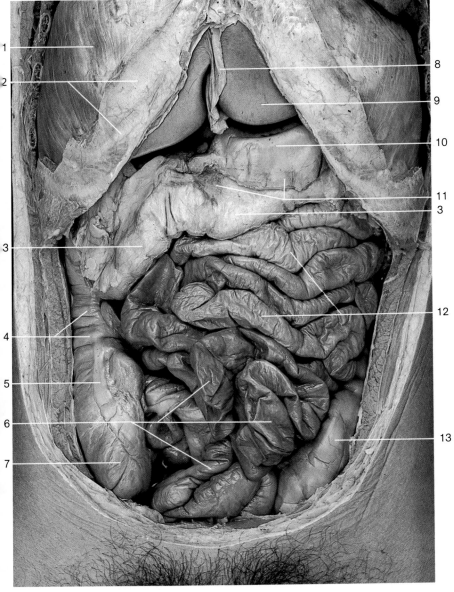

1 Diaphragm
2 Costal margin
3 Transverse colon
4 Ascending colon with haustra
5 Free taenia of cecum
6 **Ileum**
7 **Cecum**
8 **Falciform ligament of liver**
9 Liver
10 Stomach
11 Gastrocolic ligament
12 Jejunum
13 Sigmoid colon
14 **Vermiform appendix**
15 Terminal ileum
16 **Mesoappendix**
17 Mesentery

Abdominal organs in situ. The greater omentum has been removed.

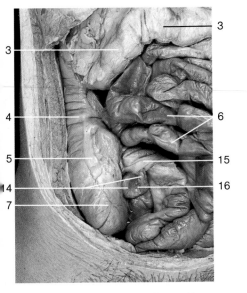

Ascending colon, cecum and vermiform appendix (detail of the preceding figure).

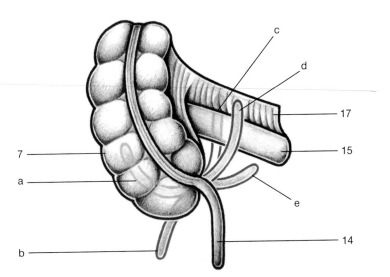

Variations in the position of the vermiform appendix.
a = retrocecal; b = paracolic; c = retroileal; d = preileal;
e = subcecal.

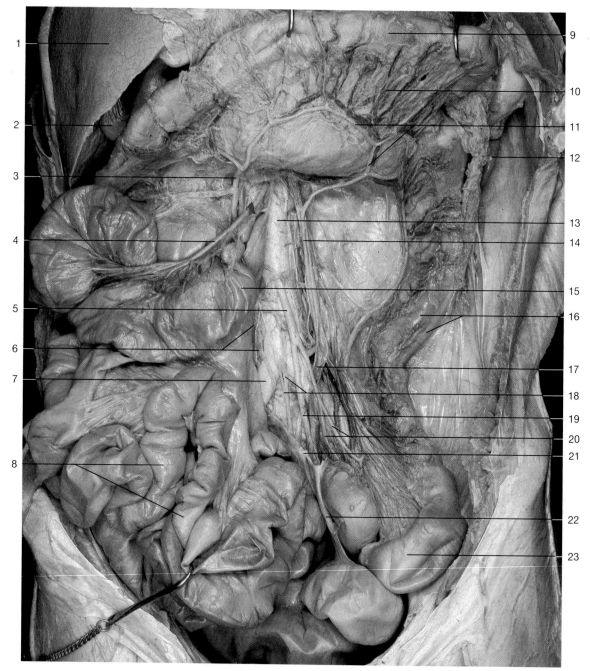

Abdominal organs. Dissection of inferior mesenteric artery and autonomic plexus. The transverse colon with mesocolon has been raised and the small intestine reflected.

1 Liver
2 Gallbladder
3 **Middle colic artery**
4 Jejunal artery
5 **Inferior mesenteric artery**
6 Sympathetic nerves and ganglia
7 Right common iliac artery
8 Small intestine (ileum)
9 Transverse colon (reflected)
10 Transverse mesocolon
11 Anastomosis between middle
     and left colic artery

12 Spleen
13 **Abdominal aorta**
14 **Left colic artery**
15 Duodenojejunal flexure
16 Descending colon (free taenia of colon)
17 Inferior mesenteric vein
18 Superior hypogastric plexus
19 **Superior rectal artery**
20 Sigmoid arteries
21 Peritoneum (cut edge)
22 Sigmoid mesocolon
23 Sigmoid colon

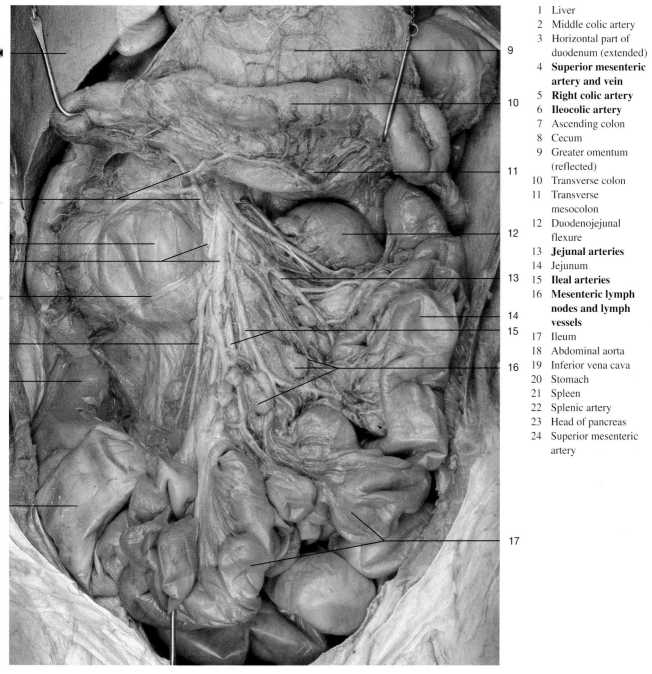

1 Liver
2 Middle colic artery
3 Horizontal part of
   duodenum (extended)
4 **Superior mesenteric
   artery and vein**
5 **Right colic artery**
6 **Ileocolic artery**
7 Ascending colon
8 Cecum
9 Greater omentum
   (reflected)
10 Transverse colon
11 Transverse
   mesocolon
12 Duodenojejunal
   flexure
13 **Jejunal arteries**
14 Jejunum
15 **Ileal arteries**
16 **Mesenteric lymph
   nodes and lymph
   vessels**
17 Ileum
18 Abdominal aorta
19 Inferior vena cava
20 Stomach
21 Spleen
22 Splenic artery
23 Head of pancreas
24 Superior mesenteric
   artery

Abdominal organs. Superior mesenteric artery. Mesenteric lymph nodes. Transverse colon reflected.

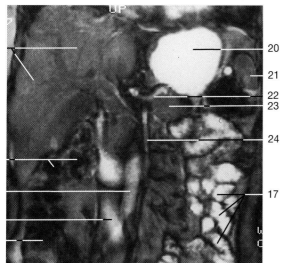

Frontal section through the abdominal cavity. (MRI scan: the intestinal tract and vessels are filled with a paramagnetic substance [Gadolinium]; courtesy of Dr. W. Rödl, Erlangen, Germany.)

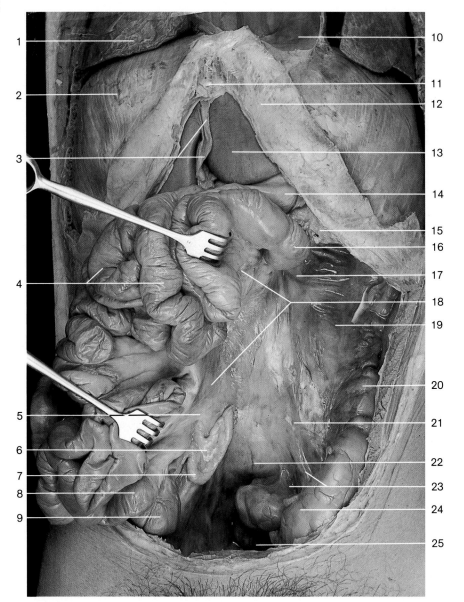

1	Lung
2	Diaphragm
3	Falciform ligament of liver
4	Jejunum
5	Ileocecal fold
6	Mesoappendix
7	Vermiform appendix
8	**Ileocecal junction**
9	**Cecum**
10	Pericardial sac
11	Xiphoid process
12	Costal margin
13	Liver
14	Stomach
15	Transverse colon
16	**Duodenojejunal flexure**
17	Inferior duodenal fold
18	Mesentery
19	Position of left kidney
20	Descending colon
21	Position of left common iliac artery
22	Sacral promontory
23	Sigmoid mesocolon
24	Sigmoid colon
25	Rectum
26	Beginning of jejunum
27	Peritoneum of posterior abdominal wall
28	Transverse mesocolon
29	Superior duodenal fold
30	Superior duodenal recess
31	Retroduodenal recess
32	Free taenia of ascending colon
33	**Ileocecal valve**
34	Frenulum of ileocecal valve
35	Orifice of vermiform appendix (probe)
36	**Ileocolic artery**
37	Vermiform appendix with appendicular artery
38	Ascending colon

Abdominal cavity. Mesenteries. The small intestine has been reflected laterally to demonstrate the mesentery.

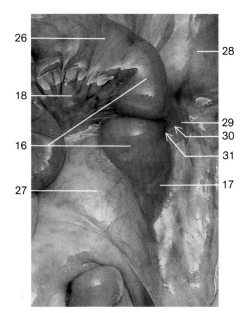

Duodenojejunal flexure
(enlargement of preceding figure).

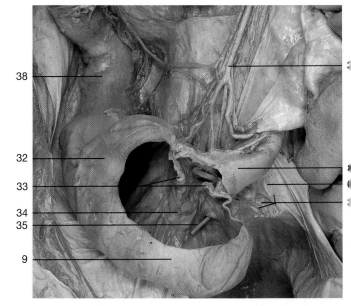

Ileocecal valve (ventral aspect). The cecum and terminal part of the ileum have been opened.

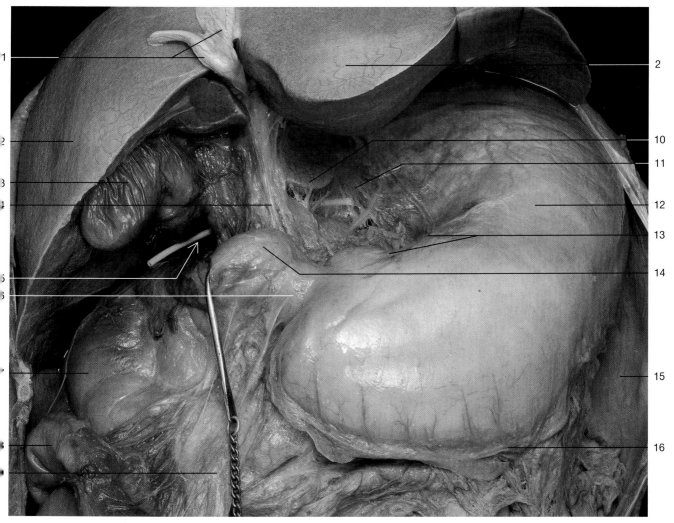

Upper abdominal organs. Thorax and anterior part of diaphragm have been removed and the liver raised to display the lesser omentum. A probe has been inserted into the epiploic foramen and lesser sac.

1   Falciform ligament and ligamentum teres
2   Liver
3   Gallbladder (fundus)
4   Hepatoduodenal ligament
5   **Epiploic foramen** (probe)
6   Pylorus
7   Descending part of duodenum
8   Right colic flexure
9   **Gastrocolic ligament**
10 Caudate lobe of liver (behind lesser omentum)
11 **Lesser omentum**
12 Stomach
13 Lesser curvature of stomach
14 Superior part of duodenum
15 Diaphragm
16 Greater curvature of stomach with gastro-omental
    vessels
17 Twelfth thoracic vertebra
18 Right kidney
19 Right suprarenal gland
20 Inferior vena cava
21 Falciform ligament of liver
22 Abdominal aorta
23 Spleen
24 Lienorenal ligament
25 Gastrosplenic ligament
26 Pancreas
27 Lesser sac

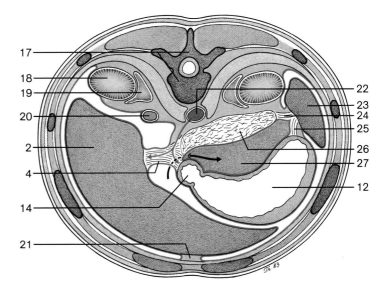

Horizontal section through omental bursa above the level of epiploic foramen (black arrow). Viewed from above. Red arrows: routes of the arterial branches of celiac trunk to liver, stomach, duodenum, and pancreas. (Schematic drawing.)

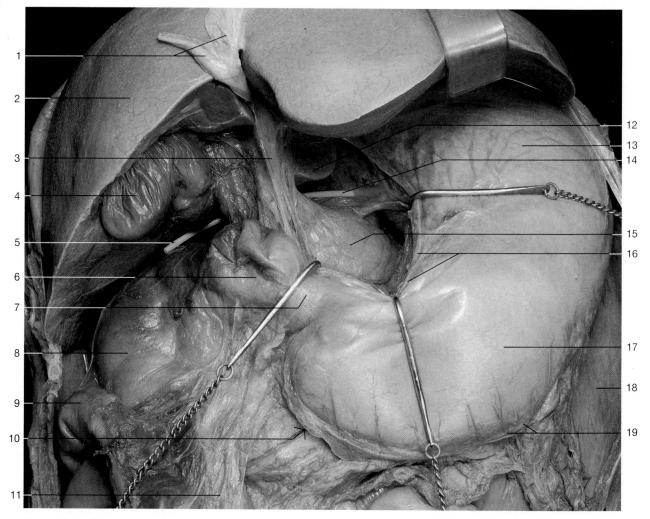

Upper abdominal organs, lesser sac, omental bursa (anterior aspect). Lesser omentum partly removed, liver and stomach slightly reflected.

1	Falciform ligament and ligamentum teres	18	Diaphragm
2	Liver	19	Greater curvature with gastro-omental vessels
3	**Hepatoduodenal ligament**		
4	Gallbladder	20	Head of pancreas and gastropancreatic fold
5	Probe within the epiploic foramen	21	**Spleen**
6	Superior part of duodenum	22	**Tail of pancreas**
7	Pylorus	23	Left colic flexure
8	Descending part of duodenum	24	Root of transverse mesocolon
9	Right colic flexure	25	Transverse mesocolon
10	Gastrocolic ligament	26	Gastrocolic ligament (cut edge)
11	**Greater omentum**	**27**	**Transverse colon**
12	Caudate lobe of liver	28	Umbilicus
13	Fundus of stomach	29	Small intestine
14	Probe at the level of the vestibule of lesser sac (through epiploic foramen)	30	Lesser omentum
		31	Lesser sac (omental bursa)
15	**Head of pancreas**	32	Duodenum
16	Lesser curvature of stomach	33	Mesentery
17	**Body of stomach**	34	Sigmoid colon

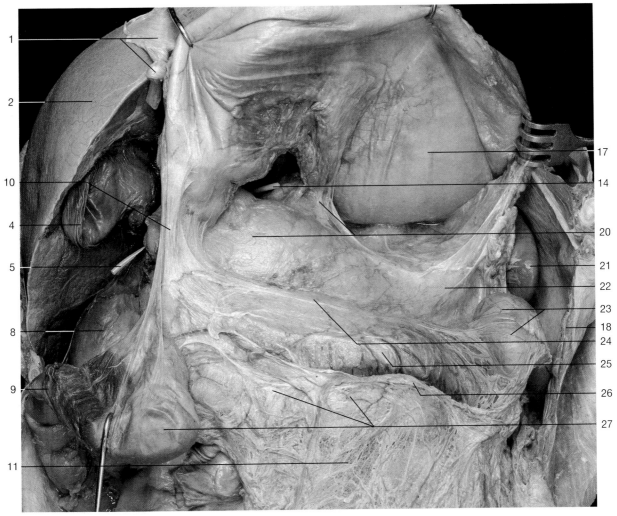

Upper abdominal organs, lesser sac, omental bursa (anterior aspect). The gastrocolic ligament has been divided and the whole stomach raised to display the posterior wall of the lesser sac.

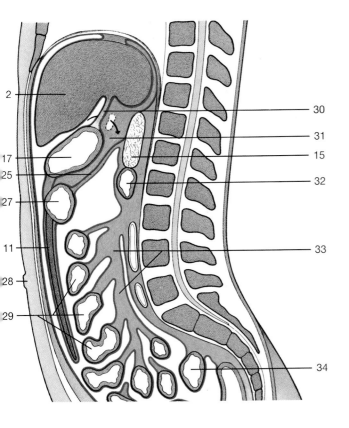

Midsagittal section through abdominal cavity, demonstrating the site of lesser sac (blue). (Schematic drawing.) The epiploic foramen, entrance to the lesser sac, is indicated by an arrow. Red = peritoneum.

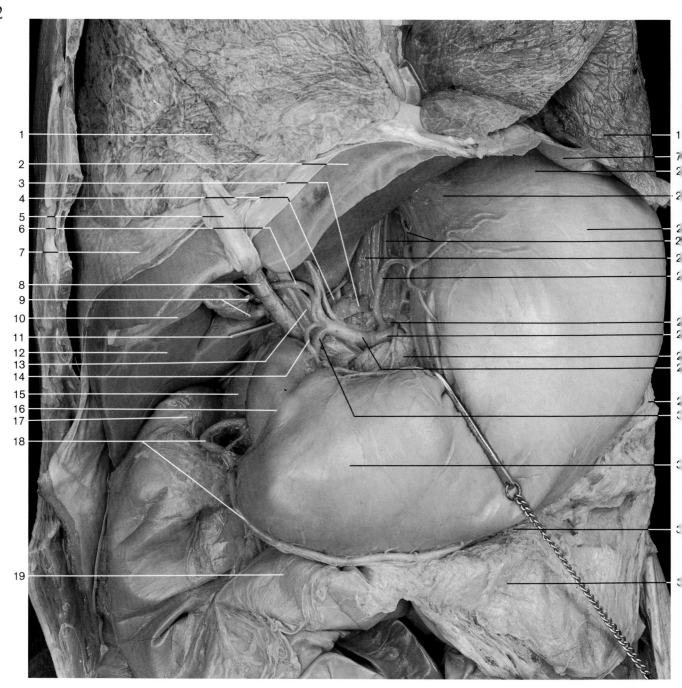

Arteries of upper abdominal organs; dissection of celiac trunk. The lesser omentum has been removed and the lesser curvature of the stomach reflected to display the branches of the celiac trunk. The probe is situated within the epiploic foramen.

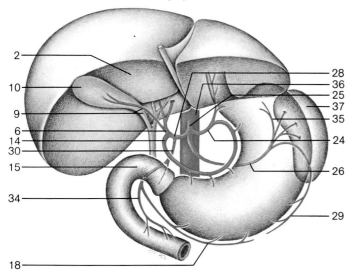

Branches of celiac trunk.
(Schematic drawing.)

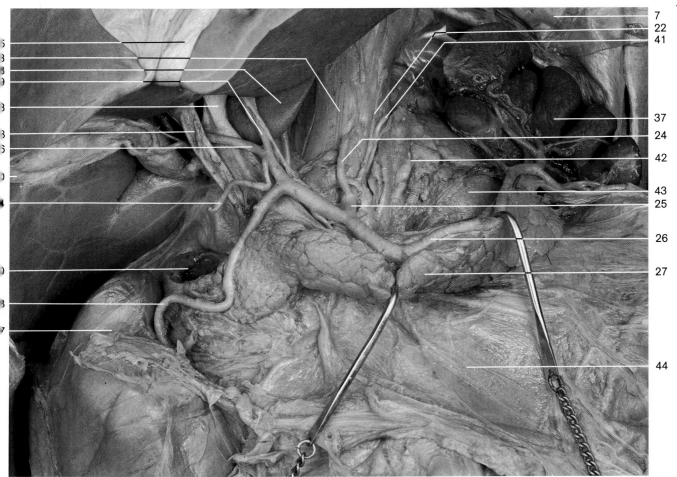

Branches of celiac trunk; blood supply of liver, pancreas and spleen. The stomach, superior part of duodenum and celiac ganglion have been removed to reveal the anterior aspect of the posterior wall of the lesser sac (omental bursa) and the vessels and ducts of the hepatoduodenal ligament. The pancreas has been slightly reflected anteriorly.

1	Lung	23	Lumbar part of diaphragm
2	Liver (visceral surface)	24	Left gastric artery
3	Lymph node	25	**Celiac trunk**
4	Inferior vena cava	26	**Splenic artery**
5	Ligamentum teres (reflected)	27	Pancreas
6	Right branch of hepatic artery proper	28	**Common hepatic artery**
7	Diaphragm	29	Left gastro-omental (gastroepiploic) artery
8	**Common hepatic duct** (dilated)	30	**Gastroduodenal artery**
9	Cystic duct and artery	31	Pyloric part of stomach
10	Gallbladder	32	Greater curvature of stomach
11	Probe in epiploic foramen	33	Gastrocolic ligament
12	Right lobe of liver	34	Superior pancreaticoduodenal artery
13	**Portal vein**	35	Short gastric arteries
14	**Right gastric artery**	36	Aorta
15	Duodenum	37	Spleen
16	Pylorus	38	Caudate lobe of liver
17	Right colic flexure	39	Left branch of hepatic artery proper
18	**Right gastro-omental** (gastroepiploic) **artery**	40	Descending part of duodenum (cut)
19	Transverse colon	41	Left inferior phrenic artery
20	Abdominal part of esophagus (cardiac part of stomach)	42	Suprarenal gland
21	Fundus of stomach	43	Kidney
22	Esophageal branches of left gastric artery	44	Transverse mesocolon

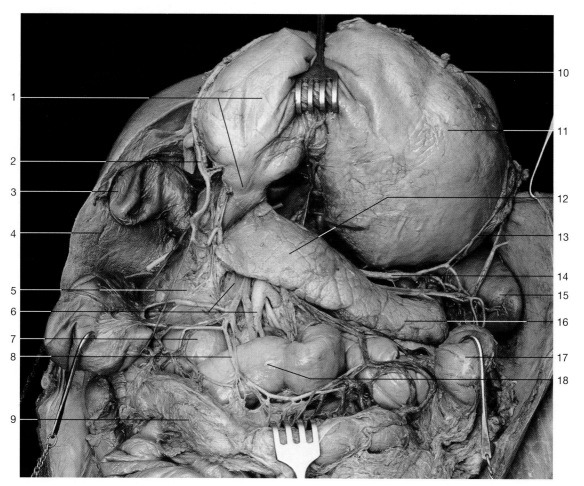

Pancreas and extrahepatic bile ducts in situ (anterior aspect). The gastrocolic ligament has been divided, the transverse colon and the stomach were replaced to display the pancreas and superior mesenteric vessels.

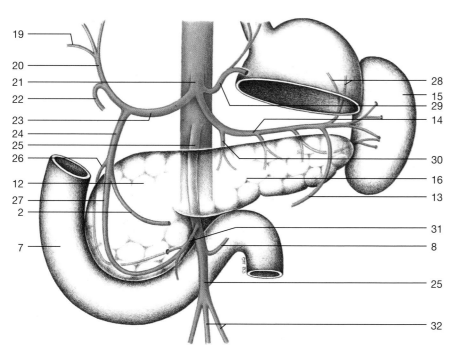

Blood supply of upper abdominal organs (branches of the celiac trunk and superior mesenteric artery). (Schematic drawing.)

1 Stomach (pyloric part) and pylorus
2 Right gastro-omental (gastroepiploic) artery
3 **Fundus of gallbladder**
4 Liver, right lobe
5 Head of pancreas
6 **Superior mesenteric artery** and **vein**
7 Duodenum
8 Middle colic artery
9 Transverse colon
10 Greater curvature of stomach
    (remnants of gastrocolic ligament)
11 **Body of stomach**
12 **Body of pancreas**
13 Left gastro-omental (gastroepiploic) artery
14 **Splenic artery**
15 **Spleen**
16 Tail of pancreas
17 Left colic flexure
18 Jejunum
19 Cystic artery
20 Hepatic artery proper
21 **Celiac trunk**
22 Right gastric artery
23 **Common hepatic artery**
24 Gastroduodenal artery
25 **Superior mesenteric artery**
26 Superior posterior pancreaticoduodenal artery
27 Superior anterior pancreaticoduodenal artery
28 Short gastric arteries
29 Left gastric artery
30 Posterior pancreatic branch of splenic artery
31 Inferior pancreaticoduodenal artery
32 Jejunal arteries

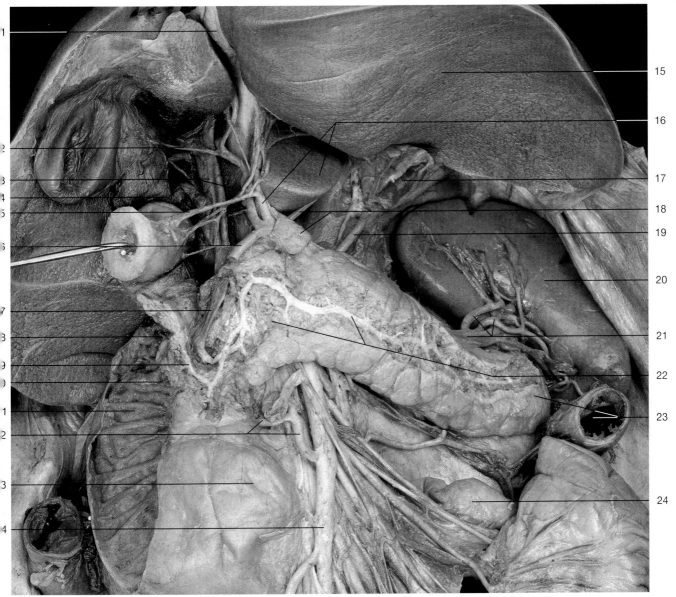

Posterior abdominal wall with duodenum, pancreas and spleen (anterior aspect). Dissection of pancreatic and common bile duct. The stomach has been removed, the liver raised and the duodenum anteriorly opened.

1   Ligamentum teres
2   Gallbladder and cystic artery
3   Common hepatic duct and portal vein
4   Cystic duct
5   Right gastric artery (pylorus with superior part of duodenum, cut and reflected)
6   Gastroduodenal artery
7   **Common bile duct**
8   Probe within the minor duodenal papilla
9   **Accessory pancreatic duct**
10 Probe within the major duodenal papilla
11 Descending part of duodenum (opened)
12 Middle colic artery and inferior pancreaticoduodenal artery

13 Horizontal part of duodenum (distended)
14 **Superior mesenteric artery**
15 Liver (left lobe)
16 Caudate lobe of liver and hepatic artery proper
17 Abdominal part of esophagus (cut)
18 Probe in epiploic foramen and lymph node
19 Left gastric artery
20 **Spleen**
21 Splenic vein and branches of splenic artery
22 **Pancreatic duct and head of pancreas**
23 Left colic flexure and tail of pancreas
24 Duodenojejunal flexure

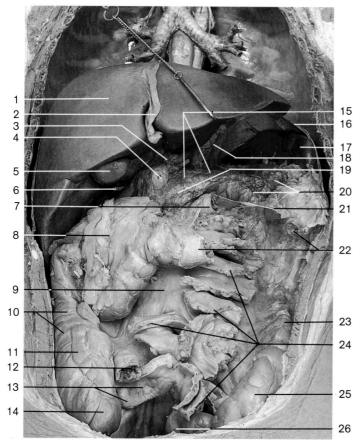

Abdominal cavity after removal of stomach, jejunum, ileum and part of the transverse colon. Liver has been slightly raised.

1 Liver
2 Falciform ligament
3 Hepatoduodenal ligament
4 Pylorus (divided)
5 Gallbladder
6 Probe within the epiploic foramen
7 Duodenojejunal flexure (divided)
8 **Greater omentum**
9 Root of mesentery
10 Ascending colon
11 Free colic taenia
12 End of ileum (divided)
13 Vermiform appendix with mesoappendix
14 Cecum
15 Pancreas and site of lesser sac
16 Diaphragm
17 Spleen
18 Cardia (part of stomach, divided)
19 Head of pancreas
20 Body and tail of pancreas
21 **Transverse mesocolon**
22 Transverse colon (divided)
23 Descending colon
24 Cut edge of mesentery
25 Sigmoid colon
26 Rectum
27 Attachment of bare area of liver
28 Inferior vena cava
29 Kidney
30 Attachment of right colic flexure
31 Root of transverse mesocolon
32 Junction between descending and horizontal parts of duodenum
33 Bare surface for ascending colon
34 **Ileocecal recess**
35 **Retrocecal recess**
36 Root of mesoappendix
37 Superior recess ⎫
38 Isthmus (opening) ⎬ of **lesser sac**
39 Splenic recess ⎭ **(omental bursa)**
40 **Superior duodenal recess**
41 **Inferior duodenal recess**
42 Bare surface for descending colon
43 **Paracolic recesses**
44 **Root of mesentery**
45 Root of mesosigmoid
46 **Intersigmoid recess**
47 Hepatic veins
48 Duodenojejunal flexure
49 Attachment of left colic flexure
50 Esophagus
51 Entrance to lesser sac through the epiploic foramen

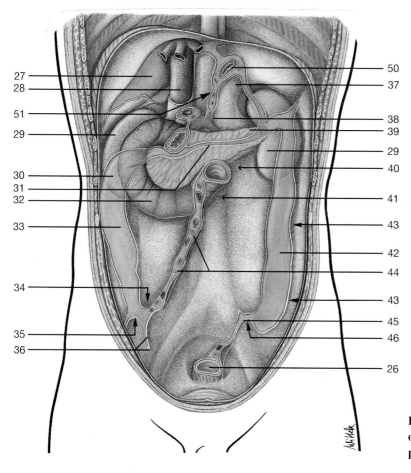

Peritoneal reflections from organs and the position of root of mesentry and peritoneal recesses on the posterior abdominal wall. (Schematic drawing.)

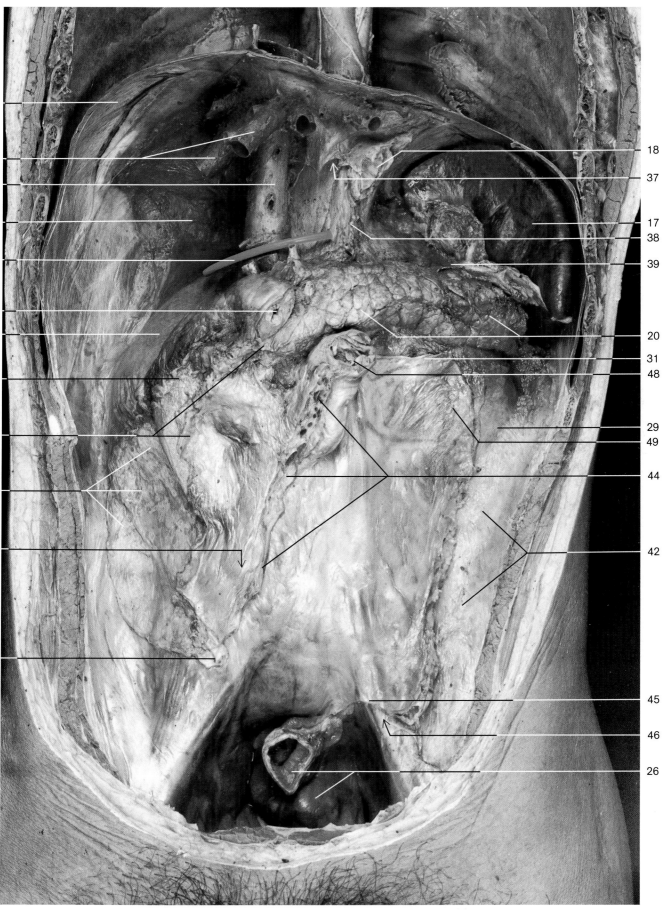

18
37
17
38
39

20
31
48

29
49

44

42

45
46
26

Peritoneal recesses on the posterior abdominal wall. The liver, stomach, jejunum, ileum, and colon have been removed. The duodenum, pancreas, and spleen have been left in place.

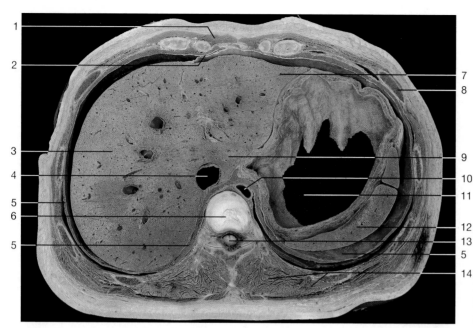

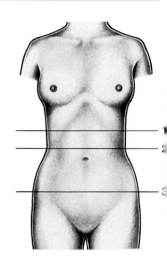

Horizontal section through the abdominal cavity at level 1 (from below).

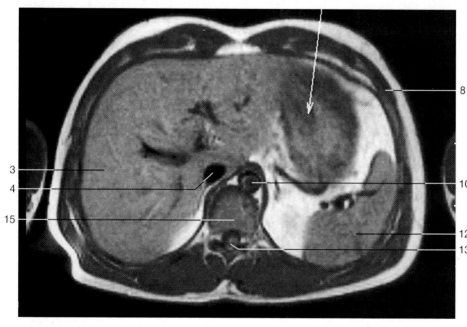

Horizontal section through the body. MRI scan, corresponding to level 1. Arrow: stomach.

1	Rectus abdominis muscle	20	**Greater duodenal papilla**
2	Falciform ligament	21	Duodenum
3	**Liver** (right lobe)	22	Suprarenal gland and ureter
4	Inferior vena cava	23	**Kidney**
5	Diaphragm	24	Round ligament of liver
6	Intervertebral disc	25	Superior mesenteric artery and vein
7	Liver (left lobe)	26	Psoas major muscle
8	Rib	27	Descending colon
9	Liver (caudate lobe)	28	Quadratus lumborum muscle
10	Abdominal (descending) aorta	29	Cauda equina
11	**Stomach**	30	Right renal vein
12	**Spleen**	31	**Small intestine**
13	Spinal cord	32	Iliacus muscle
14	Longissimus and iliocostalis muscles	33	Ilium
15	Body of vertebra	34	**Ileocecal valve**
16	Rectus abdominis muscle	35	Cecum
17	External abdominal oblique muscle	36	Common iliac artery and vein
18	Transverse colon	37	Gluteus medius muscle
19	**Head of pancreas**	38	Vertebral canal and dura mater

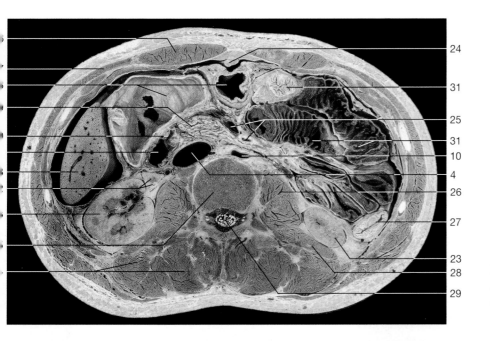

	24
	31
	25
	31
	10
	4
	26
	27
	23
	28
	29

Horizontal section through the abdominal cavity at the level of greater duodenal papilla (from below).

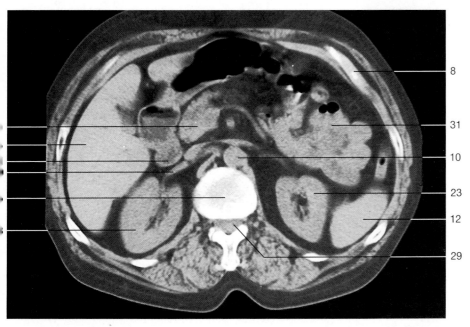

	8
	31
	10
	23
	12
	29

Horizontal section through the body. CT scan, corresponding to level 2.

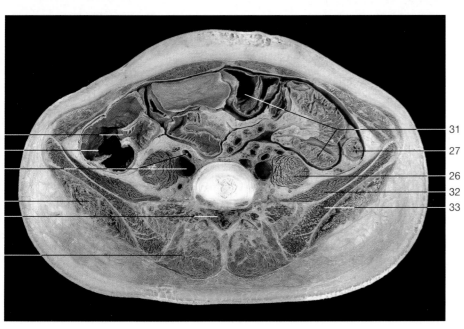

	31
	27
	26
	32
	33

Horizontal section through the abdominal cavity at level 3 (from below).

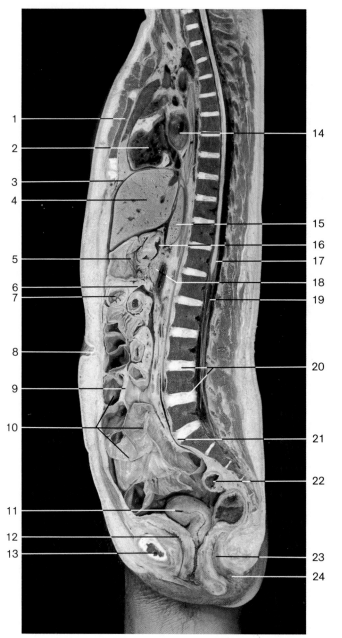

Midsagittal section through the trunk (female).

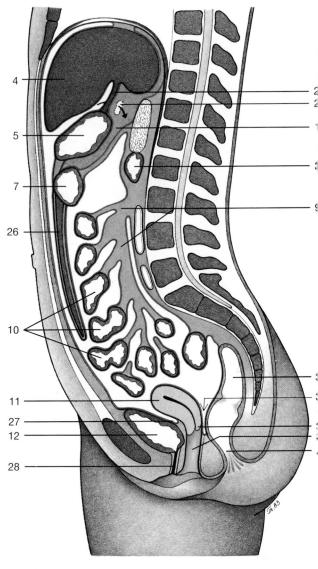

Midsagittal section through the trunk (female).
(Schematic drawing.)
Blue = omental bursa; red = peritoneum.

1	Sternum	13	Pubic symphysis
2	Right ventricle of heart	14	Left atrium of heart
3	Diaphragm	15	Caudate lobe of liver
4	Liver	16	Omental bursa or lesser sac
5	Stomach	17	Conus medullaris
6	Transverse mesocolon	18	Pancreas
7	Transverse colon	19	Cauda equina
8	Umbilicus	20	Intervertebral discs
9	Mesentery		(lumbar vertebral column)
10	Small intestine	21	Sacral promontory
11	Uterus	22	Sigmoid colon
12	Urinary bladder	23	Anal canal

24	Anus
25	Lesser omentum
26	Greater omentum
27	Vesicouterine pouch
28	Urethra
29	Epiploic (omental) foramen
30	Duodenum
31	Rectum
32	Rectouterine pouch
33	Vaginal part of
	cervix of uterus
34	Vagina

Retroperitoneal Organs

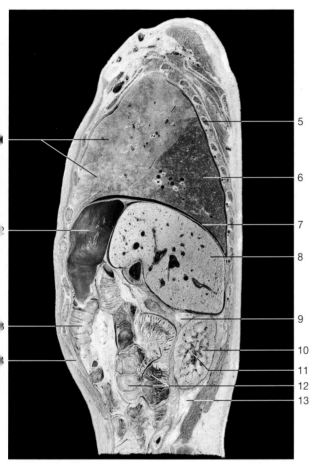

Parasagittal section through the thoracic and abdominal cavities (medial aspect, 6 cm right of median plane).

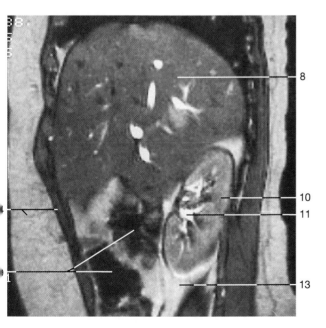

Parasagittal section through the abdominal cavity.
(MRI scan, courtesy of Prof. W. Rödl, Erlangen, Germany.)

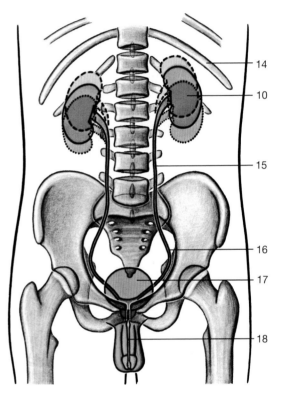

Position of kidneys and urinary system (anterior view). The excursions of the kidneys with the respiratory movements of the diaphragm are indicated. (Schematic drawing.)

1   Right lung (superior and middle lobes)
2   Transverse colon
3   Jejunum
4   Abdominal wall
5   Fourth rib
6   Right lung (inferior lobe)
7   Diaphragm
8   **Liver**
9   Suprarenal gland
10 **Kidney**
11 Renal pelvis
12 Small intestine
13 Perirenal fatty tissue
14 Eleventh rib
15 Ureter (abdominal part)
16 Ureter (pelvic part)
17 **Urinary bladder**
18 Urethra
19 Colon

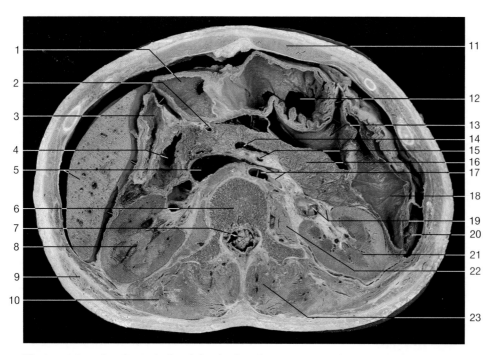

1 Pyloric antrum
2 Gastroduodenal artery
3 Descending part of
   duodenum
4 Vestibule of lesser sac
5 Inferior vena cava and liver
6 Body of first lumbar vertebra
7 Cauda equina
8 **Right kidney**
9 Latissimus dorsi muscle
10 Iliocostalis muscle
11 Rectus abdominis muscle
12 Stomach
13 Lesser sac
14 Splenic vein
15 Superior mesenteric artery
16 Pancreas
17 Aorta and left renal artery
18 Transverse colon
19 Renal artery and vein
20 Spleen
21 **Left kidney**
22 Psoas major muscle
23 Multifidus muscle
24 Margin of lung
25 Margin of pleura
26 Renal pelvis
27 **Left ureter**
28 Descending colon
29 Rectum
30 Right suprarenal gland
31 Twelfth rib
32 Ascending colon
33 **Right ureter**
34 Cecum
35 Vermiform appendix
36 Urinary bladder
37 Liver
38 Anterior layer of renal fascia
39 Duodenum
40 Perirenal fatty tissue
41 Posterior layer of renal fascia
42 Abdominal cavity

Horizontal section through the abdominal cavity at the level of the first lumbar vertebra (from below).

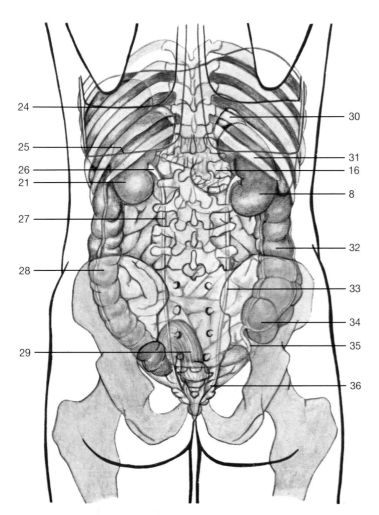

Positions of urinary organs (posterior view). Notice that the upper part of the kidney reaches the level of the margin of pleura and lung.

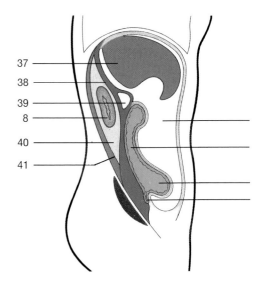

Retroperitoneal tissue, location of the right kidney. (Schematic drawing.)
Yellow = adipose capsule of kidney.

1   Scalenus anterior, medius and posterior muscles
2   Left subclavian artery
3   Left subclavian vein
4   Pulmonic valve
5   Arterial cone
6   Right ventricle of heart
7   Liver
8   Stomach
9   Transverse colon
10 Small intestine
11 Left lung
12 Left main bronchus
13 Branches of pulmonary vein
14 Left ventricle of heart
15 Spleen
16 Splenic artery and vein and pancreas
17 **Left kidney**
18 Psoas major muscle
19 Inferior vena cava
20 **Renal vein**
21 Body of twelfth thoracic vertebra and vertebral canal
22 **Right kidney**
23 Superior mesenteric artery
24 Superior mesenteric vein
25 Pancreas
26 Abdominal aorta
27 Left psoas major and quadratus lumborum muscles
28 Anterior layer of renal fascia ⎱ of Gerota
29 Posterior layer of renal fascia ⎰
30 Perirenal fatty tissue
31 Abdominal cavity
32 Descending and sigmoid colon

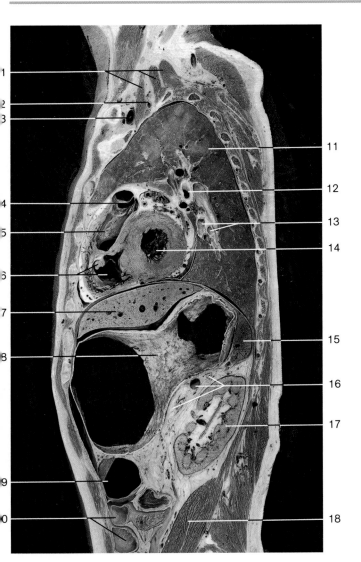

Parasagittal section through the thoracic and abdominal cavities at the level of the left kidney (5.5 cm left of median plane).

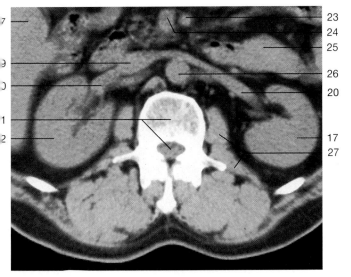

Horizontal section through the retroperitoneal region at level of 12th thoracic vertebra. (CT scan, from below.)

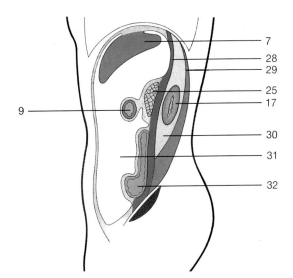

Retroperitoneal tissue, position of left kidney. (Schematic drawing.)

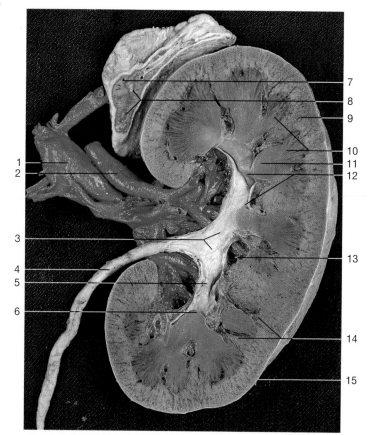

1 Renal vein
2 Renal artery
3 **Renal pelvis**
4 Abdominal part of ureter
5 **Major renal calyx**
6 Cribriform area of renal papilla
7 Cortex of suprarenal gland
8 Medulla of suprarenal gland
9 **Cortex of kidney**
10 **Medulla of kidney**
11 Renal papilla
12 **Minor renal calyx**
13 Renal sinus
14 Renal columns
15 **Fibrous capsule** of kidney

Coronal section through right kidney and suprarenal gland (posterior view). The renal pelvis has been opened and the fatty tissue removed to display the renal vessels.

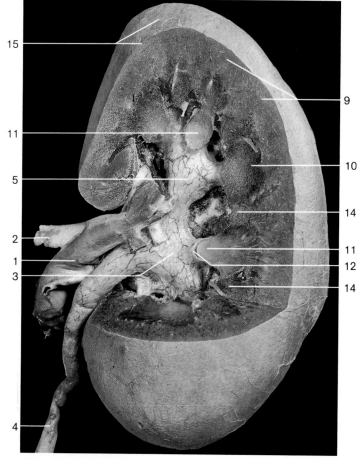

Right kidney (posterior view). Partial coronal section to expose internal aspect of the kidney.

Each kidney can be divided into five segments supplied by individual interlobar arteries considered as end arteries. Thus, obstruction leads to infarcts marking the trace of segment borders. The anterior kidney surface reveals four segments, the posterior only three (No. 1, 4 and 5).

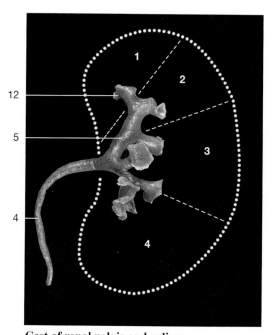

Cast of renal pelvis and calices.
1–4 = Renal segments on anterior surface.

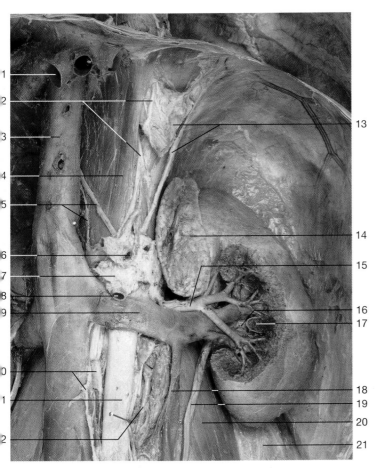

1 Hepatic vein
2 Anterior and posterior vagal trunk
3 Inferior vena cava
4 Lumbar part of diaphragm
5 Right greater and lesser splanchnic nerves
6 Celiac trunk
7 Celiac ganglion and plexus
8 Superior mesenteric artery
9 Left renal vein
10 Right sympathetic trunk and ganglion
11 Abdominal aorta
12 Left sympathetic trunk
13 Esophagus (cut),
   left greater splanchnic nerve
14 **Left suprarenal gland**
15 Left renal artery
16 Renal pelvis
17 Renal papilla with minor calyx
18 Left testicular vein
19 Left ureter
20 Psoas major muscle
21 Quadratus lumborum muscle
22 **Glomerulus**
23 Afferent arteriole of glomerulus
24 **Glomeruli**
25 Radiating cortical artery
26 Subcortical or arcuate artery
27 Subcortical or arcuate vein
28 Interlobular vein
29 Interlobular artery
30 **Interlobar artery and vein**
31 Vessels of renal capsule
32 Efferent arteriole of glomerulus
33 **Vasa recta** of renal medulla
34 Spiral arteries of renal pelvis

Left kidney and suprarenal gland in situ. The anterior cortical layer of the kidney has been removed to display the renal pelvis and papillae.

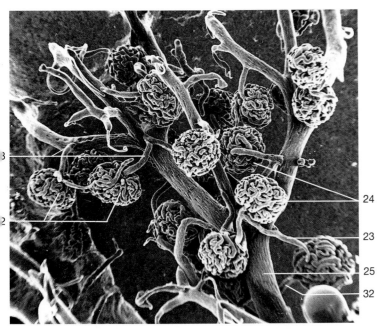

Glomeruli (210×). Scanning electron micrograph showing glomeruli and associated arteries.

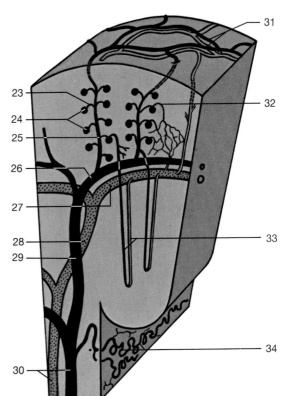

Architecture of vascular system of kidney.
(Schematic drawing.)

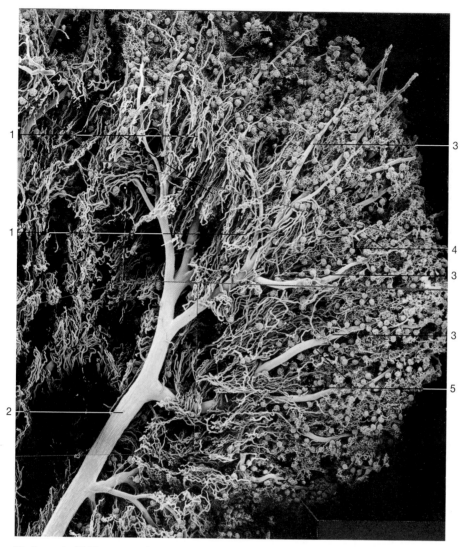

1 Arteriolae rectae of renal medulla
2 Interlobar artery
3 Interlobular arteries
4 Cortical glomeruli
5 Juxtamedullary glomeruli
6 Body of first lumbar vertebra
7 Left renal artery
8 Abdominal aorta with catheter
9 Upper pole of kidney
10 Anterior branch } of renal
11 Posterior branch } artery
12 Anterior inferior segmental artery
13 Lower pole of kidney
14 Celiac trunk
15 Superior mesenteric artery
16 Middle colic artery
17 Splenic artery

Resin cast of kidney arteries. (Scanning electron micrograph.)

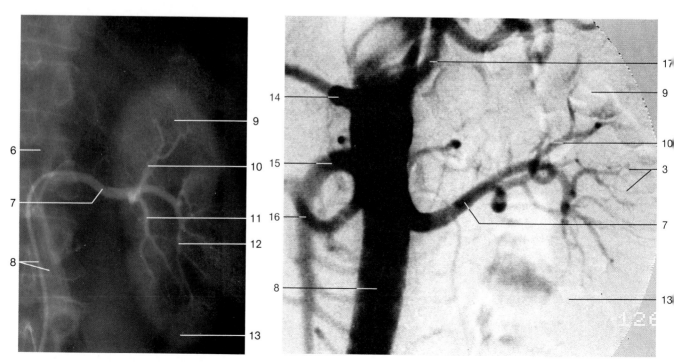

Left kidney. (Arteriogram.)

Abdominal aorta. (Subtraction angiograph.)

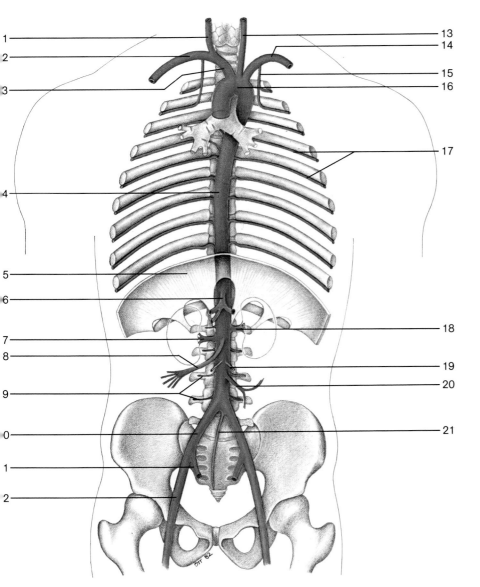

1	Right common carotid artery
2	Right subclavian artery
3	**Brachiocephalic trunk**
4	Thoracic aorta
5	Diaphragm
6	**Celiac trunk**
7	Right **renal artery**
8	**Superior mesenteric artery**
9	Lumbar arteries
10	Right **common iliac artery**
11	Internal iliac artery
12	**External iliac artery**
13	Left common carotid artery
14	Left subclavian artery
15	Highest intercostal artery
16	Aortic arch
17	**Posterior intercostal arteries**
18	Left renal artery
19	Left testicular (or ovarian) artery
20	Inferior mesenteric artery
21	Median sacral artery
22	**Superior suprarenal artery**
23	Upper capsular artery
24	Anterior branch of renal artery
25	Perforating artery
26	Lower capsular artery
27	Ureter
28	Right inferior phrenic artery
29	Left inferior phrenic artery
30	**Middle suprarenal artery**
31	**Inferior suprarenal artery**
32	Posterior branch of renal artery

Main branches of descending aorta. (Schematic drawing.)

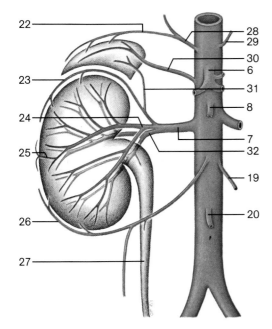

Arteries of kidney and suprarenal gland. (Schematic drawing.)

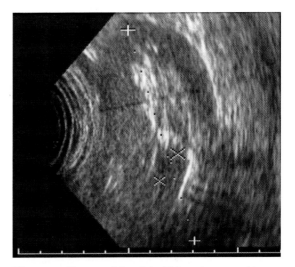

Ultrasound image of the right kidney (upper and lower border of the kidney marked by crosses; × = small cortical cyst).

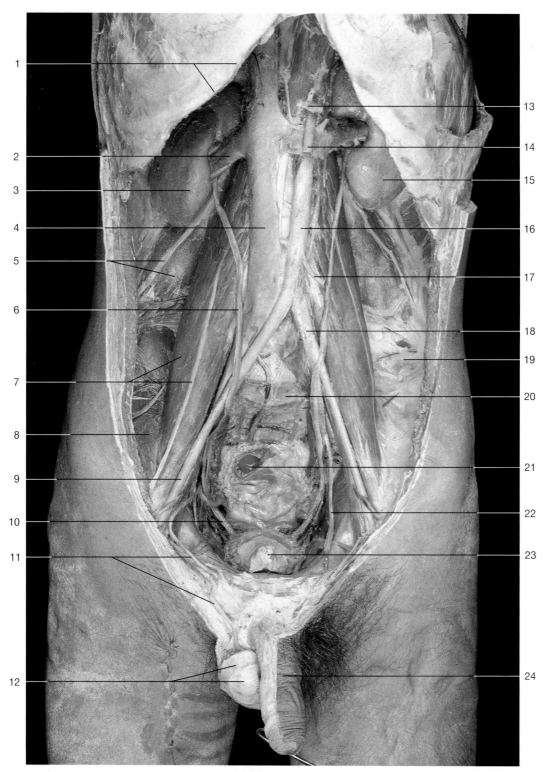

Retroperitoneal organs, urinary system in the male (anterior view). The peritoneum has been removed.

1 Costal arch	8 Iliacus muscle	17 Inferior mesenteric artery
2 Right renal vein	9 External iliac artery	18 Common iliac artery
3 **Right kidney**	10 **Ureter** (pelvic part)	19 Iliac crest
4 Inferior vena cava	11 Ductus deferens	20 Sacral promontory
5 Iliohypogastric nerve and	12 Testis and epididymis	21 Rectum (cut)
quadratus lumborum muscle	13 Celiac trunk	22 Medial umbilical ligament
6 **Ureter** (abdominal part)	14 Superior mesenteric artery	23 **Urinary bladder**
7 Psoas major muscle and	15 **Left kidney**	24 Penis
genitofemoral nerve	16 Abdominal aorta	

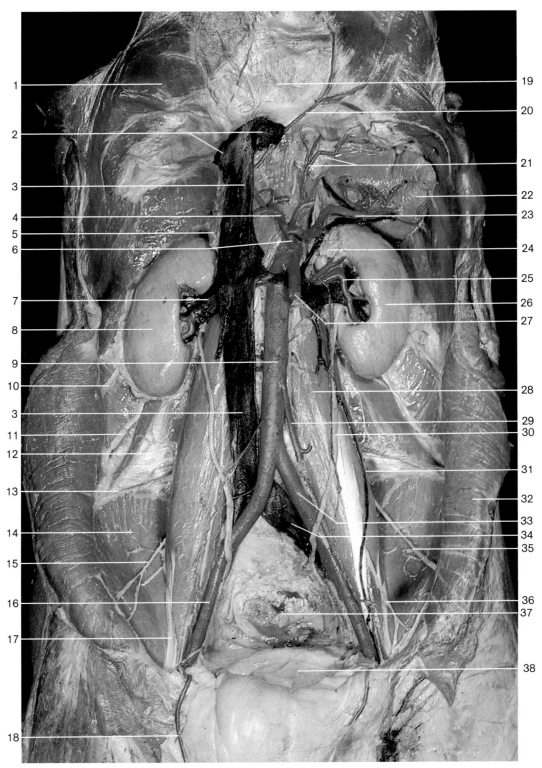

Retroperitoneal organs, urinary system in situ (anterior view). The peritoneum has been removed.
Red = arteries; blue = veins.

1	Diaphragm	12	Quadratus lumborum muscle		31	Testicular artery and vein
2	Hepatic veins	13	Iliac crest	esophageal branches of left	32	Transversus abdominis muscle
3	**Inferior vena cava**	14	Iliacus muscle	gastric artery	33	Left common iliac artery
4	Common hepatic artery	15	Right lateral femoral	22 Spleen	34	Left common iliac vein
5	Right suprarenal gland		cutaneous nerve	23 Splenic artery	35	Lateral femoral cutaneous
6	Celiac trunk	16	**External iliac artery**	24 Left subprarenal gland		nerve
7	**Right renal vein**	17	Femoral nerve	25 **Left renal artery**	36	Genitofemoral nerve
8	Right kidney	18	Right inferior epigastric artery	26 Left **kidney**	37	Rectum (cut)
9	**Abdominal aorta**	19	Central tendon of diaphragm	27 Superior mesenteric artery	38	Urinary bladder
10	Subcostal nerve	20	Inferior phrenic artery	28 Psoas major muscle		
11	Iliohypogastric nerve	21	Cardiac part of stomach and	29 Inferior mesenteric artery		
				30 **Ureter**		

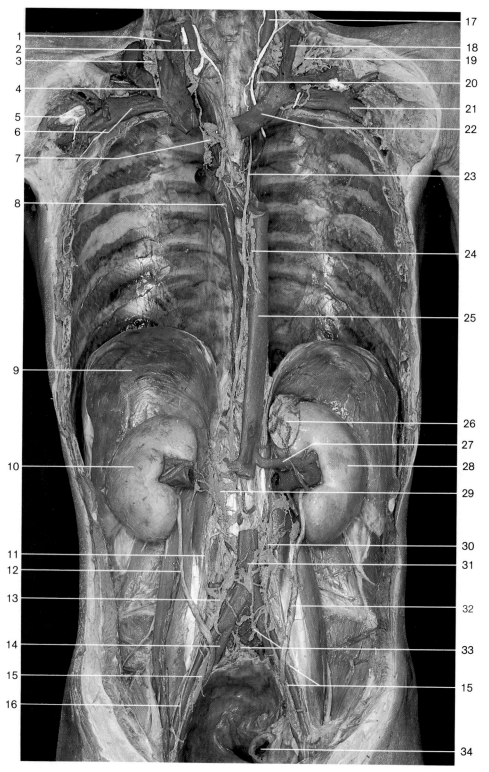

1 Internal jugular vein
2 Right common carotid
   artery and right vagus nerve
3 Jugulo-omohyoid lymph
   node
4 **Right lymphatic duct**
5 Subclavian trunk
6 Right subclavian vein
7 Bronchomediastinal trunk
8 Azygos vein
9 Diaphragm
10 Right kidney
11 Right lumbar trunk
12 Right ureter
13 Common iliac lymph nodes
14 Right internal iliac artery
15 External iliac lymph nodes
16 Right external iliac artery
17 Left common carotid artery
   and left vagus nerve
18 Internal jugular vein
19 Deep cervical lymph nodes
20 Thoracic duct entering
   left jugular angle
21 Left subclavian vein
22 Left brachiocephalic vein
23 **Thoracic duct**
24 Mediastinal lymph nodes
25 Thoracic aorta
26 Left suprarenal gland
27 Left renal artery
28 Left kidney
29 **Cisterna chyli**
30 Lumbar lymph nodes
31 Abdominal aorta
32 Left ureter
33 Sacral lymph nodes
34 Rectum (cut edge)

Lymph vessels and lymph nodes of the posterior wall of thoracic and abdominal cavities (anterior aspect). Green = lymph vessels and nodes; blue = veins; red = arteries; white = nerves.

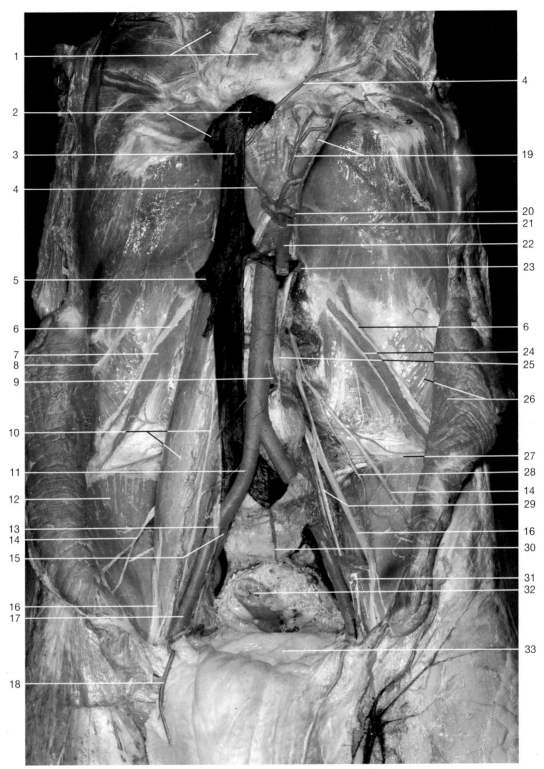

Vessels and nerves of posterior abdominal wall (anterior aspect). Part of the left psoas major muscle has been removed to display the lumbar plexus. Red = arteries, blue = veins.

1	Diaphragm	11	Common iliac artery	20	Splenic artery	31	Psoas major muscle
2	Hepatic veins	12	Iliacus muscle	21	Celiac trunk		(divided) with supplying
3	**Inferior vena cava**	13	Right ureter (divided)	22	**Superior mesenteric artery**		artery
4	Inferior phrenic artery	14	Lateral femoral cutaneous nerve	23	Left renal artery	32	Rectum (cut)
5	Right renal vein	15	Internal iliac artery	24	**Ilioinguinal nerve**	33	Urinary bladder
6	**Iliohypogastric nerve**	16	**Femoral nerve**	25	Sympathetic trunk		
7	Quadratus lumborum muscle	17	**External iliac artery**	26	Transversus abdominis muscle		
8	Subcostal nerve	18	Inferior epigastric artery	27	Iliac crest		
9	Inferior mesenteric artery	19	Cardiac part of stomach and	28	Left **genitofemoral nerve**		
10	Right genitofemoral nerve		oesophageal branches of left	29	Left **obturator nerve**		
	and psoas major muscle		gastric artery	30	Median sacral artery		

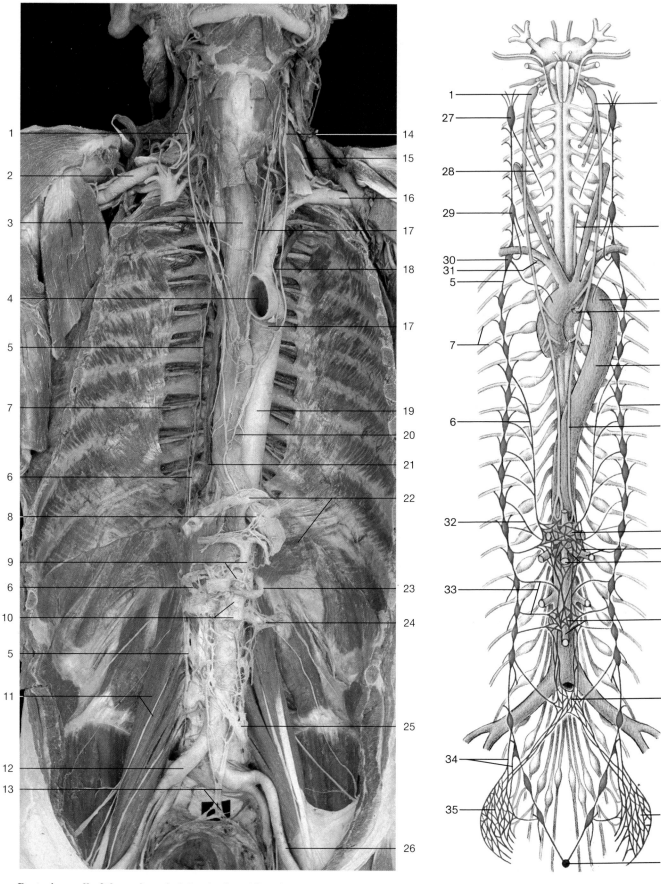

Posterior wall of thoracic and abdominal cavities with sympathetic trunk, vagus nerve and autonomic ganglia (anterior view). Thoracic and abdominal organs removed, except for the esophagus and aorta.

Organization of autonomic nervous system (after Mattuschka). (Schematic drawing.) Yellow = parasympathetic nerves; green = sympathetic nerves.

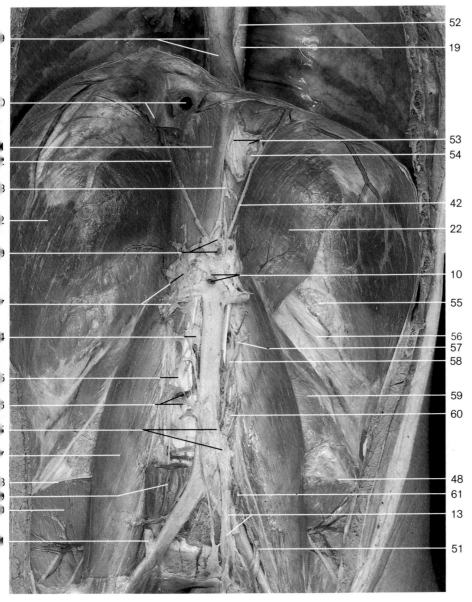

Ganglia and plexus of the autonomic nervous system within the retroperitoneal space (anterior view). The kidneys and the inferior vena cava with its tributaries have been removed (compare pp. 272 and 273).

1 **Right vagus nerve**
2 Right subclavian artery
3 Esophagus
4 Aortic arch
5 **Sympathetic trunk**
6 Greater splanchnic nerve
7 Intercostal nerve
8 Abdominal part of esophagus and vagal trunk
9 **Celiac trunk with celiac ganglion**
10 **Superior mesenteric artery and ganglion**
11 Psoas major muscle and genitofemoral nerve
12 Common iliac artery
13 **Superior hypogastric plexus and ganglion**
14 **Left vagus nerve**

15 Brachial plexus
16 Left subclavian artery
17 Left recurrent laryngeal nerve
18 Inferior cervical cardiac nerve
19 Thoracic aorta
20 Esophageal plexus
21 Azygos vein
22 Diaphragm
23 Splenic artery
24 Left renal artery and plexus
25 **Inferior mesenteric ganglion and artery**
26 Left external iliac artery
27 **Superior cervical ganglion** of sympathetic trunk
28 Superior cardiac branch of sympathetic trunk
29 Middle cervical ganglion of sympathetic trunk
30 **Inferior cervical ganglion** of sympathetic trunk
31 Right recurrent laryngeal nerve
32 Lesser splanchnic nerve
33 Lumbar splanchnic nerves
34 Sacral splanchnic nerves
35 **Inferior hypogastric ganglion and plexus**
36 Left recurrent laryngeal nerve
37 **Aorticorenal plexus** and renal artery
38 Ganglion impar
39 Esophagus with branches of vagus nerve
40 Hepatic veins
41 Right crus of diaphragm
42 Inferior phrenic artery
43 Right vagus nerve entering the celiac ganglion
44 Right lumbar lymph trunk
45 Lumbar part of right sympathetic trunk
46 Lumbar artery and vein
47 Psoas major muscle
48 Iliac crest
49 Inferior vena cava
50 Iliacus muscle
51 Ureter
52 Left vagus nerve forming the esophageal plexus
53 Left vagus nerve forming the gastric plexus
54 Esophagus continuing into the cardiac part of stomach
55 Lumbocostal triangle
56 Position of twelfth rib
57 Left lumbar lymph trunk
58 Ganglion of sympathetic trunk
59 Quadratus lumborum muscle
60 Lumbar part of left sympathetic trunk
61 Iliac lymph vessels

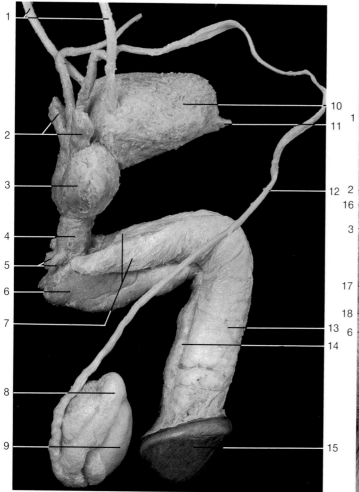

Male genital organs isolated (right lateral aspect).

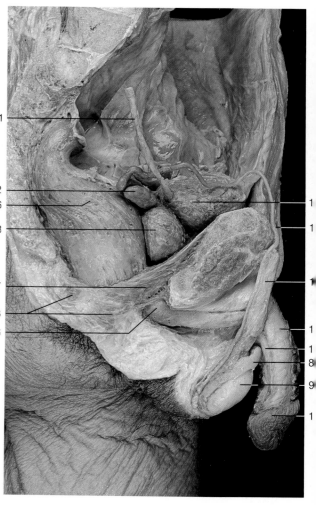

Male genital organs in situ (right lateral aspect).

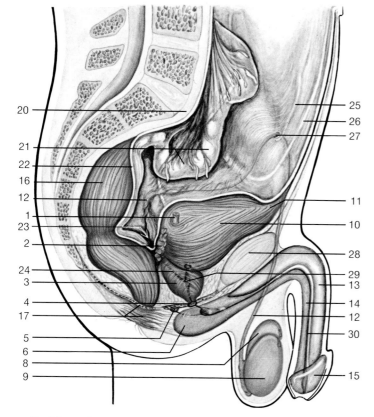

Positions of male genital organs (right lateral aspect).
(Schematic drawing.)

1 Ureter
2 **Seminal vesicle**
3 **Prostate gland**
4 Urogenital diaphragm and membranous part of urethra
5 Bulbourethral or Cowper's gland
6 Bulb of penis
7 Left and right crus penis
8 **Epididymis**
9 **Testis**
10 **Urinary bladder**
11 Apex of urinary bladder
12 **Ductus deferens**
13 **Corpus cavernosum of penis**
14 **Corpus spongiosum of penis**
15 Glans penis
16 Ampulla of rectum
17 Levator ani muscle
18 Anal canal and external anal sphincter muscle
19 Spermatic cord (cut)
20 Sacral promontory
21 Sigmoid colon
22 Peritoneum (cut edge)
23 **Rectovesical pouch**
24 Ejaculatory duct
25 Lateral umbilical fold
26 Medial umbilical fold
27 Deep inguinal ring and ductus deferens
28 Pubic symphysis
29 Prostatic part of urethra
30 Spongy urethra

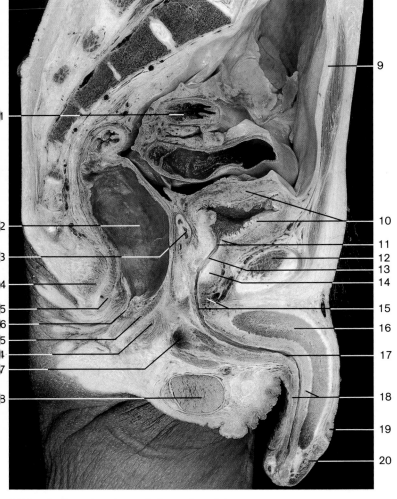

Midsagittal section through the male pelvis.

1 Sigmoid colon
2 **Ampulla of rectum**
3 Ampulla of ductus deferens
4 External anal sphincter muscle
5 Internal anal sphincter muscle
6 **Anal canal**
7 Bulb of penis
8 **Testis** (cut surface)
9 Median umbilical ligament
10 **Urinary bladder**
11 Internal urethral orifice and sphincter
   muscle (sphincter vesicae)
12 Pubic symphysis
13 Prostatic part of urethra
14 **Prostate gland**
15 Membranous urethra and external urethral
   sphincter muscle
16 **Corpus cavernosum of penis**
17 **Spongy urethra**
18 Corpus spongiosum of penis
19 Foreskin or prepuce
20 Glans penis
21 Kidney
22 Renal pelvis
23 Abdominal part of ureter
24 Pelvic part of ureter
25 Seminal vesicle
26 Ejaculatory duct
27 Bulbourethral or Cowper's gland
28 **Ductus deferens**
29 **Epididymis**
30 Umbilicus
31 Trigone of bladder and ureteric orifice
32 Navicular fossa of urethra
33 External urethral orifice
34 **Testis**

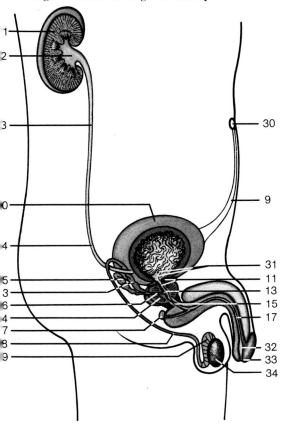

Male urogenital system. (Schematic drawing.)

The **prostate** is located between the bladder and urogenital diaphragm. The penis includes the **urethra** and thus serves for both ejaculation and micturition. The internal (involuntary) and external (voluntary) urethral sphincters are widely separated. The **ureter** having crossed the ductus deferens enters the urinary bladder at its base. The peritoneum is reflected off the posterior surface of the bladder onto the rectum, thus forming the rectovesical pouch.

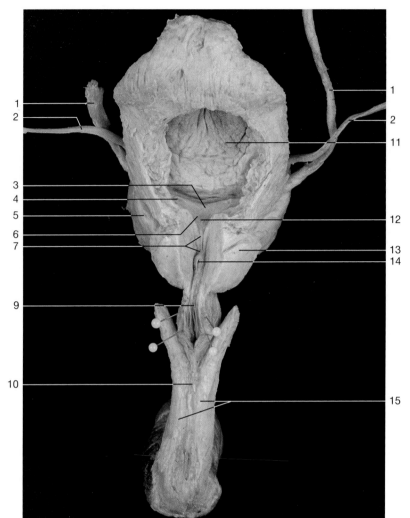

1 Ureter
2 Ductus deferens
3 Interureteric fold
4 Ureteric orifice
5 Seminal vesicle
6 Trigone of bladder
7 Prostatic urethra with seminal colliculus
   and urethral crest
8 Deep transverse perineal muscle
9 Membranous urethra
10 **Spongy urethra**
11 Mucous membrane of **urinary bladder**
12 Internal urethral orifice and uvula of bladder
13 **Prostate**
14 Prostatic utricle
15 Right and left **corpus cavernosum of penis**
16 Ejaculatory duct
17 **Sphincter urethrae muscle**
18 **Median umbilical fold** with remnant of urachus
19 Medial umbilical fold with remnant of umbilical
   artery
20 **Urinary bladder**
21 Rectovesical pouch
22 Rectum
23 Sacrum
24 Deep iliac circumflex artery
25 Deep inguinal ring and ductus deferens
26 External iliac artery and vein
27 **Femoral nerve**
28 Obturator nerve and internal iliac artery
29 Ilium and sacrum
30 Inferior epigastric artery
31 Iliopsoas muscle

Male urogenital organs, isolated (anterior view). Urinary bladder, prostate and urethra have been opened. The urinary bladder is contracted.

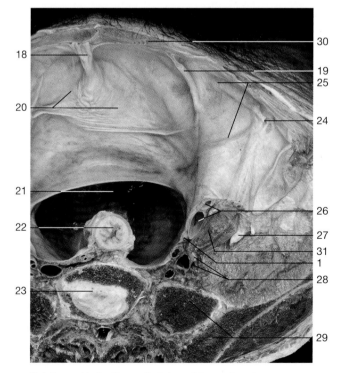

Pelvic cavity in the male (viewed from above).

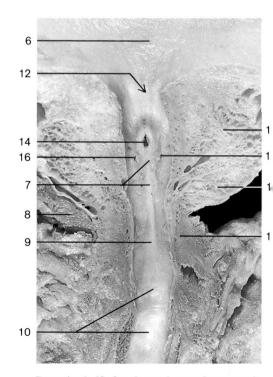

Posterior half of male urethra and prostate in continuity with neck of bladder (anterior view).

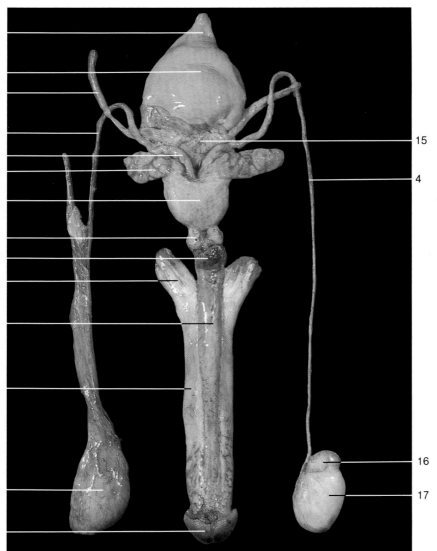

1 Apex of urinary bladder with urachus
2 **Urinary bladder**
3 Ureter
4 **Ductus deferens**
5 Ampulla of ductus deferens
6 **Seminal vesicle**
7 **Prostate**
8 **Bulbourethral or Cowper's gland**
9 **Bulb of penis**
10 Crus penis
11 **Corpus spongiosum of penis**
12 **Corpus cavernosum of penis**
13 Testis and epididymis with coverings
14 Glans penis
15 Fundus of bladder
16 **Head of epididymis**
17 **Testis**
18 Mucous membrane of bladder
19 Trigone of bladder
20 Ureteric orifice
21 Internal urethral orifice
22 Seminal colliculus
23 Prostate
24 Prostatic urethra
25 Membranous urethra
26 Spongy (penile) urethra
27 Skin of penis
28 Deep dorsal vein of penis (unpaired)
29 Dorsal artery of penis (paired)
30 **Tunica albuginea of corpora cavernosa**
31 Septum of penis
32 Deep artery of penis
33 Tunica albuginea of corpus spongiosum
34 Deep fascia of penis

Male genital organs, isolated (posterior view).

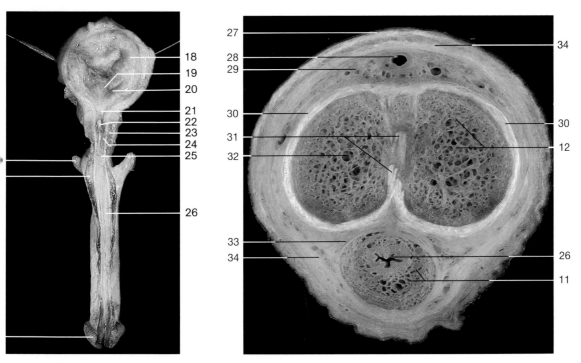

Urinary bladder, urethra and penis (anterior view, opened longitudinally).

Cross section of penis (inferior aspect).

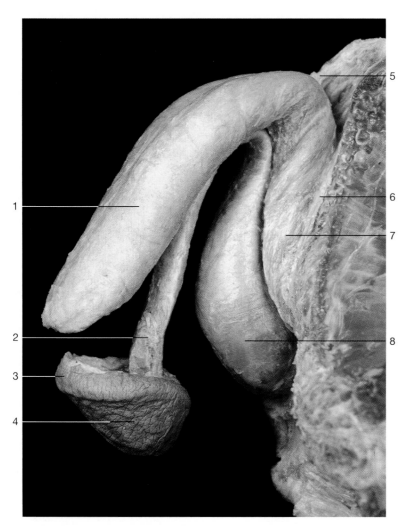

1 Corpus cavernosum of penis
2 Corpus spongiosum of penis
3 Corona of glans penis
4 Glans penis
5 Suspensory ligament of penis
6 Inferior pubic ramus
7 Crus penis
8 Bulb of penis
9 Deep dorsal vein of penis
10 Septum pectiniforme
11 Dorsal artery of penis
12 Bulbourethral or Cowper's gland
13 Urinary bladder
14 Seminal vesicle
15 Ampulla of ductus deferens
16 Ductus deferens
17 Membranous urethra
18 Prostate
19 Ureter

Male external genital organs (lateral view). The corpus spongiosum of the penis with the glans penis has been isolated and reflected.

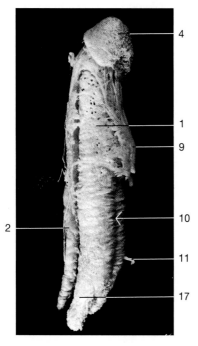

Resin cast of erected penis.

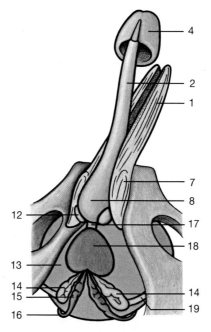

Male external genital organs and accessory glands. (Schematic drawing.)

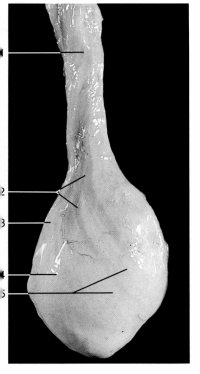

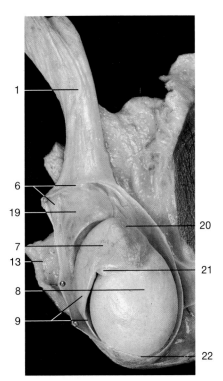

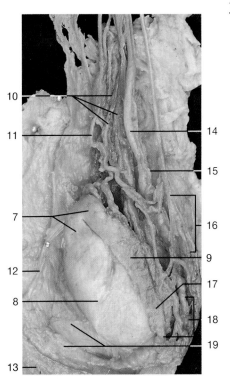

Testis and epididymis with investing layers (lateral view).

Testis and epididymis (lateral view). The tunica vaginalis has been opened.

Testis, epididymis and spermatic cord. Dissection of spermatic cord and ductus deferens (left side, posterolateral aspect).

1 Spermatic cord covered with cremasteric fascia
2 **Cremaster muscle**
3 Position of epididymis
4 Internal spermatic fascia
5 Position of testis
6 Internal spermatic fascia with adjacent investing layers of testis (cut surface)

7 **Head of epididymis**
8 **Testis with tunica vaginalis** (visceral layer)
9 Body of epididymis
10 Pampiniform venous plexus (anterior veins)
11 **Testicular artery**

12 Tunica vaginalis (parietal layer, cut edge)
13 Skin and dartos muscle (reflected)
14 **Ductus deferens**
15 Artery of ductus deferens
16 Posterior veins of pampiniform plexus
17 Tail of epididymis
18 Transition of epididymal duct to ductus deferens and venous plexus
19 Parietal layer of tunica vaginalis
20 Appendix of epididymis
21 Appendix of testis
22 Gubernaculum testis

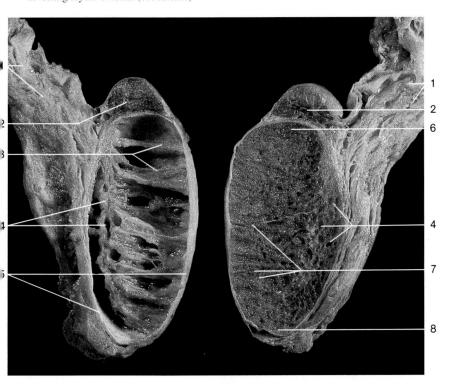

Longitudinal section through testis and epididymis. The left figure shows the testicular septa after removal of the seminiferous tubules.

1 Spermatic cord (cut surface)
2 Head of epididymis (cut surface)
3 Septa of testis
4 Mediastinum testis
5 Tunica albuginea
6 Superior pole of testis
7 Convoluted seminiferous tubules
8 Inferior pole of testis

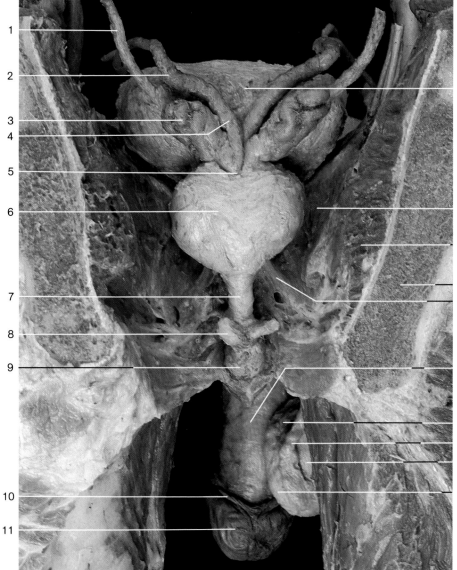

1 Ureter
2 **Ductus deferens**
3 **Seminal vesicle**
4 **Ampulla of ductus deferens**
5 Ejaculatory duct
   (proximal portion)
6 **Prostate**
7 Membranous urethra
8 **Bulbourethral or Cowper's
   gland**
9 Bulb of penis
10 Penis
11 Glans penis
12 **Urinary bladder**
13 Levator ani muscle
14 Obturator internus muscle
15 Pelvic bone (cut edge)
16 Puboprostatic ligament
17 **Corpus spongiosum
   of penis**
18 Head of epididymis
19 Beginning of ductus
   deferens
20 Testis
21 Tail of epididymis
22 Corpus cavernosum of penis
23 Spermatic cord
24 Pectineus and adductor
   muscles
25 Pubic bone
26 **Prostatic part of urethra**
   (seminal colliculus)
27 Rectum
28 Sciatic nerve
29 Great saphenous vein
30 Sartorius muscle
31 Femoral artery and vein
32 Rectus femoris muscle
33 Tensor fasciae latae muscle
34 Pectineus muscle
35 Iliopsoas muscle
36 Vastus lateralis muscle
37 Obturator externus muscle
38 Femur
39 Ischial tuberosity
40 Gluteus maximus muscle

Accessory glands of male genital organs in situ. Coronal section through the pelvic cavity. Posterior aspect of urinary bladder, prostate and seminal vesicles.

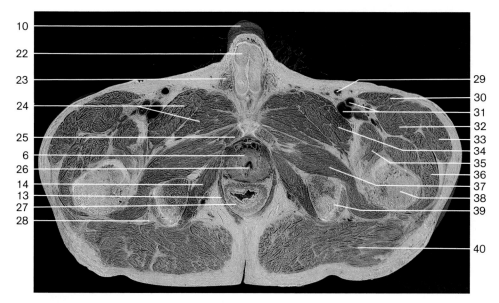

Horizontal section through pelvic cavity at level of prostate.

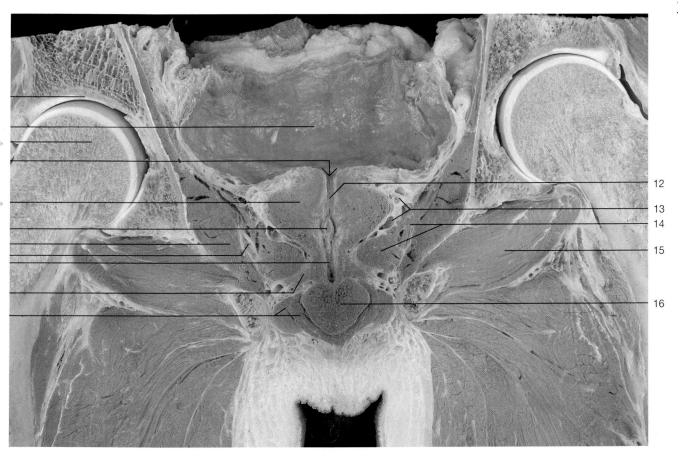

Coronal section through pelvic cavity at the level of prostate and hip joint (anterior aspect).

1	Acetabulum of hip joint	10	Deep transverse perineus muscle	19	Seminal vesicle
2	**Urinary bladder**	11	**Crus penis** and **ischiocavernosus muscle**	20	Internal anal sphincter muscle
3	Head of femur	12	Prostatic part of urethra	21	External anal sphincter muscle
4	Internal urethral orifice	13	Prostatic plexus	22	Anus
5	**Prostate**	14	Levator ani muscle	23	Psoas major muscle
6	**Seminal colliculus**	15	Obturator externus muscle	24	Intervertebral disc
7	Obturator internus muscle	16	**Bulb of penis**	25	Ilium
8	Ischiorectal fossa	17	Ampulla of rectum	26	Ligament of the head of the femur
9	Membranous urethra	18	**Anal canal**	27	Sacral promontory

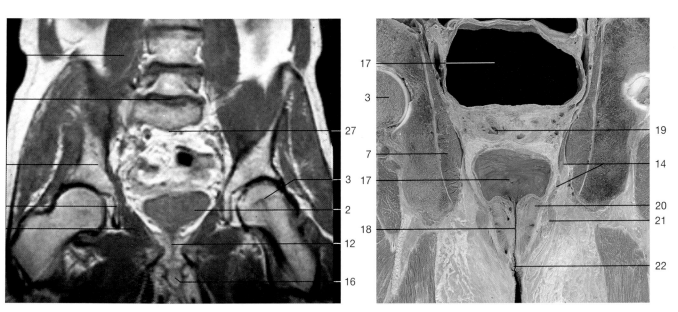

Coronal section through pelvic cavity. (MRI scan.)

Coronal section through anal canal.

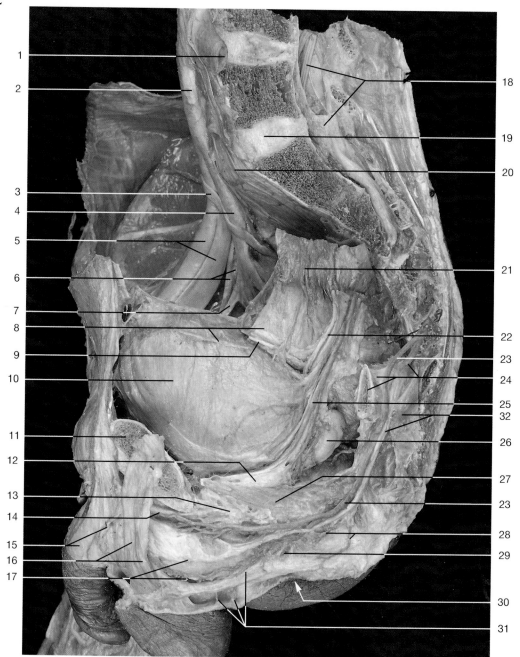

Pelvic cavity in the male (right half of parasagittal section). The arteries have been injected with red resin. The parietal layer of peritoneum has been removed. The urinary bladder is filled to a great extent.

1 Left common iliac artery
2 Right common iliac artery
3 Right **ureter**
4 Right **internal iliac artery**
5 Right external iliac artery and vein
6 Right **obturator artery and nerve**
7 Umbilical artery
8 Sigmoid and superior vesical artery
9 Left ductus deferens
10 **Urinary bladder**
11 Pubic bone (cut)
12 **Prostate**
13 Vesicoprostatic venous plexus
14 Deep dorsal vein of penis and dorsal artery of penis
15 Penis and superficial dorsal vein
16 **Spermatic cord and testicular artery**
17 **Bulb of penis** and deep artery of penis

18 Cauda equina and dura mater (divided)
19 Intervertebral disc between fifth lumbar vertebra and sacrum
20 **Sacral promontory**
21 Mesosigmoid
22 Left ureter
23 Left internal pudendal artery
24 Ischial spine (cut), sacrospinal ligament, inferior gluteal artery
25 Left **inferior vesical artery**
26 **Seminal vesicle**
27 Levator ani muscle
28 Branches of inferior rectal artery
29 Perineal artery
30 Anus
31 Posterior scrotal branches
32 **Pudendal nerve** and sacrotuberal ligament

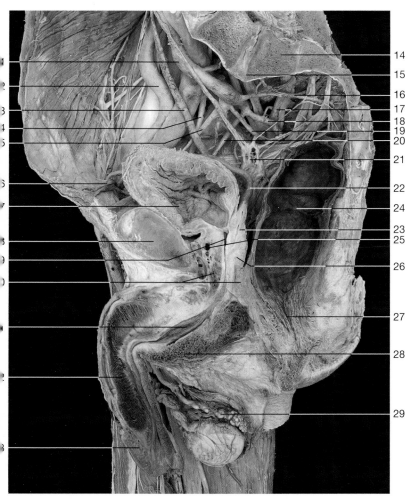

1	**Internal iliac artery**
2	External iliac artery
3	**Ureter**
4	Obturator nerve
5	Umbilical artery
6	Annulus inguinalis profundus
7	**Vesica urinaria**
8	Symphysis
9	Prostatic part of urethra
10	Sphincter muscle of urethra
11	**Urethra** (spongy part)
12	Cavernous body of penis
13	Glans penis
14	Sacrum
15	Promontorium
16	**Lateral sacral artery**
17	Plexus sacralis
18	**Inferior gluteal artery**
19	Internal pudendal artery
20	Obturator artery
21	**Inferior hypogastric plexus**
22	Ductus deferens
23	Vesicula seminalis
24	Rectum
25	Prostatic venous plexus
26	**Prostate**
27	Anal canal
28	Spongy part of penis
29	**Pampiniform plexus**
30	**Testis and epididymis**
31	Common iliac artery
32	Umbilical artery
33	Medial umbilical ligament
34	Branches of superior vesical artery
35	Urogenital diaphragm
36	Deep artery of penis
37	Dorsal artery of penis
38	**Penis**
39	Iliolumbar artery
40	**Superior gluteal artery**
41	Middle rectal artery
42	Levator ani muscle
43	Inferior rectal artery
44	Inferior vesical artery

Vessels of the pelvic cavity in the male (sagittal section, right side, medial aspect). The gluteus maximus muscle has been removed.

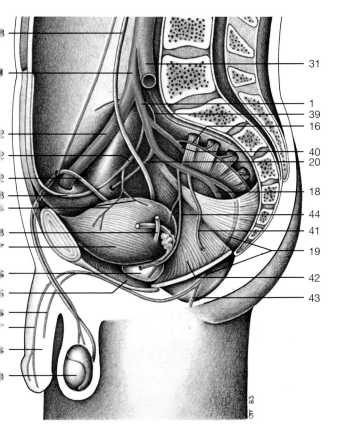

Main branches of internal iliac artery in the male. (Schematic drawing.)

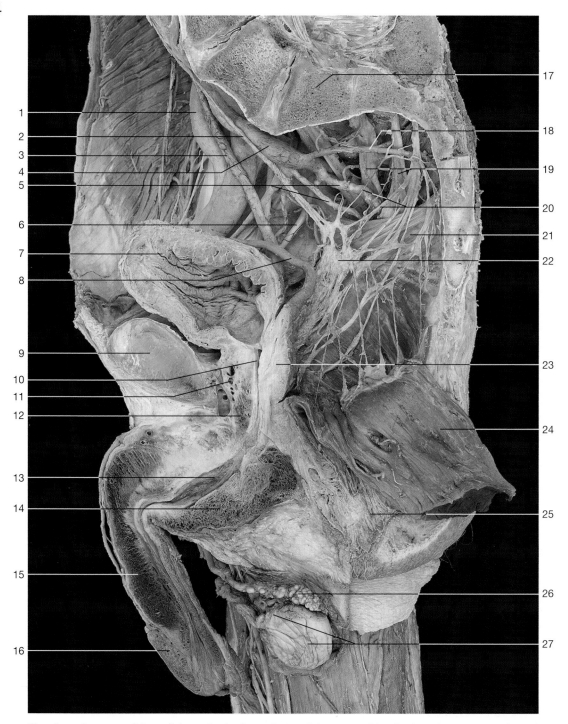

Vessels and nerves of the pelvic cavity in the male (medial aspect, midsagittal section, rectum reflected to display the inferior hypogastric plexus).

1 External iliac artery	10 Prostatic part of urethra	20 Pelvic splanchnic nerves (nervi erigentes)
2 Right hypogastric nerve	11 **Prostatic venous plexus**	21 Levator ani muscle
3 **Ureter**	12 Sphincter urethrae muscle	22 **Inferior hypogastric plexus**
4 **Internal iliac artery**	13 Spongy part of urethra	(pelvic plexus)
5 Inferior gluteal artery and internal	14 Corpus spongiosum penis	23 **Prostate**
pudendal artery	15 Corpus cavernosum penis	24 Rectum (reflected)
6 Obturator artery	16 Glans penis	25 Anal canal and external anal sphincter
7 **Urinary bladder**	17 Sacrum	26 Pampiniform plexus continuous with
8 Ductus deferens	18 Lateral sacral artery	testicular vein
9 Symphysis pubica	19 **Sacral plexus**	27 Testis and epididymis

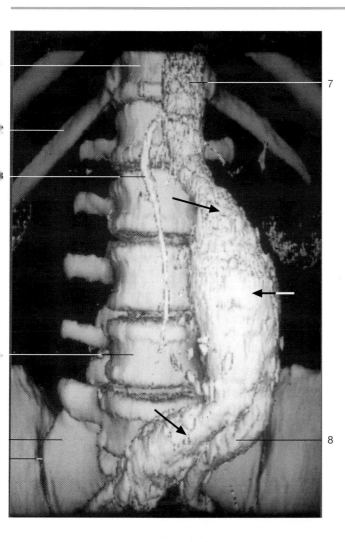

1   Twelfth thoracic vertebra (T$_{12}$)
2   Twelfth rib (rib XII)
3   Inferior mesenteric artery
4   Fourth lumbar vertebra (L$_4$)
5   Sacrum
6   Sacroiliac articulation
7   **Aorta** (abdominal part)
8   Left common iliac artery (included into the aneurysm)
9   **Aorta with aneurysm**
10 Body of lumbar vertebra
11 Intrinsic muscles of the back
12 Thrombotic part of the aneurysm (green)
13 **Inferior vena cava** (compressed, blue)
14 Iliopsoas muscle
15 Vertebral canal
16 **Aneurysm of the aorta** (red)

Abdominal part of the aorta showing an infrarenal aneurysm with involvement of both iliac arteries (arrows) (3-D reconstruction, courtesy of Prof. H. Rupprecht and Dr. M. Rexer, Klinikum Hof, Germany).

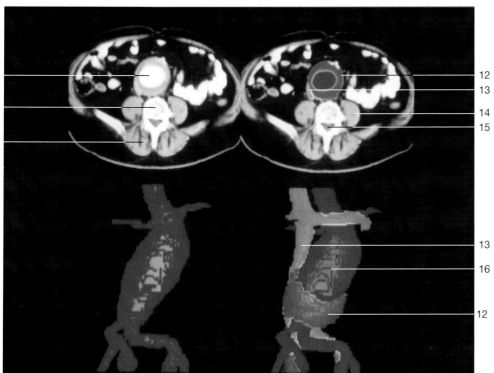

Abdominal part of the aneurysm of the aorta, after injection of contrast medium.
Above = horizontal sections through the abdominal cavity, showing different contrast medium concentrations within the aorta and the aneurysm; below = 3-D reconstruction of the aneurysm; red = aorta; green = thrombotic areas; blue = vein (vena cava inferior, partly compressed).

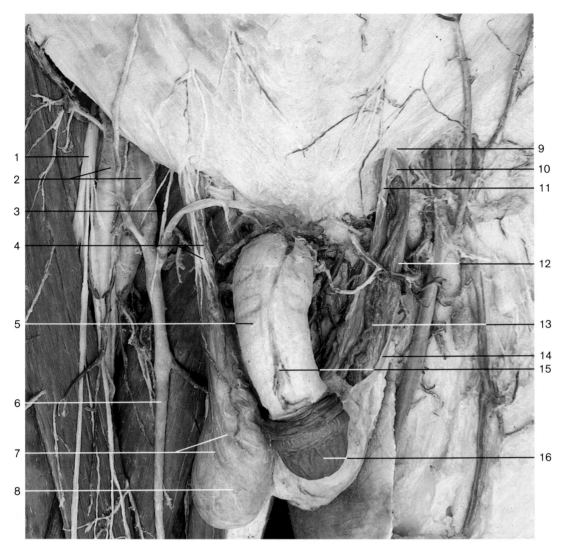

Male external genital organs with penis, testis, and spermatic cord, superficial layers (anterior view).

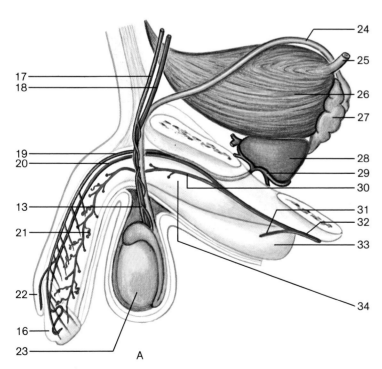

1 Femoral nerve
2 Femoral artery and vein
3 Femoral branch of genitofemoral nerve
4 **Spermatic cord** with genital branch of genitofemoral nerve
5 **Penis** with deep fascia
6 Great saphenous vein
7 Cremaster muscle
8 **Testis with cremaster muscle**
9 Superficial inguinal ring
10 Internal spermatic fascia (cut edge)
11 Ilioinguinal nerve
12 Left spermatic cord
13 Pampiniform venous plexus
14 External spermatic fascia
15 Superficial dorsal vein of penis
16 **Glans penis**

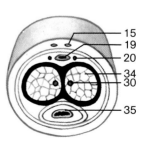

Vessels of male genital organs. (Schematic drawing.)
A = lateral aspect; B = cross section of penis.

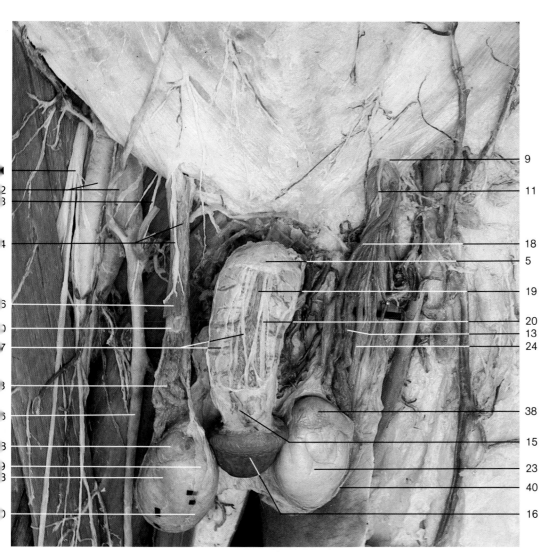

9
11
18
5
19
20
13
24
38
15
23
40
16

Male external genital organs with penis, testis and spermatic cord, deeper layers (ventral aspect).
The deep fascia of the penis has been opened to display the dorsal nerves and vessels.

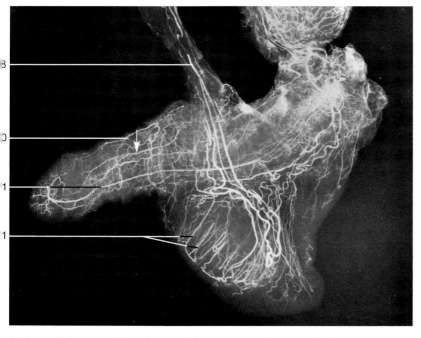

Male genital organs (lateral aspect). (Arteriogram.) Arrow = Helicine artery.

17 Testicular vein
18 Testicular artery
19 Deep dorsal vein of penis
20 **Dorsal artery of penis**
21 **Helicine arteries**
22 Prepuce
23 **Testis** with **tunica albuginea**
24 Ductus deferens
25 Ureter
26 Urinary bladder
27 **Seminal vesicle**
28 **Prostate**
29 Vesicoprostatic venous plexus
30 **Deep artery of penis**
31 Artery of bulb of penis
32 Internal pudendal artery
33 Corpus spongiosum of penis
34 Corpus cavernosum of penis
35 Urethra
36 Cremasteric fascia with cremaster muscle
37 Dorsal nerve of penis
38 **Epididymis**
39 **Tunica vaginalis** (visceral layer)
40 Tunica vaginalis (parietal layer)
41 Testis with vascular loops

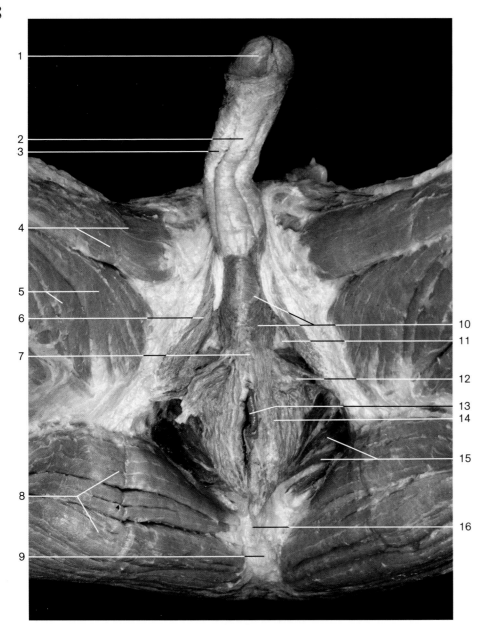

1 Glans penis
2 **Corpus spongiosum of penis**
3 **Corpus cavernosum of penis**
4 Gracilis muscle
5 Adductor muscles
6 Ischiocavernosus muscle
   overlying crus of penis
7 Perineal body
8 Gluteus maximus muscle
9 Coccyx
10 **Bulbospongiosus** muscle
11 Deep transverse perineus
   muscle covered by inferior
   fascia of urogenital diaphragm
12 Superficial transverse
   perineus muscle
13 Anus
14 **External anal sphincter
   muscle**
15 **Levator ani muscle**
16 Anococcygeal ligament
17 Obturator internus muscle
18 Urethra
19 **Deep transverse perineus
   muscle**

Muscles of urogenital and pelvic diaphragms in the male (from below).

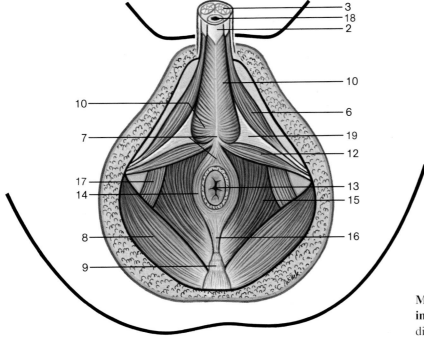

Muscles of urogenital and pelvic diaphragms in the male (from below). The penis has been divided. (Schematic drawing.)

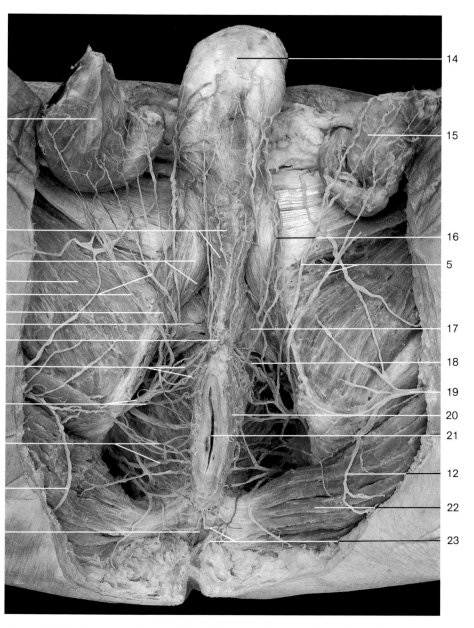

1　Right testis (reflected laterally and upward)
2　Bulbospongiosus muscle
3　Ischiocavernosus muscle
4　Adductor magnus muscle
5　**Posterior scrotal nerves** and superficial perineal arteries
6　Posterior scrotal artery and vein
7　Right artery of bulb of penis
8　Perineal body
9　Perineal branches of pudendal nerve
10　**Pudendal nerve** and **internal pudendal artery**
11　**Inferior rectal arteries** and **nerves**
12　Inferior cluneal nerve
13　Coccyx (location)
14　Penis
15　Left testis (reflected laterally)
16　Left posterior scrotal artery
17　**Deep transverse perineal muscle**
18　Left artery of bulb of penis
19　**Posterior femoral cutaneous nerve**
20　External anal sphincter muscle
21　**Anus**
22　Gluteus maximus muscle
23　Anococcygeal nerves
24　Acetabulum (femur removed)
25　Ligament of femoral head
26　Body of ischium (cut)
27　Sciatic nerve
28　Coccygeus muscle
29　**Levator ani muscle**
　　a　iliococcygeus muscle
　　b　pubococcygeus muscle
　　c　puborectalis muscle
30　Prostatic venous plexus
31　Body of pubis
32　Testis

Urogenital diaphragm and external genital organs in the male with vessels and nerves (from below). The testes have been reflected laterally.

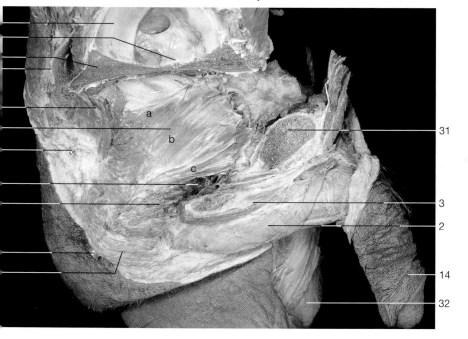

Pelvic diaphragm and external genital organs in the male. The right half of the pelvis including obturator internus muscle and femur had been removed to display the right half of levator ani muscle.

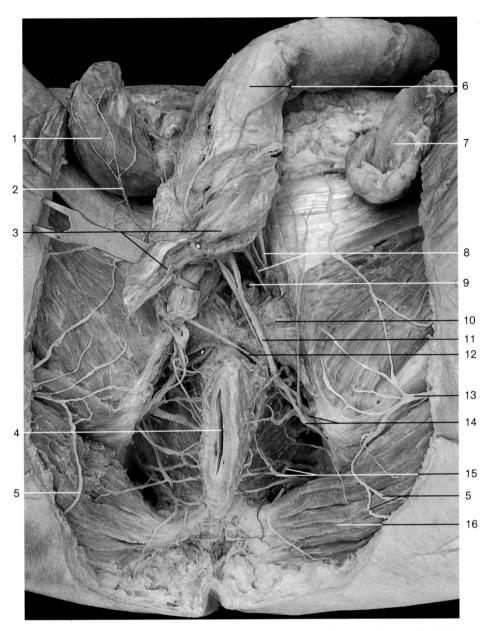

1 Right testis (reflected)
2 Posterior scrotal nerves
3 Left crus penis with ischiocavernosus muscle
4 **Anus**
5 Inferior cluneal nerves
6 **Penis**
7 Left testis (reflected)
8 Dorsal artery and nerve of penis
9 Urethra
10 **Deep transverse perineus muscle**
11 **Perineal branch of pudendal nerve**
12 Artery of bulb of penis (reflected)
13 Branch of posterior femoral cutaneous nerve
14 **Internal pudendal artery and pudendal nerve**
15 Inferior rectal arteries and nerves
16 Gluteus maximus muscle
17 Dorsal nerve of penis
18 Posterior femoral cutaneous nerve
19 Perineal branches of pudendal nerve
20 Inferior rectal nerves
21 **Bulbocavernosus muscle** (inside: dorsal artery of penis)
22 Perineal artery
23 **External anal sphincter muscle**
24 Inferior rectal artery and veins

Urogenital diaphragm and external genital organs in the male (from below). The left crus penis has been isolated and reflected laterally together with the bulb of the penis. The urethra has been cut.

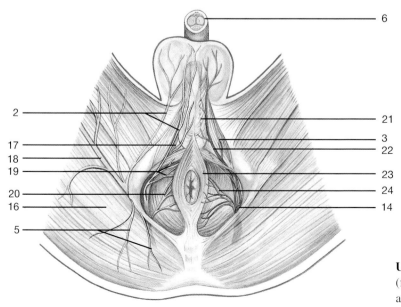

Urogenital and anal region in the male (from below). Right side: nerves; left side: arteries and veins.

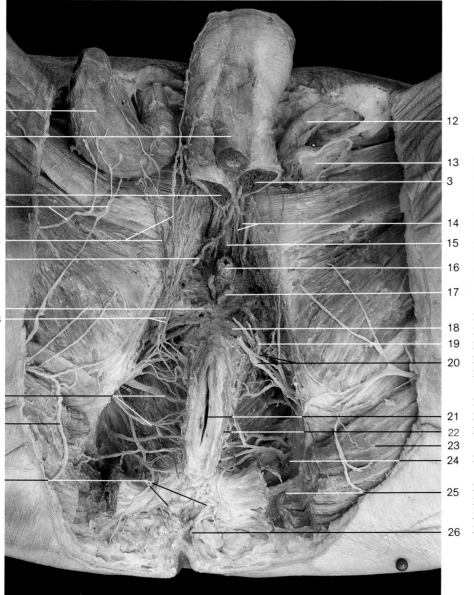

1	Right testis (reflected)
2	**Corpus spongiosum of penis**
3	**Corpus cavernosum of penis**
4	Perineal branch of posterior femoral cutaneous nerve
5	Posterior scrotal arteries and nerves
6	Deep artery of penis
7	Deep transverse perineal muscle
8	Right **perineal nerves**
9	**Inferior rectal nerves**
10	Inferior cluneal nerve
11	Anococcygeal nerves
12	Left spermatic cord
13	Left testis (cut surface)
14	Dorsal artery and nerve of penis
15	Deep dorsal vein of penis
16	**Urethra** (cut)
17	Artery of bulb of penis
18	Superficial transverse perineus muscle
19	Left artery of bulb of penis
20	Perineal branch of pudendal nerve
21	**Anus**
22	**External anal sphincter muscle**
23	Gluteus maximus muscle
24	Internal pudendal artery and pudendal nerve
25	Sacrotuberous ligament
26	Coccyx
27	Urogenital diaphragm (deep transverse perineus muscle)
28	Tendinous center of perineum (perineal body)
29	**Levator ani muscle**
30	Anococcygeal ligament
31	Obturator internus muscle
32	Dorsal artery of penis

Anal and urogenital region in the male (from below). The root of the penis has been cut. Dissection of the urogenital diaphragm.

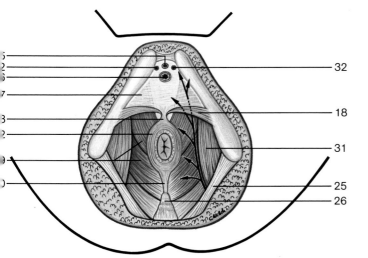

Urogenital and pelvic diaphragms in the male (from below). The penis has been removed. The arrows indicate the course of vessels and nerves. (Schematic drawing.)

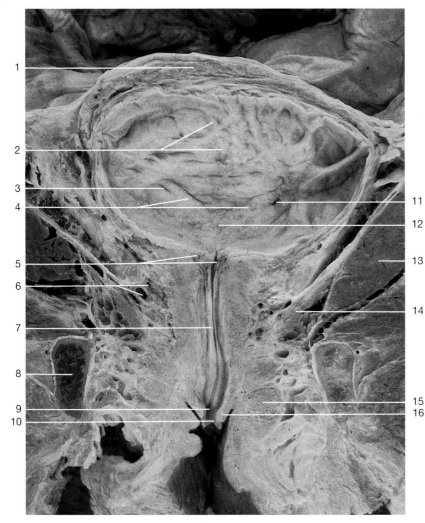

1   Muscular coat of **urinary bladder**
2   Folds of mucous membrane of urinary bladder
3   Right ureteric orifice
4   Interureteric fold
5   Internal urethral orifice
6   Vesicouterine venous plexus
7   **Urethra**
8   Pubic bone (cut edge)
9   External urethral orifice
10   Vestibule of vagina
11   Left ureteric orifice
12   Trigone of bladder
13   Obturator internus muscle
14   Levator ani muscle
15   Bulb of the vestibule
16   Left labium minus
17   **Uterine tube**
18   Mesosalpinx
19   **Ovary**
20   Sigmoid colon
21   Saphenous opening
22   Urinary bladder
23   Vesicouterine pouch
24   **Fundus of uterus**
25   Rectouterine pouch (of Douglas)
26   Ampulla of rectum
27   Kidney
28   Abdominal part of ureter
29   Pelvic part of ureter
30   Anal canal
31   Perineum (perineal body)
32   Umbilicus
33   Infundibulum of uterine tube
34   Vaginal portion of cervix of uterus
35   Vagina
36   Pubic symphysis
37   Clitoris
38   Deep transverse perineus muscle

Coronal section through the female urinary bladder and urethra (anterior view).

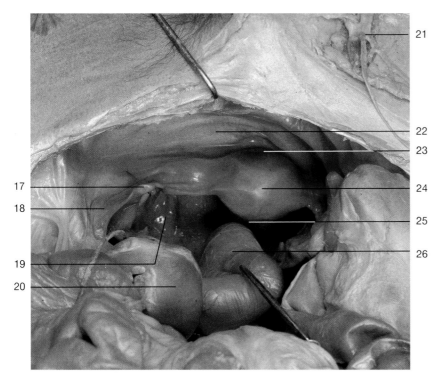

Female internal genital organs. Pelvic cavity (from above).

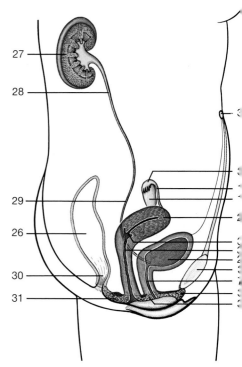

Female urogenital system (midsagittal section). (Schematic drawing.)

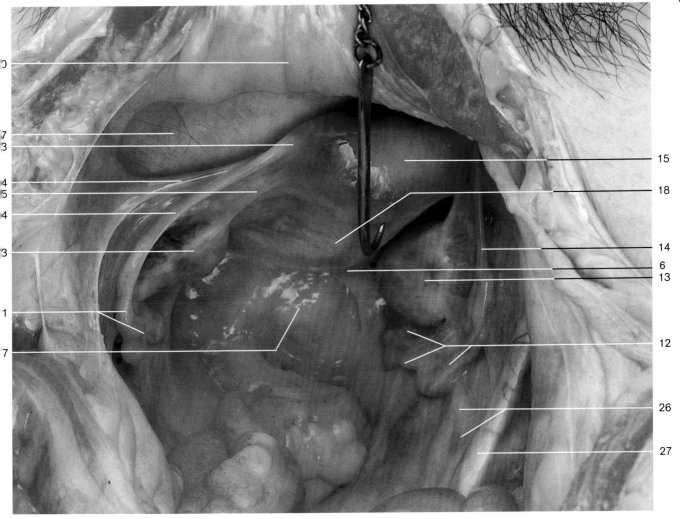

Female internal genital organs. Pelvic cavity, seen from above. The uterus has been reflected to the right.

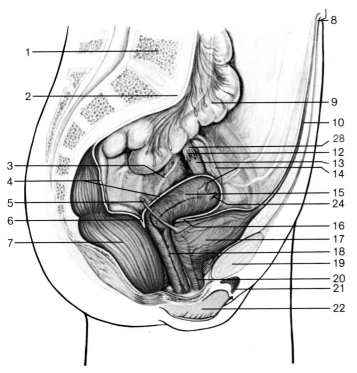

Regional relations of female internal genital organs (medial aspect). (Schematic drawing.)

1 Body of fifth lumbar vertebra
2 Sacral promontory
3 Left ureter
4 Peritoneum (cut edge)
5 Right ureter (divided)
6 **Rectouterine pouch** (of Douglas)
7 Rectum
8 Umbilicus
9 Sigmoid colon
10 Median umbilical fold with urachus
11 Ampulla of uterine tube
12 Fimbriae of uterine tube
13 **Ovary**
14 **Uterine tube** (isthmus)
15 **Uterus**
16 **Vesicouterine pouch**
17 Urinary bladder
18 Vagina
19 Pubic symphysis
20 Urethra
21 Clitoris
22 Labium minus
23 Insertion of uterine tube at fundus of uterus
24 Round ligament of uterus
25 Ligament of the ovary
26 Suspensory ligament of ovary
27 Right common iliac artery (covered by peritoneum)
28 Infundibulum of uterine tube

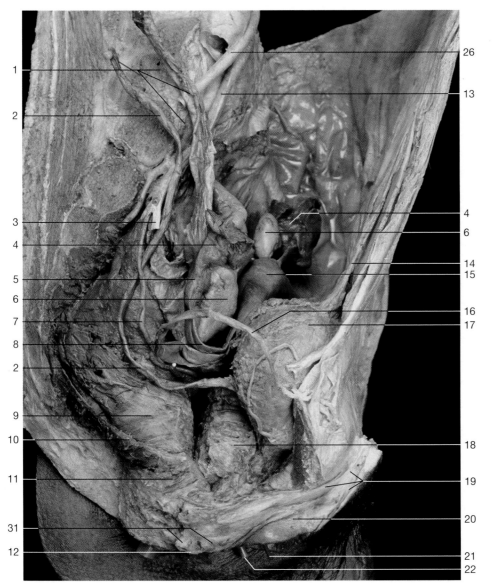

1 Body of fifth lumbar vertebra, **suspensory ligament of ovary** and sacral promontory
2 Ureter
3 Medial umbilical ligament (remnant of umbilical artery) (cut)
4 Infundibulum of uterine tube
5 Ampulla of uterine tube
6 **Ovary**
7 **Uterine artery**
8 **Uterine tube**
9 Rectum
10 Levator ani muscle (pelvic diaphragm – cut edge)
11 External anal sphincter muscle
12 Anus (probe)
13 Internal iliac artery
14 Remnant of urachus (median umbilical ligament)
15 **Uterus**
16 Round ligament of uterus
17 **Urinary bladder**
18 **Vagina**
19 **Clitoris**
20 Labium minus
21 External orifice of urethra (red probe)
22 Vaginal orifice (green probe)
23 Lateral umbilical ligament
24 Inferior epigastric artery
25 Obturator artery, vein and nerve
26 External iliac artery
27 **Rectouterine pouch** (of Douglas)
28 Rectouterine fold
29 Vesicouterine pouch
30 Suspensory ligament of ovary
31 Greater vestibular gland and bulb of the vestibule

Female internal genital organs in situ. Right half of the pelvis and sacrum have been removed.

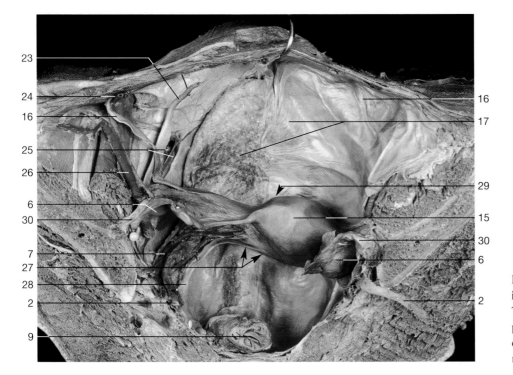

Female internal genital organs in situ (seen from above).
The peritoneum at the left half of pelvic cavity has been removed to display uterine tube, vessels, and nerves.

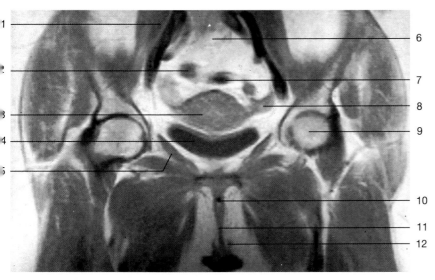

Coronal section through the pelvic cavity of the female. (MRI scan.)

1 Psoas major muscle
2 Ampulla of rectum
3 **Uterus**
4 **Urinary bladder**
5 Obturator internus muscle
6 Promontory
7 Sigmoid colon
8 **Uterine tube**
9 Head of femur
10 Urethra
11 Vagina
12 Labium minus
13 Umbilicus
14 Duodenum
15 Ascending part of duodenum
16 Root of mesentery
17 Mesentery
18 Vesicouterine pouch
19 **Urinary bladder** (collapsed)
20 Pubic symphysis
21 Anterior fornix of vagina
22 Clitoris
23 Labium minus
24 Labium majus
25 Vertebral canal with cauda equina
26 Intervertebral disc
27 Body of fifth lumbar vertebra
28 Sacral promontory
29 Mesosigmoid
30 **Rectouterine pouch** (of Douglas)
31 Posterior fornix of vagina
32 Cervix of uterus
33 External anal sphincter muscle
34 Anal canal
35 Internal anal sphincter muscle
36 Anus
37 Hymen
38 Small intestine
39 Rectus abdominis muscle

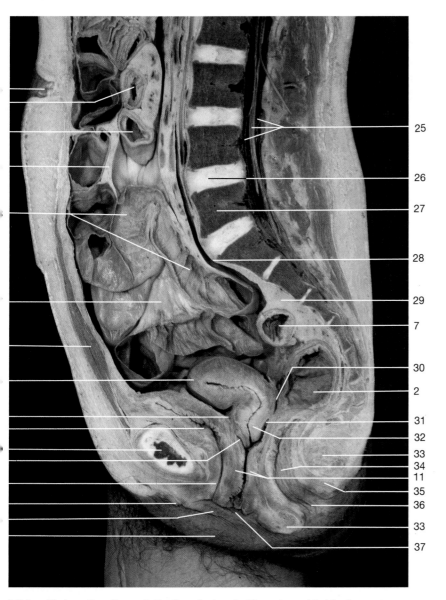

Midsagittal section through the female trunk. The urinary bladder is empty; the position and shape of the uterus are normal.

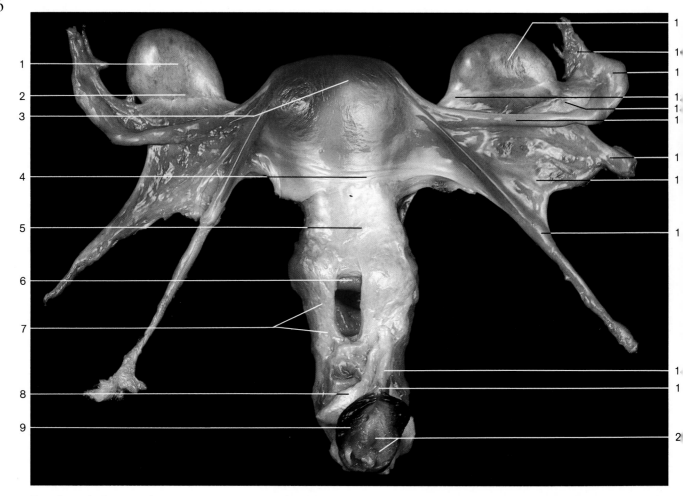

Female genital organs, isolated (anterior view). The anterior wall of the vagina has been opened to display the vaginal portion of the cervix.

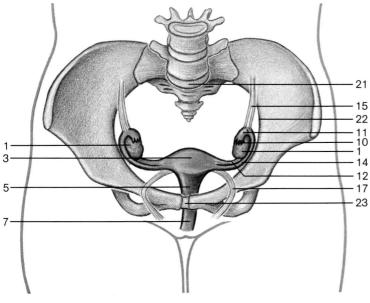

Female internal genital organs. (Schematic drawing.)

1 **Ovary**
2 Mesovarium
3 **Fundus of uterus**
4 Vesicouterine pouch
5 **Cervix of uterus**
6 Vaginal portion of cervix
7 **Vagina**
8 Crus of clitoris
9 Labium minus
10 Fimbriae of uterine tube
11 Infundibulum of uterine tube
12 Ligament of the ovary
13 Mesosalpinx
14 Uterine tube
15 Suspensory ligament of ovary
    (caudally displaced)
16 Broad ligament of uterus
17 Round ligament of uterus
18 Corpus cavernosum of clitoris
19 Glans of clitoris
20 **Hymen, vaginal orifice**
21 Promontory
22 Linea terminalis of pelvis
23 Pubic symphysis

1 **Fundus of uterus**
2 Uterine tube
3 **Ligament of the ovary**
4 **Ovary**
5 Infundibulum of uterine tube
6 Fimbriae of uterine tube
7 **Ureter**
8 Rectum
9 Apex of urinary bladder and median umbilical ligament
10 Urinary bladder
11 Round ligament of uterus
12 **Mesosalpinx**
13 **Mesovarium**
14 **Rectouterine pouch** (of Douglas)
15 Suspensory ligament of ovary
16 Scarring of ovary (following ovulation)
17 Abdominal opening of uterine tube
18 Body of uterus
19 **Cervical canal**
20 Vaginal portion of cervix of uterus (congestion)
21 Vagina
22 Mucous membrane of uterus
23 Anterior fornix of vagina

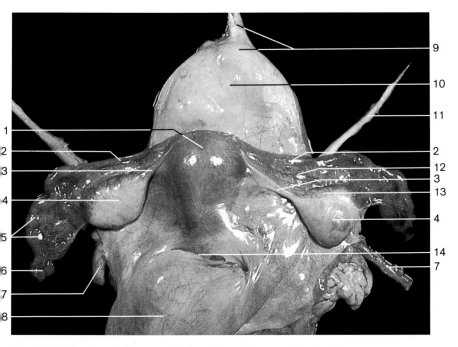

Female internal genital organs, isolated (superior-posterior view).

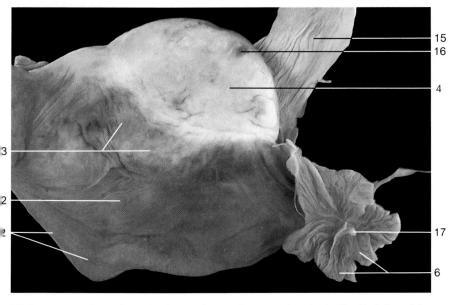

Right ovary and uterine tube, isolated (superior-posterior view). The fimbriae of the uterine tube have been reflected to show the abdominal ostium.

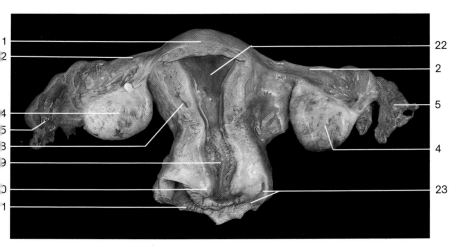

Uterus and related organs (posterior view). The posterior wall of the uterus has been opened.

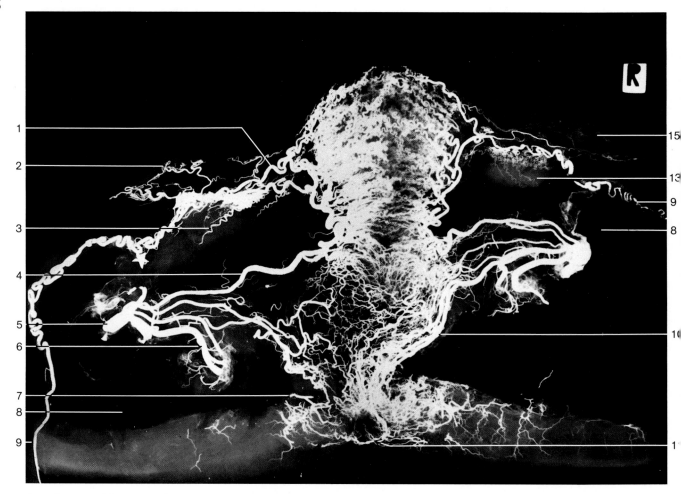

Arteriogram of female genital organs (anterior-posterior view). Notice the helicine arteries supplying uterus and ovary.

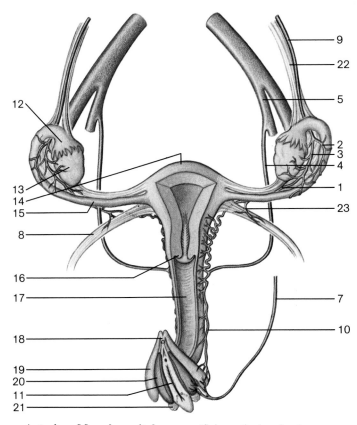

Arteries of female genital organs. (Schematic drawing.)

1 Ovarian branch of uterine artery
   (anastomoses with ovarian artery)
2 Tubal branch of ovarian artery
3 Ovarian branch of ovarian artery
4 **Uterine artery**
5 Internal iliac artery
6 Inferior gluteal artery
7 **Internal pudendal artery**
8 Round ligament of uterus
9 **Ovarian artery**
10 Vaginal artery
11 Vaginal orifice
12 Infundibulum of uterine tube
13 Ovary
14 Fundus of uterus
15 Uterine tube
16 Vaginal portion of cervix of uterus
17 Vagina
18 Clitoris
19 Corpus cavernosum of clitoris
20 Bulb of vestibule
21 Greater vestibular gland
22 Suspensory ligament of ovary
23 Artery of round ligament

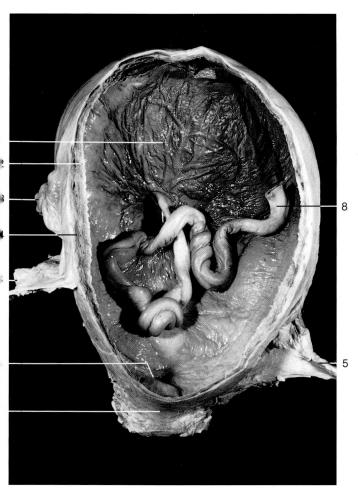

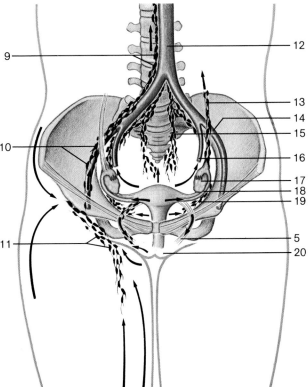

Main drainage routes of lymph vessels of uterus and its adnexa (indicated by arrows). (Schematic drawing.) Red = arteries; black = lymph vessels and nodes; yellow = internal genital organs.

Full term uterus with placenta (anterior view). The anterior wall of the uterus has been removed to show the location of the placenta.

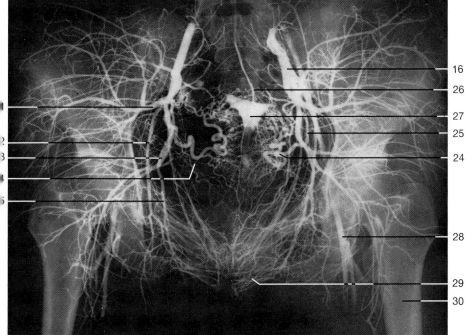

Pelvic vessels in the female (anterior-posterior view). (Arteriogram.)

1 Placenta
2 Amnion and chorion
3 Adnexa of uterus
    (uterine tube and ovaries)
4 Myometrium
5 Round ligament of uterus
6 Internal orifice of uterus
7 Cervix of uterus
8 **Umbilical cord**
9 Lumbar lymph nodes
10 External iliac lymph nodes
11 Inguinal lymph nodes
12 Abdominal aorta
13 Suspensory ligament of ovary
14 External iliac artery
15 Sacral lymph nodes
16 Internal iliac artery
17 Ovary
18 Uterine tube
19 Internal iliac lymph nodes
20 External genital organs
21 Superior gluteal artery
22 **Obturator artery**
23 Inferior gluteal artery
24 **Uterine artery**
25 **Internal pudendal artery**
26 Middle sacral artery
27 **Uterine cavity**
28 Femoral artery
29 Vessels of labium majus
30 Femur

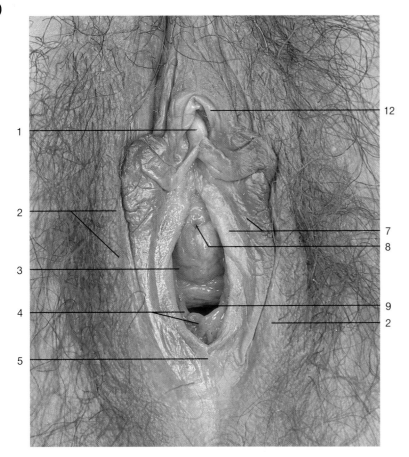

External genital organs in the female (anterior aspect). Labia reflected.

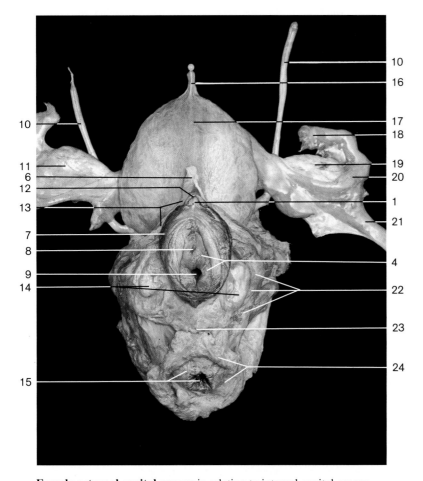

Female external genital organs in relation to internal genital organs and urinary system (isolated, anterior aspect).

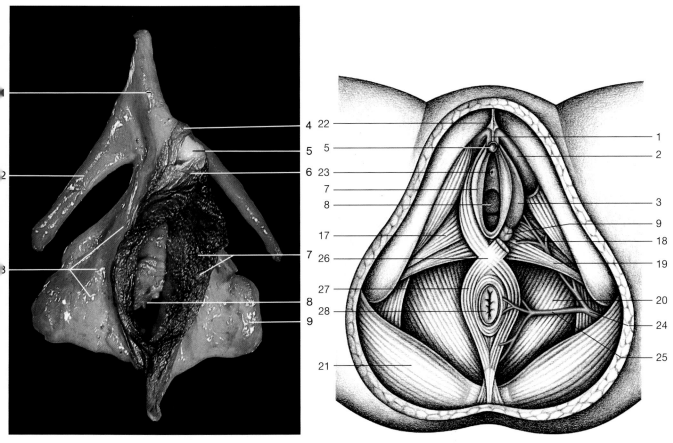

Cavernous tissue of female external genital organs,
isolated (anterior aspect).

Urogenital and pelvic diaphragms (anterior aspect).
(Schematic drawing.)
Blue = cavernous tissue of clitoris and bulb of vestibule.

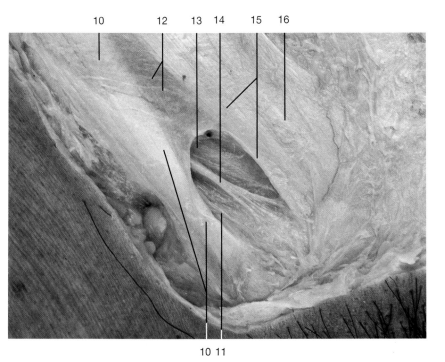

Inguinal canal and round ligament of uterus in situ
(right side, ventral aspect).

1 Body of clitoris
2 Crus of clitoris
3 Bulb of vestibule
4 Prepuce of clitoris
5 **Glans of clitoris**
6 Frenulum of clitoris
7 **Labium minus**
8 **Vaginal orifice**
9 **Greater vestibular gland**
10 Lateral crus of superficial inguinal ring
11 Ilioinguinal nerve
12 Intercrural fibers
13 Superficial inguinal ring
14 **Round ligament of uterus**
15 Medial crus of superficial inguinal ring
16 Aponeurosis of external abdominal
   oblique muscle
17 Deep transverse perineal muscle with
   fascia
18 Deep artery of clitoris
19 Superficial transverse perineus muscle
20 Levator ani muscle
21 Gluteus maximus muscle
22 Suspensory ligament of clitoris
23 External orifice of urethra
24 **Internal pudendal artery**
25 Inferior rectal artery
26 Perineal body
27 External anal sphincter muscle
28 Anus

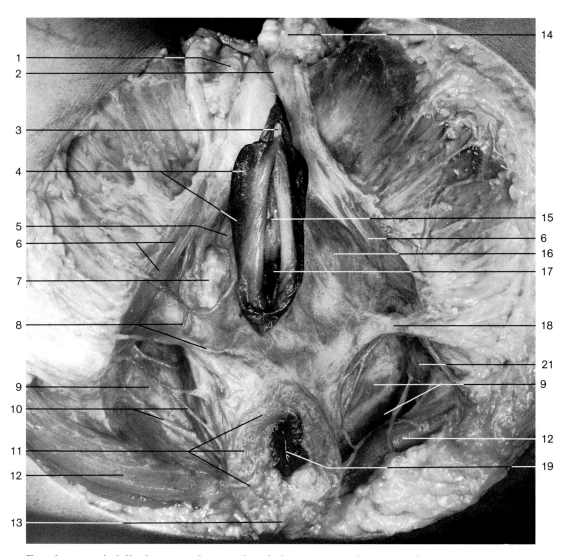

Female urogenital diaphragm and external genital organs, superficial layer (from below).

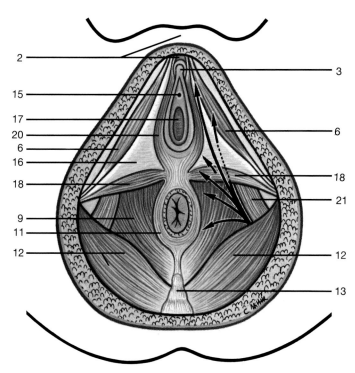

Muscles of pelvic and urogenital diaphragms (from below).
(Schematic drawing.)

1   Fatty tissue encasing round ligament
2   Position of pubic symphysis
3   Clitoris
4   Labium minus
5   Bulb of vestibule
6   Ischiocavernosus muscle
7   **Greater vestibular gland**
8   Perineal branches of pudendal nerve
9   Levator ani muscle
10 Inferior rectal nerves
11 External anal sphincter muscle
12 Gluteus maximus muscle
13 Coccyx
14 Fatty tissue of mons pubis
15 **External orifice of urethra**
16 Urogenital diaphragm with fascia of deep transverse perineus muscle
17 **Vaginal orifice**
18 Superficial transverse perineal muscle
19 **Anus**
20 Bulbospongiosus muscle
21 Obturator internus muscle

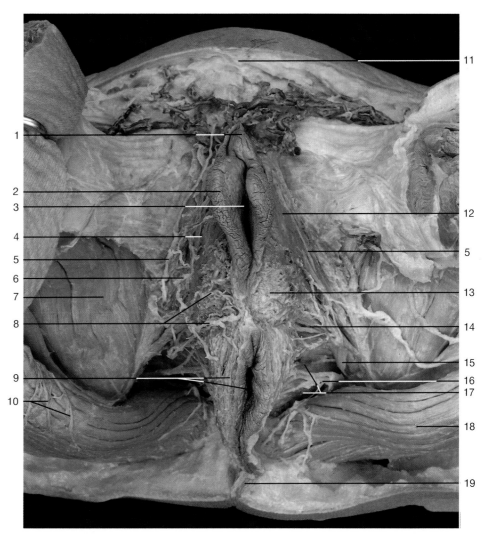

Urogenital diaphragm and external genital organs in the female, superficial layer (from below). On the right side the bulb of vestibule has been removed.

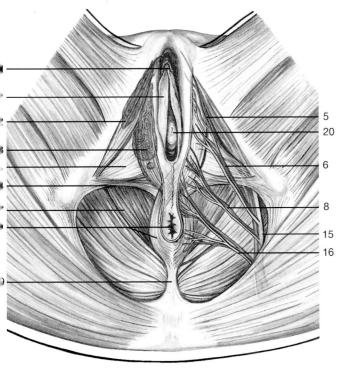

External female genital organs. Position of arteries and nerves; bulb of vestibule in blue. (Schematic drawing.)

1 **Prepuce of clitoris**
2 Labium minus
3 **Vaginal orifice**
4 Deep transverse perineus muscle
5 Dorsal nerve of clitoris
6 Posterior labial nerves
7 Great adductor muscle
8 Perineal branches of pudendal nerve
9 **Anus** and **external anal sphincter muscle**
10 Inferior cluneal nerves
11 Mons pubis
12 Crus of clitoris with ischiocavernosus muscle
13 Bulb of vestibule
14 Superficial transverse perineus muscle
15 **Pudendal nerve** and **internal pudendal artery**
16 Inferior rectal nerves
17 Levator ani muscle
18 Gluteus maximus muscle
19 Anococcygeal ligament
20 External urethral orifice
21 Glans of clitoris

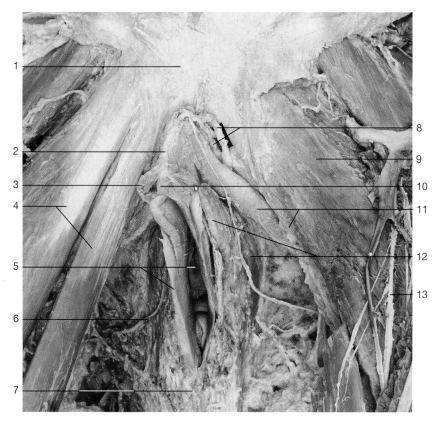

1   Position of pubic symphysis
2   Body of clitoris
3   Prepuce of clitoris
4   Adductor longus and gracilis muscles
5   External orifice of vagina and
      labium minus
6   Posterior labial nerve
7   Perineal body
8   Deep artery of clitoris and
      dorsal nerve of clitoris
9   Adductor brevis muscle
10   **Glans of clitoris**
11   Crus of clitoris and
      ischiocavernosus muscle
12   **Bulb of vestibule** and
      bulbospongiosus muscle
13   Anterior branch of obturator nerve
14   Labium minus
15   **Vaginal orifice**
16   Posterior labial nerves
17   Branches of pudendal nerve
18   External sphincter of anus
19   **Anus**
20   Bulb of vestibule (divided)
21   Dorsal artery of clitoris
22   Superficial transverse perineus muscle
23   Perineal branch of posterior femoral
      cutaneous nerve
24   Levator ani muscle
25   **Pudendal nerve** and
      internal pudendal artery
26   Inferior rectal nerves
27   Gluteus maximus muscle
28   Anococcygeal ligament

External female genital organs (inferior aspect). The clitoris has been dissected and slightly reflected to the right. The prepuce of clitoris has been divided to display the glans.

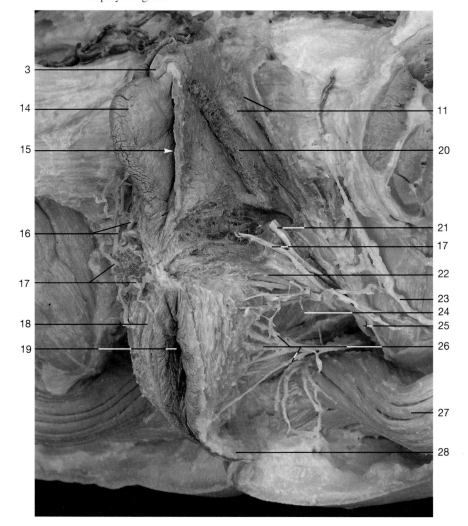

Urogenital diaphragm and external genital organs in the female (lateral inferior view). The bulb of vestibule has partly been removed; the left labium minus was cut away.

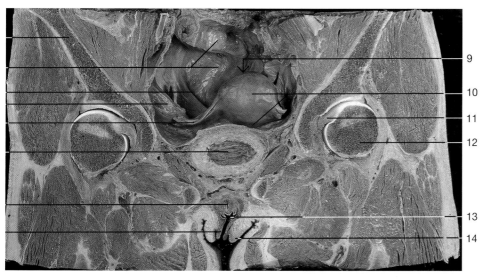

1 Ilium
2 Rectum
3 Rectouterine fold
4 **Ovary**
5 **Uterine tube**
6 **Urinary bladder**
7 **Urethra**
8 Labium minus
9 Rectouterine pouch of
   Douglas
10 **Uterus** (uterovesical
   pouch)
11 Ligament of the head of
   the femur
12 Head of femur
13 Vestibule of vagina
14 Labium majus
15 Anal cleft
16 Coccyx
17 Rectum
18 Myometrium of uterus
19 Uterine cavity
20 Obturator internus
   muscle
21 Iliopsoas muscle
22 Sartorius muscle
23 Sciatic nerve and
   gluteus maximus muscle
24 Uterine venous plexus
25 Broad ligament
26 Small intestine
27 Femoral artery and vein
28 Femoral nerve
29 Pyramidalis muscle
30 Rectum (anal canal)
31 Vagina
32 Urethral sphincter muscle
   (base of urinary bladder)
33 Pubic symphysis
34 Levator ani muscle
35 Obturator externus
   muscle
36 Mons pubis
37 Pectineus muscle

Coronal section through the pelvic cavity of the female (cf. MRI scan on page 345).

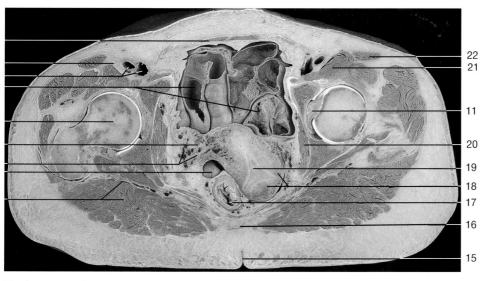

Horizontal section through pelvic cavity at level of uterus (from below). The uterus is retroverted to the left.

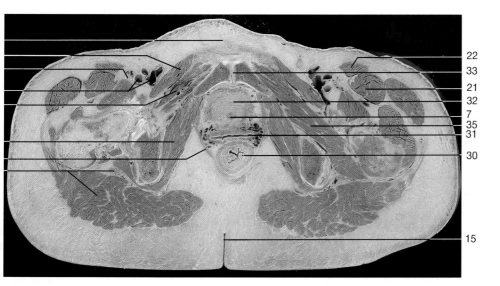

Horizontal section through the pelvic cavity at level of the urethral sphincter and vagina (from below).

Upper Limb

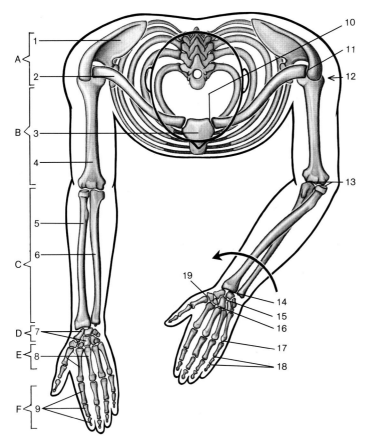

A Shoulder girdle
B Arm
C Forearm
D Wrist
E Palm of hand
F Finger

Bones
1 Scapula
2 Clavicle
3 Sternum
4 Humerus
5 Radius
6 Ulna
7 Carpal bones
8 Metacarpal bones
9 Phalanges

Joints
10 Sternoclavicular joint
11 Acromioclavicular joint
12 Shoulder joint
13 Elbow joint
14 Radiocarpal joint
15 Midcarpal joint
16 Carpometacarpal joint
17 Metacarpophalangeal joint
18 Interphalangeal joints of fingers
19 Carpometacarpal joint of thumb

Organization of shoulder girdle and upper limb (superior aspect). The two positions of the forearm essential to manual skills in the human, supination (right arm) and pronation (left arm) are shown.

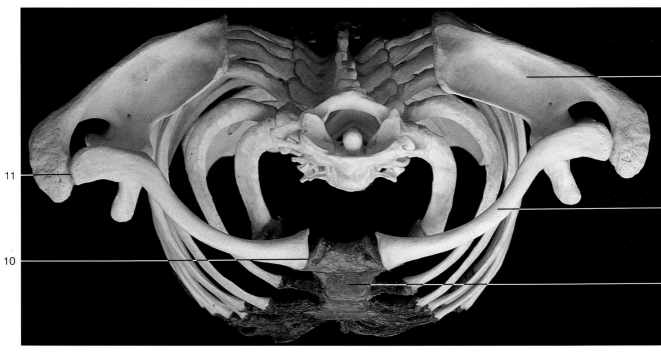

Bones of shoulder girdle articulated with the thorax (superior aspect).

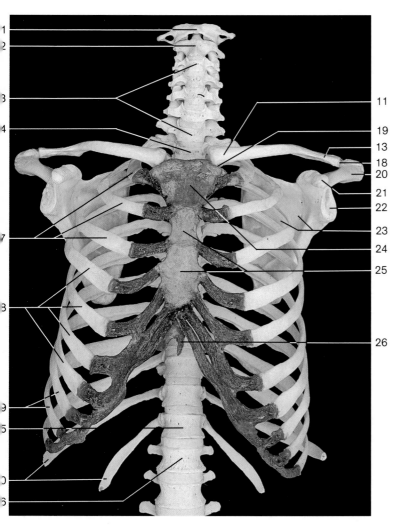

Vertebral column

1 Atlas
2 Axis
3 Third–seventh cervical vertebrae
4 First thoracic vertebra
5 Twelfth thoracic vertebra
6 First lumbar vertebra

Ribs

7 First–third ribs ⎫
8 Fourth–seventh ribs ⎬ True ribs
9 Eighth–tenth ribs ⎫
10 Eleventh and twelfth ribs ⎬ False ribs
   (floating ribs)

Clavicle

11 Sternal end
12 Articular facet for sternum
13 Acromial end
14 Articular facet for acromion
15 Impression for costoclavicular ligament
16 Conoid tubercle
17 Trapezoid line
18 Site of acromioclavicular joint
19 Site of sternoclavicular joint

Scapula

20 Acromion
21 Coracoid process
22 Glenoid cavity
23 Costal surface

Sternum

24 Manubrium
25 Body
26 Xiphoid process

Skeleton of shoulder girdle and thorax (anterior aspect).
The cartilaginous parts of the ribs appear dark brown.

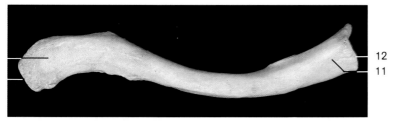

Right clavicle (superior aspect).

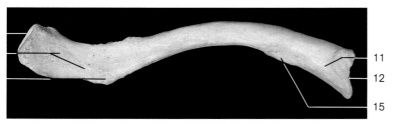

Right clavicle (inferior aspect).

Because of his upright posture, man's upper limb has developed a high degree of mobility. The shoulder girdle is to a great extent movable in the thorax and is connected with the trunk only by the sternoclavicular joint. A further characteristic of man's forearm is the capacity for rotation (i.e., pronation and supination).

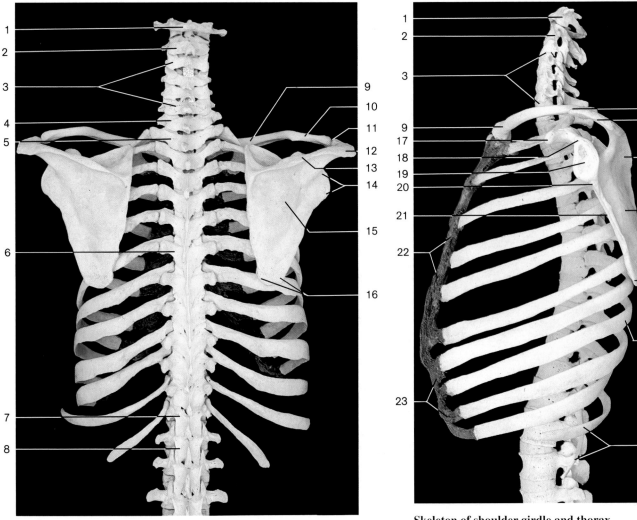

Skeleton of shoulder girdle and thorax (posterior view).

Skeleton of shoulder girdle and thorax
(lateral view).

Vertebral column
1 Atlas
2 Axis
3 Third–sixth cervical vertebrae
4 Seventh vertebra (vertebra prominens)
5 First thoracic vertebra
6 Sixth thoracic vertebra
7 Twelfth thoracic vertebra
8 First lumbar vertebra

Clavicle
9 Sternal end
10 Acromial end
11 Site of acromioclavicular joint

Scapula
12 Acromion
13 Spine of scapula

14 Lateral angle
15 Posterior surface
16 Inferior angle
17 Coracoid process
18 Supraglenoid tubercle
19 Glenoid cavity
20 Infraglenoid tubercle
21 Lateral margin

Thorax
22 Body of sternum
23 Costal arch
24 Angle of ribs
25 Free ribs

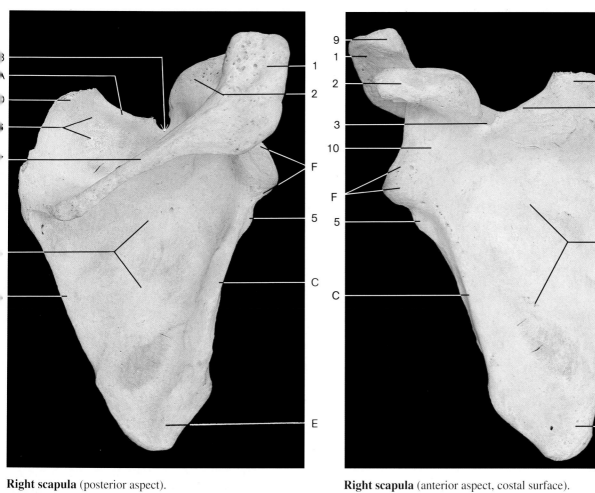

Right scapula (posterior aspect).

Right scapula (anterior aspect, costal surface).

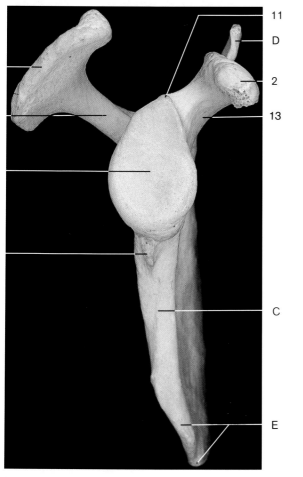

Right scapula (lateral aspect).

Scapula

A   Superior border
B   Medial border
C   Lateral border
D   Superior angle
E   Inferior angle
F   Lateral angle

1   Acromion
2   Coracoid process
3   Scapular notch
4   Glenoid cavity
5   Infraglenoid tubercle
6   Supraspinous fossa
7   Spine
8   Infraspinous fossa
9   Articular facet for acromion
10   Neck
11   Supraglenoid tubercle
12   Costal (anterior) surface
13   Base of coracoid process

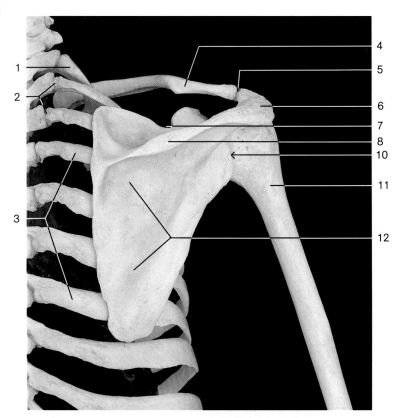

1 1st rib
2 Position of costotransverse joints
3 Fourth–seventh ribs
4 **Clavicle**
5 Position of acromioclavicular joint
6 Acromion
7 Scapular notch
8 Spine of scapula
9 Head of humerus
10 Glenoid cavity
11 Surgical neck of humerus
12 Posterior surface of **scapula**
13 Coracoid process
14 Infraglenoid tubercle
15 Greater tubercle of **humerus**
16 Anatomical neck of humerus

Bones of shoulder joint (posterior aspect).

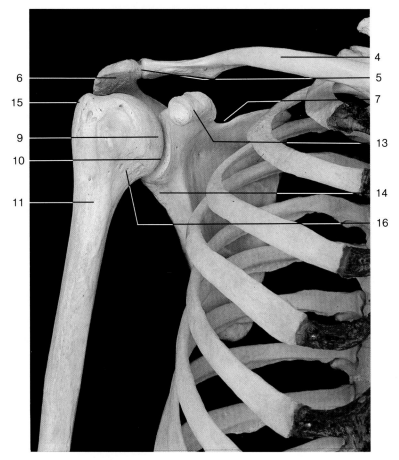

Bones of shoulder joint (anterior aspect).

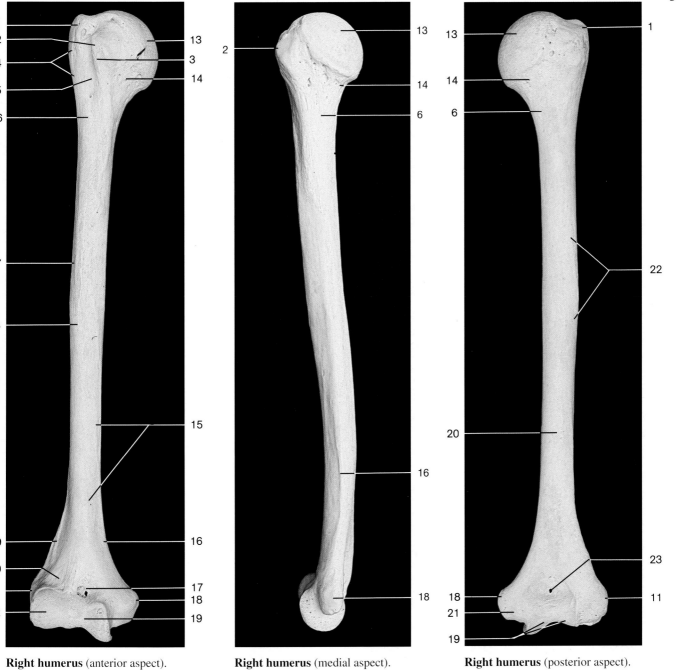

Right humerus (anterior aspect).   **Right humerus** (medial aspect).   **Right humerus** (posterior aspect).

Humerus

1	Greater tubercle	7	Deltoid tuberosity	13 Head
2	Lesser tubercle	8	Anterolateral surface	14 Anatomical neck
3	Crest of lesser tubercle	9	Lateral supracondylar ridge	15 Anteromedial surface
4	Crest of greater tubercle	10	Radial fossa	16 Medial supracondylar ridge
5	Intertubercular sulcus	11	Lateral epicondyle	17 Coronoid fossa
6	Surgical neck	12	Capitulum	18 Medial epicondyle
				19 Trochlea
				20 Posterior surface
				21 Groove for ulnar nerve
				22 Groove for radial nerve
				23 Olecranon fossa

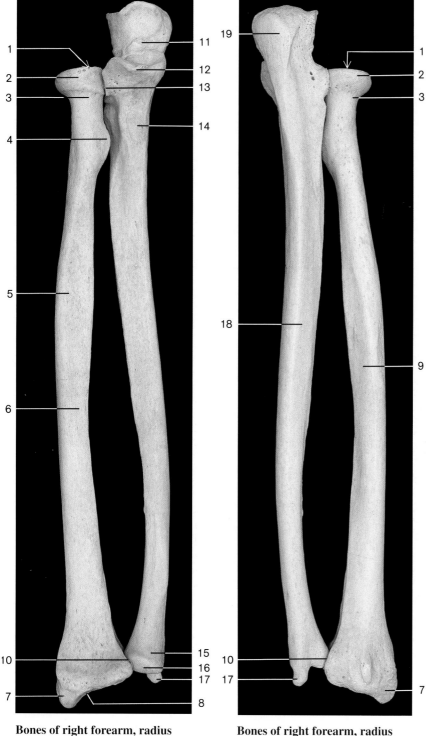

Radius
1 Head
2 Articular circumference
3 Neck
4 Radial tuberosity
5 Shaft
6 Anterior surface
7 Styloid process
8 Articular surface
9 Posterior surface
10 Ulnar notch

Ulna
11 Trochlear notch
12 Coronoid process
13 Radial notch
14 Ulnar tuberosity
15 Head
16 Articular circumference
17 Styloid process
18 Posterior surface
19 Olecranon

Bones of right forearm, radius and ulna (anterior aspect).

Bones of right forearm, radius and ulna (posterior aspect).

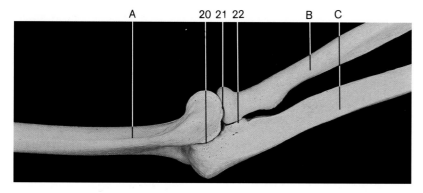

Bones of right elbow joint (lateral aspect).

Articulations at the right elbow
20 Site of humeroulnar joint
21 Site of humeroradial joint
22 Site of proximal radioulnar joint

A Humerus
B Radius
C Ulna

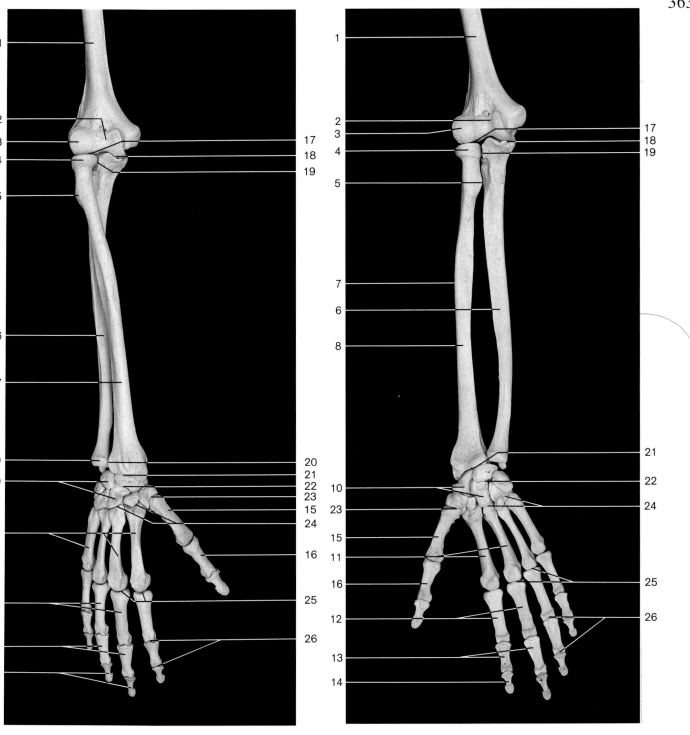

Skeleton of right forearm and hand in pronation.

Skeleton of right forearm and hand in supination.

1	Humerus	11	**Metacarpal bones**		**Sites of joints**
2	Trochlea of humerus	12	Proximal phalanges	17	Humeroradial joint
3	Capitulum of humerus	13	Middle phalanges	18	Humeroulnar joint
4	Articular circumference of radius	14	Distal phalanges	19	Proximal radioulnar joint
5	Radial tuberosity	15	Metacarpal bone of thumb	20	Distal radioulnar joint
6	Anterior surface of **ulna**	16	Proximal phalanx of thumb	21	Radiocarpal joint
7	Posterior surface of **radius**			22	Midcarpal joint
8	Anterior surface of radius			23	Carpometacarpal joint of thumb
9	Articular circumference of ulna			24	Carpometacarpal joints
10	**Carpal bones**			25	Metacarpophalangeal joints
				26	Interphalangeal joints of fingers

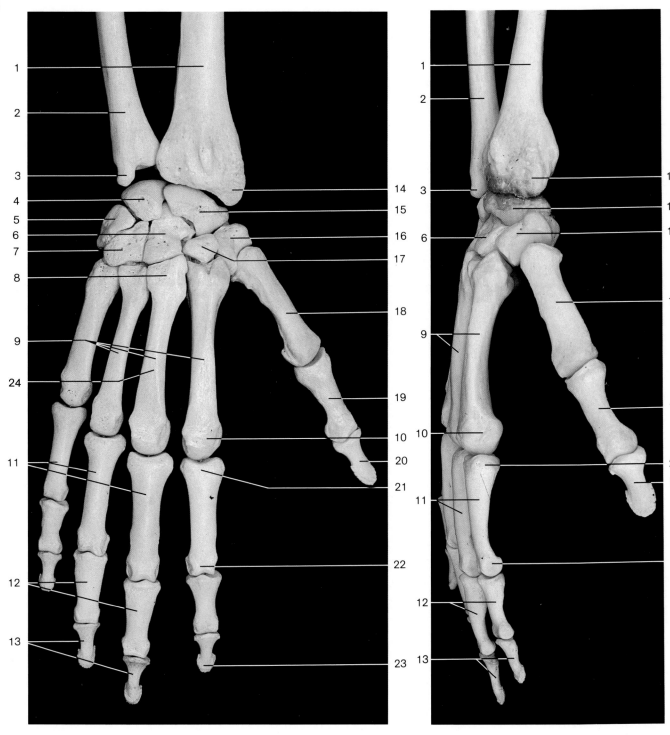

Skeleton of right wrist and hand (dorsal aspect).

Skeleton of right wrist and hand
(medial aspect).

1	**Radius**	8	Base of third metacarpal bone	15	Scaphoid bone
2	**Ulna**	9	**Metacarpal bones**	16	Trapezium bone
3	Styloid process of ulna	10	Head of metacarpal bone	17	Trapezoid bone
4	Lunate bone	11	Proximal phalanges of hand	18	Metacarpal bone of thumb
5	Triquetral bone	12	Middle phalanges of hand	19	Proximal phalanx of thumb
6	Capitate bone	13	Distal phalanges of hand	20	Distal phalanx of thumb
7	Hamate bone	14	Styloid process of radius	21	Base of second proximal phalanx

15 Scaphoid bone ⎫
16 Trapezium bone ⎬ **Carpal bones**
17 Trapezoid bone ⎭

4 Lunate bone ⎫
5 Triquetral bone ⎬ **Carpal bones**
6 Capitate bone ⎪
7 Hamate bone ⎭

22 Head of second
  proximal phalanx
23 Tuberosity of distal
  phalanx
24 Body of
  third metacarpal
  bone

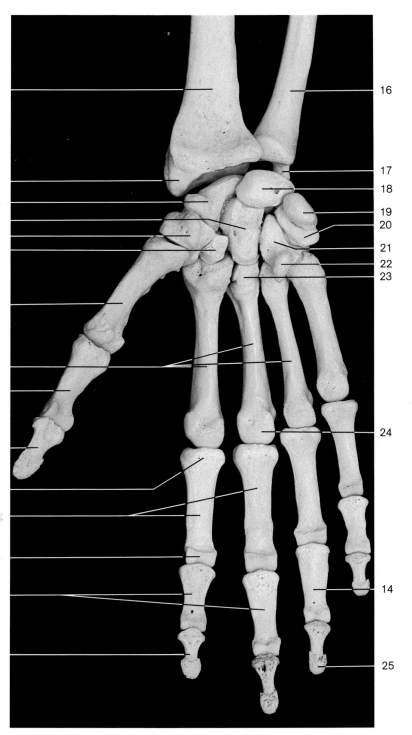

Skeleton of right wrist and hand (palmar aspect).

1 Radius
2 Styloid process of radius
3 Scaphoid bone ⎫
4 Capitate bone ⎪
5 Trapezium ⎬ **Carpal bones**
6 Trapezoid bone ⎭
7 First metacarpal bone
8 Second to fourth metacarpal bones
9 Proximal phalanx of thumb
10 Distal phalanx of thumb
11 Base of second proximal phalanx
12 Proximal phalanges
13 Head of second proximal phalanx
14 Middle phalanges
15 Distal phalanx
16 Ulna
17 Styloid process of ulna
18 Lunate bone ⎫
19 Pisiform bone ⎪
20 Triquetral bone ⎪
21 Hamate bone ⎬ **Carpal bones**
22 Hamulus or hook ⎪
   of hamate bone ⎭
23 Base of third metacarpal bone
24 Head of metacarpal bone
25 Tuberosity of distal phalanx

The human hand is one of the most admirable structures of the human body. The carpometacarpal joint of the thumb, a saddle joint, enjoys wide mobility, so that the thumb can get in contact with all other fingers, thus enabling the hand to become an instrument for grasping and psychologic expression. During evolution these newly developed functions appeared after the erect posture of the human body was achieved. An inevitable prerequisite for the development of human cultures is not only the differentiation of the brain but also the development of an organ capable of realizing its ideas: the human hand.

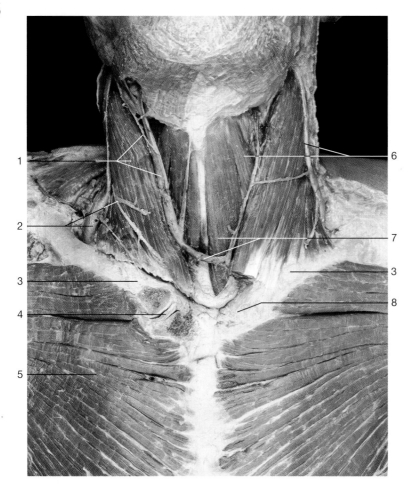

1 Sternocleidomastoid muscle, cervical branch of
    facial nerve and anterior jugular vein
2 External jugular vein and transverse cervical nerve
    (inferior branch)
3 Clavicle
4 **Sternoclavicular joint** (opened) with articular disk
5 Pectoralis major muscle
6 Omohyoid muscle and external jugular vein
7 Jugular venous arch and sternohyoid muscle
8 Sternoclavicular joint (not opened)
9 Acromial end of clavicle
10 **Acromioclavicular joint**
11 Acromion
12 Tendon of supraspinatus muscle
    (attached to the articular capsule)
13 Coracoacromial ligament
14 Tendon of long head of biceps brachii muscle
15 Tendon of subscapularis muscle
    (attached to the articular capsule)
16 Intertubercular sulcus
17 Articular capsule of shoulder joint
18 Humerus
19 Trapezoid ligament
20 Coracoid process
21 Glenoid labrum
22 **Shoulder joint** (joint cavity)
23 Scapula
24 Supraspinatus muscle
25 Cartilage of glenoid cavity
26 Tendon of long head of triceps brachii muscle
27 Head of humerus (articular cartilage)
28 Epiphyseal line

Right sternoclavicular joint (anterior aspect). On the right side the joint has been opened by a coronal section. Note the articular disc.

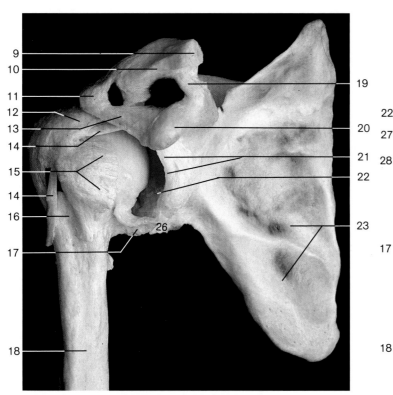

Right shoulder joint. The anterior part of the articular capsule has been removed and the head of the humerus has been slightly rotated outward to show the cavity of the joint.

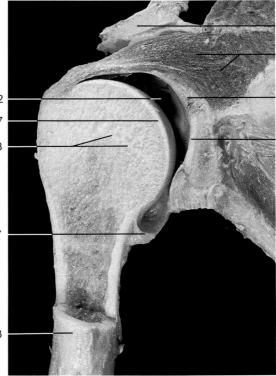

Coronal section of the right shoulder joint (anterior aspect).

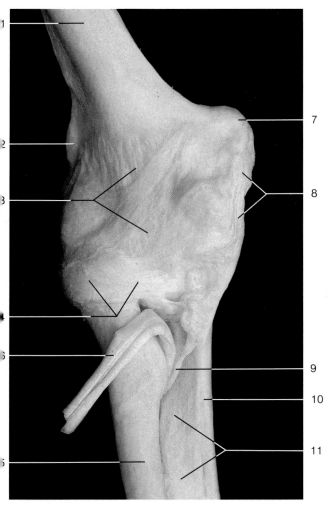

1   Humerus
2   Lateral epicondyle of humerus
3   Articular capsule
4   Annular ligament of proximal radioulnar joint
5   Radius
6   Tendon of biceps brachii muscle
7   Medial epicondyle of humerus
8   Ulnar collateral ligament
9   Oblique cord
10   Ulna
11   Interosseous membrane
12   Radial fossa
13   Capitulum of humerus
14   Head of radius
15   Radial collateral ligament
16   Coronoid fossa
17   Trochlea of humerus
18   Coronoid process of ulna
19   Olecranon
20   Radial tuberosity

Ligaments of elbow joint (anterior aspect).

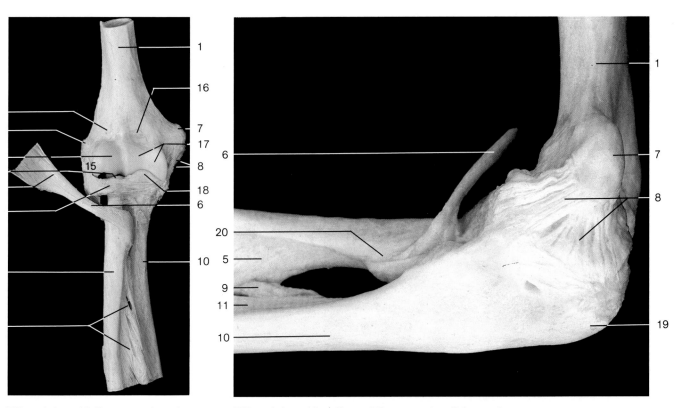

Elbow joint with ligaments (anterior aspect). Articular capsule has been removed to show the annular ligament.

Elbow joint with collateral ligaments (medial aspect).

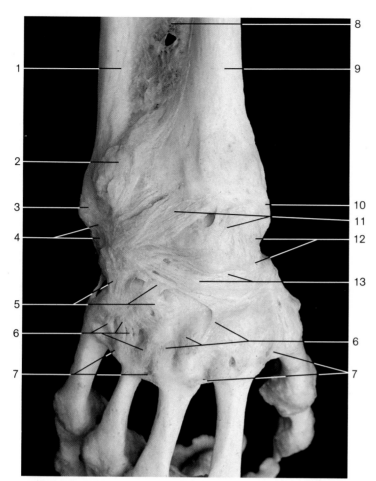

Ligaments of hand and wrist (dorsal aspect).

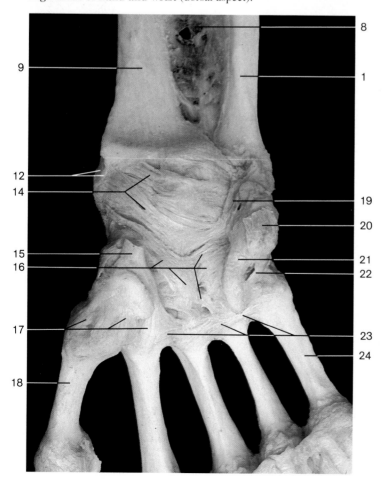

Ligaments of hand and wrist (palmar aspect).

1 Ulna
2 Exostosis (pathological)
3 Head of ulna
4 **Ulnar carpal collateral ligament**
5 Deep intercarpal ligaments
6 Dorsal carpometacarpal ligaments
7 Dorsal metacarpal ligaments
8 Interosseous membrane
9 Radius
10 Styloid process of radius
11 **Dorsal radiocarpal ligament**
12 Radial collateral ligament
13 Articular capsule and dorsal intercarpal ligaments
14 **Palmar radiocarpal ligament**
15 Tendon of flexor carpi radialis muscle (cut)
16 Radiating carpal ligament
17 Palmar carpometacarpal ligaments
18 First metacarpal bone
19 Palmar ulnocarpal ligament
20 Tendon of flexor carpi ulnaris muscle (cut)
21 **Pisohamate ligament**
22 **Pisometacarpal ligament**
23 Palmar metacarpal ligaments
24 Fifth metacarpal bone

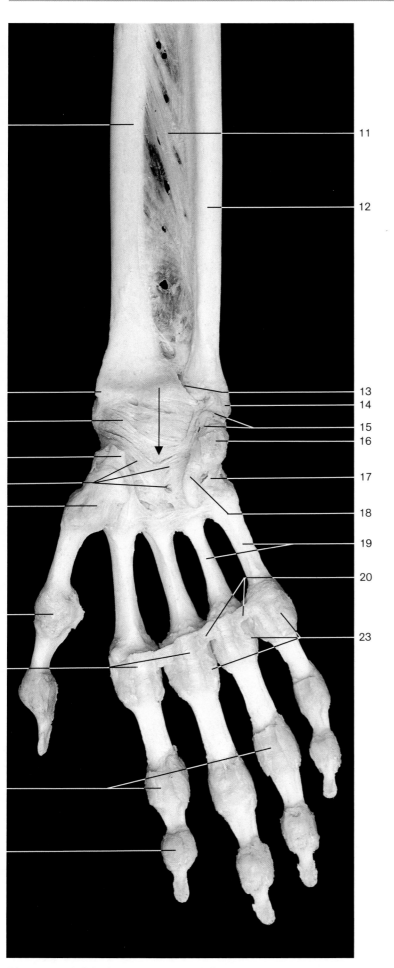

1 Radius
2 Styloid process of radius
3 Palmar radiocarpal ligament
4 Tendon of flexor carpi radialis muscle (cut)
5 Radiating carpal ligament
6 Articular capsule of **carpometacarpal joint of thumb**
7 Articular capsule of **metacarpophalangeal joint of thumb**
8 Palmar ligaments and articular capsule of metacarpophalangeal joints
9 Palmar ligaments and articular capsule of interphalangeal joints
10 Articular capsule
11 Interosseous membrane
12 Ulna
13 **Distal radioulnar joint**
14 Styloid process of ulna
15 Palmar ulnocarpal ligament
16 Pisiform bone with tendon of flexor carpi ulnaris muscle
17 Pisometacarpal ligament
18 Pisohamate ligament
19 Metacarpal bone
20 Deep transverse metacarpal ligament
21 Tendons of extensor muscles and articular capsule
22 Collateral ligament of **interphalangeal joint**
23 Collateral ligaments of **metacarpophalangeal joints**
24 Second metacarpal bone

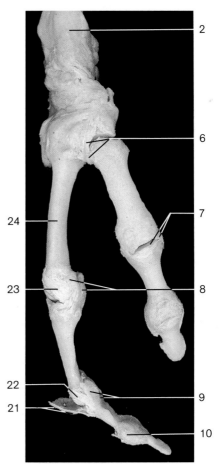

Ligaments of right forearm, hand and fingers (palmar aspect).
The arrow indicates the location of the carpal tunnel.

Ligaments of fingers
(lateral aspect).

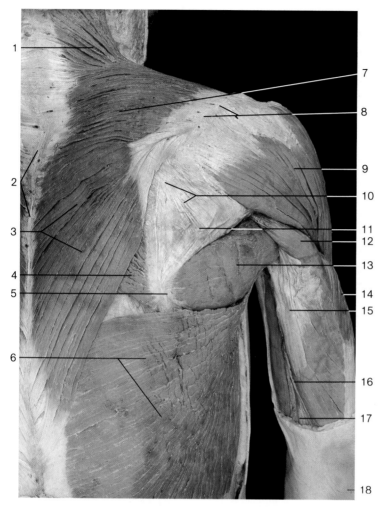

1   Descending fibers of **trapezius muscle**
2   Spinous processes of thoracic vertebrae
3   Ascending fibers of trapezius muscle
4   Rhomboid major muscle
5   Inferior angle of scapula
6   **Latissimus dorsi muscle**
7   Transverse fibers of trapezius muscle
8   Spine of scapula
9   Posterior fibers of **deltoid muscle**
10 Infraspinatus muscle and infraspinous fascia
11 Teres minor muscle and fascia
12 Long head of triceps brachii muscle
13 **Teres major muscle**
14 Lateral head of triceps brachii muscle
15 Medial head of triceps brachii muscle
16 Medial intermuscular septum
17 Ulnar nerve
18 Olecranon

Muscles of shoulder and arm, superficial layer (dorsal aspect).

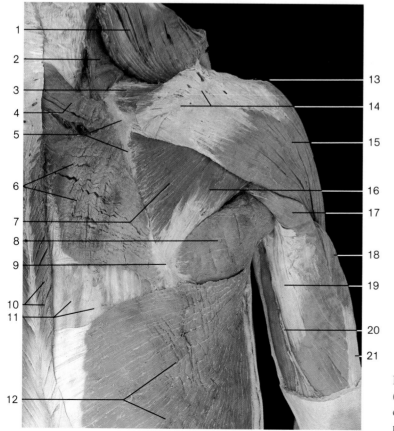

1   Trapezius muscle (reflected)
2   Levator scapulae muscle
3   Supraspinatus muscle
4   Rhomboid minor muscle
5   Medial border of scapula
6   **Rhomboid major muscle**
7   **Infraspinatus muscle**
8   **Teres major muscle**
9   Inferior angle of scapula
10 Cut edge of trapezius muscle
11 Intrinsic muscles of back with fascia
12 **Latissimus dorsi muscle**
13 Acromion
14 Spine of scapula
15 **Deltoid muscle**
16 Teres minor muscle
17 Long head of triceps brachii muscle
18 Lateral head of triceps brachii muscle
19 Medial head of triceps brachii muscle
20 Medial intermuscular septum
21 Tendon of triceps brachii muscle

Muscles of shoulder and arm, deeper layer
(right side, dorsal aspect). The trapezius has been
cut near its origin at the vertebral column and
reflected upward.

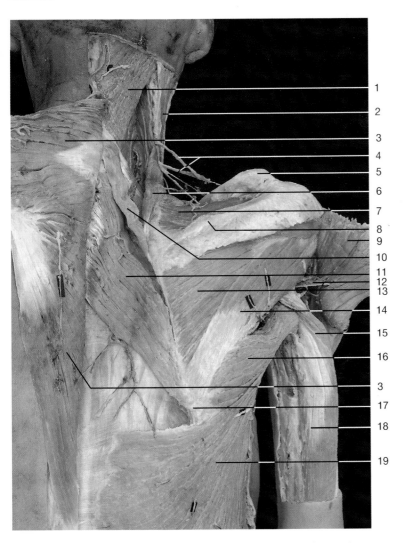

1 **Splenius capitis muscle**
2 Sternocleidomastoid muscle
3 Trapezius muscle (reflected)
4 **Lateral supraclavicular nerves**
5 Clavicle
6 Levator scapulae muscle
7 Supraspinatus muscle
8 Spine of scapula
9 Deltoid muscle (reflected)
10 Rhomboid minor muscle
11 **Rhomboid major muscle**
12 **Axillary nerve and posterior circumflex humeral artery**
13 **Infraspinatus muscle**
14 **Teres minor muscle**
15 Long head of triceps brachii muscle
16 **Teres major muscle**
17 Inferior angle of scapula
18 Triceps brachii muscle
19 **Latissimus dorsi muscle**

Muscles of shoulder and arm, deeper layer, right side (dorsal aspect). The trapezius and deltoid muscles have been divided and reflected.

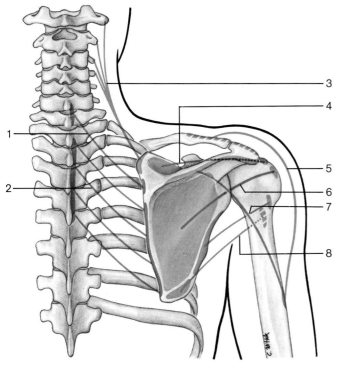

Shoulder muscles, schematic diagram illustrating the course of the main muscles of the dorsal aspect of the shoulder.

1 Rhomboid minor muscle (red)
2 Rhomboid major muscle (red)
3 Levator scapulae muscle (red)
4 Supraspinatus muscle (blue)
5 Deltoid muscle (red)
6 Infraspinatus muscle (blue)
7 Teres minor muscle (red)
8 Teres major muscle (red)

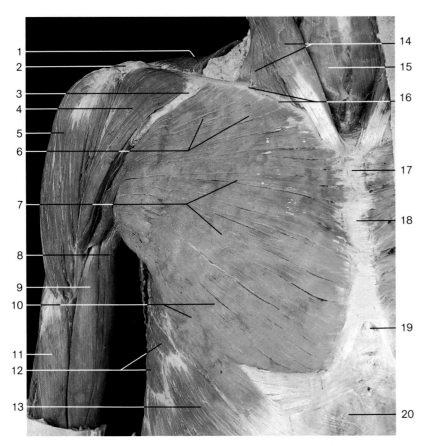

1 Trapezius muscle
2 Acromion
3 Deltopectoral triangle
4 Clavicular part of deltoid muscle
   (anterior fibers)
5 Acromial part of deltoid muscle
   (central fibers)
6 Clavicular part of pectoralis major muscle
7 Sternocostal part of pectoralis major muscle
8 Short head of biceps brachii muscle
9 Long head of biceps brachii muscle
10 Abdominal part of pectoralis major muscle
11 Brachialis muscle
12 Serratus anterior muscle
13 External abdominal oblique muscle
14 Sternocleidomastoid muscle
15 Infrahyoid muscles
16 Clavicle
17 Manubrium sterni
18 Body of sternum
19 Xiphoid process
20 Anterior layer of sheath of rectus
   abdominis muscle

Muscles of shoulder and arm, superficial layer (ventral aspect).

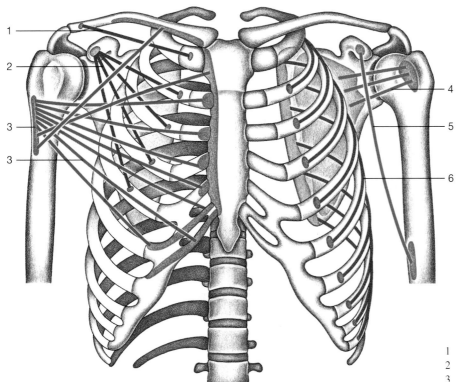

Arrangement of pectoral and shoulder muscles (ventral aspect).
(Schematic drawing.)

1 Subclavius muscle (blue)
2 Pectoralis minor muscle (blue)
3 Pectoralis major muscle (red)
4 Subscapularis muscle (red)
5 Coracobrachialis muscle (red)
6 Serratus anterior muscle (green)

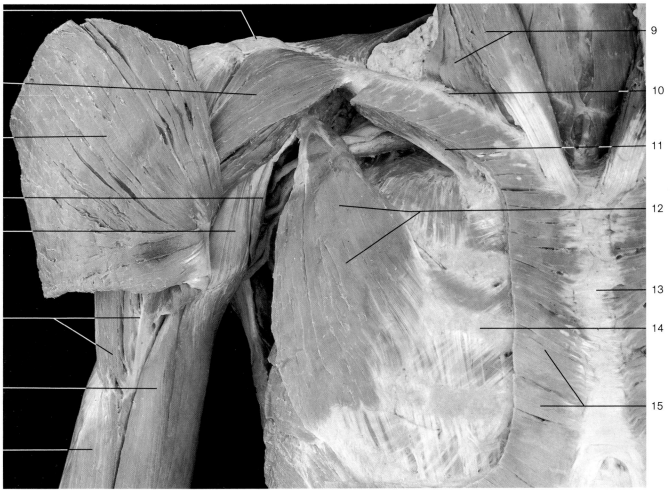

Muscles of shoulder and arm, deep layer (ventral aspect).

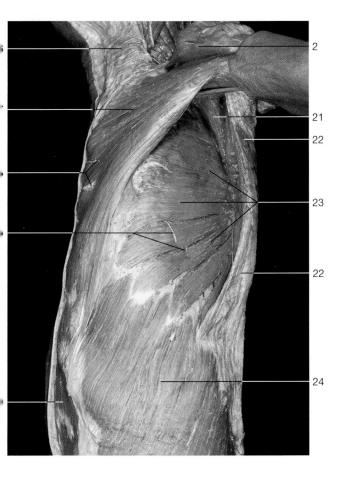

1 Acromion
2 Clavicular part of deltoid muscle
3 Pectoralis major muscle (reflected)
4 Coracobrachialis muscle
5 Short head of biceps brachii muscle
6 Deltoid muscle (insertion on humerus)
7 Long head of biceps brachii muscle
8 Brachialis muscle
9 Sternocleidomastoid muscle
10 Clavicle
11 Subclavius muscle
12 Pectoralis minor muscle
13 Sternum
14 Third rib
15 Pectoralis major muscle
16 Platysma muscle
17 Pectoralis major muscle forming the anterior axillary fold
18 Anterior cutaneous branches of intercostal nerves
19 Lateral cutaneous branches of intercostal nerves
20 Rectus abdominis muscle
21 Subscapularis muscle
22 **Latissimus dorsi muscle** forming the posterior axillary fold
23 **Serratus anterior muscle** forming the medial wall of the axilla
24 External abdominal oblique muscle

Axillary fossa and serratus anterior muscle
(left side, lateral aspect).

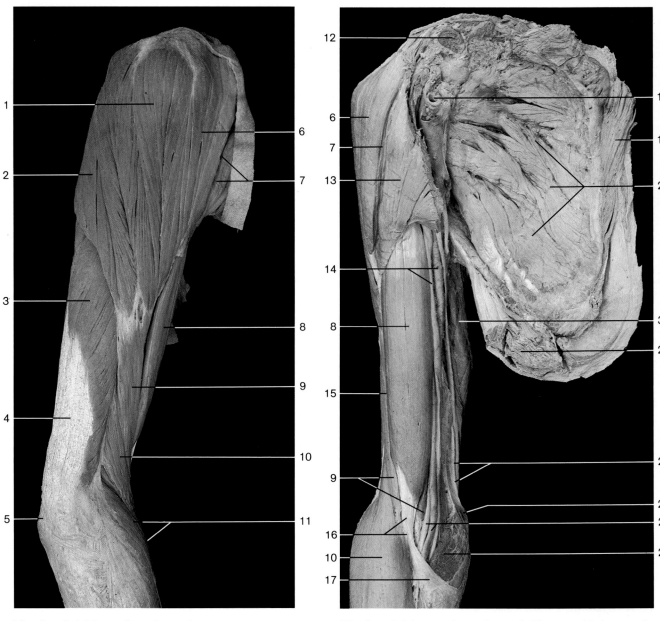

Muscles of right arm (lateral aspect).

Muscles of right arm (ventral aspect). The arm with the scapula and attached muscles has been removed from the trunk.

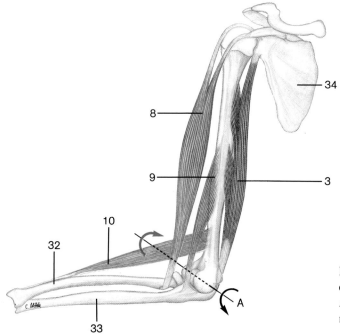

Diagram illustrating the position of the **flexor and extensor muscles of the arm** and their effect on the elbow joint. A = axis; arrows = direction of movements; red = flexion; black = extension.

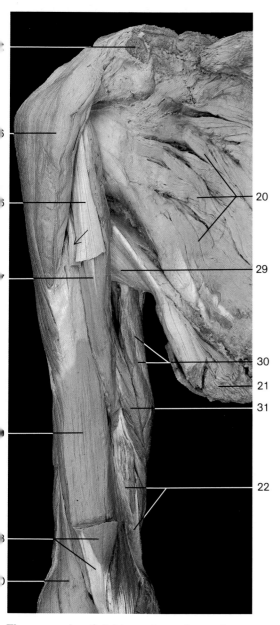

Flexor muscles of right arm (ventral aspect).
Part of the biceps brachii muscle has been
removed. Arrow: tendon of long head of biceps
brachii muscle.

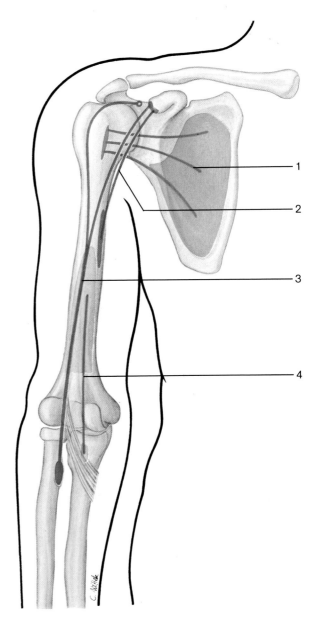

Position and course of flexors of arm. (Schematic drawing.)

1	Subscapularis muscle (red)	3	Biceps brachii muscle (red)
2	Coracobrachialis muscle (blue)	4	Brachialis muscle (blue)

1	Acromial part of deltoid muscle (central fibers)	18	Axillary artery
2	Scapular part of deltoid muscle (posterior fibers)	19	Rhomboid major muscle
3	Triceps brachii muscle	20	**Subscapularis muscle**
4	Tendon of triceps brachii muscle	21	Latissimus dorsi muscle (divided)
5	Olecranon	22	Medial intermuscular septum
6	Clavicular part of deltoid muscle (anterior fibers)	23	Medial epicondyle of humerus
7	Deltopectoral groove	24	Brachial artery and median nerve
8	**Biceps brachii muscle**	25	Pronator teres muscle
9	**Brachialis muscle**	26	Tendon of short head of biceps brachii muscle
10	**Brachioradialis muscle**	27	Coracobrachialis muscle
11	Extensor carpi radialis longus muscle	28	Distal part of biceps brachii muscle
12	Clavicle (divided)	29	Teres major muscle
13	Pectoralis major muscle	30	Long head of triceps brachii muscle
14	Medial intermuscular septum with vessels and nerves	31	Medial head of triceps brachii muscle
15	Lateral intermuscular septum	32	Radius
16	Tendon of biceps brachii muscle	33	Ulna
17	Bicipital aponeurosis	34	Scapula

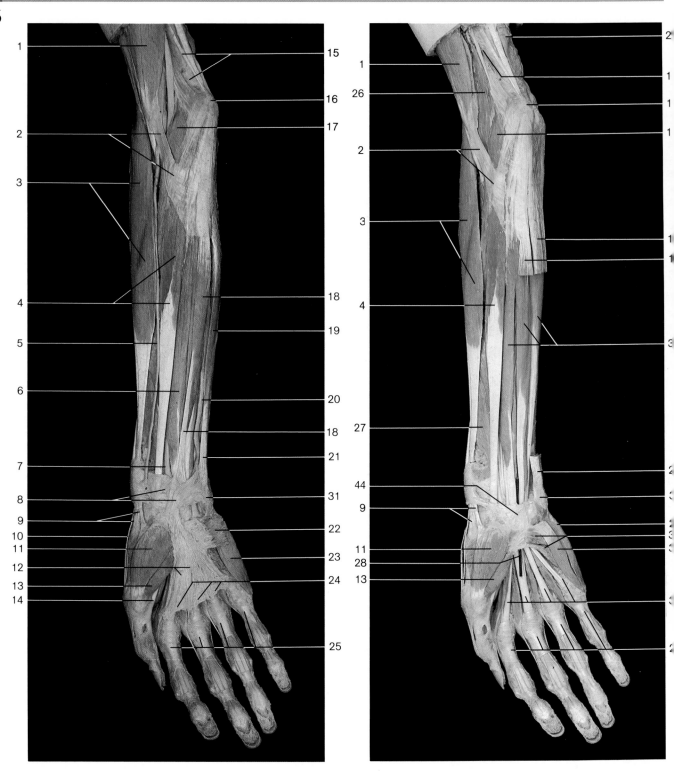

Forearm muscles, superficial layer (ventral aspect).

Forearm muscles, superficial layer (ventral aspect). The palmaris longus and flexor carpi ulnaris muscles have been removed.

1   Biceps brachii muscle
2   Bicipital aponeurosis
3   **Brachioradialis muscle**
4   **Flexor carpi radialis muscle**
5   Radial artery
6   **Flexor digitorum superficialis muscle**
7   Median nerve
8   Antebrachial fascia and tendon of palmaris longus muscle
9   Tendon of abductor pollicis longus muscle
10 Tendon of extensor pollicis brevis muscle
11 Abductor pollicis brevis muscle

12 **Palmar aponeurosis**
13 Superficial head of flexor pollicis brevis muscle
14 Tendon of flexor pollicis longus muscle
15 Medial intermuscular septum
16 Medial epicondyle of humerus
17 Humeral head of pronator teres muscle
18 **Palmaris longus muscle**
19 **Flexor carpi ulnaris muscle**
20 **Ulnar artery**
21 Tendon of flexor carpi ulnaris muscle
22 Palmaris brevis muscle

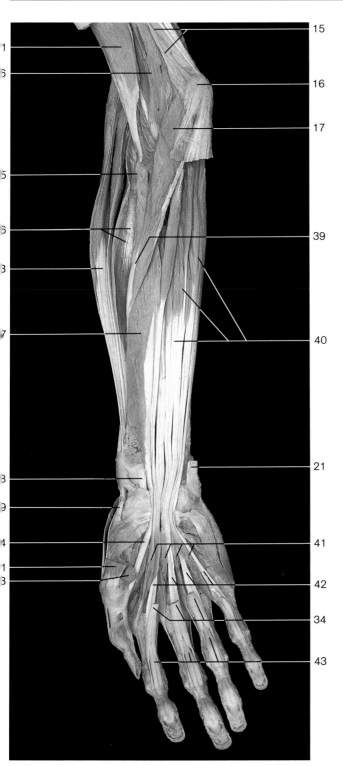

1
6
5
6
3
7

8
9
4
1
3

15
16
17
39
40
21
41
42
34
43

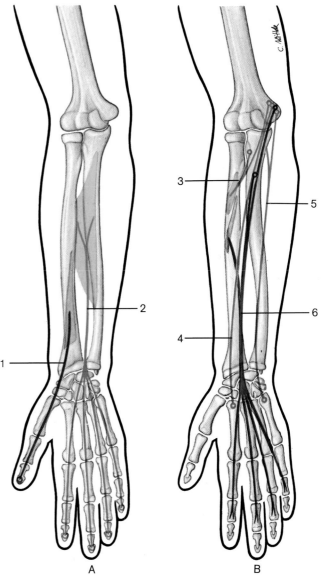

A

B

Position of flexors of fingers and hand.
(Schematic drawing.)

A   Deep layer
B   Superficial layer

△
1   Flexor pollicis longus muscle (blue)
2   Flexor digitorum profundus muscle (red)
3   Pronator teres muscle (red)
4   Flexor carpi radialis muscle (red)
5   Flexor carpi ulnaris muscle (red)
6   Flexor digitorum superficialis muscle (blue)

Forearm muscles, middle layer (ventral aspect). The palmaris
longus, flexor carpi radialis and ulnaris muscles have been
partly removed. The flexor retinaculum has been divided.

23   Abductor digiti minimi muscle
24   Transverse fasciculi of palmar aponeurosis
25   Digital fibrous sheaths of tendons of flexor digitorum muscle
26   Brachialis muscle
27   Flexor pollicis longus muscle
28   Carpal tunnel (canalis carpi, probe)
29   Triceps brachii muscle
30   Flexor digitorum superficialis muscle
31   Pisiform bone
32   Opponens digiti minimi muscle
33   Flexor digiti minimi brevis muscle
34   Tendons of flexor digitorum superficialis muscle

35   Supinator muscle
36   Extensor carpi radialis brevis muscle
37   **Flexor pollicis longus muscle**
38   Tendon of flexor carpi radialis muscle
39   **Pronator teres muscle** (insertion of radius)
40   **Flexor digitorum profundus muscle**
41   **Lumbrical muscles**
42   Tendons of flexor digitorum profundus muscle
43   Tendons of flexor digitorum profundus muscle having passed
       through the divided tendons of the flexor digitorum superficialis
       muscle
44   Flexor retinaculum

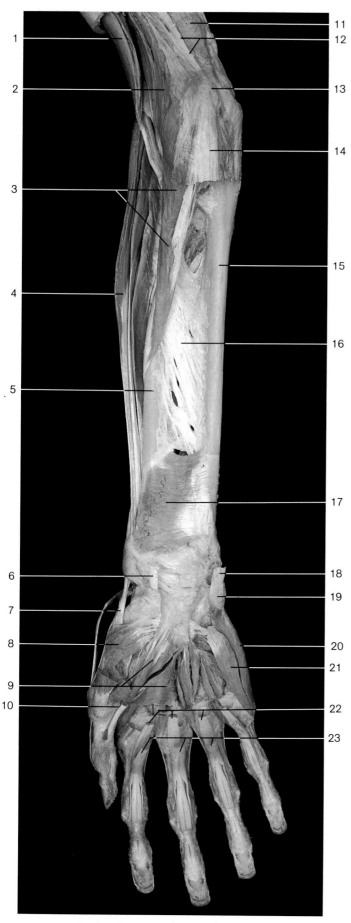

1 Biceps brachii muscle
2 Brachialis muscle
3 **Pronator teres muscle**
4 Brachioradialis muscle
5 **Radius**
6 Tendon of flexor carpi radialis muscle
7 Tendon of abductor pollicis longus muscle
8 Opponens pollicis muscle
9 Adductor pollicis muscle
10 Tendon of flexor pollicis longus muscle
11 Triceps brachii muscle
12 Medial intermuscular septum
13 Medial epicondyle of humerus
14 Common flexor mass (divided)
15 **Ulna**
16 **Interosseous membrane**
17 **Pronator quadratus muscle**
18 Tendon of flexor carpi ulnaris muscle
19 Pisiform bone
20 Abductor digiti minimi muscle
21 Flexor digiti minimi brevis muscle
22 Tendons of flexor digitorum profundus muscle
23 Tendons of flexor digitorum superficialis muscle
24 Flexor retinaculum
25 Hypothenar muscles
26 Thenar muscles
27 Common synovial sheath of flexor tendons
28 Synovial sheath of tendon of flexor pollicis longus muscle
29 Digital synovial sheaths of flexor tendons

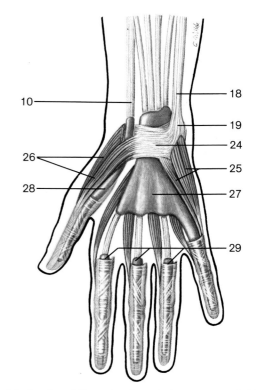

Muscles of the forearm, deep layer (ventral aspect). All flexors have been removed to display the pronator quadratus and pronator teres muscles together with the interosseous membrane. Forearm in supination.

Synovial sheaths of flexor tendons (palmar aspect of right hand). (Semischematic drawing.)

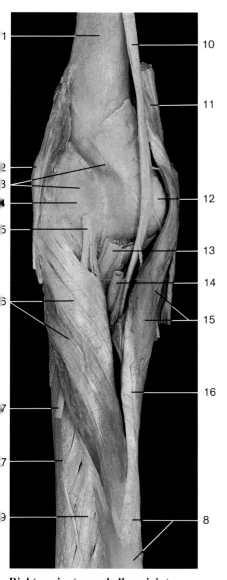

1 Humerus
2 Lateral epicondyle of humerus
3 Articular capsule
4 Position of capitulum of humerus
5 Deep branch of radial nerve
6 **Supinator muscle**
7 Entrance of deep branch of radial nerve to extensor muscles
8 Radius and insertion of pronator teres muscle
9 Interosseous membrane
10 Median nerve
11 Triceps brachii muscle
12 Trochlea of humerus
13 Tendon of biceps brachii muscle
14 Brachial artery
15 **Pronator teres muscle**
16 Tendon of pronator teres muscle
17 Ulna
18 **Pronator quadratus muscle**
19 Tendon of flexor carpi radialis muscle
20 Thenar muscles
21 Synovial sheath of tendon of flexor pollicis longus muscle
22 Fibrous sheath of flexor tendons
23 **Digital synovial sheath of flexor tendons**
24 Flexor digitorum superficialis muscle
25 Tendon of flexor carpi ulnaris muscle
26 **Common synovial sheath of flexor tendons**
27 Position of pisiform bone
28 Flexor retinaculum
29 Hypothenar muscles

Right supinator and elbow joint
(anterior aspect). Forearm in pronation.

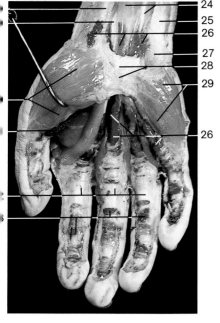

Synovial sheaths of flexor muscles
(palmar aspect of right hand). Blue PVA
solution has been injected into the sheaths.

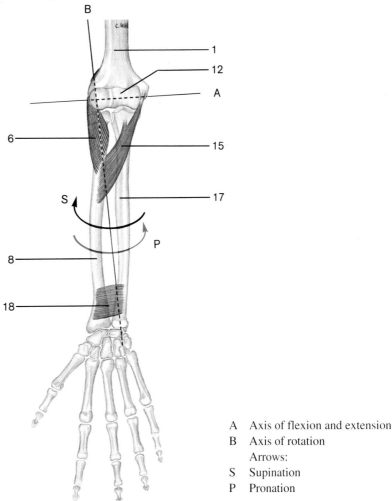

A Axis of flexion and extension
B Axis of rotation
Arrows:
S Supination
P Pronation

Diagram illustrating the two **axes of the elbow joint.**

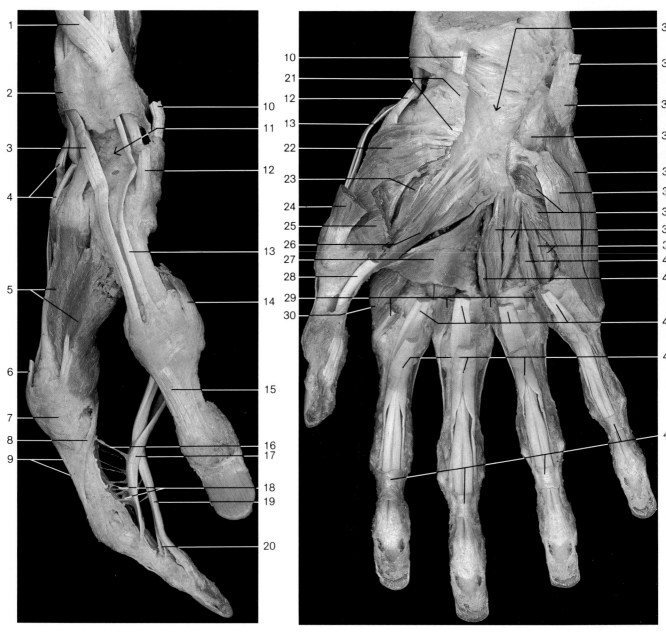

Muscles of thumb and index finger (medial aspect). The tendons of the extensor muscles of the thumb and the insertion of the flexor tendons of the index finger are displayed.

Muscles of hand (palmar aspect). The tendons of the flexor muscles and parts of the thumb muscles have been removed. The carpal tunnel has been opened.

1	Tendons of extensor pollicis brevis and abductor pollicis longus muscle	
2	Extensor retinaculum	
3	Tendon of extensor pollicis longus muscle	
4	Tendons of extensor carpi radialis longus and brevis muscles	
5	First dorsal interosseous muscle	
6	Tendon of extensor digitorum muscle for index finger	
7	Location of metacarpophalangeal joint	
8	Tendon of lumbrical muscle	
9	Extensor expansion of index finger	
10	Tendon of flexor carpi radialis muscle (cut)	
11	**Anatomical snuffbox**	
12	Tendon of abductor pollicis longus muscle	
13	Tendon of extensor pollicis brevis muscle	
14	Tendon of abductor pollicis brevis muscle	

15	Extensor expansion of extensor of thumb
16	Vinculum longum
17	Tendons of flexor digitorum superficialis muscle dividing to allow passage of deep tendons
18	Vincula of flexor tendons
19	Tendon of flexor digitorum profundus muscle
20	Vinculum breve
21	Radial carpal eminence (cut edge of flexor retinaculum)
22	Opponens pollicis muscle
23	Deep head of flexor pollicis brevis muscle
24	Abductor pollicis brevis muscle (cut)
25	Superficial head of flexor pollicis brevis muscle (cut)
26	Oblique head of adductor pollicis muscle
27	Transverse head of adductor pollicis muscle
28	Tendon of flexor pollicis longus muscle (cut)

29	Lumbrical muscles (cut)
30	First dorsal interosseous muscle
31	**Position of carpal tunnel**
32	Tendon of flexor carpi ulnaris muscle
33	Location of pisiform bone
34	Hook of hamate bone
35	Abductor digiti minimi muscle
36	Flexor digiti minimi brevis muscle
37	Opponens digiti minimi muscle
38	Second palmar interosseous muscle
39	Third palmar interosseous muscle
40	Fourth dorsal interosseous muscle
41	Third dorsal interosseous muscle
42	Tendon of flexor digitorum profundus muscle (cut)
43	Tendons of flexor digitorum superficialis muscle (cut)
44	Fibrous flexor sheaths

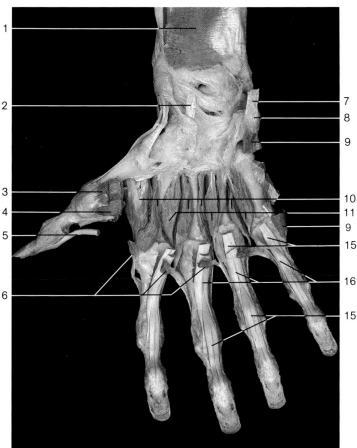

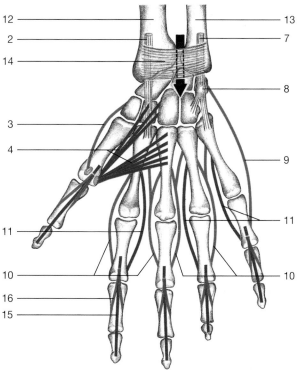

Muscles of right hand, deep layer (palmar aspect). The thenar and hypothenar muscles have been removed to display the interosseous muscles.

Actions of interosseous muscles in abduction and adduction of fingers (palmar aspect, schematic drawing). Arrow: carpal tunnel.

Red = **abduction**
(dorsal interosseous muscles, abductor digiti minimi and abductor pollicis brevis muscles).

Blue = **adduction**
(palmar interosseous muscles, adductor pollicis muscle).

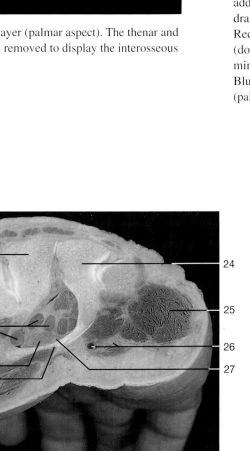

Transverse section through the right hand, showing the carpal tunnel (canalis carpi).

1 Pronator quadratus muscle
2 Tendon of flexor carpi radialis muscle
3 Abductor pollicis brevis muscle (divided)
4 Adductor pollicis muscle (divided)
5 Tendon of flexor pollicis longus muscle
6 Lumbrical muscles (cut)
7 Tendon of flexor carpi ulnaris muscle
8 Pisiform bone
9 Abductor digiti minimi muscle (divided)
10 **Dorsal interosseous muscles**
11 **Palmar interosseous muscles**
12 Radius
13 Ulna
14 **Flexor retinaculum**
15 Tendons of flexor digitorum
    profundus muscle
16 Tendons of flexor digitorum
    superficialis muscle
17 Capitate bone
18 Trapezium bone and trapezoid bone
19 Radial artery
20 Tendon of flexor muscles
21 First metacarpal bone
22 **Median nerve**
23 Thenar muscles
24 Hamate bone
25 Hypothenar muscles
26 Ulnar artery and nerve
27 **Carpal tunnel** (canalis carpi)

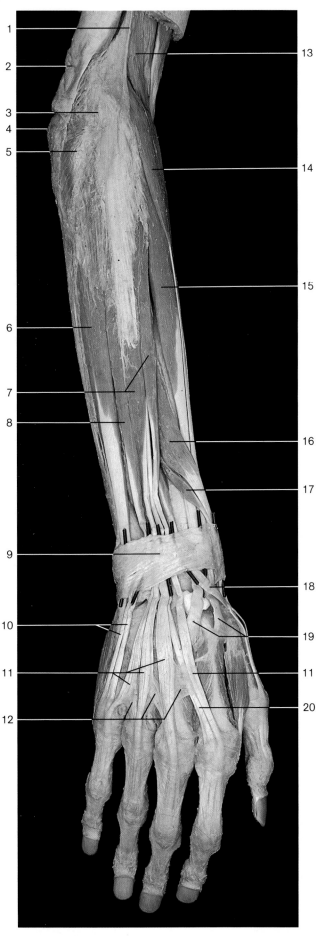

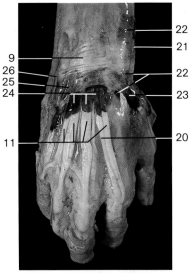

Synovial sheaths of extensor tendons. The sheaths have been injected with blue gelatin.

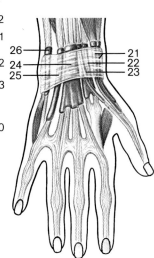

Synovial sheaths of extensor tendons on the back of the right wrist (indicated in blue).
Notice the six tunnels for the passage of the extensor tendons beneath the extensor retinaculum. (Semischematic drawing.)

1 Lateral intermuscular septum
2 Tendon of triceps brachii muscle
3 Lateral epicondyle of humerus
4 Olecranon
5 Anconeus muscle
6 Extensor carpi ulnaris muscle
7 Extensor digitorum muscle
8 Extensor digiti minimi muscle
9 Extensor retinaculum
10 Tendons of extensor digiti minimi muscle
11 Tendons of extensor digitorum muscle
12 Intertendinous connections
13 Brachioradialis muscle
14 Extensor carpi radialis longus muscle
15 Extensor carpi radialis brevis muscle
16 Abductor pollicis longus muscle
17 Extensor pollicis brevis muscle
18 Tendon of extensor pollicis longus muscle
19 Tendons of both extensor carpi radialis longus
   and extensor carpi radialis brevis muscles
20 Tendon of extensor indicis muscle
21 First tunnel: Abductor pollicis longus muscle
                  Extensor pollicis brevis muscle
22 Second tunnel: Extensor carpi radialis longus and brevis muscles
23 Third tunnel: Extensor pollicis longus muscle
24 Fourth tunnel: Extensor digitorum muscle
                  Extensor indicis muscle
25 Fifth tunnel: Extensor digiti minimi muscle
26 Sixth tunnel: Extensor carpi ulnaris muscle

Extensor muscles of forearm and hand, superficial layer (dorsal aspect). Tunnels for extensor tendons indicated by probes.

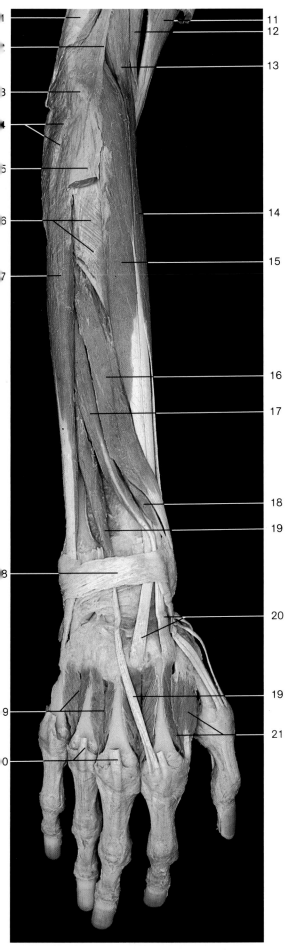

1

11
12

13

3

4

5

6

7

14

15

16

17

18

19

8

20

9

19

0

21

1   Triceps brachii muscle
2   Lateral intermuscular septum
3   Lateral epicondyle of humerus
4   Anconeus muscle
5   Extensor digitorum and extensor digiti minimi muscles (cut)
6   Supinator muscle
7   Extensor carpi ulnaris muscle
8   Extensor retinaculum
9   Third and fourth dorsal interosseous muscles
10 Tendons of extensor digitorum muscle (cut)
11 Biceps brachii muscle
12 Brachialis muscle
13 Brachioradialis muscle
14 Extensor carpi radialis longus muscle
15 Extensor carpi radialis brevis muscle
16 Abductor pollicis longus muscle
17 Extensor pollicis longus muscle
18 Extensor pollicis brevis muscle
19 Extensor indicis muscle
20 Tendons of the extensor carpi radialis longus
    and extensor carpi radialis brevis muscles
21 First dorsal interosseous muscle

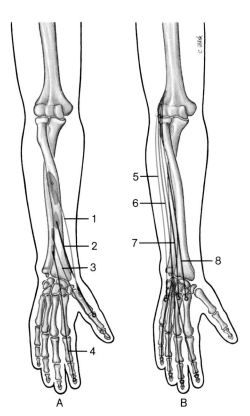

A   B

Position of extensor muscles of forearm and hand.
(Semischematic drawing.)

A Extensors of thumb   B Extensors of fingers and hand

1 Abductor pollicis longus muscle   5 Extensor carpi ulnaris muscle
   (red)   (blue)
2 Extensor pollicis brevis muscle   6 Extensor digitorum muscle
   (blue)   (red)
3 Extensor pollicis longus muscle   7 Extensor carpi radialis brevis
   (red)   muscle (blue)
4 Extensor indicis muscle   8 Extensor carpi radialis longus
   (blue)   muscle (blue)

Extensor muscles of forearm and hand, deep layer
(dorsal aspect).

Main branches of right subclavian and axillary arteries (anterior aspect). Pectoralis muscles have been reflected, clavicle and anterior wall of thorax removed and right lung divided. Left lung with pleura and thyroid gland have been reflected laterally to display aortic arch and common carotid artery with their branches.

1 Pectoralis minor muscle (reflected)	22 Thyroid gland	43 Radial collateral artery
2 Anterior circumflex humeral artery	23 Inferior thyroid artery	44 Radial recurrent artery
3 Musculocutaneous nerve (divided)	24 Internal thoracic artery	45 **Radial artery**
4 **Axillary artery**	25 Right subclavian artery	46 Anterior and posterior interosseous
5 Posterior circumflex humeral artery	26 Brachiocephalic trunk	arteries
6 **Profunda brachii artery**	27 Left brachiocephalic vein (divided)	47 Princeps pollicis artery
7 Median nerve (var.)	28 Left vagus nerve	48 **Deep palmar arch**
8 **Brachial artery**	29 Superior vena cava (divided)	49 Common palmar digital arteries
9 Biceps brachii muscle	30 **Ascending aorta**	50 Ulnar recurrent artery
10 Thoracoacromial artery	31 Median nerve (divided)	51 Recurrent interosseous artery
11 Suprascapular artery	32 Phrenic nerve	52 Common interosseous artery
12 Descending scapular artery	33 Right lung (divided) and pulmonary pleura	53 **Ulnar artery**
13 Brachial plexus (middle trunk)	34 Thoracodorsal artery	54 **Superficial palmar arch**
14 Transverse cervical artery	35 Subscapular artery	55 Median nerve and brachial artery
15 Scalenus anterior muscle and phrenic nerve	36 Lateral mammary branches (variant)	56 Biceps brachii muscle
16 Right internal carotid artery	37 Lateral thoracic artery	57 Ulnar nerve
17 Right external carotid artery	38 **Thyrocervical trunk**	58 Flexor pollicis longus muscle
18 Carotid sinus	39 Superior thoracic artery	59 Palmar digital arteries
19 Superior thyroid artery	40 Superior ulnar collateral artery	60 Anterior interosseous artery
20 Right common carotid artery	41 Inferior ulnar collateral artery	61 Flexor carpi ulnaris muscle
21 Ascending cervical artery	42 Middle collateral artery	62 Superficial palmar branch of radial artery

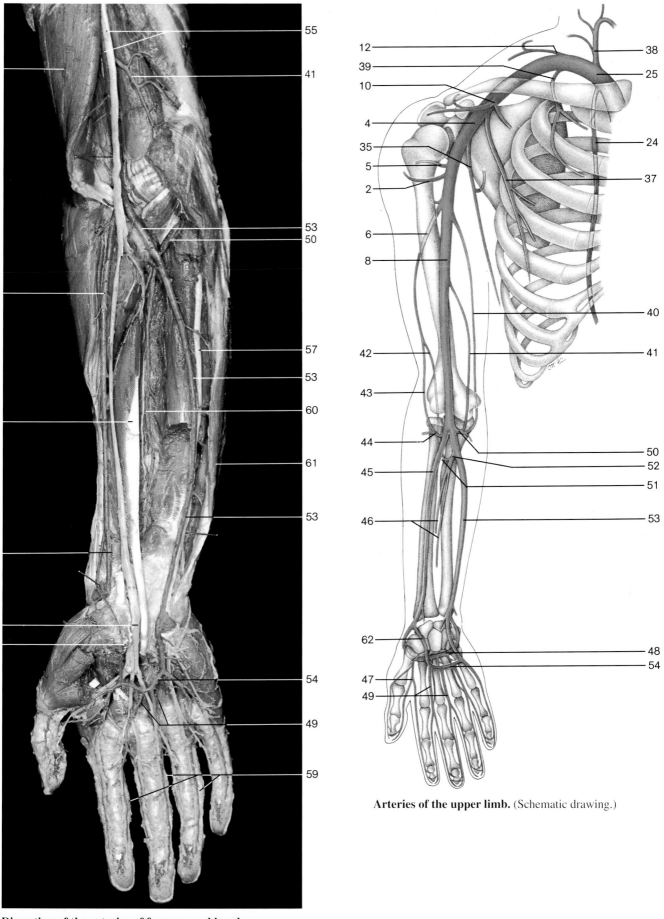

55
41
53
50
57
53
60
61
53
54
49
59

12
39
10
4
35
5
2
6
8
42
43
44
45
46
62
47
49

38
25
24
37
40
41
50
52
51
53
48
54

Arteries of the upper limb. (Schematic drawing.)

Dissection of the arteries of forearm and hand.
The superficial flexor muscles have been removed,
the carpal tunnel opened and the flexor retinaculum cut.
The arteries have been filled with colored resin.

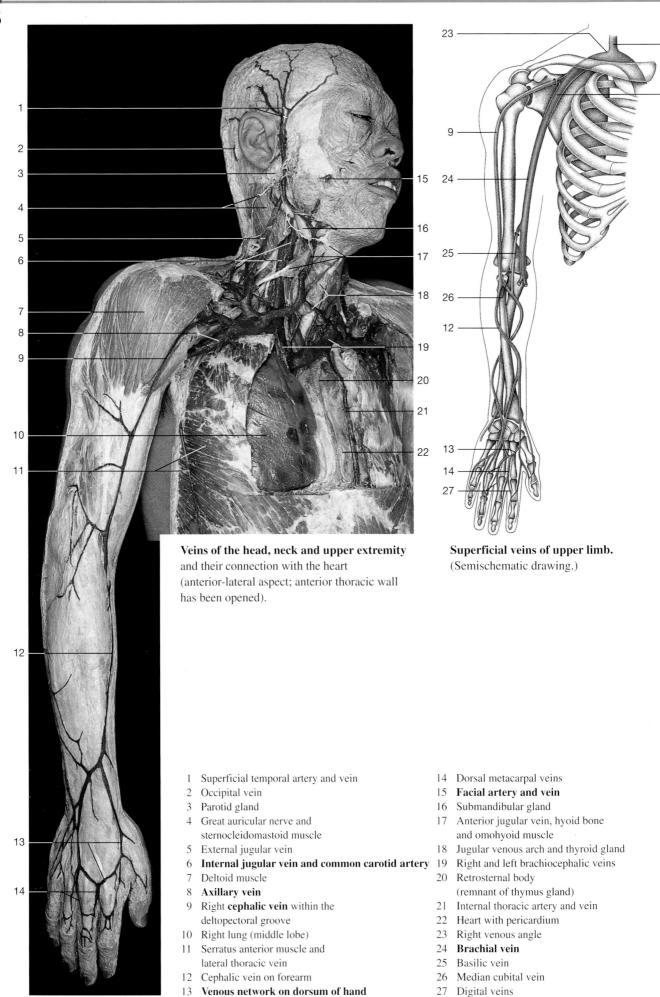

Veins of the head, neck and upper extremity and their connection with the heart (anterior-lateral aspect; anterior thoracic wall has been opened).

Superficial veins of upper limb. (Semischematic drawing.)

1 Superficial temporal artery and vein
2 Occipital vein
3 Parotid gland
4 Great auricular nerve and sternocleidomastoid muscle
5 External jugular vein
6 **Internal jugular vein and common carotid artery**
7 Deltoid muscle
8 **Axillary vein**
9 Right **cephalic vein** within the deltopectoral groove
10 Right lung (middle lobe)
11 Serratus anterior muscle and lateral thoracic vein
12 Cephalic vein on forearm
13 **Venous network on dorsum of hand**

14 Dorsal metacarpal veins
15 **Facial artery and vein**
16 Submandibular gland
17 Anterior jugular vein, hyoid bone and omohyoid muscle
18 Jugular venous arch and thyroid gland
19 Right and left brachiocephalic veins
20 Retrosternal body (remnant of thymus gland)
21 Internal thoracic artery and vein
22 Heart with pericardium
23 Right venous angle
24 **Brachial vein**
25 Basilic vein
26 Median cubital vein
27 Digital veins

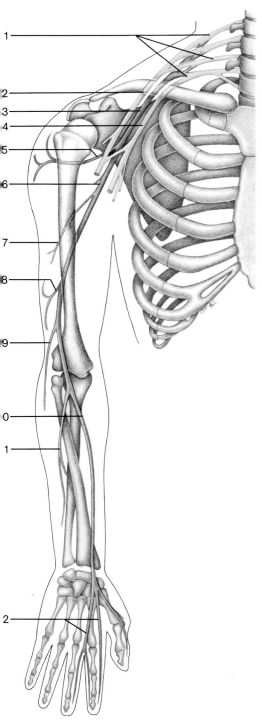

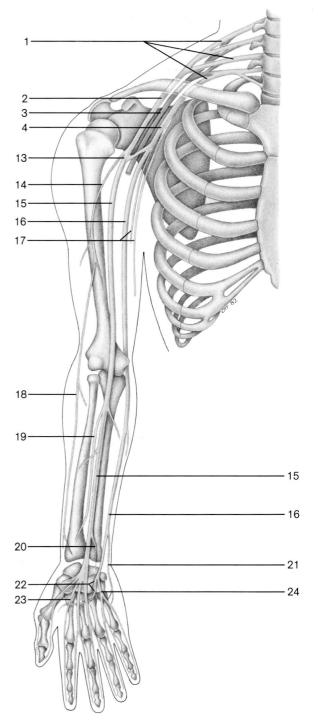

Main branches of radial nerve.
(Schematic drawing.) Posterior divisions of trunks and posterior cord and its branches are indicated in green.

Main branches of musculocutaneous, median and ulnar nerves. (Schematic drawing.)
Anterior divisions of the trunks and all the components arising from them are indicated in yellow.

1 Brachial plexus
2 Lateral cord of brachial plexus
3 Posterior cord of brachial plexus
4 Medial cord of brachial plexus
5 **Axillary nerve**
6 **Radial nerve**
7 Posterior cutaneous nerve of arm
8 Lower lateral cutaneous nerve of arm
9 Posterior cutaneous nerve of forearm
10 Superficial branch of radial nerve
11 Deep branch of radial nerve
12 Dorsal digital nerves

13 Roots of median nerve
14 Musculocutaneous nerve
15 **Median nerve**
16 **Ulnar nerve**
17 Medial cutaneous nerves of arm and forearm
18 Lateral cutaneous nerve of forearm
19 Anterior interosseous nerve
20 Palmar branch of median nerve
21 Dorsal branch of ulnar nerve
22 Deep branch of ulnar nerve
23 Common palmar digital nerves of median nerve
24 Superficial branch of ulnar nerve

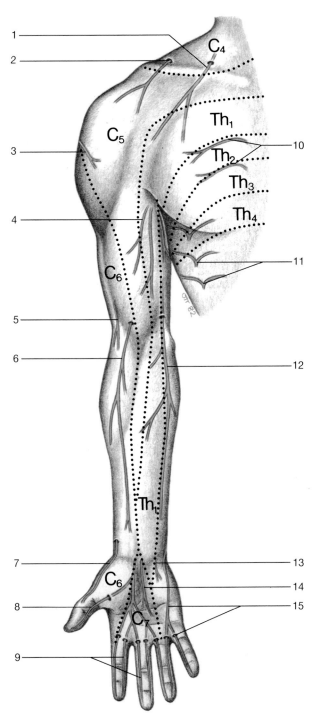

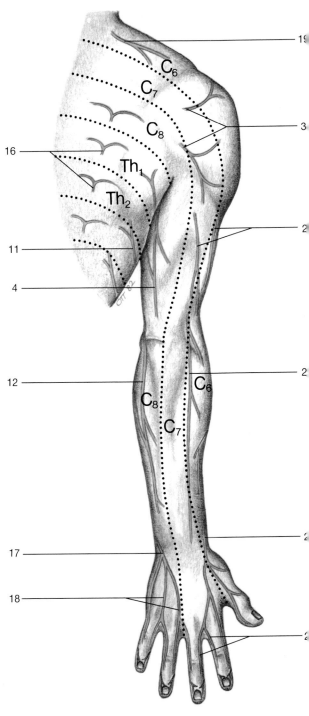

Cutaneous nerves of right upper limb (ventral aspect). (Semischematic drawing.)

Cutaneous nerves of the upper limb (dorsal aspect). (Semischematic drawing.)

1   Medial supraclavicular nerve
2   Intermediate supraclavicular nerve
3   Upper lateral cutaneous nerve of arm
4   Terminal branches of intercostobrachial nerves
5   Lower lateral cutaneous nerve of arm
6   Lateral cutaneous nerve of forearm
7   Terminal branch of superficial branch of radial nerve
8   Palmar digital nerve of thumb (branch of median nerve)
9   Palmar digital branches of median nerve
10   Anterior cutaneous branches of intercostal nerves
11   Lateral cutaneous branches of intercostal nerves
12   Medial cutaneous nerve of forearm

13   Palmar cutaneous branch of ulnar nerve
14   Palmar branch of median nerve
15   Palmar digital branches of ulnar nerve
16   Cutaneous branches of dorsal rami of spinal nerves
17   Dorsal branch of ulnar nerve
18   Dorsal digital nerves
19   Posterior supraclavicular nerve
20   Posterior cutaneous nerve of arm
21   Posterior cutaneous nerve of forearm
22   Superficial branch
23   Dorsal digital branches

} from radial nerve

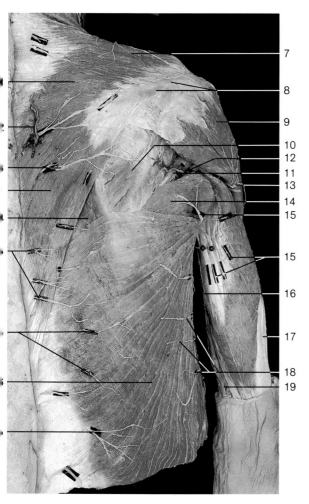

Dorsal region of shoulder, superficial layer. Note the segmental arrangement of the cutaneous nerves of the back.

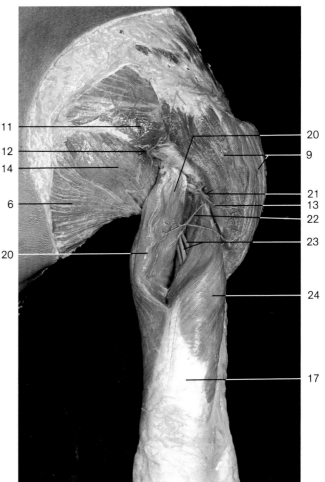

Shoulder and arm (dorsal aspect). Dissection of the quadrangular and triangular spaces of the axillary region.

1 Trapezius muscle
2 Dorsal branches of posterior intercostal artery and vein (medial cutaneous branches)
3 Medial branches of dorsal rami of spinal nerves
4 Rhomboid major muscle
5 Lateral branches of dorsal rami of spinal nerves
6 Latissimus dorsi muscle
7 Posterior supraclavicular nerves
8 Spine of scapula
9 Deltoid muscle
10 Infraspinatus muscle
11 Teres minor muscle
12 **Triangular space** with circumflex scapular artery and vein
13 Upper lateral cutaneous nerve of arm with artery
14 Teres major muscle
15 Terminal branches of intercostobrachial nerve
16 Medial cutaneous nerve of arm
17 Tendon of triceps brachii muscle
18 Lateral cutaneous branches of intercostal nerves
19 Medial cutaneous nerve of forearm
20 Long head of triceps brachii muscle
21 **Quadrangular space** with axillary nerve and posterior humeral circumflex artery
22 Anastomosis between profunda brachii artery and posterior humeral circumflex artery
23 Course of radial nerve and profunda brachii artery
24 Lateral head of triceps brachii muscle
25 Course of descending scapular artery and dorsal scapular nerve
26 Course of suprascapular nerve, artery and vein

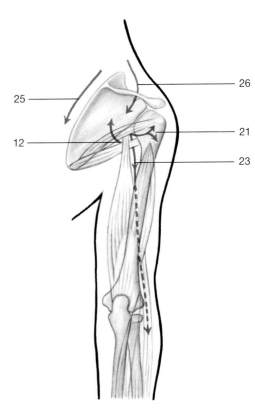

Course of vessels and nerves to shoulder and upper limb. (Schematic drawing.)

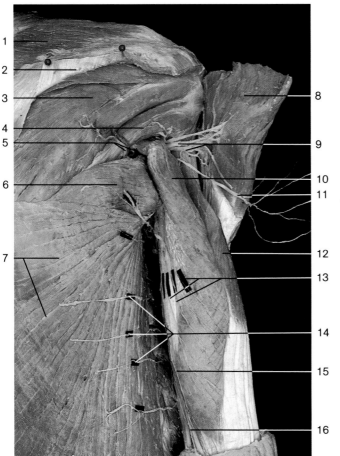

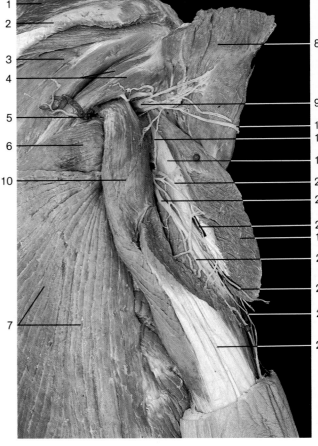

Scapular region, arm and shoulder, deep layer (dorsal aspect). Part of deltoid muscle has been cut and reflected to display the quadrangular and triangular spaces of the axillary region.

Scapular region and posterior brachial region, arm and shoulder, deep layer (dorsal aspect). The lateral head of the triceps brachii muscle has been cut to display the radial nerve and accompanying vessels.

1 Trapezius muscle
2 Spine of scapula
3 Infraspinatus muscle
4 Teres minor muscle
5 **Triangular space** containing circumflex scapular artery and vein
6 Teres major muscle
7 Latissimus dorsi muscle
8 Deltoid muscle (cut and reflected)
9 **Quadrangular space** containing axillary nerve and posterior circumflex humeral artery and vein
10 Long head of triceps brachii muscle
11 Cutaneous branch of axillary nerve
12 Lateral head of triceps brachii muscle
13 Terminal branches of intercostobrachial nerve
14 Lateral cutaneous branches of intercostal nerves
15 Medial cutaneous nerve of arm
16 Medial cutaneous nerve of forearm
17 Upper lateral cutaneous nerve of arm
18 Anastomosis between profunda brachii artery and posterior humeral circumflex artery
19 Humerus
20 **Profunda brachii artery**
21 **Radial nerve**
22 Radial collateral artery
23 Middle collateral artery
24 Lower lateral cutaneous nerve of arm
25 Posterior cutaneous nerve of forearm
26 Tendon of triceps brachii muscle

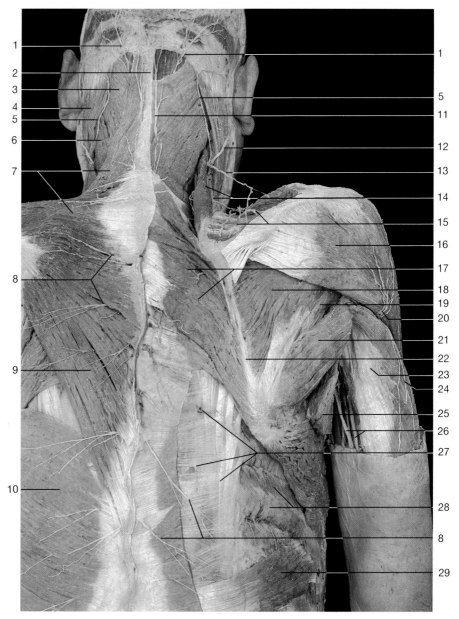

Dorsal regions of neck and shoulder (dorsal aspect). Left side: superficial layer.
Right side: trapezius and latissimus dorsi muscles have been removed. Dissection of
dorsal branches of spinal nerves.

1 **Greater occipital nerve**
2 Ligamentum nuchae
3 Splenius capitis muscle
4 Sternocleidomastoid muscle
5 Lesser occipital nerve
6 Splenius cervicis muscle
7 Descending and transverse fibers of trapezius muscle
8 **Medial cutaneous branches of dorsal rami of spinal nerves**
9 Ascending fibers of trapezius muscle
10 Latissimus dorsi muscle
11 Cutaneous branch of third occipital nerve
12 Great auricular nerve
13 Accessory nerve (n. XI)
14 Posterior supraclavicular nerve and levator scapulae muscle
15 Branches of suprascapular artery

16 Deltoid muscle
17 Rhomboid major muscle
18 Infraspinatus muscle
19 Teres minor muscle
20 Upper lateral cutaneous nerve of arm (branch of axillary nerve)
21 Teres major muscle
22 Medial margin of scapula
23 Long head of triceps muscle
24 Posterior cutaneous nerve of arm (branch of radial nerve)
25 Latissimus dorsi muscle (divided)
26 Ulnar nerve and brachial artery
27 **Lateral cutaneous branches of dorsal rami of spinal nerves** and iliocostalis thoracis muscle
28 External intercostal muscle and seventh rib
29 Serratus posterior inferior muscle

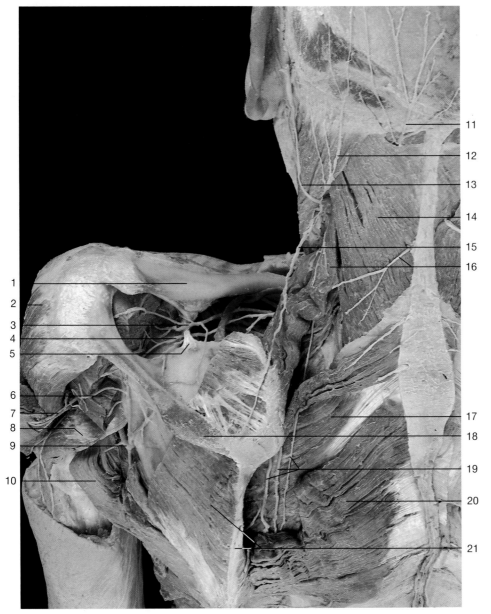

1 Clavicle
2 Deltoid muscle
3 **Suprascapular artery**
4 Suprascapular nerve
5 Superior transverse scapular ligament
6 Teres minor muscle
7 Axillary nerve and posterior circumflex humeral artery
8 Long head of triceps muscle
9 **Circumflex scapular artery**
10 Teres major muscle
11 Greater occipital nerve
12 Lesser occipital nerve
13 Great auricular nerve
14 Splenius capitis muscle
15 Accessory nerve (n. XI)
16 Third occipital nerve and levator scapulae muscle
17 Serratus posterior superior muscle
18 Spine of scapula
19 Descending scapular artery and dorsal scapular nerve
20 Rhomboid major muscle
21 Infraspinatus muscle and medial margin of scapula
22 Radial nerve and profunda brachii artery
23 Thoracodorsal artery
24 Thyrocervical trunk
25 Roots of brachial plexus

Dorsal region of shoulder; deepest layer. Rhomboid and scapular muscles fenestrated; posterior part of deltoid muscle reflected.

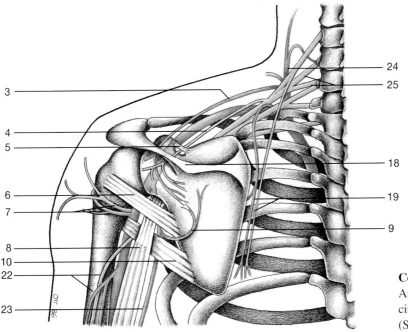

Collateral circulation of shoulder.
Anastomosis of suprascapular and circumflex scapular arteries.
(Semischematic drawing.)

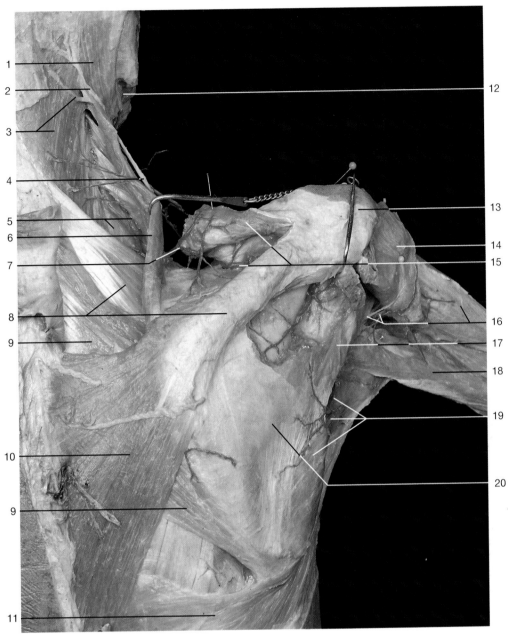

Scapular region, arm and shoulder (dorsal aspect). Arteries of scapular region are injected. Trapezius, deltoid and infraspinatus muscles are partially removed or reflected.

1 Sternocleidomastoid muscle
2 Lesser occipital nerve
3 Splenius capitis muscle and third occipital nerve
4 **Accessory nerve** (n. XI)
5 Splenius cervicis muscle and transverse cervical artery (deep branch)
6 Levator of scapula muscle
7 **Transverse cervical artery** (superficial branch)
8 Spine of scapula and serratus posterior superior muscle
9 Rhomboid major muscle
10 Trapezius muscle
11 Latissimus dorsi muscle
12 Facial artery
13 Acromion
14 Deltoid muscle
15 **Suprascapular artery** and supraspinatus muscle (reflected)
16 **Axillary nerve,** posterior circumflex humeral artery and lateral head of triceps brachii muscle
17 Teres minor muscle
18 Long head of triceps brachii muscle
19 **Circumflex scapular artery** and teres major
20 Infraspinatus muscle

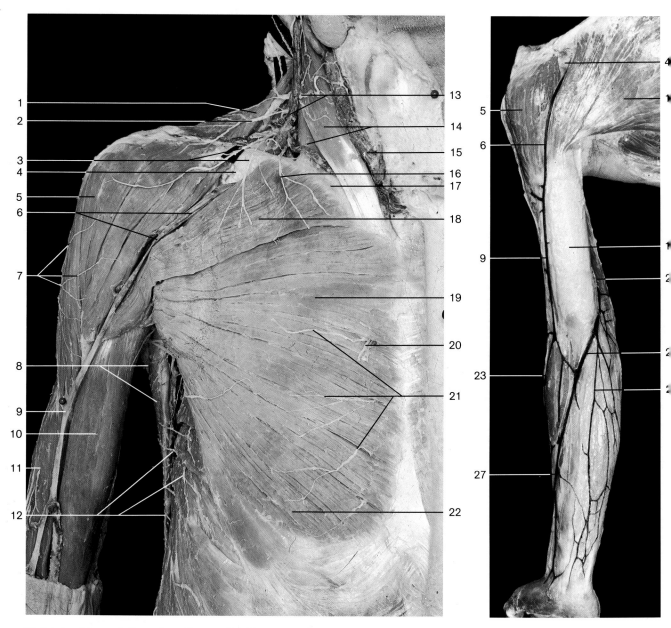

Right shoulder and thoracic wall, superficial layer (anterior aspect). Dissection of the cutaneous nerves and veins.

Superficial veins of right arm have been injected with blue gelatin.

1 Trapezius muscle	14 Sternocleidomastoid muscle
2 Posterior supraclavicular nerve	15 **Anterior jugular vein**
3 Middle supraclavicular nerve	16 Anterior supraclavicular nerve
4 Deltopectoral triangle	17 Clavicle
5 Deltoid muscle	18 Clavicular part of pectoralis major muscle
6 Cephalic vein within the deltopectoral groove	19 Sternocostal part of pectoralis major muscle
7 Upper lateral cutaneous nerve of arm	20 Perforating branch of internal thoracic artery
(branch of axillary nerve)	21 **Anterior cutaneous branches of intercostal nerves**
8 Latissimus dorsi muscle	22 Abdominal part of pectoralis major muscle
9 **Cephalic vein**	23 Accessory cephalic vein
10 Biceps brachii muscle	24 **Basilic vein**
11 Triceps brachii muscle	25 **Median cubital vein**
12 Lateral cutaneous branches of intercostal nerves	26 Median vein of forearm
13 Transverse cervical nerve and external jugular vein	27 Cephalic vein in the forearm

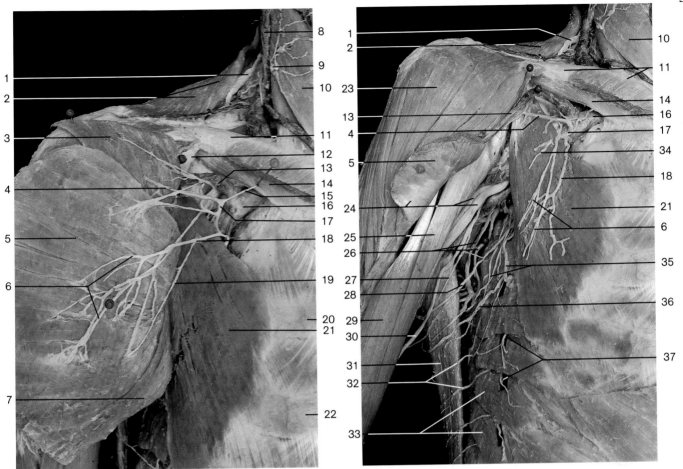

Right deltopectoral triangle, infraclavicular region (anterior aspect). The pectoralis major muscle has been cut and reflected.

Thoracic wall and shoulder, deep layer. **Right axillary region** (anterior aspect). The pectoralis major muscle has been cut and partly removed.

1	Accessory nerve	21	Pectoralis minor muscle
2	Trapezius muscle	22	Third rib
3	Pectoralis major muscle (clavicular part)	23	Deltoid muscle
4	Acromial branch of thoracoacromial artery	24	Pectoralis major muscle (reflected), **brachial artery** and **median nerve**
5	Pectoralis major muscle	25	Short head of biceps brachii muscle
6	**Lateral pectoral nerves**	26	Thoracodorsal artery and nerve
7	Abdominal part of pectoralis major muscle	27	Medial cutaneous nerve of arm
8	External jugular vein	28	Intercostobrachial nerve (T_2)
9	Cutaneous branches of cervical plexus	29	Long head of biceps brachii muscle
10	Sternocleidomastoid muscle	30	Medial cutaneous nerve of forearm
11	Clavicle	31	Latissimus dorsi muscle
12	Clavipectoral fascia	32	Lateral cutaneous branches of intercostal nerves (posterior branches)
13	**Cephalic vein**	33	Serratus anterior muscle
14	Subclavius muscle	34	Medial pectoral nerve
15	Clavicular branch of thoracoacromial artery	35	**Long thoracic nerve and lateral thoracic artery**
16	**Subclavian vein**	36	Intercostobrachial nerve (T_3)
17	**Thoracoacromial artery**	37	**Lateral cutaneous branches of intercostal nerves** (anterior branches)
18	Pectoral branch of thoracoacromial artery		
19	Medial pectoral nerve		
20	Second rib		

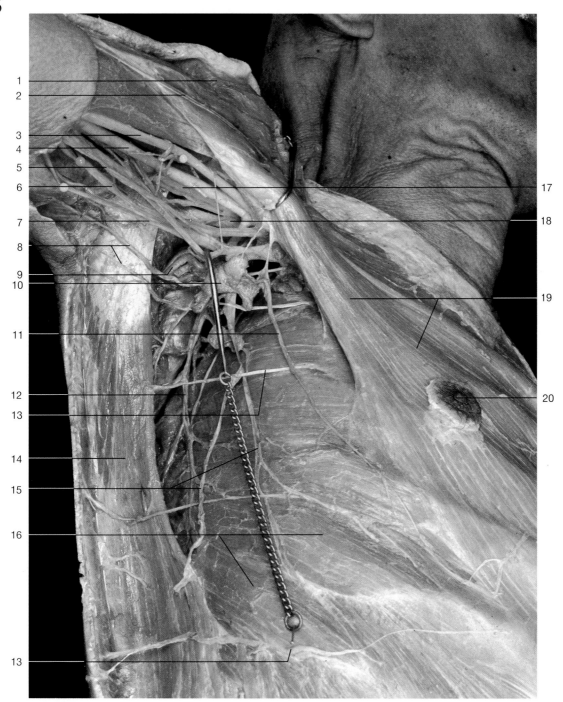

Right axillary region (inferior aspect). **Dissection of superficial axillary nodes and lymphatic vessels.**
The pectoralis major muscle has been slightly elevated.

1 Deltoid muscle	12 Thoracodorsal artery
2 Cephalic vein	13 Lateral cutaneous branch of intercostal nerve
3 Median nerve	14 Latissimus dorsi muscle
4 Brachial artery	15 Thoracoepigastric vein
5 Medial cutaneous nerves of arm and forearm	16 Serratus anterior muscle
6 Ulnar nerve	17 Musculocutaneous nerve
7 Basilic vein	18 Radial nerve
8 Intercostobrachial nerves	19 Pectoralis major muscle
9 Circumflex scapular artery	20 Nipple
10 **Superficial axillary nodes**	
11 Lateral thoracic artery	

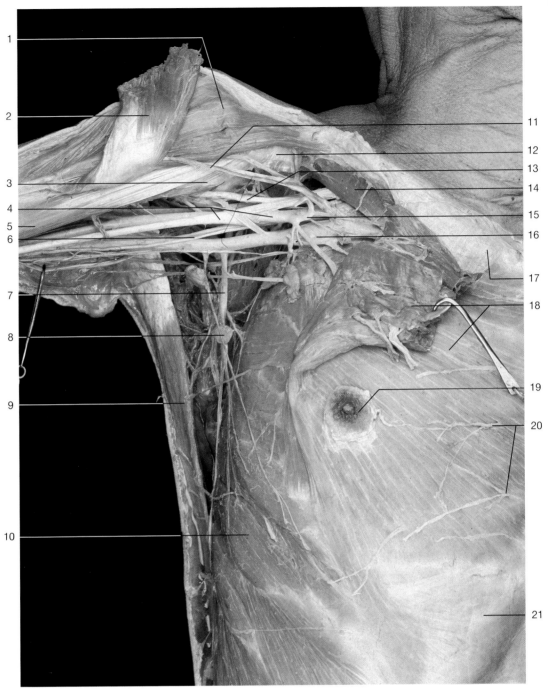

Axillary region (anterior aspect). Dissection of deep axillary nodes. Pectoralis major and minor divided and reflected. Shoulder girdle and arm elevated and reflected.

1 Deltoid muscle
2 Insertion of pectoralis major muscle
3 Coracobrachialis muscle
4 Roots of **median nerve, axillary artery**
5 Short head of biceps brachii muscle
6 **Ulnar nerve** and medial cutaneous nerve of forearm
7 Thoracoepigastric vein
8 Deep axillary node
9 Latissimus dorsi muscle
10 Serratus anterior muscle

11 Cephalic vein
12 Insertion of pectoralis minor muscle (coracoid process)
13 **Musculocutaneous nerve**
14 Subclavius muscle
15 Thoracoacromial artery
16 **Axillary vein**
17 Clavicle
18 Pectoralis major and minor muscles (reflected)
19 Nipple
20 Anterior cutaneous branches of intercostal nerves
21 Anterior layer of rectus sheath

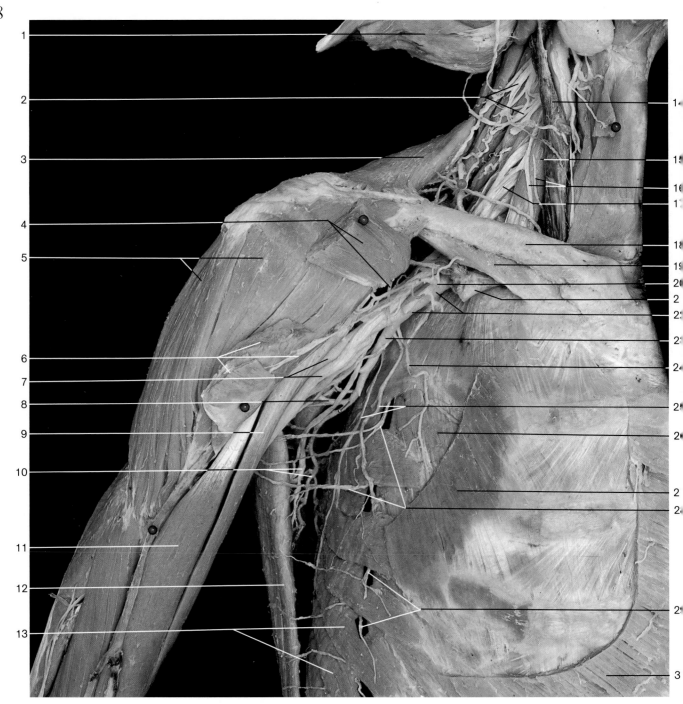

Right axillary region (anterior aspect). The pectoralis major and minor muscles have been cut and reflected to display the vessels and nerves of the axilla.

1 Sternocleidomastoid muscle (cut and reflected)
2 Cervical plexus
3 Trapezius muscle
4 Pectoralis minor muscle and medial pectoral nerve
5 Deltoid muscle
6 Pectoralis major muscle and lateral pectoral nerve
7 **Median nerve and brachial artery**
8 Circumflex scapular artery
9 Short head of biceps brachii muscle
10 **Thoracodorsal artery and nerve**
11 Long head of biceps brachii muscle
12 Latissimus dorsi muscle
13 Serratus anterior muscle
14 Internal jugular vein
15 **Scalenus anterior muscle**

16 Phrenic nerve and ascending cervical artery
17 Brachial plexus (at the levels of the trunks)
18 Clavicle
19 Subclavius muscle
20 **Thoracoacromial artery**
21 Subclavian vein (cut)
22 **Axillary artery**
23 Subscapular artery
24 Superior thoracic artery
25 **Lateral thoracic artery and long thoracic nerve**
26 External intercostal muscle
27 Insertion of pectoralis minor muscle
28 Intercostobrachial nerves
29 Lateral cutaneous branches of intercostal nerves
30 Insertion of pectoralis major muscle

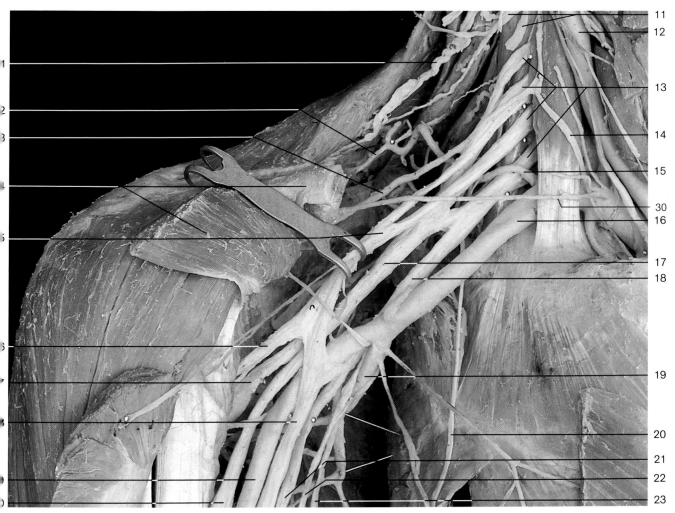

Brachial plexus (anterior aspect). Clavicle and the two pectoralis muscles have been partly removed.

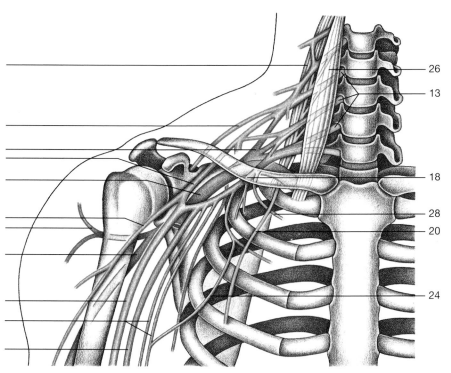

Main branches of brachial plexus. Posterior cord in purple, lateral cord in orange and medial cord in green. (Schematic drawing.)

1   Accessory nerve
2   Dorsal scapular artery
3   Suprascapular nerve
4   Clavicle and pectoralis minor muscle
5   **Lateral cord** of brachial plexus
6   Musculocutaneous nerve
7   Axillary nerve
8   Median nerve
9   Brachial artery
10 Radial nerve
11 Cervical plexus
12 Common carotid artery
13 Roots of brachial plexus (C_5–T_1)
14 Phrenic nerve
15 Transverse cervical artery
16 Subclavian artery
17 **Posterior cord** of brachial plexus
18 **Medial cord** of brachial plexus
19 Subscapular artery
20 Long thoracic nerve
21 Ulnar nerve
22 Medial cutaneous nerve of forearm
23 Thoracodorsal nerve
24 Intercostobrachial nerve
25 Medial cutaneous nerves of arm and forearm
26 Scalenus anterior muscle
27 Scalenus medius muscle
28 Intercostal nerve (T_1)
29 Axillary artery
30 Suprascapular artery

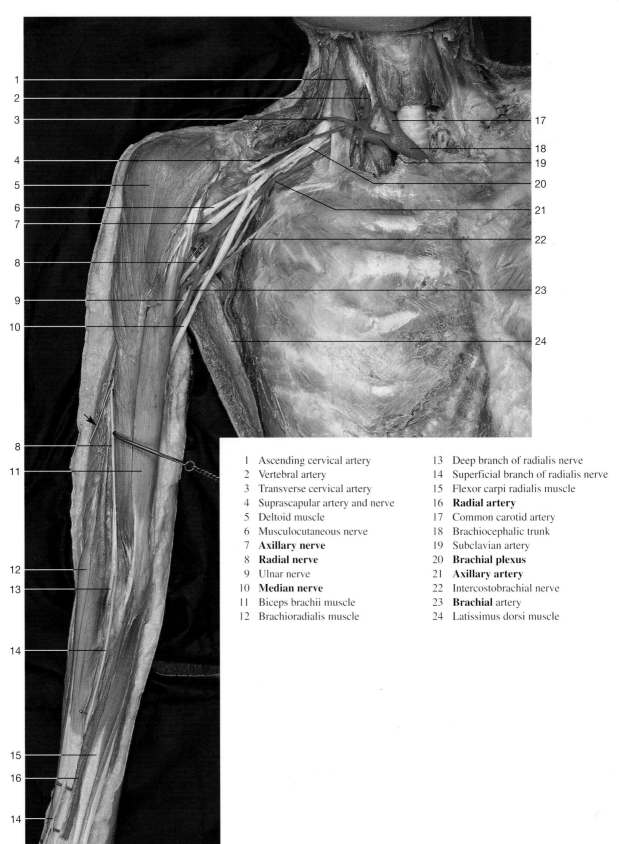

1	Ascending cervical artery	13	Deep branch of radialis nerve
2	Vertebral artery	14	Superficial branch of radialis nerve
3	Transverse cervical artery	15	Flexor carpi radialis muscle
4	Suprascapular artery and nerve	16	**Radial artery**
5	Deltoid muscle	17	Common carotid artery
6	Musculocutaneous nerve	18	Brachiocephalic trunk
7	**Axillary nerve**	19	Subclavian artery
8	**Radial nerve**	20	**Brachial plexus**
9	Ulnar nerve	21	**Axillary artery**
10	**Median nerve**	22	Intercostobrachial nerve
11	Biceps brachii muscle	23	**Brachial** artery
12	Brachioradialis muscle	24	Latissimus dorsi muscle

Nerves and arteries of neck and upper limb
(anterior aspect). Arteries are colored in red. The course of
the radial nerve is indicated by a wire probe (arrow).

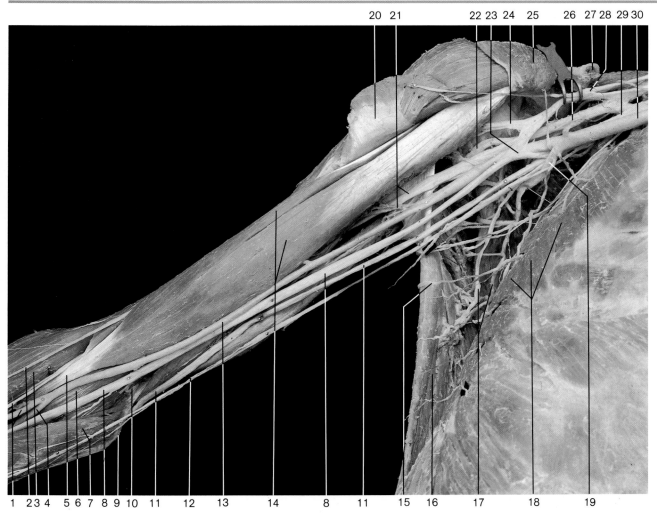

20 21   22 23 24   25   26 27 28 29 30

1 2 3 4   5 6 7 8 9 10   11   12   13   14   8   11   15   16   17   18   19

Right arm. Dissection of vessels and nerves (medial aspect). Shoulder girdle has been reflected slightly.

1 Radial artery and superficial branch
   of radial nerve
2 Lateral cutaneous nerve of forearm
3 Brachioradialis muscle
4 Ulnar artery
5 Tendon of biceps brachii muscle
6 Brachialis muscle
7 Pronator teres muscle
8 **Median nerve**
9 Medial epicondyle of humerus
10 Inferior ulnar collateral artery
11 **Ulnar nerve**
12 Medial cutaneous nerve of forearm
13 **Brachial artery**
14 Biceps brachii muscle
15 Intercostobrachial nerve (T_3)
16 Latissimus dorsi muscle
17 Thoracodorsal nerve and artery
18 Serratus anterior muscle
19 Subscapular artery
20 Pectoralis major muscle (reflected) and lateral pectoral nerve
21 Radial nerve and profunda brachii artery
22 Axillary nerve
23 Roots of the median nerve with axillary artery
24 **Musculocutaneous nerve**
25 Pectoralis minor muscle (reflected) and medial pectoral nerve
26 Posterior cord of brachial plexus
27 Clavicle (cut)
28 Lateral cord of brachial plexus
29 Medial cord of brachial plexus
30 Subclavian artery
31 Brachial vein

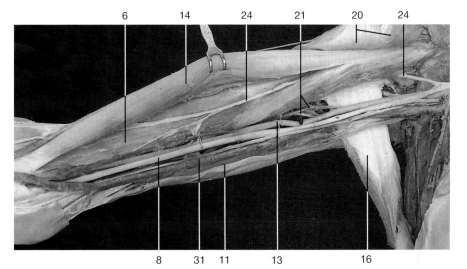

6   14   24   21   20   24

8   31   11   13   16

Right arm. Dissection of vessels and nerves, deeper layer.
Biceps muscle has been reflected.

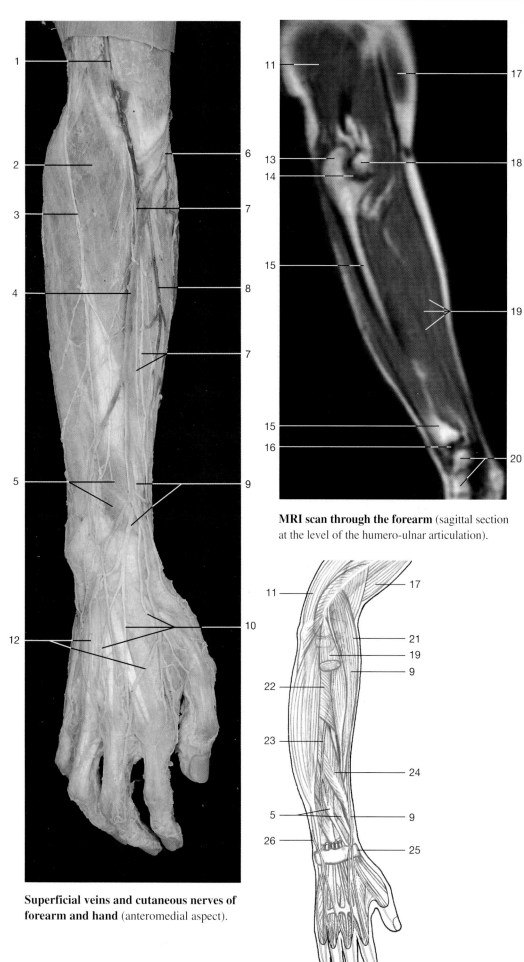

1 **Cephalic vein**
2 Brachioradialis muscle
   covered by its fascia
3 **Posterior cutaneous nerve
   of forearm**
   (branch of radialis nerve)
4 Cephalic vein of forearm
5 Extensor pollicis longus and
   brevis muscles covered by
   their fascia
6 **Median cubital vein**
7 Lateral cutaneous nerves of
   forearm (branch of
   musculocutaneous nerve)
8 Intermedian vein of forearm
9 Superficial branch of radial
   nerve
10 **Dorsal digital branches of
   radial nerve**
11 Triceps brachii muscle
12 Venous network on the
   dorsum of the hand
13 Olecranon
14 **Humeroulnar articulation**
15 Ulna
16 Radiocarpal articulation
17 Biceps brachii muscle
18 Trochlea of humerus
19 Flexor muscles of forearm
20 Carpal bones
21 Brachioradialis muscle
22 Supinator muscle
23 **Deep branch of
   radial nerve**
   (ramus profundus of
   radial nerve)
24 Abductor pollicis
   longus muscle
25 Extensor retinaculum
26 Ulnar nerve

MRI scan through the forearm (sagittal section
at the level of the humero-ulnar articulation).

**Superficial veins and cutaneous nerves of
forearm and hand** (anteromedial aspect).

Course of the nerves to forearm and hand
(dorsal aspect).

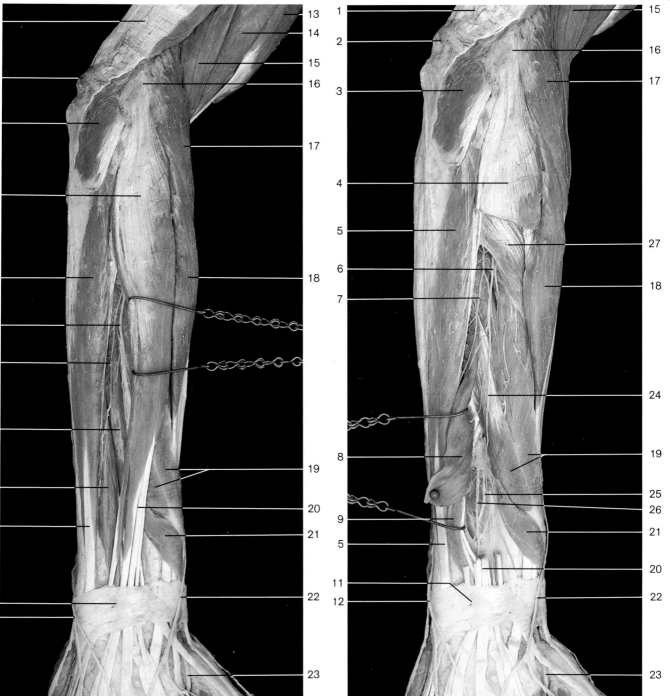

Vessels and nerves of right forearm, superficial layer
(dorsal aspect).

Vessels and nerves of right forearm, deep layer
(dorsal aspect).

1	Tendon of triceps brachii muscle	11	Extensor retinaculum
2	Olecranon	12	Dorsal branch of ulnar nerve
3	Anconeus muscle	13	Biceps brachii muscle
4	Extensor digitorum muscle	14	Brachialis muscle
5	Extensor carpi ulnaris muscle	15	Brachioradialis muscle
6	Deep branch of radial nerve	16	Lateral epicondyle of humerus
7	Posterior interosseous artery	17	Extensor carpi radialis longus muscle
8	Extensor pollicis longus muscle	18	Extensor carpi radialis brevis muscle
9	Extensor indicis muscle	19	Abductor pollicis longus muscle
10	Tendon of extensor carpi ulnaris muscle	20	Tendons of extensor digitorum muscle

21	Extensor pollicis brevis muscle
22	Superficial branch of radial nerve
23	Radial artery
24	Posterior interosseous nerve
25	Posterior interosseous branch of radial nerve
26	Posterior branch of anterior interosseous artery
27	Supinator muscle

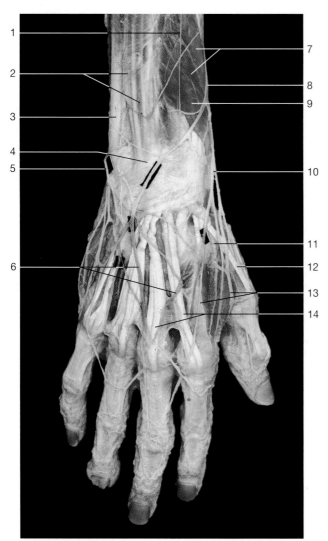

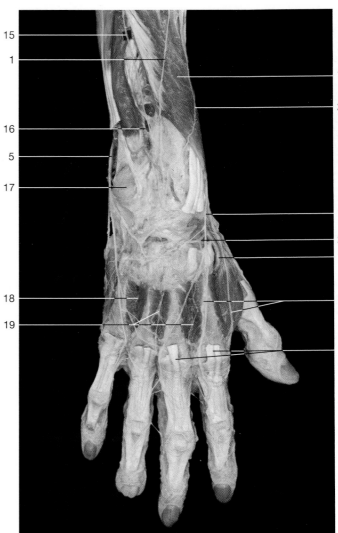

Cutaneous nerves and veins of forearm and hand
(superficial layer, dorsal aspect).

Dorsal region of forearm and hand (deeper layer).
Extensor digitorum muscle has been partly removed.

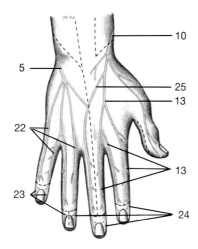

Innervation pattern of dorsal surfaces of hand
2½ digits by radial nerve, 2½ digits by ulnar nerve. Note
that the terminal branches to the dorsal surfaces of the
distal phalanges are derived from the palmar digital
nerves. The cutaneous distribution varies; often 3½ digits
are innervated by the radial and 1½ digits by the ulnar
nerve.

1 **Posterior cutaneous nerve of forearm** (branch of radial nerve)
2 Extensor digitorum muscle
3 Tendon of extensor carpi ulnaris muscle
4 Extensor retinaculum
5 **Ulnar nerve**
6 **Venous network of dorsum of hand**
7 Abductor pollicis longus muscle
8 Cephalic vein
9 Extensor pollicis brevis muscle
10 **Radial nerve,** superficial branch
11 **Radial artery**
12 Tendon of extensor pollicis longus muscle
13 Dorsal digital branches of radial nerve
14 Tendons of extensor digitorum muscle with intertendinous connections
15 Posterior interosseus nerve (branch of the deep radial nerve)
16 Posterior interosseous artery
17 Styloid process of ulna
18 Dorsal interosseus muscle IV
19 Dorsal carpal branch of radial artery
20 **Lateral cutaneous nerve of forearm**
   (branch of musculocutaneous nerve)
21 Dorsal metacarpal artery
22 Proper dorsal digital branches of ulnar nerve
23 Regions supplied by palmar digital nerves (ulnar nerve)
24 Regions supplied by palmar digital nerves (median nerve)
25 Communicating branch with ulnar nerve

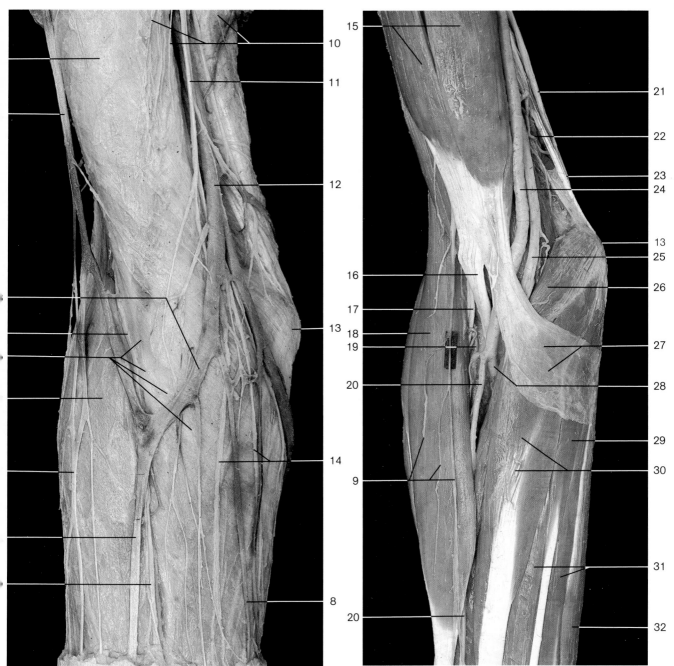

Cubital region (anterior aspect), dissection of cutaneous nerves and veins.

Cubital region, superficial layer (anterior aspect). The fasciae of the muscles have been removed.

1 Biceps brachii muscle with fascia	16 Tendon of biceps brachii muscle
2 **Cephalic vein**	17 Radial nerve
3 **Median cubital vein**	18 Brachioradialis muscle
4 Lateral cutaneous nerve of forearm	19 Radial recurrent artery
5 Tendon and aponeurosis of biceps brachii muscle	20 **Radial artery**
(covered by the antebrachial fascia)	21 **Ulnar nerve**
6 Brachioradialis muscle with fascia	22 Superior ulnar collateral artery
7 Accessory cephalic vein	23 Medial intermuscular septum
8 Median vein of forearm	24 **Brachial artery**
9 Branches of lateral cutaneous nerve of forearm	25 **Median nerve**
10 Terminal branches of medial cutaneous nerve of arm	26 Pronator teres muscle
11 **Medial cutaneous nerve of forearm**	27 Bicipital aponeurosis
12 **Basilic vein**	28 Ulnar artery
13 Medial epicondyle of humerus	29 Palmaris longus muscle
14 Terminal branches of medial cutaneous nerve	30 Flexor carpi radialis muscle
of forearm	31 Flexor digitorum superficialis muscle
15 Biceps brachii muscle	32 Flexor carpi ulnaris muscle

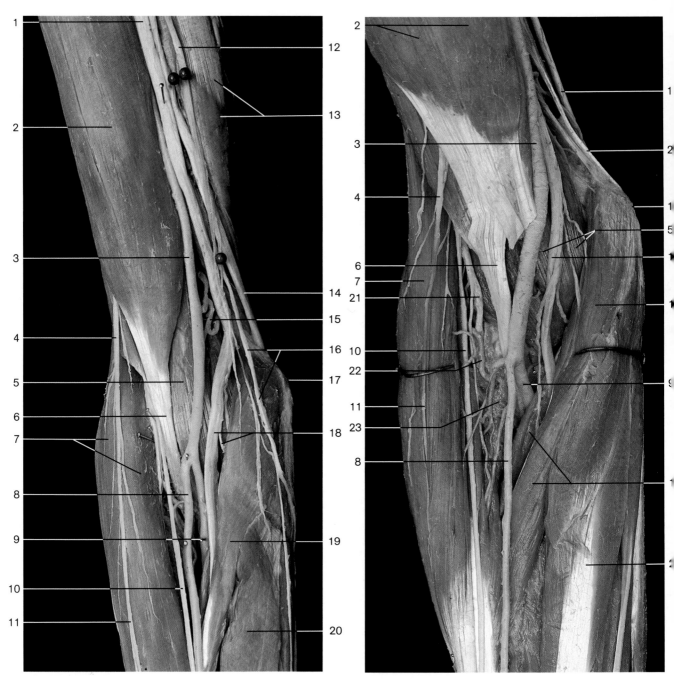

Cubital region, middle layer (anterior aspect).
The bicipital aponeurosis has been removed.

Cubital region, middle layer (anterior aspect).
The pronator teres and brachioradialis muscles
have been slightly reflected.

1 Median nerve
2 Biceps brachii muscle
3 Brachial artery
4 Lateral cutaneous nerve of forearm
   (terminal branch of **musculocutaneous nerve)**
5 Brachialis muscle
6 Tendon of biceps brachii muscle
7 Brachioradialis muscle
8 **Radial artery**
9 **Ulnar artery**
10 Superficial branch of radial nerve
11 Lateral cutaneous nerve of forearm
12 Medial cutaneous nerve of forearm

13 Triceps brachii muscle
14 **Ulnar nerve**
15 Inferior ulnar collateral artery
16 Anterior branch of medial cutaneous nerve of forearm
17 Medial epicondyle of humerus
18 **Median nerve** with branches to pronator teres muscle
19 Pronator teres muscle
20 Flexor carpi radialis muscle
21 Deep branch of radial nerve
22 Radial recurrent artery
23 Supinator muscle
24 Medial intermuscular septum of arm

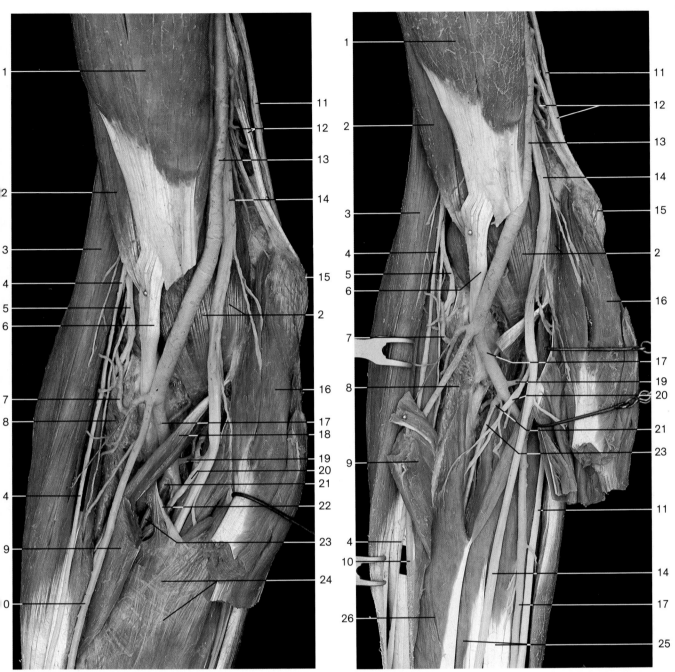

Cubital region, deep layer (anterior aspect). The pronator teres and flexor carpi ulnaris muscles have been cut and reflected.

Cubital region, deepest layer (anterior aspect). The flexor digitorum superficialis and the ulnar head of the pronator teres have been cut and reflected.

1 Biceps brachii muscle
2 Brachialis muscle
3 Brachioradialis muscle
4 Superficial branch of radial nerve
5 Deep branch of radial nerve
6 Tendon of biceps brachii muscle
7 **Radial recurrent artery**
8 Supinator muscle
9 Insertion of pronator teres muscle
10 **Radial artery**
11 **Ulnar nerve**
12 Medial intermuscular septum of arm and superior ulnar collateral artery
13 **Brachial artery**

14 **Median nerve**
15 Medial epicondyle of humerus
16 Humeral head of pronator teres muscle
17 **Ulnar artery**
18 Ulnar head of pronator teres muscle
19 **Ulnar recurrent artery**
20 Anterior interosseous nerve
21 Common interosseous artery
22 Tendinous arch of flexor digitorum superficialis muscle
23 Anterior interosseous artery
24 Flexor digitorum superficialis muscle
25 Flexor digitorum profundus muscle
26 Flexor pollicis longus muscle

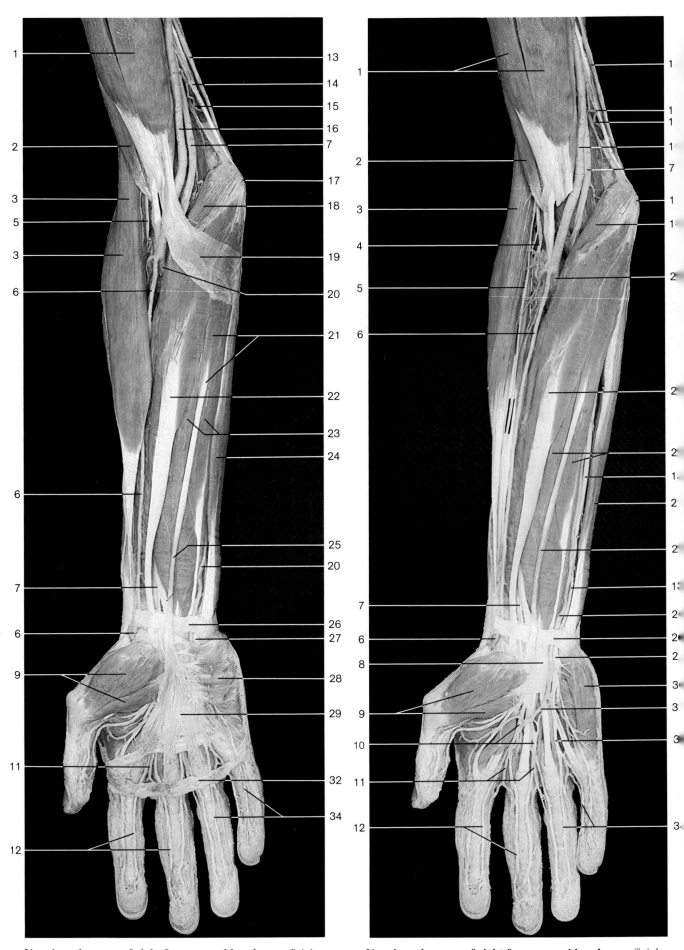

Vessels and nerves of right forearm and hand, superficial layer (palmar aspect).

Vessels and nerves of right forearm and hand, superficial layer (palmar aspect). The palmar aponeurosis of the hand and the bicipital aponeurosis have been removed.

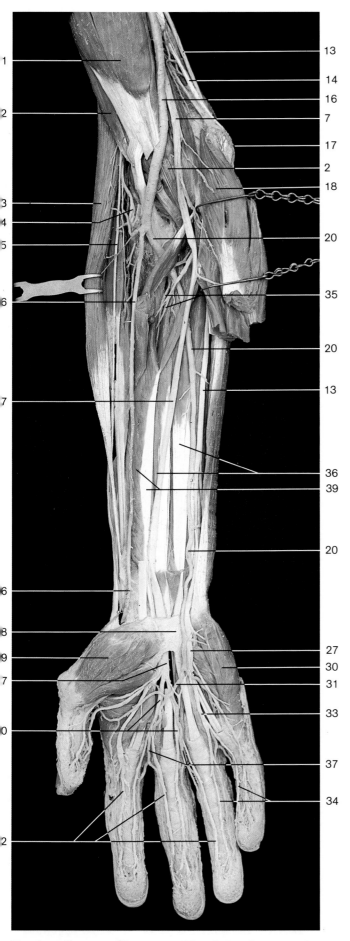

1 Biceps brachii muscle
2 Brachialis muscle
3 Brachioradialis muscle
4 **Deep branch of radial nerve**
5 **Superficial branch of radial nerve**
6 **Radial artery**
7 **Median nerve**
8 Flexor retinaculum
9 Thenar muscles
10 Common palmar digital branches of median nerve
11 Common palmar digital arteries
12 Proper palmar digital nerves (median nerve)
13 **Ulnar nerve**
14 Medial intermuscular septum of arm
15 Superior ulnar collateral artery
16 Brachial artery
17 Medial epicondyle of humerus
18 Pronator teres muscle
19 Bicipital aponeurosis
20 **Ulnar artery**
21 Palmaris longus muscle
22 Flexor carpi radialis muscle
23 Flexor digitorum superficialis muscle
24 Flexor carpi ulnaris muscle
25 Tendon of palmaris longus muscle
26 Remnant of antebrachial fascia
27 Superficial branch of ulnar nerve
28 Palmaris brevis muscle
29 Palmar aponeurosis
30 Hypothenar muscles
31 **Superficial palmar arch**
32 Superficial transverse metacarpal ligament
33 Common palmar digital branch of ulnar nerve
34 Proper palmar digital branches of ulnar nerve
35 Anterior interosseous artery and nerve
36 Flexor digitorum profundus muscle
37 Common palmar digital arteries
38 Palmar branch of median nerve
39 Flexor pollicis longus muscle
40 Palmar branch of ulnar nerve

Vessels and nerves of forearm and hand, deep layer (anterior aspect). The superficial layer of the flexor muscles has been removed.

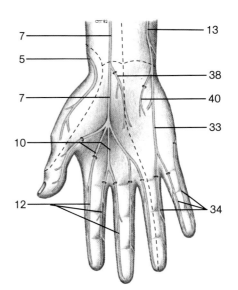

Cutaneous innervation of hand (palmar aspect). (Schematic drawing.)
Cutaneous innervation of palmar surface:
3½ digits by median nerve,
1½ digits by ulnar nerve.

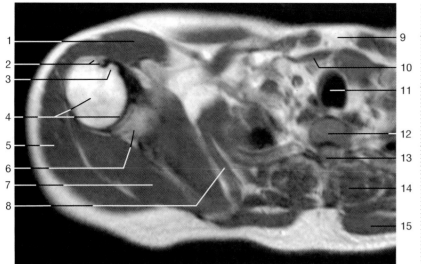

Horizontal section through shoulder joint (section 1; MRI scan; inferior aspect).

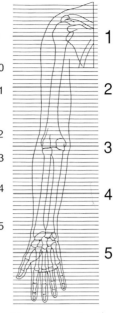

Upper extremity, location of sections 1–5 (MRI scans, courtesy of Prof. Dr. A. Heuck, Munich, Germany).

1 Pectoralis major muscle
2 Greater tubercle and tendon of biceps muscle
3 Lesser tubercle
4 Head of humerus and articular cavity of shoulder joint
5 Deltoid muscle
6 Scapula
7 Infraspinatus muscle
8 Serratus anterior muscle
9 Sternum
10 Infrahyoid muscles
11 Trachea
12 Body of thoracic vertebra
13 Vertebral canal and spinal cord
14 Deep muscles of the back
15 Trapezius muscle
16 Brachialis muscle
17 Radial nerve and profunda brachii vessels

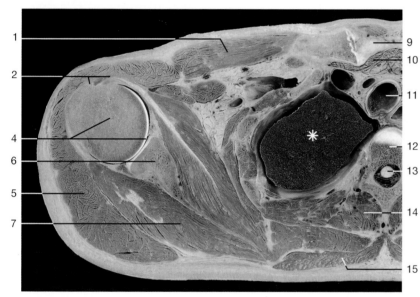

Horizontal section through the right shoulder at the level of T₁
(section 1; inferior aspect). * = Upper lobe of lung.

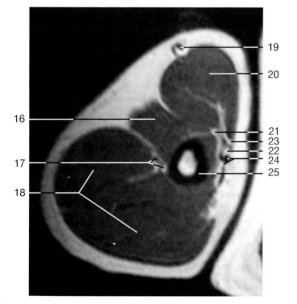

Axial section through the middle of the right arm (section 2; MRI scan, inferior aspect).

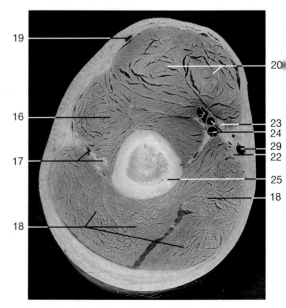

Axial section through the middle of the right arm (section 2; inferior aspect).

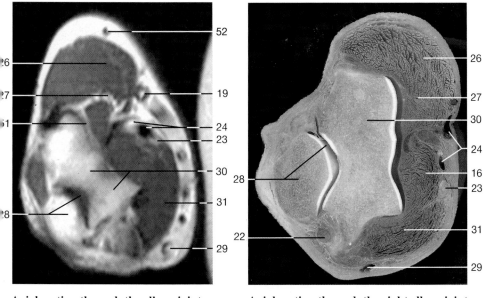

18 Triceps brachii muscle
19 Cephalic vein
20 Biceps brachii muscle
21 Musculocutaneous nerve
22 **Ulnar nerve**
23 **Medianus nerve**
24 Brachial artery and vein
25 Shaft of humerus
26 Brachioradialis muscle
27 **Radial nerve**
28 Olecranon and articular cavity of elbow joint
29 Basilic vein
30 Humerus
31 Pronator teres muscle
32 Extensor muscles of forearm
33 Ramus profundus of radialis nerve
34 Anterior interosseus vessels and nerve
35 Interosseous membrane
36 Ulna
37 Radius
38 Radial artery and superficial branch of radial nerve
39 Flexor pollicis longus muscle
40 Flexor digitorum superficialis and profundus muscles
41 Ulnar nerve, ulnar artery and vein
42 Flexor carpi ulnaris muscle
43 Radial artery
44 Metacarpal bones III and IV
45 **Carpal canal** with tendons of flexor digitorum muscles
46 Hypothenar muscle
47 Median nerve
48 Interosseous muscles
49 First metacarpal bone
50 Thenar muscles
51 Articular cavity of humeroradial joint
52 Accessory cephalic vein

Axial section through the elbow joint (section 3; MRI scan; inferior aspect).

Axial section through the right elbow joint (section 3; inferior aspect).

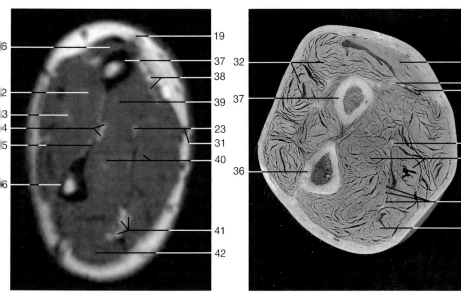

Axial section through the middle of the forearm (section 4; MRI scan; inferior aspect).

Axial section through the right forearm (section 4; inferior aspect).

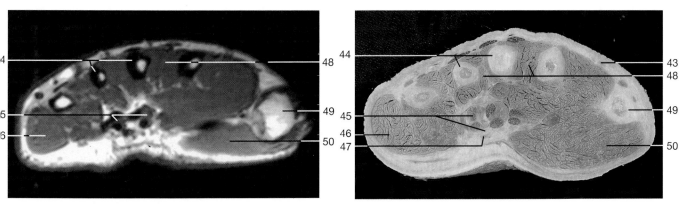

Axial section through the right hand (metacarpus; MRI scan; section 5; inferior aspect).

Axial section through the right hand at the level of the metacarpus (section 5; inferior aspect).

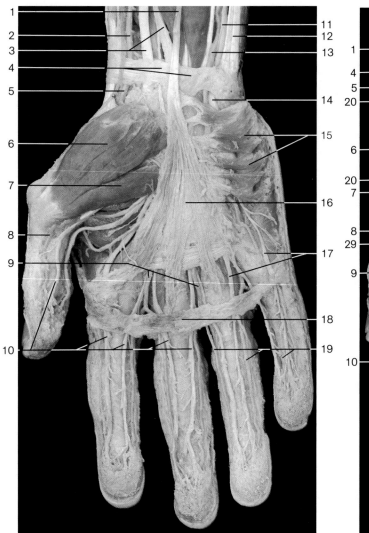

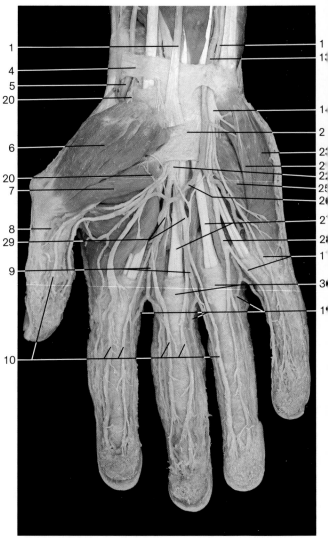

Right hand, superficial layer, dissection of vessels and nerves (palmar aspect).

Right hand, superficial layer, dissection of vessels and nerves (palmar aspect). The palmar aponeurosis has been removed to display the superficial palmar arch.

1   Tendon of palmaris longus muscle
2   **Radial artery**
3   Tendon of flexor carpi radialis muscle and median nerve
4   Distal part of antebrachial fascia
5   Radial artery passing into the anatomical snuffbox
6   Abductor pollicis brevis muscle
7   Superficial head of flexor pollicis brevis muscle
8   Palmar digital artery of thumb
9   Common palmar digital arteries
10 Proper palmar digital nerves (median nerve)
11 **Ulnar nerve**
12 Tendon of flexor carpi ulnaris muscle
13 **Ulnar artery**
14 Superficial branch of ulnar nerve
15 Palmaris brevis muscle
16 Palmar aponeurosis

17 Palmar digital nerves (ulnar nerve)
18 Superficial transverse metacarpal ligament
19 Proper palmar digital arteries
20 Superficial palmar branch of radial artery (contributing to the superficial palmar arch)
21 Flexor retinaculum
22 **Median nerve**
23 Abductor digiti minimi muscle
24 Flexor digiti minimi brevis muscle
25 Opponens digiti minimi muscle
26 **Superficial palmar arch**
27 Tendons of flexor digitorum superficialis muscle
28 Common palmar digital branch of ulnar nerve
29 Common palmar digital branch of median nerve
30 Fibrous sheath of flexor tendons

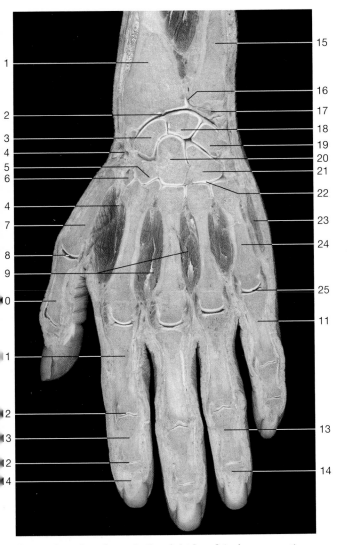

Coronal section through the right hand (palmar aspect).

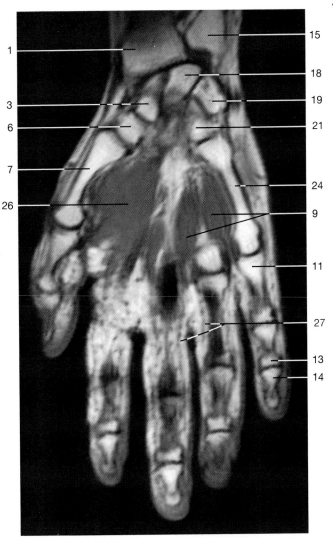

Coronal section through the right hand (palmar aspect) (MRI scan, courtesy of Prof. Dr. A. Heuck, Munich).

1 Radius	15 **Ulna**
2 **Radiocarpal articulation**	16 Distal radioulnar articulation
3 **Scaphoid** (navicular) **bone**	17 Articular disc
4 **Radial artery**	18 **Lunate bone**
5 Trapezoid bone	19 **Triangular bone**
6 **Trapezium bone**	20 **Capitate bone**
7 First metacarpal bone	21 **Hamate bone**
8 Metacarpophalangeal articulation of thumb	22 Carpometacarpal articulations
9 Interosseous muscles	23 Abductor digiti minimi muscle
10 Proximal phalanx of thumb	24 Fifth metacarpal bone
11 Proximal phalanx of fingers	25 Metacarpophalangeal articulation
12 Interphalangeal articulations	26 Adductor pollicis muscle
13 Middle phalanx	27 Proper palmar digital arteries
14 Distal phalanx	

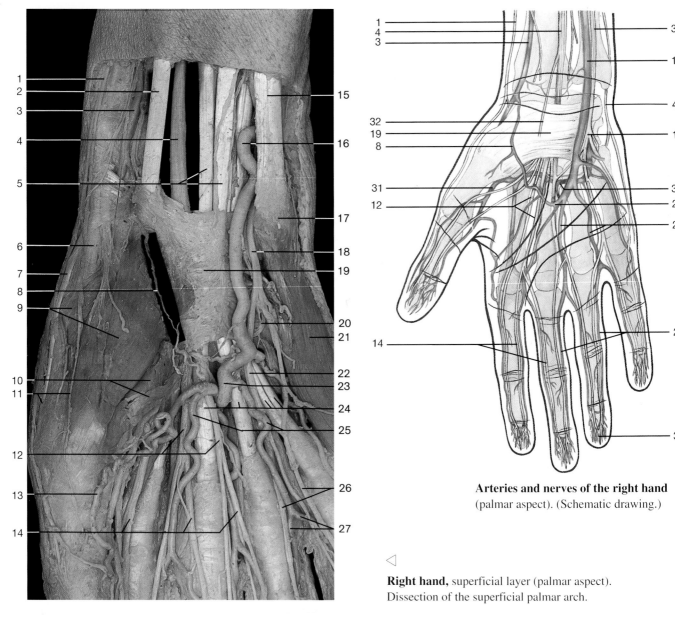

1
2
3
4
5
6
7
8
9
10
11
12
13
14

15
16
17
18
19
20
21
22
23
24
25
26
27

1
4
3

32
19
8

31
12

14

3
1
4
1

3
2
2

2

3

Arteries and nerves of the right hand
(palmar aspect). (Schematic drawing.)

◁

Right hand, superficial layer (palmar aspect).
Dissection of the superficial palmar arch.

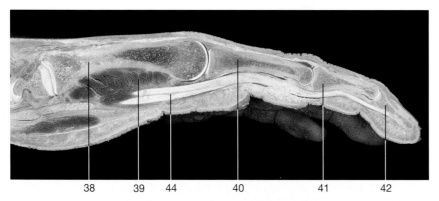

38   39   44   40   41   42

Longitudinal section through the hand
at the level of the third finger.

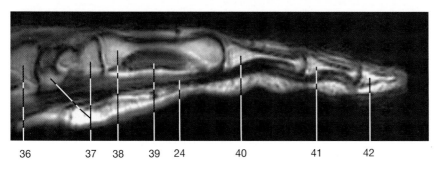

36   37   38   39   24   40   41   42

Longitudinal section through the hand
at the level of the third finger (MRI scan,
courtesy of Prof. Dr. A. Heuck, Munich).

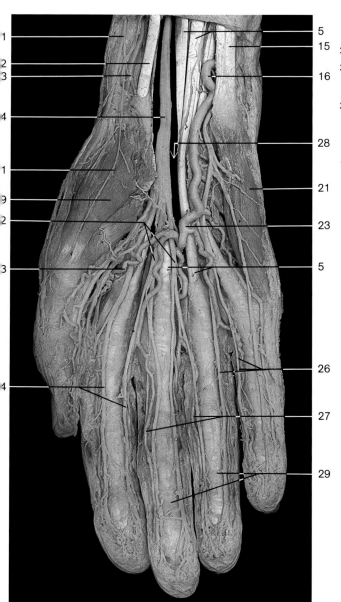

Right hand, middle layer (palmar aspect). The flexor retinaculum has been removed.

Arteriogram of the right hand (palmar aspect).

1   Superficial branch of radial nerve
2   Tendon of flexor carpi radialis muscle
3   **Radial artery**
4   **Median nerve**
5   Tendon of flexor digitorum superficialis muscle
6   Tendon of abductor pollicis longus muscle
7   Tendon of extensor pollicis brevis muscle
8   Superficial palmar branch of radial artery
9   Abductor pollicis brevis muscle
10 Superficial head of flexor pollicis brevis muscle
11 Terminal branches of superficial branch of radial nerve
12 Common palmar digital nerves (median nerve)
13 Proper palmar digital arteries of thumb
14 Proper palmar digital nerves (median nerve)
15 Tendon of flexor carpi ulnaris muscle
16 **Ulnar artery**
17 Position of pisiform bone
18 Superficial branch of ulnar nerve
19 Flexor retinaculum
20 Deep branch of ulnar nerve

21 Abductor digiti minimi muscle
22 Common palmar digital nerves (ulnar nerve)
23 **Superficial palmar arch**
24 Tendons of flexor digitorum muscles
25 Common palmar digital arteries
26 **Palmar digital nerves (ulnar nerve)**
27 **Proper palmar digital arteries**
28 **Carpal tunnel**
29 Fibrous sheaths for the tendons of flexor digitorum
    muscles
30 **Deep palmar arch**
31 Princeps pollicis artery
32 Palmar branch of median nerve
33 Common digital palmar artery
34 Ulnar nerve
35 Capillary network of finger
36 Radius
37 Carpal bones
38 Metacarpal bone
39 Interosseous muscles
40 Proximal phalanx
41 Middle phalanx
42 Distal phalanx
43 Dorsal branch of ulnar nerve
44 Tendons of flexor digitorum profundus (upper)
    and superficialis (lower) muscles

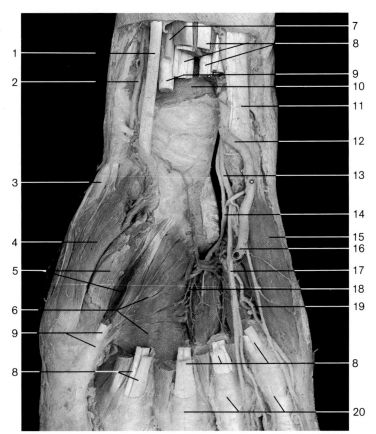

1. Tendon of flexor carpi radialis muscle
2. Radial artery
3. Tendon of abductor pollicis longus muscle
4. Abductor pollicis brevis muscle
5. Superficial and deep heads of flexor pollicis brevis muscle
6. Oblique and transverse heads of adductor pollicis muscle
7. Median nerve
8. Tendons of flexor digitorum superficialis and profundus muscles
9. Tendon of flexor pollicis longus muscle
10. Pronator quadratus muscle
11. Tendon of flexor carpi ulnaris muscle
12. Ulnar artery
13. Superficial branch of ulnar nerve
14. Deep branch of ulnar nerve
15. Abductor digiti minimi muscle
16. **Superficial palmar arch** (cut end)
17. Common palmar digital nerves (ulnar nerve)
18. Palmar metacarpal arteries of deep palmar arch
19. Palmar digital artery of the fifth finger
20. Fibrous sheaths of tendons of flexor muscles
21. Palmar interosseous muscles
22. Opponens pollicis muscle (cut)
23. **Deep palmar arch**
24. First dorsal interosseous muscle
25. First lumbrical muscle

Right hand, deep layer (palmar aspect). The carpal tunnel has been opened, the tendons of the flexor muscles have been removed and the superficial palmar arch has been cut.

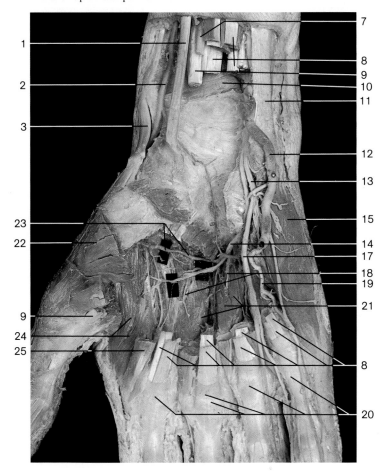

Right hand, deep layer (palmar aspect). Dissection of the deep palmar arch.

Lower Limb

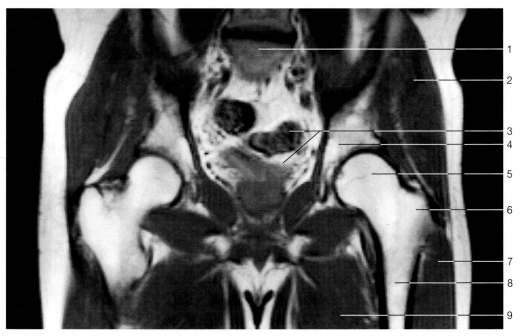

Coronal section through pelvis and thighs (MRI scan of the male after Heuck A, Luttke G, Rohen JW. MR-Atlas der Extremitäten. Stuttgart: Schattauer, 1994).

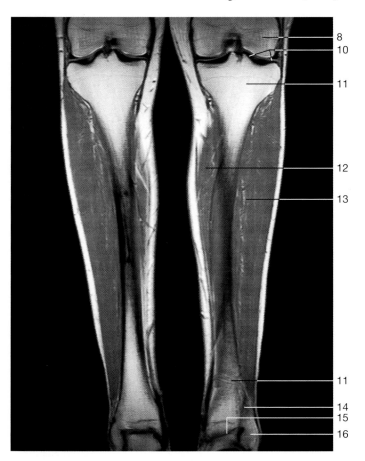

Coronal section through the legs
(MRI scan after Heuck A, Luttke G, Rohen JW, 1994).

1 Sacral promontory
2 Gluteus medius muscle
3 Small intestine and urinary bladder
4 Acetabulum
5 **Head of femur**
6 Greater trochanter of femur
7 Vastus lateralis muscle
8 **Femur**
9 Adductor muscles
10 **Knee joint** with menisci
11 **Tibia**
12 Soleus muscle
13 Tibialis anterior muscle
14 Distal tibiofibular articulation
15 **Talocrural articulation**
16 Fibula (lateral malleolus)

The lower limb (extremity) is specialized for support of the upright posture, locomotion and maintaining balance. In contrast to the upper limb, the lower limb is more restricted in its movements, and the joints are more tight and fixed by strong ligaments. The hip joint is a ball and socket type of synovial joint between the head of the femur and acetabulum. The knee joint is a hinge type of synovial joint that permits only limited rotation. The talocrural joint is a hinge joint between talus, fibula, and tibia, only allowing movements of flexion and extension.
The long axis of the foot is at right angle to that of the leg, thus forming an effective arch for the upright stance of man.

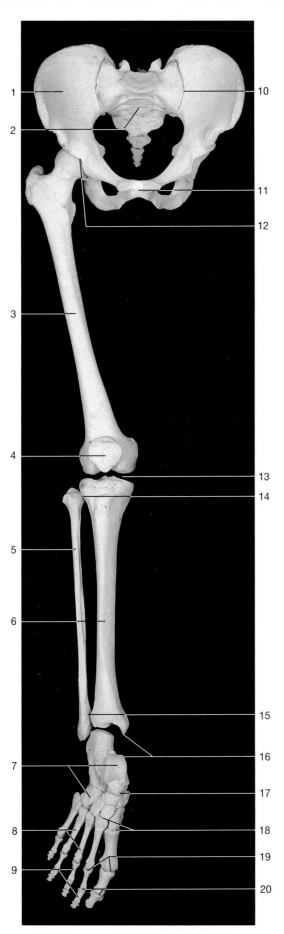

A Pelvic girdle	9 Phalanges
B Thigh	10 Sacroiliac joint
C Leg	11 Pubic symphysis
D Foot	12 Hip joint
1 Right hip bone	13 Knee joint
2 Sacrum	14 Proximal tibiofibular joint
3 Femur	15 Distal tibiofibular joint
4 Patella	16 Talocrural joint
5 Fibula	17 Talocalcaneonavicular joint
6 Tibia	18 Tarsometatarsal joints
7 Tarsal bones	19 Metatarsophalangeal joints
8 Metatarsal bones	20 Interphalangeal joints

The pelvic girdle is firmly connected to the vertebral column at the sacroiliac joint. Therefore the body can be kept upright more easily even if only one limb is used for support (as in walking). The mobility of the lower limb is more limited than that of the upper limb.

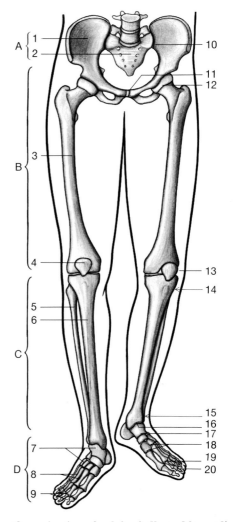

Skeleton of pelvic girdle and lower limb
(anterior aspect). The talocrural joint has been dislocated.

Organization of pelvic girdle and lower limb.

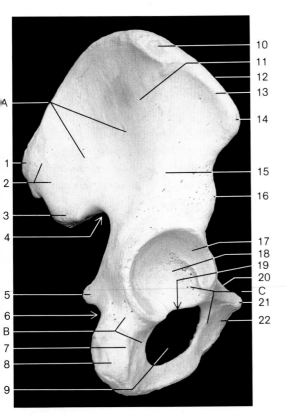

10
11
12
13
14

15
16

17
18
19
20
C
21
22

A
1
2
3
4

5
6
B
7
8
9

Right hip bone (lateral aspect).

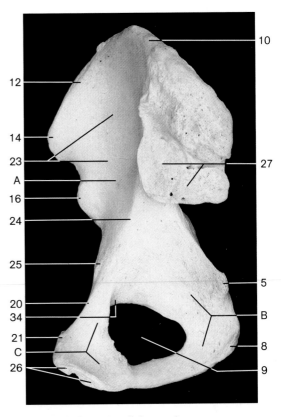

10

12
14
23
A
16
24

25

20
34
21
C
26

27

5
B
8
9

Right hip bone (medial aspect).

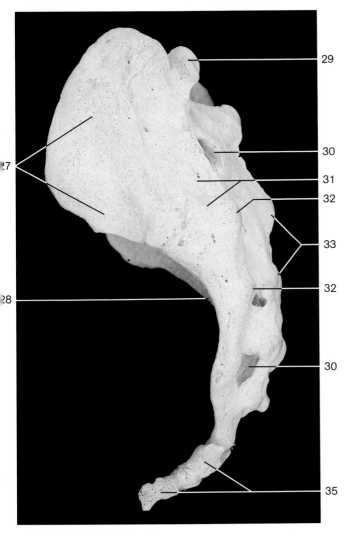

29

30

31
32

33

32

30

35

27

28

Sacrum and coccyx (lateral aspect).

A   Ilium
B   Ischium
C   Pubis

1   Posterior superior iliac spine
2   Posterior gluteal line
3   Posterior inferior iliac spine
4   Greater sciatic notch
5   Ischial spine
6   Lesser sciatic notch
7   Body of ischium
8   Ischial tuberosity
9   Obturator foramen
10 Iliac crest
11 Anterior gluteal line
12 Internal lip of iliac crest
13 External lip of iliac crest
14 Anterior superior iliac spine
15 Inferior gluteal line
16 Anterior inferior iliac spine
17 Lunate surface of acetabulum
18 Acetabular fossa
19 Acetabular notch
20 Pecten pubis
21 Pubic tubercle
22 Body of pubis
23 Iliac fossa
24 Arcuate line
25 Iliopubic eminence
26 Symphyseal surface of pubis
27 Auricular surface
28 Pelvic surface of sacrum
29 Superior articular process of sacrum
30 Dorsal sacral foramina
31 Sacral tuberosity
32 Lateral sacral crest
33 Median sacral crest
34 Obturator groove
35 Coccyx

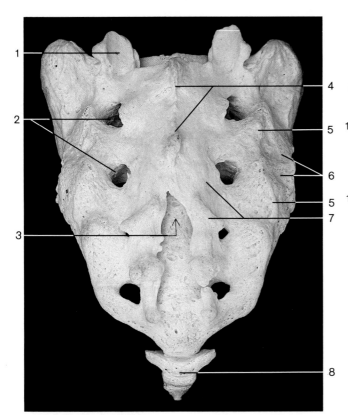

Sacrum (posterior aspect).

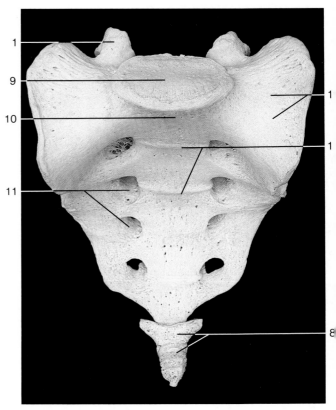

Sacrum (anterior aspect).

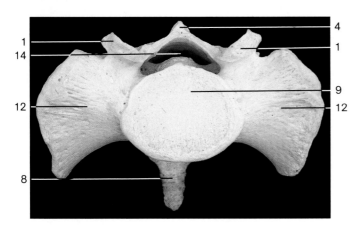

Sacrum (superior aspect).

1   Superior articular process of sacrum
2   Dorsal sacral foramina
3   Sacral hiatus
4   Median sacral crest
5   Lateral sacral crest
6   Sacral tuberosity
7   Intermediate sacral crest
8   Coccyx
9   Base of sacrum
10 Sacral promontory
11 Anterior sacral foramina
12 Lateral part of sacrum (ala)
13 Transverse line of sacrum
14 Sacral canal
15 Linea terminalis
16 True conjugate
17 Diagonal conjugate
18 Transverse diameter
19 Oblique diameter
20 Inferior pelvic aperture or outlet

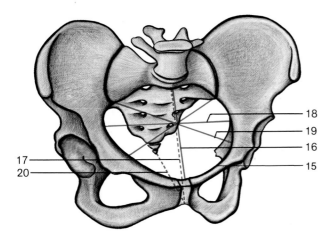

Diameters of pelvis (oblique superior aspect).
(Schematic drawing.)

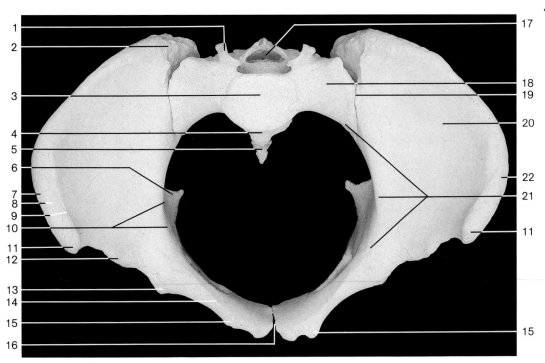

Female pelvis (superior aspect). Note the differences between the male and the female pelvis, predominantly in the form and dimensions of the sacrum, the superior and inferior apertures and the alae of the ilium.

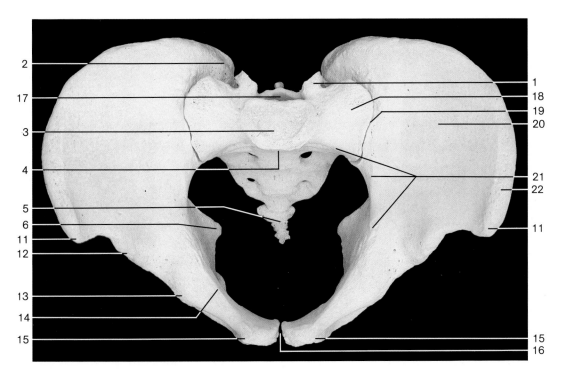

Male pelvis (superior aspect). Compare with the female pelvis (depicted above).

1	Superior articular process of sacrum	12	Anterior inferior iliac spine
2	Posterior superior iliac spine	13	Iliopubic eminence
3	Base of sacrum	14	Pecten pubis
4	Sacral promontory	15	Pubic tubercle
5	Coccyx	16	Pubic symphysis
6	Ischial spine	17	Sacral canal
7	External lip ⎫ of iliac	18	Ala of sacrum
8	Intermediate line ⎬ crest	19	Position of sacroiliac joint
9	Internal lip ⎭	20	Iliac fossa
10	Arcuate line	21	Linea terminalis
11	Anterior superior iliac spine	22	Iliac crest

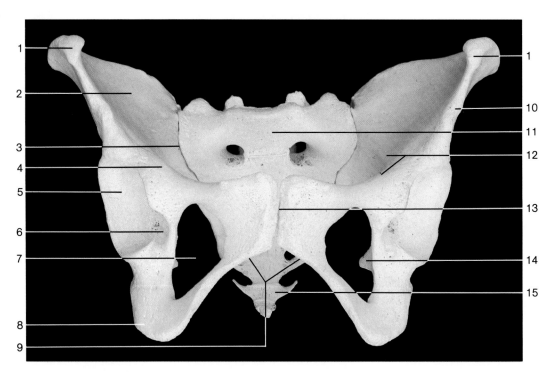

Female pelvis (anterior aspect). Note the differences between the form and dimensions of the male and the female pelvis. The female pubic arch is wider than the male. The obturator foramen in the female pelvis is triangular, while that in the male pelvis is ovoid.

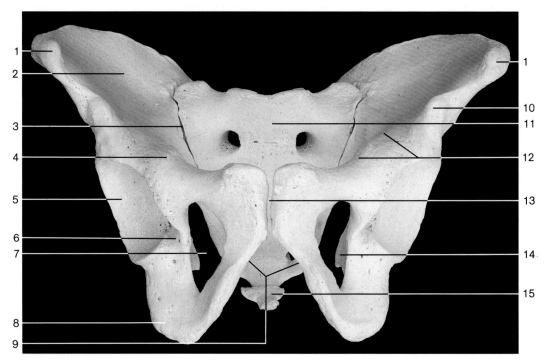

Male pelvis (anterior aspect). Compare with foregoing figure.

1	Anterior superior iliac spine	9	Pubic arch
2	Iliac fossa	10	Anterior inferior iliac spine
3	Position of sacroiliac joint	11	Sacrum
4	Iliopubic eminence	12	Linea terminalis (at margin of superior aperture)
5	Lunate surface of acetabulum	13	Pubic symphysis
6	Acetabular notch	14	Ischial spine
7	Obturator foramen	15	Coccyx
8	Ischial tuberosity		

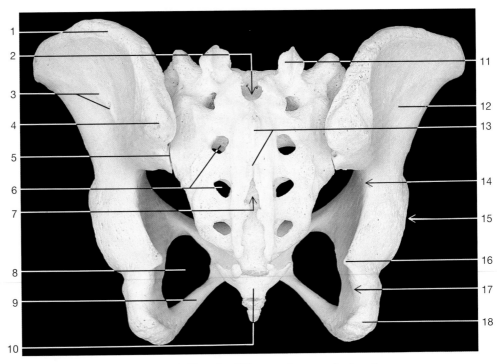

Female pelvis (posterior aspect). Note the differences between the female and male pelvis, especially with respect to the inferior aperture, the shape of the sacrum, the two sciatic notches and the pubic arch.

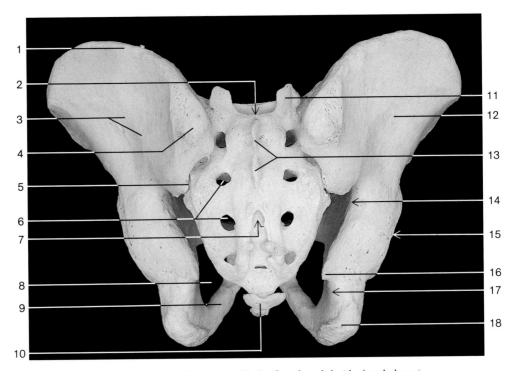

Male pelvis (posterior aspect). Compare with the female pelvis (depicted above).

1	Iliac crest	10	Coccyx
2	Sacral canal	11	Superior articular process of sacrum
3	Posterior gluteal line	12	Gluteal surface of ilium
4	Posterior superior iliac spine	13	Median sacral crest
5	Position of sacroiliac joint	14	Greater sciatic notch
6	Dorsal sacral foramina	15	Position of acetabulum
7	Sacral hiatus	16	Ischial spine
8	Obturator foramen	17	Lesser sciatic notch
9	Ramus of ischium	18	Ischial tuberosity

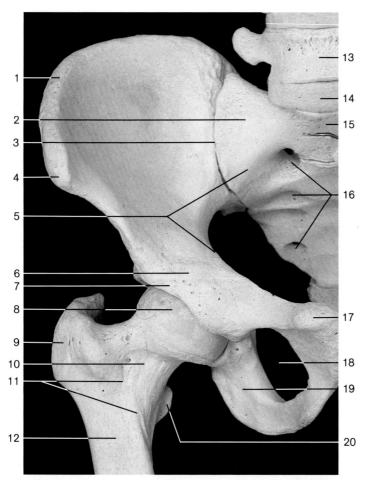

Bones of right hip joint (anterior aspect).

1 Iliac crest
2 Lateral part of sacrum (ala)
3 Position of sacroiliac joint
4 Anterior superior iliac spine
5 Linea terminalis
6 Iliopubic eminence
7 Bony margin of acetabulum
8 Head of femur
9 Greater trochanter
10 Neck of femur
11 Intertrochanteric line
12 Shaft of femur
13 Fifth lumbar vertebra
14 Imitation intervertebral disc between fifth lumbar
   vertebra and sacrum
15 Sacral promontory
16 Anterior sacral foramina
17 Pubic tubercle
18 Obturator foramen
19 Ramus of ischium
20 Lesser trochanter
21 Dorsal sacral foramina
22 Greater sciatic notch
23 Ischial spine
24 Pubic symphysis
25 Pubis
26 Ischial tuberosity
27 Intertrochanteric crest
28 Symphysial surface

Diameters of the pelvis

A True conjugate (11–11.5 cm) (Conjugata vera)
B Diagonal conjugate (12.5–13 cm)
C Largest diameter of pelvis
D Inferior pelvic aperture
E Pelvic inclination (60°)

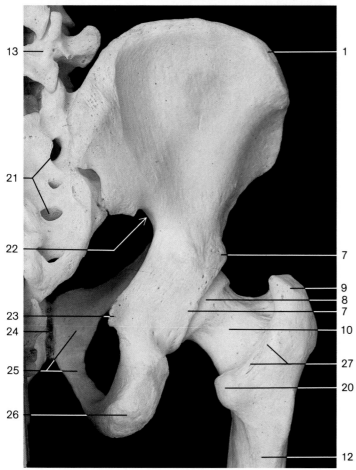

Bones of right hip joint (posterior aspect).

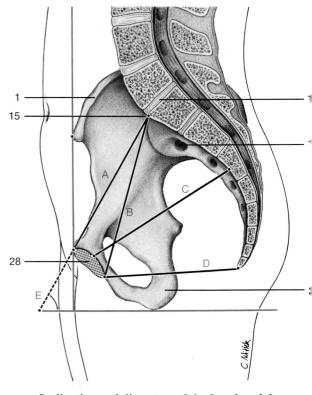

Inclination and diameters of the female pelvis,
right half (medial aspect).

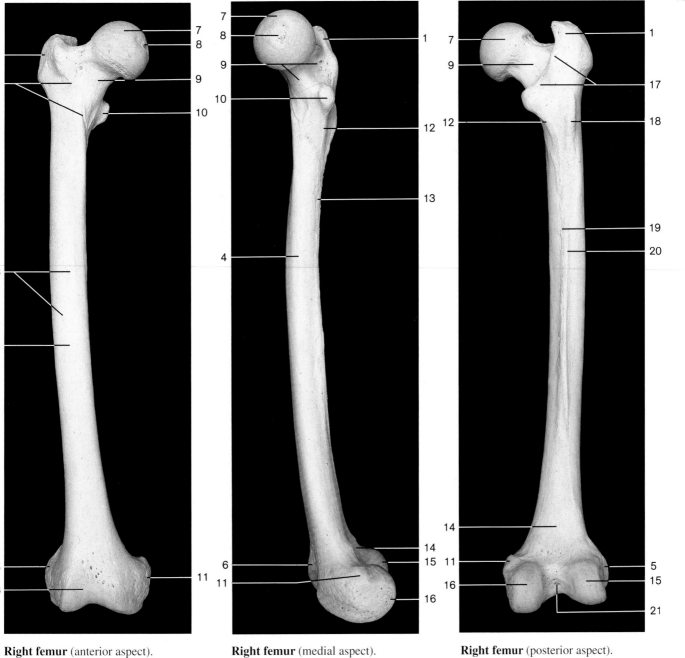

Right femur (anterior aspect).

Right femur (medial aspect).

Right femur (posterior aspect).

1	Greater trochanter	8	Fovea of head	15	Lateral condyle
2	Intertrochanteric line	9	Neck	16	Medial condyle
3	Nutrient foramina	10	Lesser trochanter	17	Intertrochanteric crest
4	Shaft of femur (diaphysis)	11	Medial epicondyle	18	Third trochanter
5	Lateral epicondyle	12	Pectineal line	19	Medial lip of linea aspera
6	Patellar surface	13	Linea aspera	20	Lateral lip of linea aspera
7	Head	14	Popliteal surface	21	Intercondylar fossa

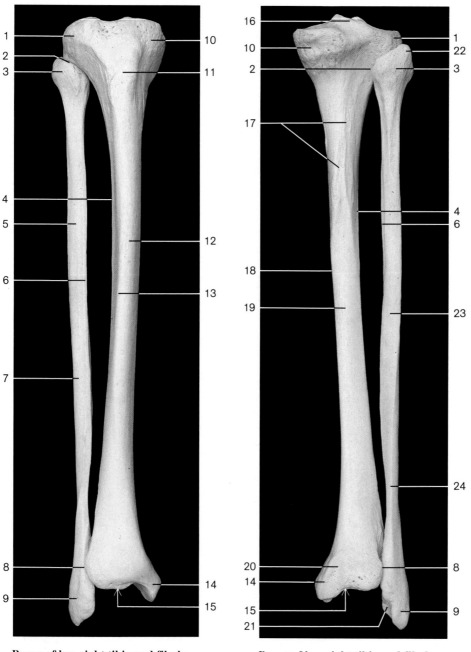

1 Lateral condyle of tibia
2 Position of tibiofibular joint
3 Head of fibula
4 Interosseous border of tibia
5 Shaft of fibula
6 Interosseous border of fibula
7 Lateral surface of fibula
8 Position of tibiofibular joint
9 Lateral malleolus
10 Medial condyle of tibia
11 Tuberosity of tibia
12 Shaft of tibia (diaphysis)
13 Anterior margin of tibia
14 Medial malleolus
15 Inferior articular surface
   of tibia
16 Intercondylar eminence
17 Soleal line
18 Medial border of tibia
19 Posterior surface of tibia
20 Malleolar sulcus of tibia
21 Malleolar articular surface
   of fibula
22 Apex of head of fibula
23 Posterior surface of fibula
24 Posterior border of fibula
25 Medial intercondylar tubercle
26 Posterior intercondylar area
27 Anterior intercondylar area
28 Lateral intercondylar tubercle

Bones of leg, right tibia and fibula
(anterior aspect).

Bones of leg, right tibia and fibula
(posterior aspect).

Upper end of right tibia with fibula
(from above), anterior margin of tibia above.
Superior articular surface of tibia.

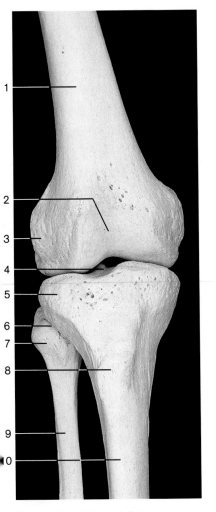

Bones of right knee joint
(anterior aspect).

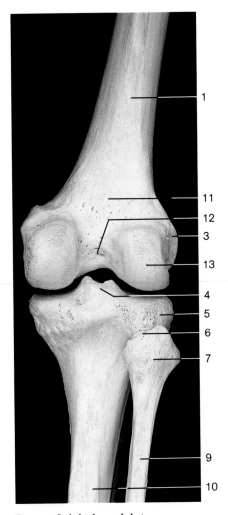

Bones of right knee joint
(posterior aspect).

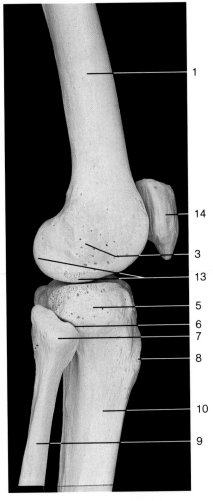

Bones of right knee joint
(lateral aspect).

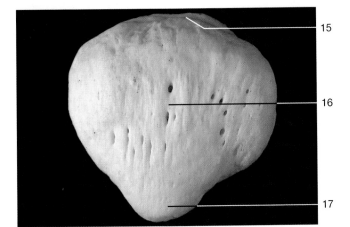

Right patella (anterior aspect).

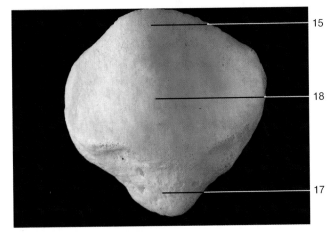

Right patella (posterior aspect).

1	**Femur**	10	Shaft of tibia
2	Patellar surface of femur	11	Popliteal surface of femur
3	Lateral epicondyle of femur	12	Intercondylar fossa of femur
4	Intercondylar eminence of tibia	13	Lateral condyle of femur
5	Lateral condyle of tibia	14	**Patella**
6	Position of tibiofibular joint	15	Base of patella
7	Head of fibula	16	Anterior surface of patella
8	Tuberosity of **tibia**	17	Apex of patella
9	**Fibula**	18	Articular surface of patella

428

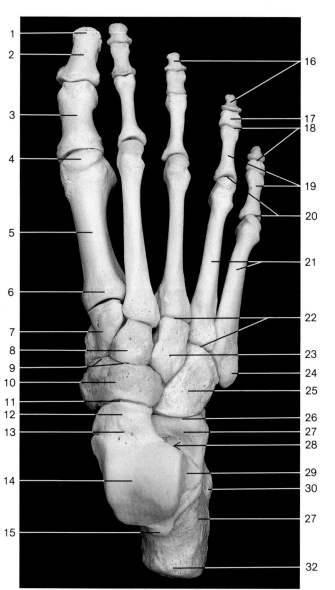

Bones of right foot (dorsal aspect).

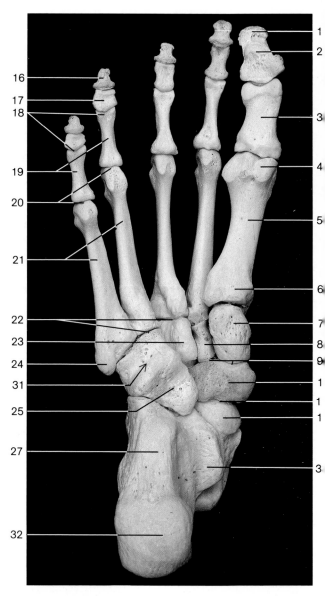

Bones of right foot (plantar aspect).

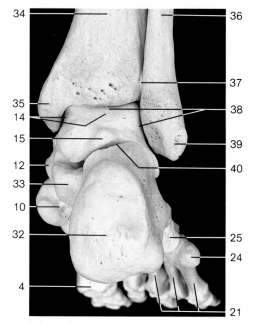

Bones of right foot together with tibia
and fibula (posterior aspect).

1 Tuberosity of distal phalanx of great toe
2 Distal phalanx of great toe
3 Proximal phalanx of great toe
4 Head of first metatarsal bone
5 First metatarsal bone
6 Base of first metatarsal bone
7 Medial cuneiform bone
8 Intermediate cuneiform bone
9 Position of **cuneonavicular joint**
10 Navicular bone

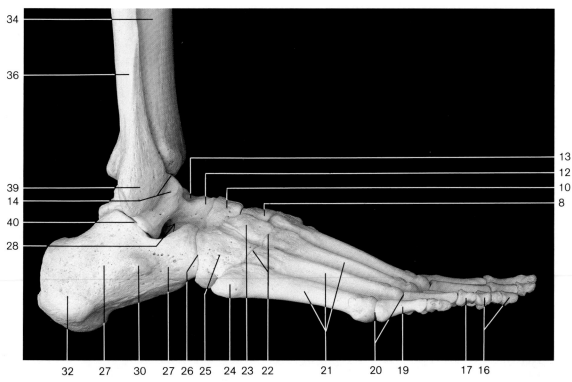

Bones of right foot, tibia and fibula (lateral aspect).

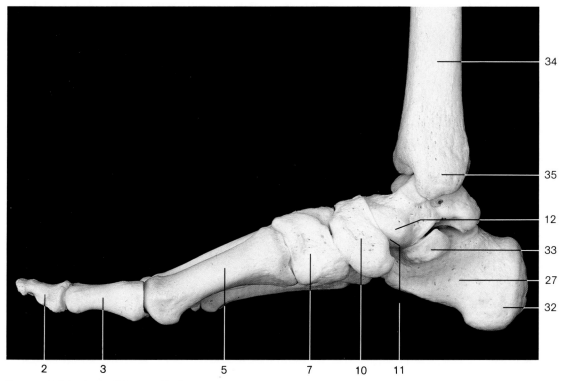

Bones of right foot, tibia and fibula (medial aspect).

11 Position of **talocalcaneonavicular joint**	21 Metatarsal bones	31 Groove for tendon of peroneus longus
12 Head of talus	22 Position of **tarsometatarsal joints**	32 Calcaneal tuberosity
13 Neck of talus	23 Lateral cuneiform bone	33 Sustentaculum tali
14 Trochlea of talus	24 Tuberosity of fifth metatarsal bone	34 Tibia
15 Posterior talar process	25 Cuboid bone	35 Medial malleolus
16 Distal phalanges	26 Position of **calcaneocuboid joint**	36 Fibula
17 Middle phalanges	27 Calcaneus	37 Position of tibiofibular syndesmosis
18 Position of **interphalangeal joints**	28 Tarsal sinus	38 Position of **talocrural joint**
19 Proximal phalanges	29 Lateral malleolar surface of talus	39 Lateral malleolus
20 Position of **metatarsophalangeal joints**	30 Peroneal trochlea of calcaneus	40 Position of **subtalar joint**

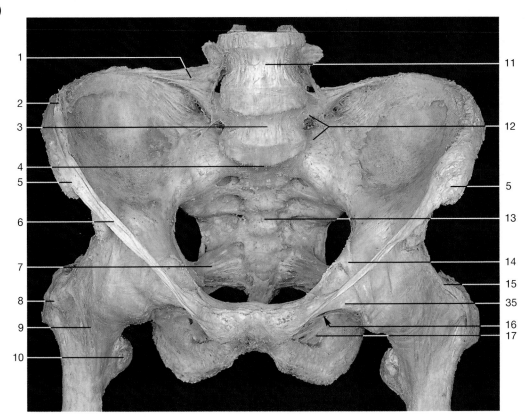

**Ligaments of pelvis
and hip joint**
(anterior aspect).

1 **Iliolumbar ligament**	13 Sacrum	26 Articular capsule of hip joint
2 Iliac crest	14 Iliopectineal arch	27 Dorsal sacroiliac ligaments
3 Fifth lumbar vertebra	15 **Iliofemoral ligament** (horizontal band)	28 Coccyx with superficial dorsal
4 Sacral promontory	16 Obturator canal	sacrococcygeal ligament
5 Anterior superior iliac spine	17 Obturator membrane	29 Head of femur
6 Inguinal ligament	18 **Greater sciatic foramen**	30 Articular cartilage of head of femur
7 Sacrospinous ligament	19 Sacrospinous ligament	31 Articular cavity of hip joint
8 Greater trochanter	20 Sacrotuberous ligament	32 Acetabular lip
9 **Iliofemoral ligament** (vertical band)	21 **Lesser sciatic foramen**	33 Spongy bone
10 Lesser trochanter	22 Ischial tuberosity	34 Ligament of head of femur
11 Fourth lumbar vertebra	23 **Ischiofemoral ligament**	35 Pubofemoral ligament
12 Iliolumbar and ventral sacroiliac	24 Intertrochanteric crest	36 Zona orbicularis
ligaments	25 Femur	

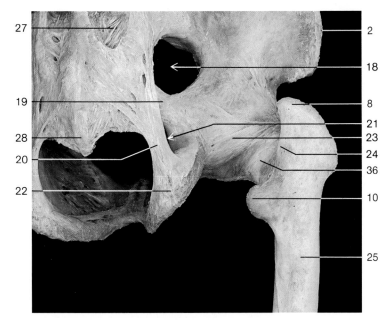

Ligaments of pelvis and hip joint (right posterior aspect).

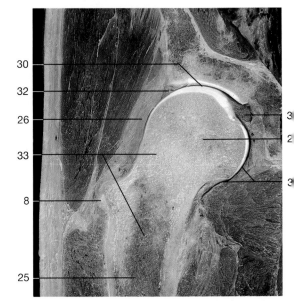

Coronal section of right hip joint (anterior view).

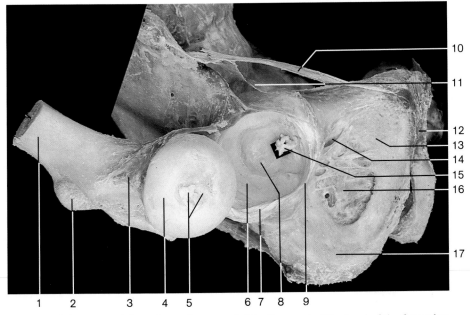

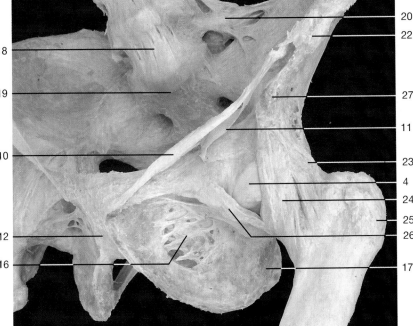

1 Femur
2 Lesser trochanter
3 Neck of femur
4 Head of femur
5 Fovea of head with cut edge of ligament of head
6 Lunate surface of acetabulum
7 Acetabular lip
8 Acetabular fossa
9 Transverse acetabular ligament
10 Inguinal ligament
11 Iliopectineal arch
12 Pubic symphysis
13 Pubic bone
14 Obturator canal
15 Ligament of head of femur
16 Obturator membrane
17 Ischium
18 Anterior longitudinal ligament (level of fifth lumbar vertebra)
19 Sacral promontory
20 Iliolumbar ligament
21 Iliac crest
22 Anterior superior iliac spine
23 Iliofemoral ligament (horizontal band)
24 Iliofemoral ligament (vertical band)
25 Greater trochanter
26 Pubofemoral ligament
27 Anterior inferior iliac spine
28 Ventral sacroiliac ligaments
29 **Sacrospinous ligament**
30 **Sacrotuberous ligament**
31 Intertrochanteric line
32 **Ischiofemoral ligament**
33 Zona orbicularis

Right hip joint, opened (lateral anterior aspect). The ligament of the head of the femur has been divided and the femur has been posteriorly reflected.

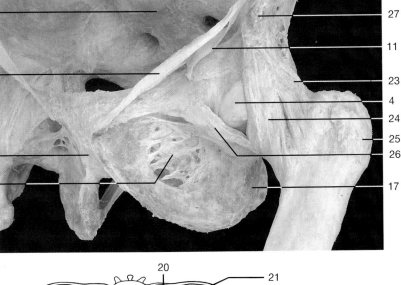

Ligaments of the pelvis and hip joint (antero lateral aspect).

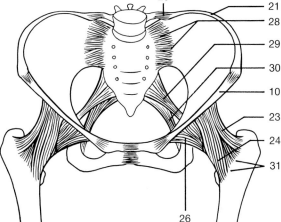

Ligaments of hip joint (anterior aspect). (Schematic drawing.)

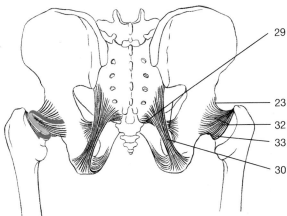

Ligaments of hip joint (posterior aspect). (Schematic drawing.)

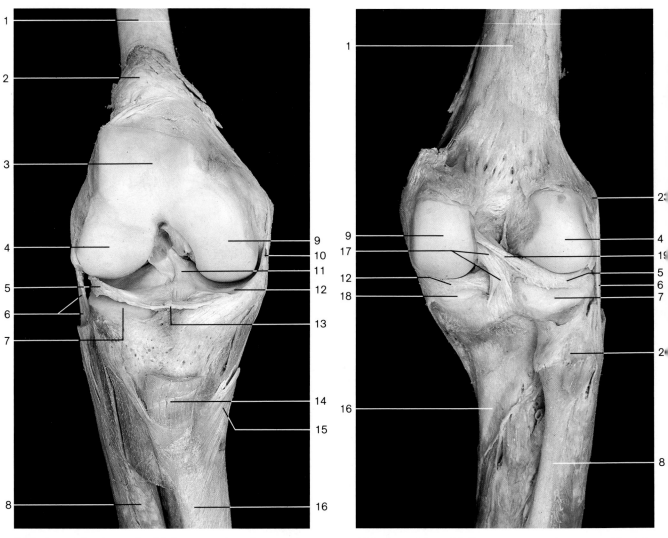

Right knee joint (opened) **with ligaments** (anterior aspect). The patella and articular capsule have been removed and the femur slightly flexed.

Right knee joint with ligaments (posterior aspect). The joint is extended and the articular capsule has been removed.

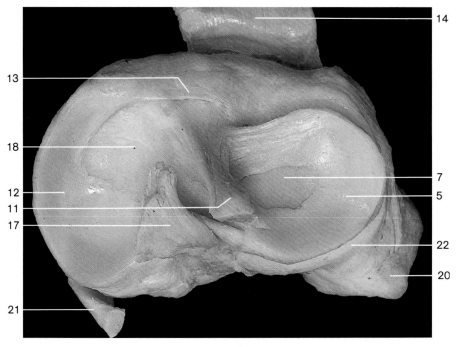

Articular surface of right tibia, menisci, and cruciate ligaments (superior aspect). Anterior margin of tibia above.

1   Femur
2   Articular capsule with **suprapatellar bursa**
3   Patellar surface
4   Lateral condyle of femur
5   **Lateral meniscus of knee joint**
6   Fibular collateral ligament
7   Lateral condyle of tibia (superior articular surface)
8   Fibula
9   Medial condyle of femur
10 Tibial collateral ligament
11 **Anterior cruciate ligament**
12 **Medial meniscus of knee joint**
13 Transverse ligament of knee
14 Patellar ligament
15 Common tendon of sartorius, semitendinosus and gracilis muscles
16 Tibia
17 **Posterior cruciate ligament**
18 Medial condyle of tibia (superior articular surface)
19 Posterior meniscofemoral ligament
20 Head of fibula
21 Tendon of semimembranosus muscle
22 Posterior attachment of articular capsule of knee joint
23 Lateral epicondyle of femur

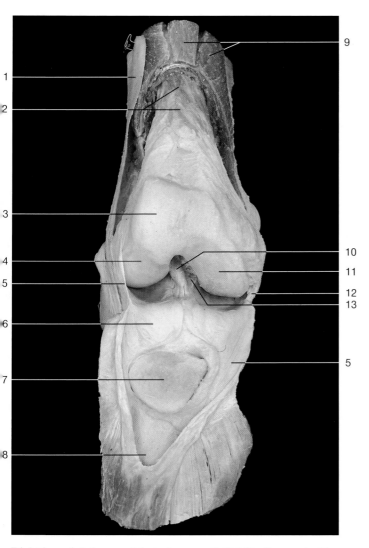

1 Iliotibial tract
2 Articular muscle of knee
3 Patellar surface
4 Lateral condyle of femur
5 Articular capsule
6 Infrapatellar fat pad
7 **Patella** (articular surface)
8 **Suprapatellar bursa**
9 Quadriceps muscle of thigh (divided)
10 **Anterior cruciate ligament**
11 Medial condyle of femur
12 Fibular collateral ligament
13 **Posterior cruciate ligament**
14 Medial epicondyle of femur
15 Intercondylar fossa of femur
16 Tibial collateral ligament
17 **Medial meniscus** of knee joint
18 Medial intercondylar tubercle
19 Femur
20 Lateral epicondyle of femur
21 **Lateral meniscus** of knee joint
22 Epiphyseal line of tibia
23 Tibia

Right knee joint, opened (anterior aspect). Patellar ligament with patella reflected.

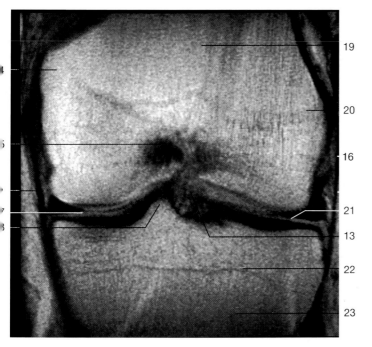

Right knee joint. Frontal section through the central part of the joint (posterior aspect, MRI scan). (See also p. 10.)

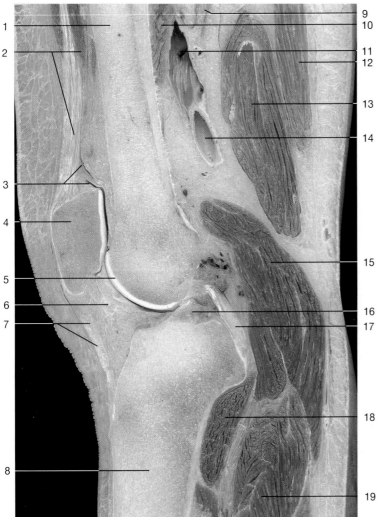

1	**Femur**
2	Quadriceps femoris muscle
3	Suprapatellar bursa and articular cavity
4	**Patella**
5	Patellar surface (articular cartilage)
6	Infrapatellar fat pad
7	Patellar ligament
8	**Tibia**
9	Tibial nerve
10	Adductor magnus muscle
11	Popliteal vein
12	Semitendinosus muscle
13	Semimembranosus muscle
14	**Popliteal artery**
15	Gastrocnemius muscle
16	Anterior cruciate ligament
17	Posterior cruciate ligament
18	Popliteus muscle
19	Soleus muscle
20	Deep flexor muscles of leg
21	Calcaneal tendon
22	Epiphyseal line of tibia
23	Calcaneus
24	**Talocrural joint**
25	Talus
26	Lateral meniscus
27	Epiphysial line of femur

Sagittal section through the knee joint. Anterior surface to the left.

Talocrural joint. Sagittal section; anterior part to the left. (MRI scan.)

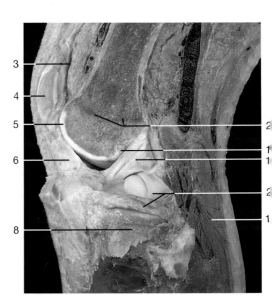

Left knee joint. Anterior cruciate ligament (lateral aspect).

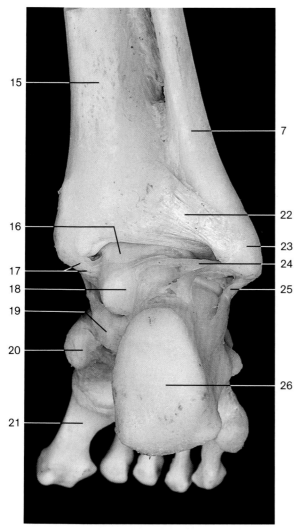

Ligaments of talocrural joint, right leg (posterior aspect).

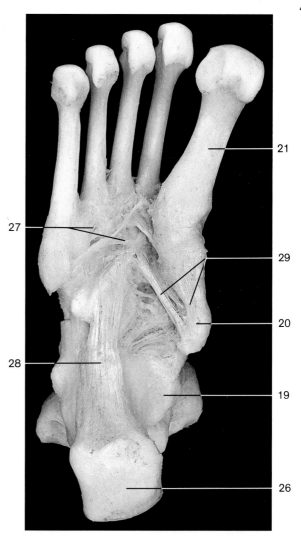

Deep ligaments of the foot, right foot (plantar aspect). The toes have been removed.

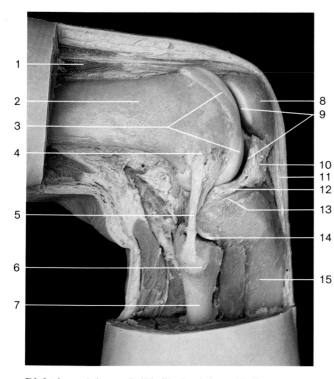

Right knee joint and tibiofibular joint with ligaments.
Note the position of the lateral meniscus.

1 Quadriceps femoris muscle
2 Femur
3 Patellar surface
4 Lateral epicondyle of femur
5 **Fibular collateral ligament**
6 Head of fibula
7 **Fibula**
8 **Patella**
9 Articular cavity of knee joint
10 Infrapatellar fat pad
11 **Patellar ligament**
12 **Lateral meniscus of knee joint**
13 Lateral condyle of tibia (superior articular facet)
14 **Tibiofibular joint**
15 Tibia
16 Trochlea of talus (superior surface)
17 Deltoid ligament of ankle (posterior tibiotalar part)
18 Talus
19 **Sustentaculum tali**
20 Navicular bone
21 First metatarsal bone
22 **Posterior tibiofibular ligament**
23 Lateral malleolus
24 Posterior talofibular ligament
25 Calcaneofibular ligament
26 Calcaneal tuberosity
27 Plantar tarsometatarsal ligaments
28 **Long plantar ligament**
29 Plantar cuneonavicular ligaments

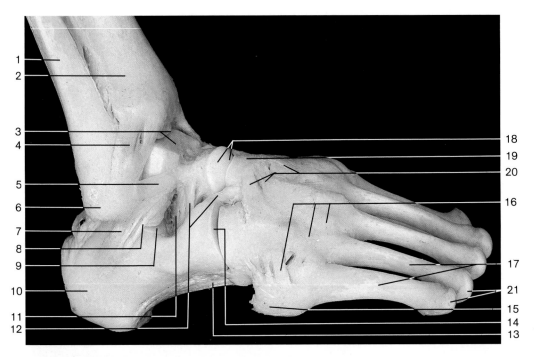

Ligaments of right foot (lateral aspect).

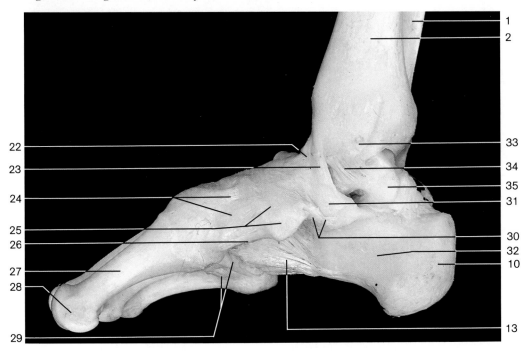

Ligaments of right foot (medial aspect).

1	Fibula	18	Head of talus and **talocalcaneonavicular joint**
2	Tibia	19	Navicular bone
3	Trochlea of talus and **talocrural joint**	20	Dorsal cuneonavicular ligaments
4	Anterior tibiofibular ligament	21	Heads of metatarsal bones
5	Anterior talofibular ligament	22	Medial or deltoid ligament of ankle (tibionavicular part)
6	Lateral malleolus	23	Medial or deltoid ligament of ankle (tibiocalcaneal part)
7	Calcaneofibular ligament	24	Dorsal cuneonavicular ligaments
8	Lateral talocalcaneal ligament	25	Navicular bone
9	**Subtalar joint**	26	Plantar cuneonavicular ligament
10	Tuber calcanei	27	First metatarsal bone
11	Interosseous talocalcaneal ligament	28	Head of first metatarsal bone
12	Bifurcate ligament	29	Plantar tarsometatarsal ligaments
13	Long plantar ligament	30	Plantar calcaneonavicular ligament
14	**Calcaneocuboid joint**	31	Sustentaculum tali
15	Tuberosity of fifth metatarsal bone	32	Calcaneus
16	Dorsal tarsometatarsal ligaments	33	Medial malleolus
17	Metatarsal bones	34	Medial or deltoid ligament of ankle (posterior part)
		35	Talus

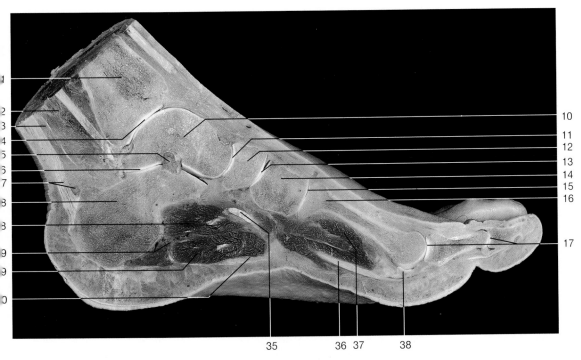

Longitudinal section through the foot at the level of first phalanx.

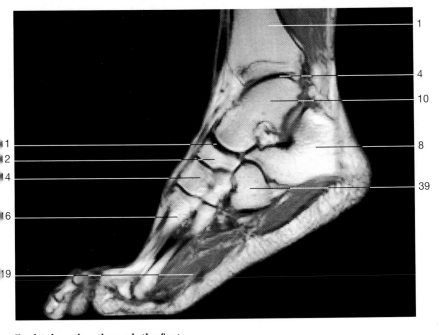

Sagittal section through the foot
(MRI scan after Heuck A, Luttke G, Rohen JW, 1994).

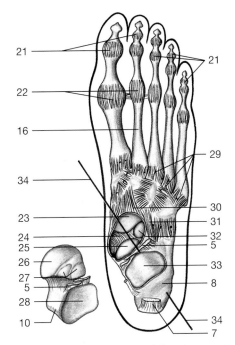

Talocalcaneonavicular joint.
The talus has been rotated to show
the articular surfaces of the joint.

1	Tibia
2	Deep flexor muscles
3	Superficial flexor muscles
4	**Talocrural joint**
5	Interosseous talocalcaneal ligament
6	**Subtalar joint**
7	Calcaneal or Achilles tendon and bursa
8	Calcaneus
9	Vessels and nerves of foot
10	Talus
11	**Talocalcaneonavicular joint**
12	Navicular bone
13	**Cuneonavicular joint**
14	Intermediate cuneiform bone
15	**Tarsometatarsal joints**
16	Metatarsal bones
17	**Metatarsophalangeal** and **interphalangeal joints**
18	Quadratus plantae muscle with flexor tendons
19	Flexor digitorum brevis muscle
20	Plantar aponeurosis
21	Articular capsules of interphalangeal joints
22	Articular capsules of metatarsophalangeal joints
23	Articular surface of navicular bone
24	Plantar calcaneonavicular ligament
25	Middle talar articular surface of calcaneus
26	Navicular articular surface of talus
27	Anterior and middle calcaneal surfaces of talus
28	Posterior calcaneal surface of talus
29	Dorsal tarsometatarsal ligaments
30	Talonavicular ligament
31	Bifurcate ligament
32	Anterior talar articular surface of calcaneus
33	Posterior talar articular surface of calcaneus
34	Axis for inversion and eversion
35	Tendon of tibialis posterior muscle
36	Tendon of flexor hallucis longus muscle
37	Flexor hallucis brevis muscle
38	Sesamoid bone
39	Cuboid bone

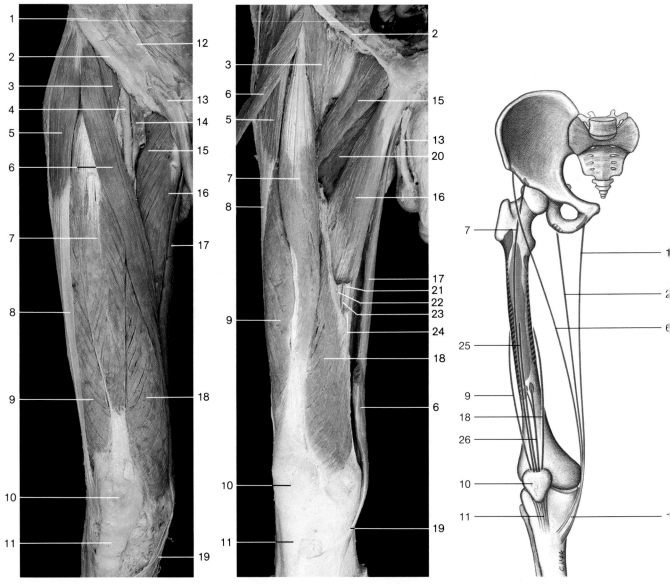

Extensor and adductor muscles of thigh, right thigh (anterior aspect).

Quadriceps muscle and superficial layer of adductor muscles, right thigh (anterior aspect). The sartorius muscle has been divided.

Course of extensor muscles of thigh and muscles inserting with common tendon on tibia.

1 Anterior superior iliac spine	15 **Pectineus muscle**
2 Inguinal ligament	16 **Adductor longus muscle**
3 Iliopsoas muscle	17 Gracilis muscle
4 Femoral artery	18 Vastus medialis muscle
5 Tensor fasciae latae muscle	19 Common tendon of sartorius, gracilis, and semitendinosus muscles
6 Sartorius muscle	(pes anserinus)
7 **Rectus femoris muscle**	20 **Adductor brevis muscle**
8 Iliotibial tract	21 Femoral artery
9 Vastus lateralis muscle	22 Femoral vein entering the adductor canal
10 Patella	23 Saphenous nerve
11 Patellar ligament	24 Fascia of adductor canal
12 Aponeurosis of external abdominal oblique muscle	25 Vastus intermedius muscle
13 Spermatic cord	26 Articularis genus muscle
14 Femoral vein	27 Semitendinosus muscle

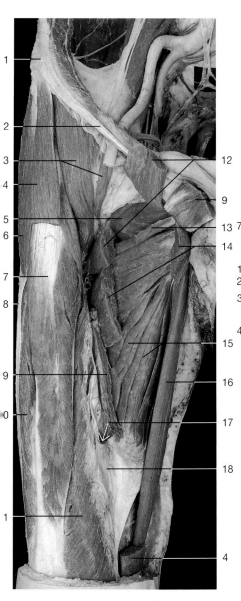

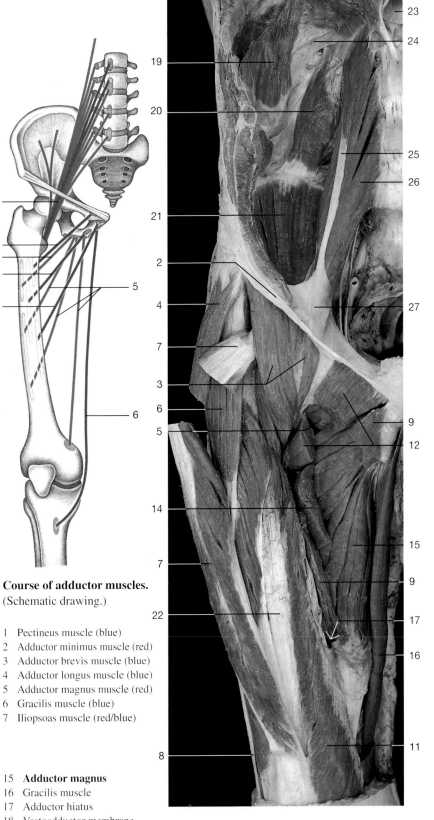

Deep layer of adductor muscles.
Adductor magnus muscle (anterior aspect). Pectineus, adductor longus and brevis muscles have been divided.

Course of adductor muscles.
(Schematic drawing.)

1 Pectineus muscle (blue)
2 Adductor minimus muscle (red)
3 Adductor brevis muscle (blue)
4 Adductor longus muscle (blue)
5 Adductor magnus muscle (red)
6 Gracilis muscle (blue)
7 Iliopsoas muscle (red/blue)

Iliopsoas and adductor muscles, deepest layer (anterior aspect). Pectineus, adductor longus and brevis, rectus femoris muscles have been divided.

1 Anterior superior iliac spine
2 Inguinal ligament
3 **Iliopsoas muscle**
4 Sartorius muscle
5 Obturator externus muscle
6 Tensor fasciae latae muscle
7 Rectus femoris muscle
8 Iliotibial tract
9 Adductor longus muscle (divided)
10 Vastus lateralis muscle
11 Vastus medialis muscle
12 Pectineus muscle (divided)
13 Adductor minimus muscle
14 Adductor brevis muscle (cut)

15 **Adductor magnus**
16 Gracilis muscle
17 Adductor hiatus
18 Vastoadductor membrane
19 Diaphragm
20 Quadratus lumborum muscle
21 **Iliacus muscle**
22 Vastus intermedius muscle
23 Aorta in aortic hiatus
24 Twelfth rib
25 **Psoas minor muscle**
26 **Psoas major muscle**
27 Iliopectineal arch

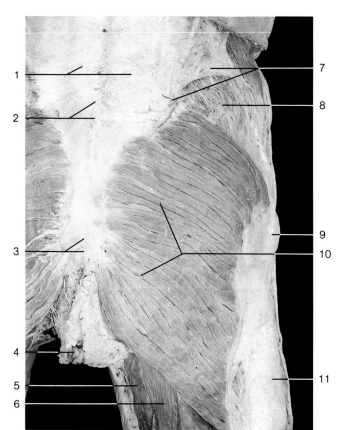

1
2

3

4
5
6

7
8

9
10

11

Gluteal muscles, superficial layer (posterior aspect).

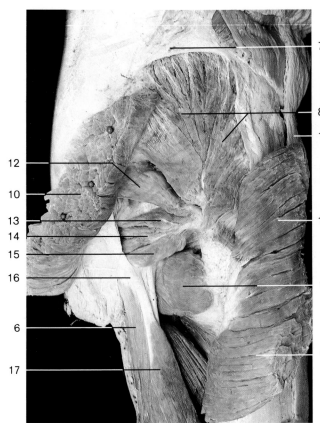

12

10

13
14
15

16

6

17

7

8

Gluteal muscles, deeper layer (posterior aspect).

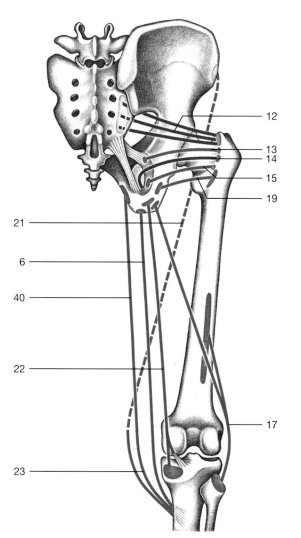

12

13
14

15

19

21

6

40

22

17

23

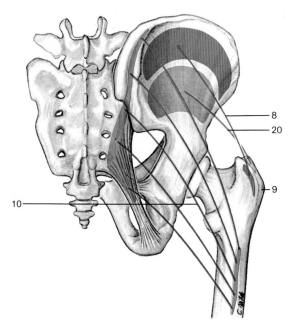

8
20

10

9

Course of gluteal muscles
(posterior aspect; schematic drawing).

◁

Course of gluteal muscles (deeper layer) **and of
ischiocrural muscles** (posterior aspect).
Sartorius muscle is indicated by dotted line (schematic drawing).

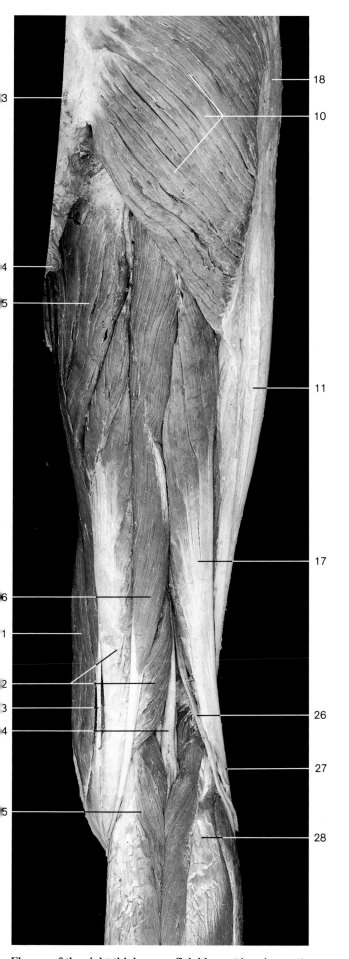

1 Thoracolumbar fascia
2 Spinous processes of lumbar vertebrae
3 Coccyx
4 Anus
5 Adductor magnus muscle
6 Semitendinosus muscle
7 Iliac crest
8 **Gluteus medius muscle**
9 Greater trochanter
10 **Gluteus maximus muscle**
11 Iliotibial tract
12 Piriformis muscle
13 Superior gemellus muscle
14 Obturator internus muscle
15 Inferior gemellus muscle
16 Ischial tuberosity
17 **Biceps femoris muscle**
18 Tensor fasciae latae muscle
19 Quadratus femoris muscle
20 **Gluteus minimus muscle**
21 Sartorius muscle
22 Semimembranosus muscle
23 Tendon of gracilis muscle
24 Tibial nerve
25 Medial head of gastrocnemius muscle
26 Common peroneal nerve
27 Tendon of biceps femoris muscle
28 Lateral head of gastrocnemius muscle
29 Rectus femoris muscle
30 Vastus medialis muscle
31 Vastus intermedius muscle
32 Vastus lateralis muscle
33 Sciatic nerve
34 Gluteus maximus muscle (insertion)
35 Great saphenous vein
36 Femoral artery
37 Femoral vein
38 Adductor longus muscle
39 Femur
40 Gracilis muscle
41 Septum between semitendinosus
   and semimembranosus muscles

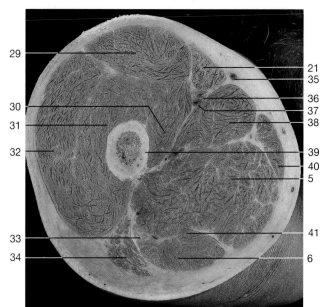

Flexors of the right thigh, superficial layer (dorsal aspect).

Cross section of right thigh (inferior aspect).
Anterior side on top.

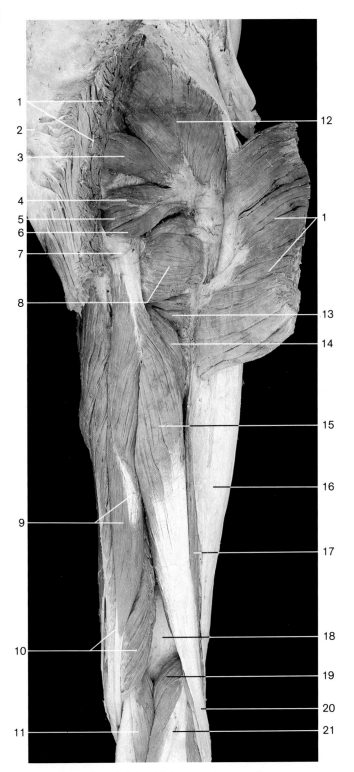

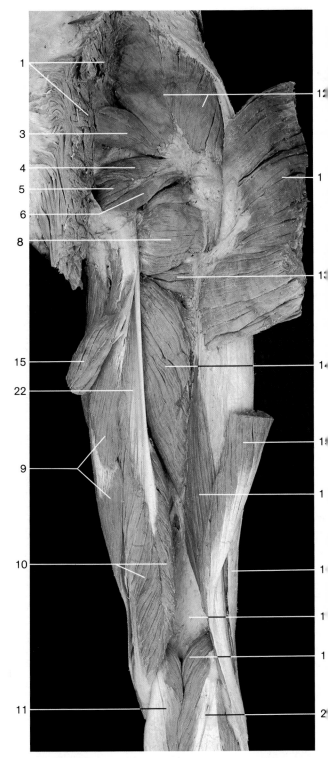

Dorsal muscles of right thigh (posterior aspect).
The gluteus maximus muscle has been cut and reflected.

Dorsal muscles of right thigh (posterior aspect).
The gluteus maximus muscle and the long head of biceps
femoris muscle have been divided and displaced.

1 Gluteus maximus muscle (divided)	9 Semitendinosus muscle with intermediate tendon	17 Short head of biceps femoris muscle
2 Position of coccyx	10 Semimembranosus muscle	18 Popliteal surface of femur
3 Piriformis muscle	11 Medial head of gastrocnemius muscle	19 Plantaris muscle
4 Superior gemellus muscle	12 Gluteus medius muscle	20 Tendon of biceps femoris muscle
5 Obturator internus muscle	13 Adductor minimus muscle	21 Lateral head of gastrocnemius muscle
6 Inferior gemellus muscle	14 Adductor magnus muscle	22 Membranous part of
7 Ischial tuberosity	15 Long head of biceps femoris muscle	semimembranosus muscle
8 Quadratus femoris muscle	16 Iliotibial tract	

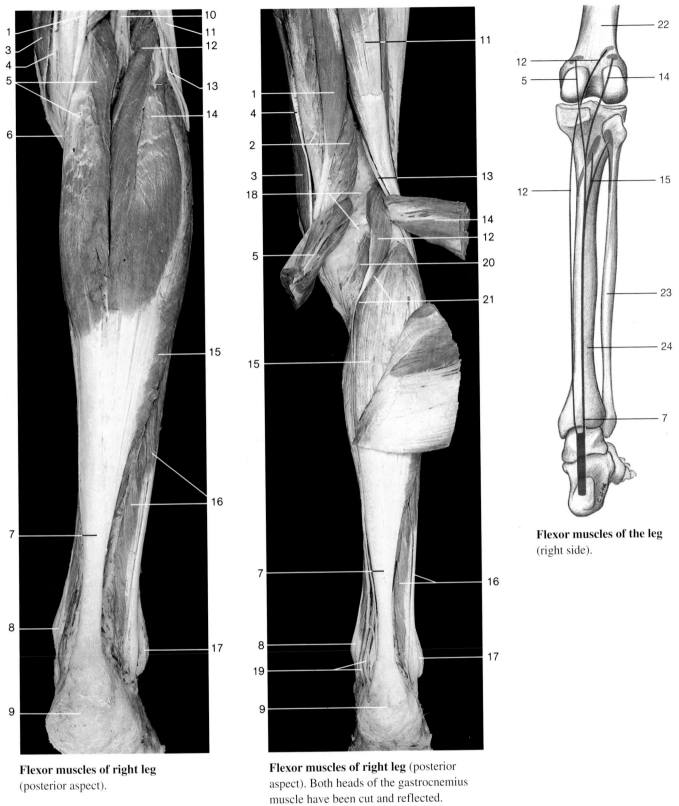

Flexor muscles of right leg
(posterior aspect).

Flexor muscles of right leg (posterior
aspect). Both heads of the gastrocnemius
muscle have been cut and reflected.

Flexor muscles of the leg
(right side).

1	Semitendinosus muscle		9	Calcaneal tuberosity	18	Popliteal fossa
2	Semimembranosus muscle		10	Tibial nerve	19	Tibial nerve and posterior tibial artery
3	Sartorius muscle		11	Biceps femoris muscle	20	Popliteus muscle
4	Tendon of gracilis muscle		12	Plantaris muscle	21	Tendinous arch of soleus muscle
5	**Medial head of gastrocnemius muscle**		13	Common peroneal nerve	22	Femur
6	Common tendon of gracilis,		14	**Lateral head of gastrocnemius muscle**	23	Fibula
	sartorius, and semitendinosus muscles		15	**Soleus muscle**	24	Tibia
7	Calcaneal or Achilles tendon		16	Peroneus longus and brevis muscles		
8	Medial malleolus		17	Lateral malleolus		

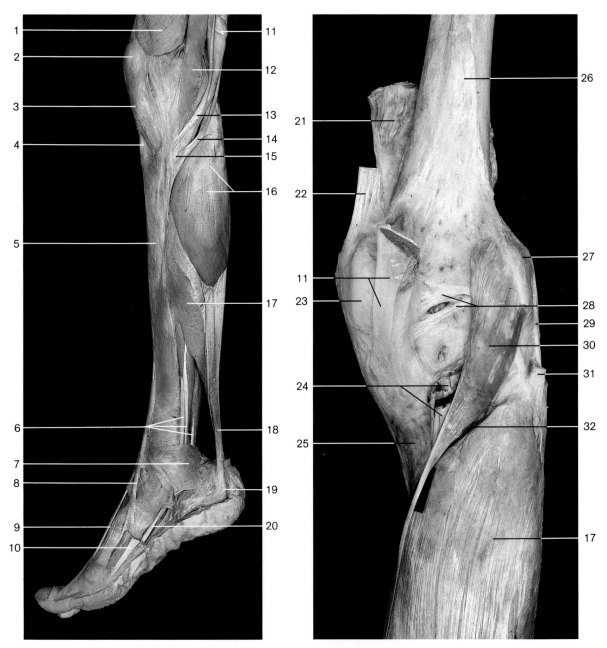

Muscles of right leg and foot (medial aspect).

Popliteal region with plantaris and soleus, right side (dorsal aspect). Notice the insertion of the tendon of semimembranosus.

1 Vastus medialis muscle
2 Patella
3 Patellar ligament
4 Tibial tuberosity
5 Tibia
6 Tendons of deep flexor muscles (from anterior to posterior: 1. tibialis posterior; 2. flexor digitorum longus; 3. flexor hallucis longus muscles)
7 Flexor retinaculum
8 Tendon of tibialis anterior muscle
9 Tendon of extensor hallucis longus muscle
10 Abductor hallucis muscle
11 Semimembranosus muscle
12 Sartorius muscle
13 Tendon gracilis muscle
14 Tendon of semitendinosus muscle
15 Common tendon of gracilis, semitendinosus and sartorius muscles

16 **Medial head of gastrocnemius muscle**
17 **Soleus muscle**
18 Calcaneal or Achilles tendon
19 Calcaneus muscle
20 Tendon of flexor hallucis longus muscle
21 Quadriceps femoris muscle (divided)
22 Tendon of adductor magnus muscle (divided)
23 Medial condyle of femur
24 Popliteal artery and vein, tibial nerve
25 Tibia
26 Femur
27 Lateral epicondyle of femur
28 Oblique popliteal ligament
29 Lateral (fibular) collateral ligament
30 **Plantaris muscle**
31 Tendon of biceps femoris muscle (divided)
32 Tendinous arch of soleus muscle

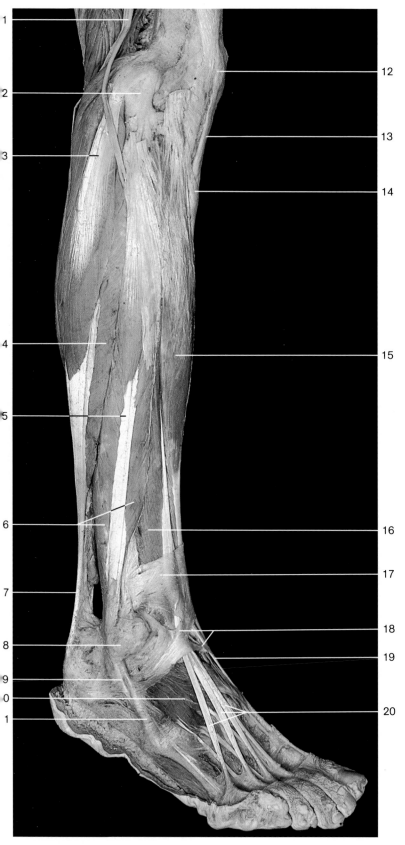

Muscles of right leg and foot (lateral aspect).

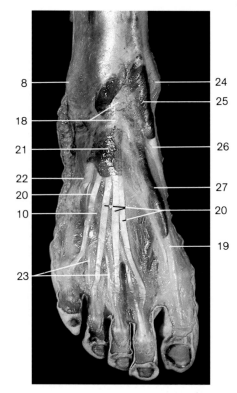

Right foot with synovial sheaths of extensor muscles (dorsal aspect). The synovial sheaths have been injected with blue solution.

1 Common peroneal nerve
2 Head of fibula
3 Lateral head of gastrocnemius muscle
4 Soleus muscle
5 Peroneus longus muscle
6 Peroneus brevis muscle
7 Calcaneal or Achilles tendon
8 Lateral malleolus muscle
9 Tendon of peroneus longus muscle
10 Extensor digitorum brevis muscle
11 Tendon of peroneus brevis muscle
12 Patella
13 Patellar ligament
14 Tuberosity of tibia
15 Tibialis anterior muscle
16 Extensor digitorum longus muscle
17 Superior extensor retinaculum
18 Inferior extensor retinaculum
19 Tendon of extensor hallucis longus muscle
20 Tendons of extensor digitorum longus muscle
21 Common synovial sheath of extensor digitorum longus muscle
22 Tendon of peroneus tertius muscle to the lateral margin of foot
23 Tendons of extensor digitorum brevis muscle
24 Medial malleolus
25 Synovial sheath of tendon of tibialis anterior muscle
26 Tendon of tibialis anterior muscle
27 Synovial sheath of tendon of extensor hallucis longus muscle

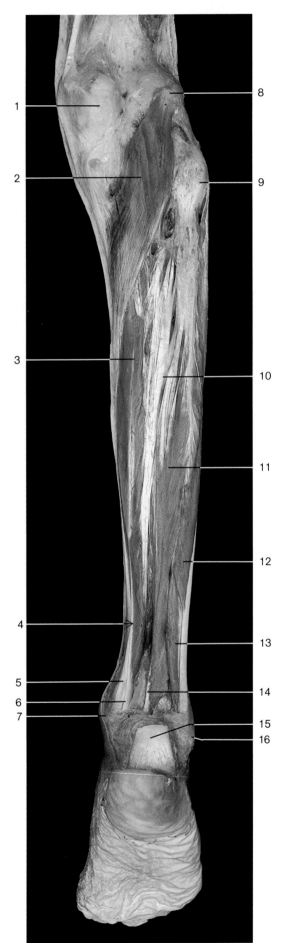

1 Medial condyle of femur
2 Popliteus muscle
3 Flexor digitorum longus muscle
4 Crossing of tendons in leg
5 Tendon of tibialis posterior muscle
6 Tendon of flexor digitorum longus muscle
7 Medial malleolus
8 Lateral condyle of femur
9 Head of fibula
10 Tibialis posterior muscle
11 Flexor hallucis longus muscle
12 Peroneus longus muscle
13 Peroneus brevis muscle
14 Tendon of flexor hallucis longus muscle
15 Calcaneal tendon (divided)
16 Lateral malleolus

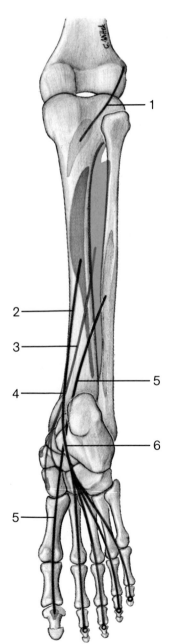

1 Popliteus muscle (blue)
2 Flexor digitorum longus muscle (blue)
3 Tibialis posterior muscle (red)
4 Crossing of tendons in leg
5 Flexor hallucis longus muscle (blue)
6 Crossing of tendons in sole

Deep flexor muscles of right leg
(posterior aspect).

Course of deep flexor muscles of leg. (Schematic drawing.)

1 Medial condyle of femur
2 Tibia
3 Flexor digitorum longus muscle
4 Crossing of tendons in leg
5 Tendon of tibialis posterior muscle
6 Abductor hallucis muscle
7 Tendon of flexor hallucis longus muscle
8 Lateral condyle of femur
9 Head of fibula
10 Tibialis posterior muscle
11 Tendon of flexor digitorum longus muscle
12 Flexor retinaculum
13 Calcaneal tendon
14 Calcaneal tuberosity
15 Crossing of tendons in sole
16 Quadratus plantae muscle
17 Tendons of flexor digitorum longus muscle
18 Tendon of tibialis anterior muscle
19 Area of insertion of tibialis posterior muscle
20 Lumbrical muscles
21 Flexor hallucis longus muscle

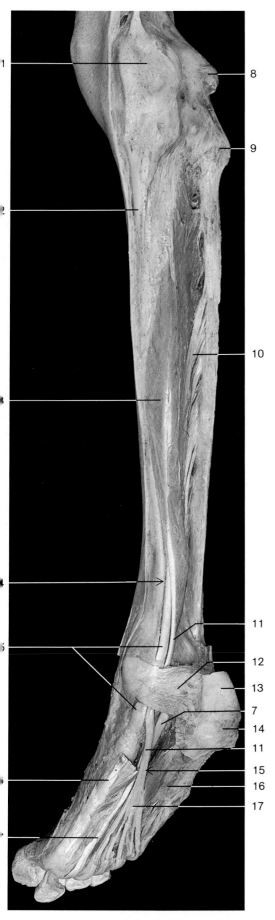

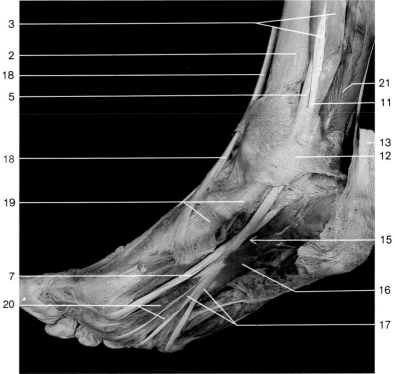

Deep flexor muscles of right leg and foot
(posterior oblique medial aspect). Flexor
digitorum brevis and flexor hallucis longus
muscles have been removed.

Sole of foot; tendons of long flexor muscles (oblique medial and inferior
aspect).

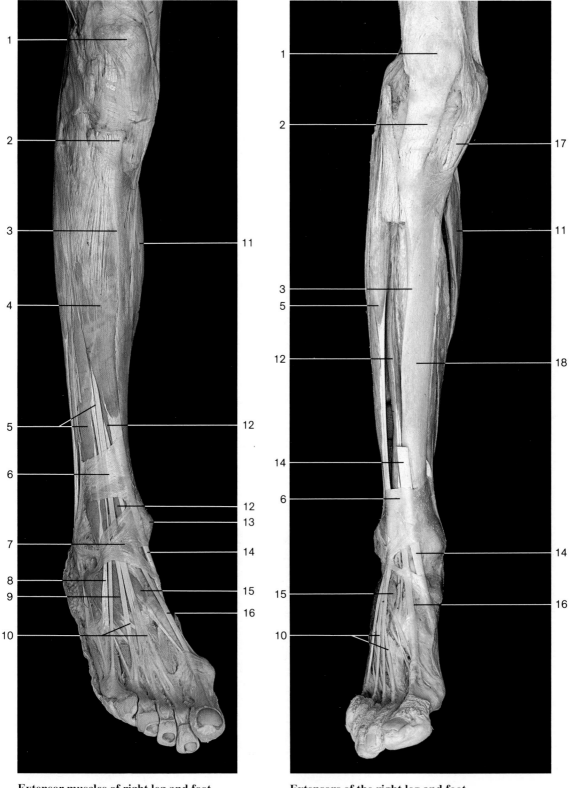

Extensor muscles of right leg and foot
(oblique anterolateral aspect).

Extensors of the right leg and foot
(anterior aspect). Part of the tibialis anterior muscle
has been removed.

1 Patella	8 Tendon of peroneus tertius muscle	14 Tendon of tibialis anterior muscle
2 Patellar ligament	9 Extensor digitorum brevis muscle	15 Extensor hallucis brevis muscle
3 Anterior margin of tibia	10 Tendons of extensor digitorum	16 Tendon of extensor hallucis
4 Tibialis anterior muscle	longus muscle	longus muscle
5 Extensor digitorum longus muscle	11 Gastrocnemius muscle	17 Common tendon of gracilis,
6 Superior extensor retinaculum	12 Extensor hallucis longus muscle	semitendinosus and sartorius muscles
7 Inferior extensor retinaculum	13 Medial malleolus	18 Tibia

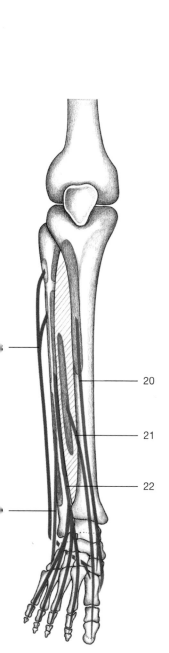

Extensor muscles of the leg (right side).

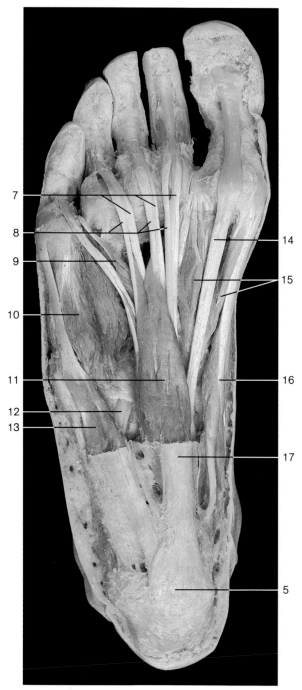

Sole of foot, first layer of muscles (from below). The plantar aponeurosis and the fasciae of the superficial muscles have been removed.

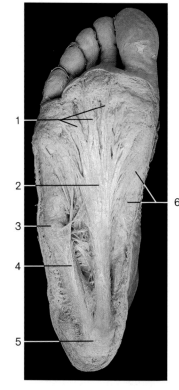

Sole of foot, plantar aponeurosis (from below).

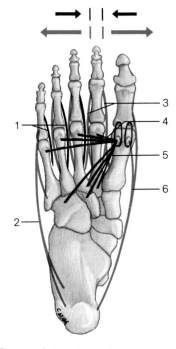

Course of abductor and adductor muscles of foot.
(Schematic drawing.)
Red arrows = abduction.
Black arrows = adduction.

1 Plantar interossei muscles (black)
2 Abductor digiti minimi muscle (red)
3 Dorsal interosseous muscles (red)
4 Transverse head of adductor muscle (black)
5 Oblique head of adductor muscle (black)
6 Abductor hallucis muscle (red)

1 Longitudinal bands of plantar aponeurosis
2 Plantar aponeurosis
3 Position of tuberosity of fifth metatarsal bone
4 Muscles of fifth toe with fascia
5 Calcaneal tuberosity
6 Muscles of great toe with fascia
7 Tendons of flexor digitorum longus muscle
8 Tendons of flexor digitorum brevis muscle
9 Lumbrical muscle
10 Flexor digiti minimi brevis muscle
11 Flexor digitorum brevis muscle

12 Tendon of peroneus longus muscle
13 Abductor digiti minimi muscle
14 Tendon of flexor hallucis longus muscle
15 Flexor hallucis brevis muscle
16 Abductor hallucis muscle
17 Plantar aponeurosis (cut)
18 Peroneus longus muscle
19 Peroneus brevis muscle
20 Tibialis anterior muscle
21 Extensor hallucis longus muscle
22 Extensor digitorum longus muscle

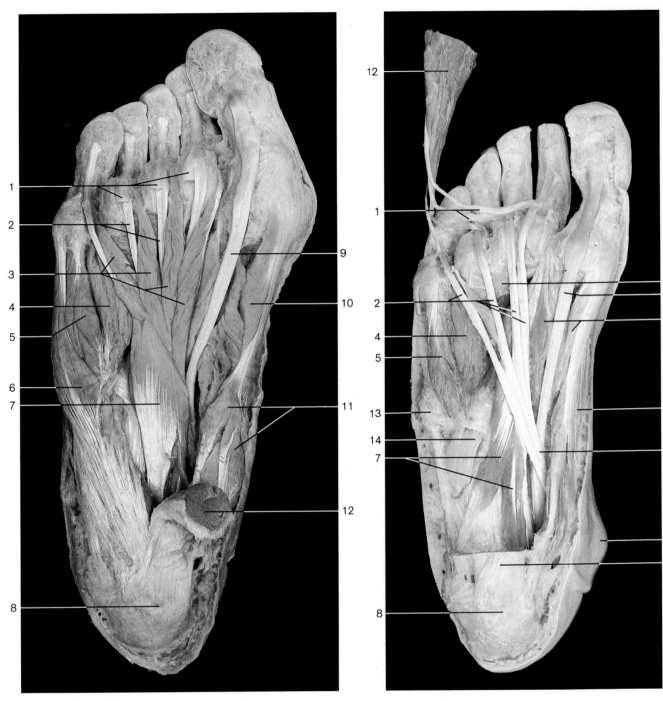

Muscles of sole of foot, second layer (from below).
The flexor digitorum brevis muscle has been divided.

Muscles of sole of foot, second layer (from below).
The tendons of the flexor muscles and the crossing of
tendons are displayed. The flexor digitorum brevis
muscle has been divided and reflected.

1 Tendons of flexor digitorum brevis muscle	6 Abductor digiti minimi muscle	13 Tuberosity of fifth metatarsal bone
2 Tendons of flexor digitorum longus muscle	7 Quadratus plantae muscle	14 Tendon of peroneus longus muscle
3 Lumbrical muscles	8 Calcaneal tuberosity	15 Transverse head of adductor hallucis muscle
4 Interossei muscles	9 Tendon of flexor hallucis longus muscle	16 Crossing of tendons in sole of foot
5 Flexor digiti minimi brevis muscle	10 Flexor hallucis brevis muscle	17 Medial malleolus
	11 Abductor hallucis muscle	18 Plantar aponeurosis (divided)
	12 Flexor digitorum brevis muscle (divided)	

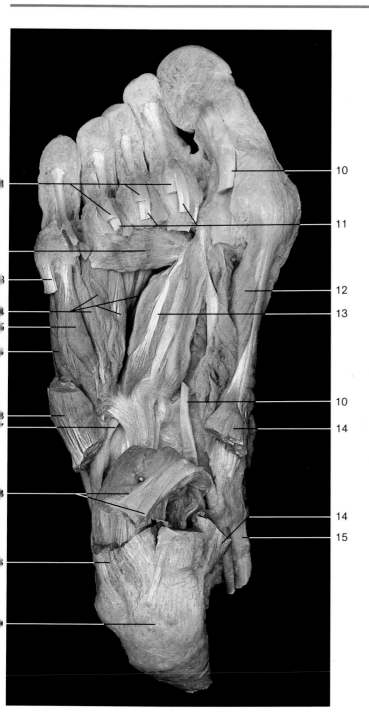

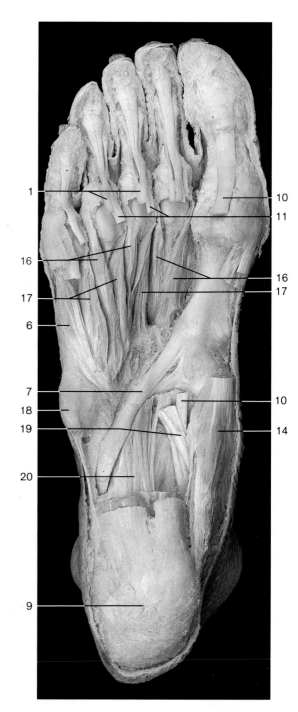

Muscles of sole of foot, third layer (from below). The flexor digitorum brevis muscle has been removed, and the quadratus plantae muscle and the abductor hallucis and digiti minimi muscles have been divided.

Muscles of sole of foot, fourth layer (from below). The interosseous muscles and the canal for the tendon of peroneus longus muscle are shown.

1 Tendons of flexor digitorum brevis muscle
2 Transverse head of adductor hallucis muscle
3 Abductor digiti minimi muscle
4 Interossei muscles
5 Flexor digiti minimi brevis muscle
6 Opponens digiti minimi muscle
7 Tendon of peroneus longus muscle

8 Quadratus plantae muscle with tendon of flexor digitorum longus muscle
9 Calcaneal tuberosity
10 Tendons of flexor hallucis longus muscle (divided)
11 Tendon of flexor digitorum longus muscle
12 Flexor hallucis brevis muscle
13 Oblique head of adductor hallucis muscle
14 Abductor hallucis muscle (cut)

15 Tendon of tibialis posterior muscle
16 Dorsal interossei muscles
17 Plantar interossei muscles
18 Tuberosity of fifth metatarsal bone
19 Tendon of flexor digitorum longus muscle (crossing of plantar tendons)
20 Long plantar ligament

452

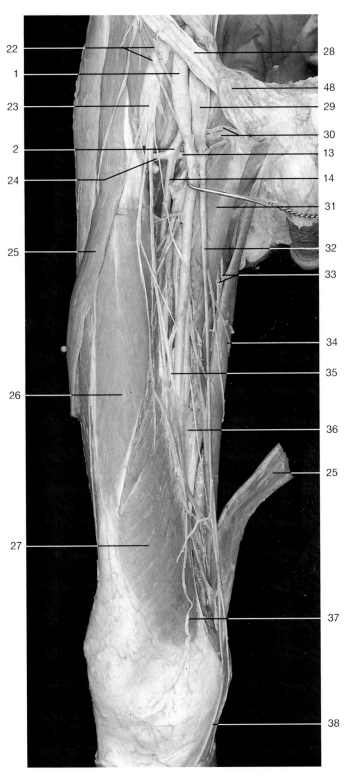

22		28
1		48
23		29
2		30
24		13
		14
		31
25		32
		33
26		34
		35
27		36
		25
		37
		38

Main arteries and nerves of right thigh (anterior aspect).
Sartorius muscle has been divided and reflected.
The femoral vein has been partly removed to show the
deep femoral artery. Notice: the vessels enter the adductor
canal to reach the popliteal fossa.

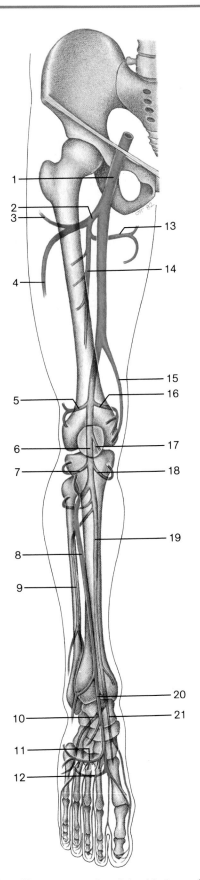

Main arteries of lower extremity, right side (ventral aspect).
(Schematic drawing.)

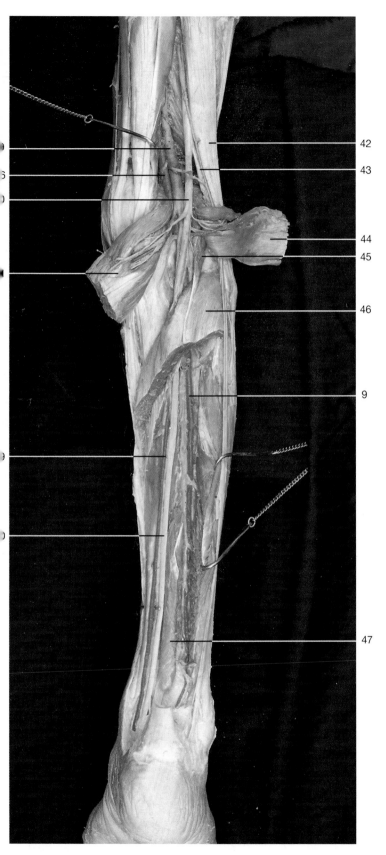

Arteries of the right leg (posterior aspect).

1 **Femoral artery**
2 **Profunda femoris artery**
3 Ascending branch of lateral circumflex femoral artery
4 Descending branch of lateral circumflex femoral artery
5 Lateral superior genicular artery
6 Popliteal artery
7 Lateral inferior genicular artery
8 **Anterior tibial artery**
9 **Peroneal artery**
10 **Lateral plantar artery**
11 Arcuate artery with dorsal metatarsal arteries
12 **Plantar arch** with plantar metatarsal arteries
13 Medial circumflex femoral artery
14 Profunda femoris artery with perforating arteries
15 Descending genicular artery
16 Medial superior genicular artery
17 Middle genicular artery
18 Medial inferior genicular artery
19 **Posterior tibial artery**
20 **Dorsalis pedis artery**
21 **Medial plantar artery**
22 Superficial and deep circumflex iliac arteries
23 **Femoral nerve**
24 Lateral circumflex femoral artery
25 Sartorius muscle (cut and reflected)
26 Rectus femoris muscle
27 Vastus medialis muscle
28 Inguinal ligament
29 **Femoral vein** (cut)
30 External pudendal artery and vein
31 Adductor longus muscle
32 Great saphenous vein
33 Obturator artery and nerve
34 Gracilis muscle
35 Saphenous nerve
36 Tendinous wall of adductor canal
37 Anterior cutaneous branch of femoral nerve
38 Infrapatellar branch of saphenous nerve
39 Popliteal vein
40 **Tibial nerve**
41 Medial head of gastrocnemius muscle
42 Biceps femoris muscle
43 Common peroneal nerve
44 Lateral head of gastrocnemius muscle
45 Plantaris muscle
43 Soleus muscle
47 Flexor hallucis longus muscle
48 Spermatic cord

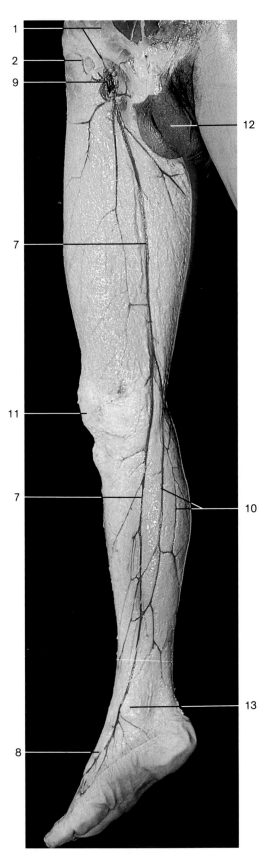

Main veins of lower limb, right side (anterior aspect).
(Schematic drawing.)

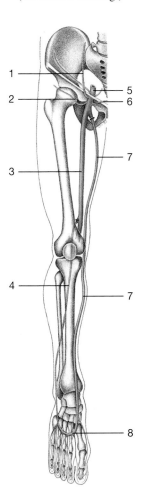

1 Superficial epigastric vein
2 Superficial circumflex iliac vein
3 Femoral vein
4 **Small saphenous vein**
5 External iliac vein
6 External pudendal vein
7 **Great saphenous vein**
8 Dorsal venous arch
9 Saphenous opening with femoral vein
10 Venous anastomoses of small saphenous
   vein with great saphenous vein
11 Patella
12 Penis
13 Medial malleolus
14 Popliteal fossa
15 Perforating veins
16 Lateral malleolus
17 Dorsal digital veins of foot
18 Dorsal venous arch of foot
19 Dorsal metatarsal veins of foot
20 Anterior tibial artery and veins
21 Tibia
22 **Posterior tibial artery and veins**
23 Fibula
24 Peroneal artery and vein
25 Deep layer of crural fascia
26 Superficial layer of crural fascia
27 Perforating veins I–III (of Cockett)
28 **Tibial nerve**
29 **Arcuate vein**
30 **Saphenous nerve**
31 Medial dorsal cutaneous nerve
   (branch of superficial peroneal nerve)
32 Posterior tibial vein

Superficial veins of lower limb, right side
(medial anterior aspect). The veins have
been injected with red solution.

▷

Medial malleolar region. Dissection of
tibial nerve, posterior tibial vessels, and
great saphenous vein (veins injected with
blue resin).

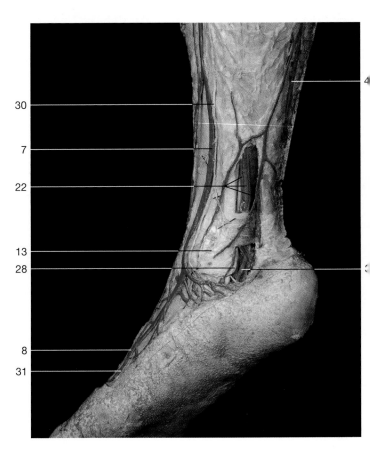

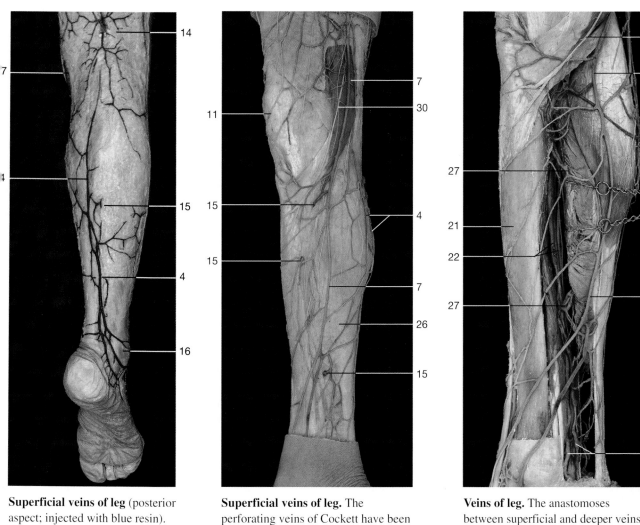

Superficial veins of leg (posterior aspect; injected with blue resin).

Superficial veins of leg. The perforating veins of Cockett have been dissected (left side, medial aspect).

Veins of leg. The anastomoses between superficial and deeper veins are dissected (left side, medial aspect).

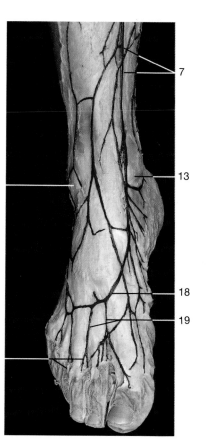

Anastomoses between superficial and deep veins of the leg (after Aigner). (Schematic drawing.) Arrows: directions of blood flow. ▷

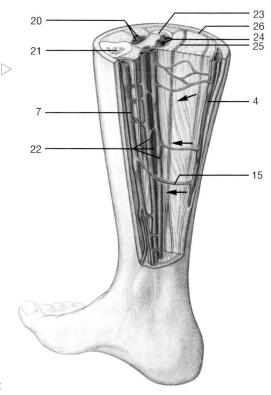

◁

Superficial veins on dorsum of foot (injected with blue resin).

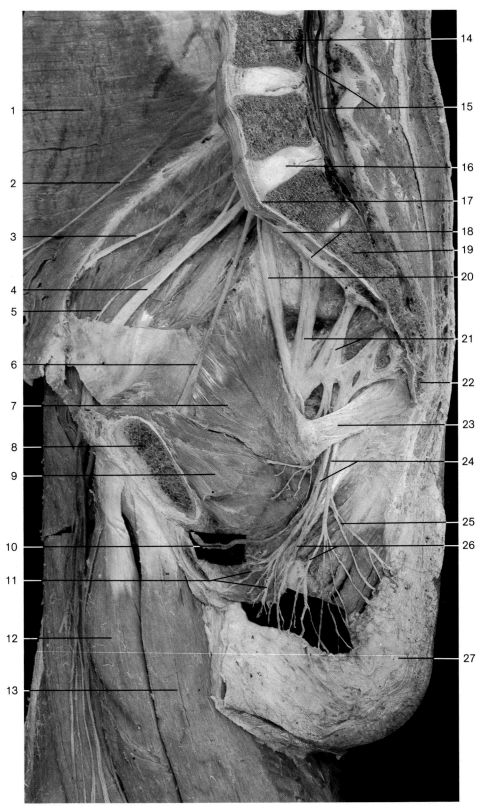

1 Transversus abdominis muscle
2 Iliohypogastric nerve
3 Ilioinguinal nerve
4 **Femoral nerve**
5 Lateral femoral cutaneous nerve
6 Obturator nerve
7 Obturator internus muscle
8 Pubic bone (cut edge)
9 Levator ani muscle (remnant)
10 Dorsal nerve of penis
11 Posterior scrotal nerves
12 Adductor longus muscle
13 Gracilis muscle
14 Body of fourth lumbar vertebra
15 Cauda equina
16 Intervertebral disc
17 Sacral promontory
18 Sympathetic trunk
19 Sacrum
20 **Lumbosacral trunk**
21 **Sacral plexus**
22 Coccyx
23 Sacrospinous ligament
24 **Pudendal nerve**
25 Inferior rectal nerves
26 Perineal nerves
27 Subcutaneous fat tissue
    of gluteal region

Lumbosacral plexus in situ, right side (medial aspect).
Pelvic organs with peritoneum and part of the levator ani muscle have been removed.

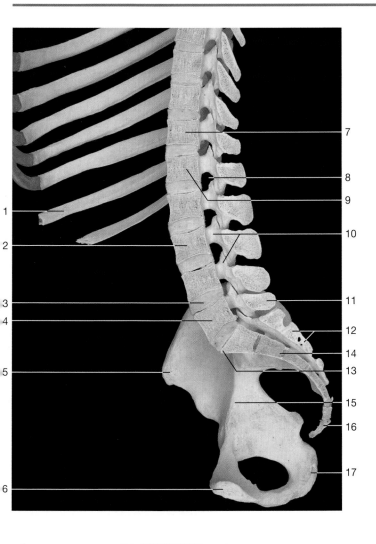

Lumbar part of vertebral column with pelvis
(sagittal section, medial aspect).

1   Eleventh rib
2   Body of third lumbar vertebra
3   Intervertebral disc
4   Body of fifth lumbar vertebra
5   Anterior superior iliac spine
6   Symphyseal surface
7   Body of twelfth thoracic vertebra
8   Intervertebral foramen
9   Body of first lumbar vertebra
10 **Vertebral canal**
11 Spinous process of fifth lumbar vertebra
12 Sacrum (median sacral crest)
13 Promontory (Promontorium)
14 Sacrum
15 Arcuate line
16 Coccyx
17 Ischial tuberosity
18 Sympathetic trunk with ganglia
19 Ureter
20 Iliohypogastric nerve (Th_{12}, L_1)
21 Ilioinguinal nerve (L_1)
22 **Femoral nerve** (L_2–L_4)
23 Genitofemoral nerve (L_1, L_2)
24 **Inferior hypogastric plexus**
25 Ductus deferens
26 Urinary bladder
27 Medullary cone of spinal cord
28 Root filaments of spinal nerves
29 Subarachnoidal cavity
    (filled with cerebrospinal fluid) (blue)
30 Terminal filament of spinal cord
31 **Sacral plexus**
32 Pelvic splanchnic nerves (nervi erigentes)
33 Rectum

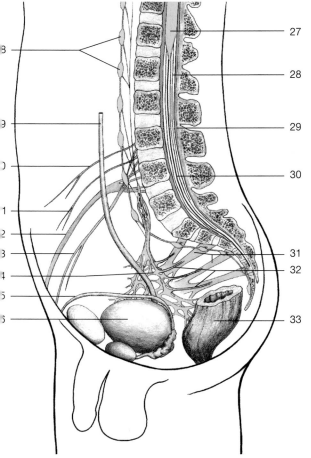

Vertebral canal with spinal cord and root filaments.
Note the high location of the medullary cone.
Sacral plexus and inferior hypogastric plexus are
schematically shown.

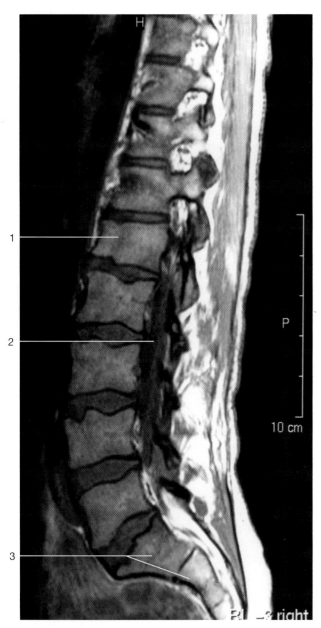

MRI scan of lumbar part of vertebral canal (paramedian section).

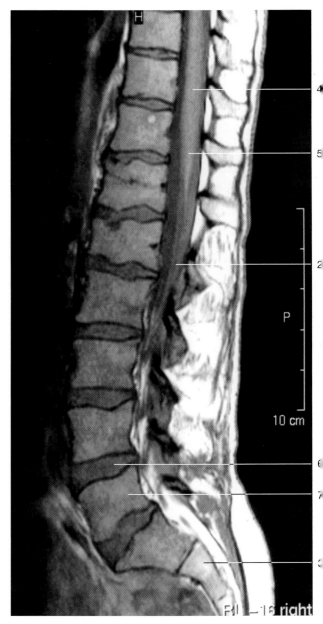

MRI scan of lumbar part of vertebral canal at the level of the medullary cone (median section).

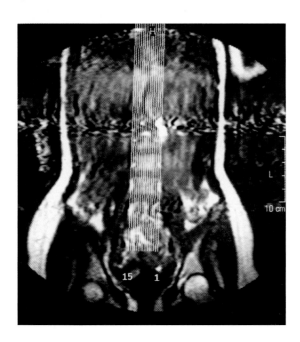

1 First lumbar vertebra
2 Root filaments of spinal nerves
3 Sacrum
4 **Spinal cord**
5 Medullary cone of spinal cord
6 Intervertebral disk between fourth and fifth lumbar vertebra
7 Fifth lumbar vertebra

Location of the sagittal sections through the vertebral canal. (Sections 7 and 11 are depicted above; courtesy of Prof. W. Bautz, Erlangen, Germany).

1 Subcostal nerve
2 Iliohypogastric nerve
3 Ilioinguinal nerve
4 Lateral femoral cutaneous nerve
5 Genitofemoral nerve
6 **Pudendal nerve**
7 **Femoral nerve**
8 Obturator nerve
9 **Sciatic nerve**
10 Lumbar plexus (L_1–L_4)
11 Sacral plexus (L_4–S_4)   } lumbosacral plexus
12 "Pudendal" plexus (S_2–S_4)
13 Inferior cluneal nerve
14 Posterior femoral cutaneous nerve
15 Common peroneal nerve
16 **Tibial nerve**
17 Lateral sural cutaneous nerve
18 Medial and lateral plantar nerves
19 Saphenous nerve
20 Infrapatellar branch of saphenous nerve
21 **Deep peroneal nerve**
22 **Superficial peroneal nerve**
23 Anterior cutaneous branch of iliohypogastric nerve
24 Lateral cutaneous branch of iliohypogastric nerve
25 Femoral branch of genitofemoral nerve
26 Lateral cutaneous branches of intercostal nerve
27 Anterior cutaneous branches of intercostal nerve
28 Genital branch of genitofemoral nerve
29 Anterior scrotal nerve

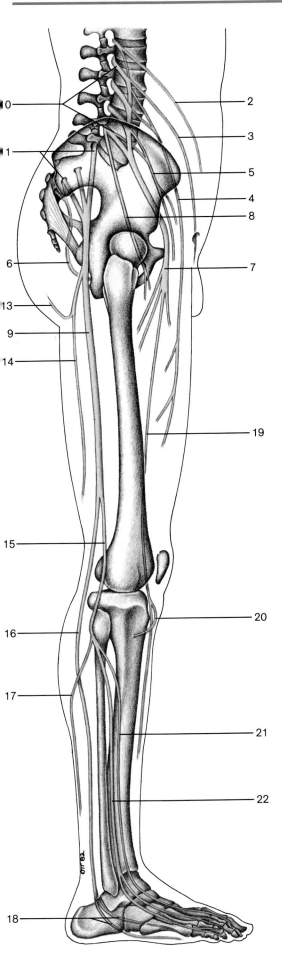

Nerves of lower limb, right side (lateral aspect).
(Schematic drawing.)

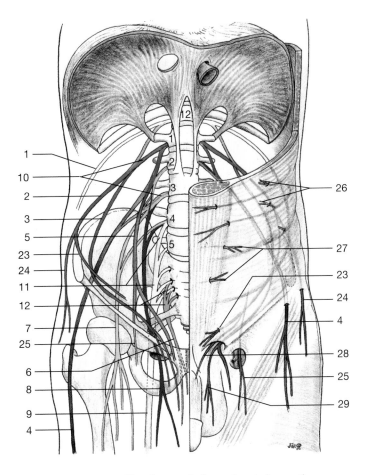

Main branches of lumbosacral plexus (ventral aspect).
(Schematic drawing.)

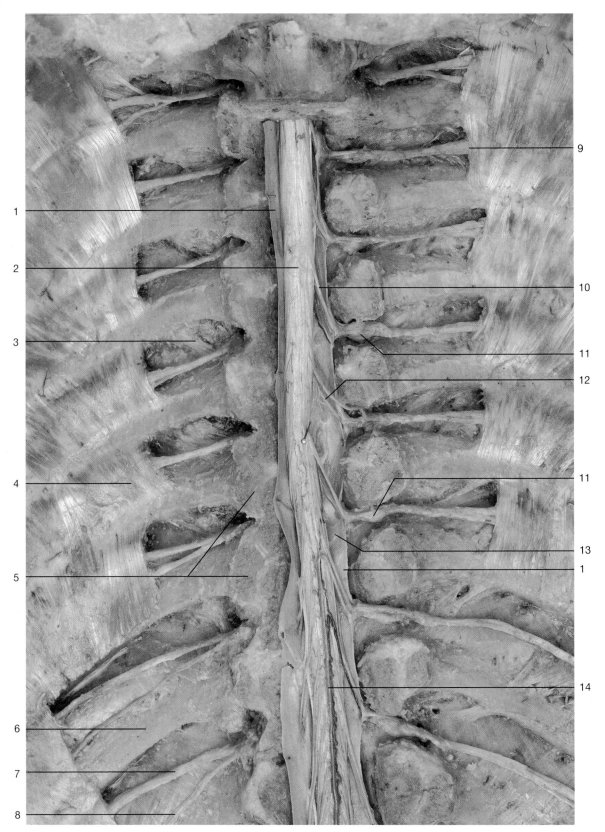

Spinal cord with intercostal nerves. Inferior thoracic region (anterior aspect). Anterior portion of thoracic vertebrae removed, dural sheath opened and spinal cord slightly reflected to the right to display the dorsal and ventral roots.

1 Dura mater	6 Eleventh rib	10 Anterior root filaments
2 **Spinal cord**	7 **Intercostal nerve**	11 Spinal (dorsal root) ganglion
3 Costotransverse ligament	8 Collateral branch of intercostal nerve	12 Posterior root filaments
4 Innermost intercostal muscle	9 Intercostal nerve (entering the	13 Arachnoid mater and denticulate ligament
5 Vertebral arches (cut surfaces)	intermuscular interval)	14 Anterior spinal artery

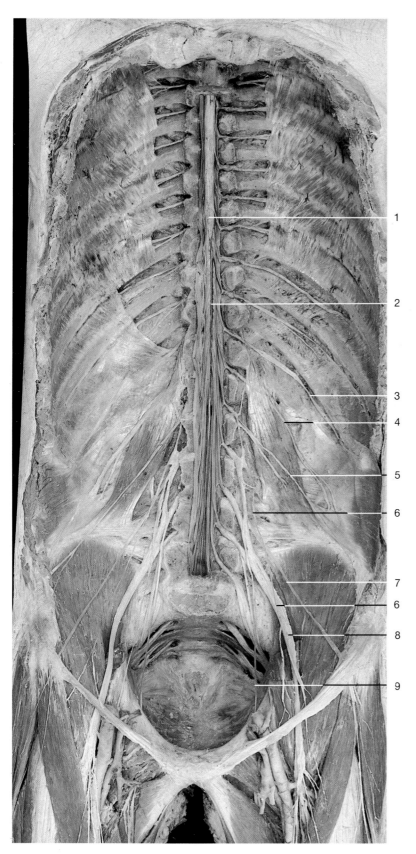

Spinal cord and lumbar plexus in situ (anterior aspect).

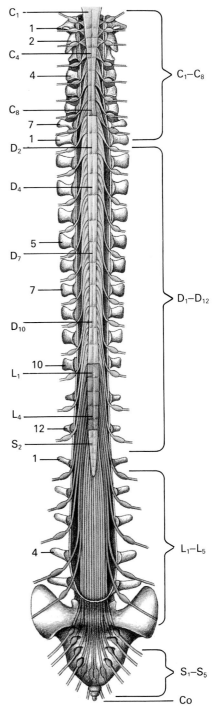

Organization of spinal cord segments in relation to the vertebral column (anterior aspect). C = cervical; D = thoracic; L = lumbar; S = sacral segments; Co = coccygeal bone. Numbers indicate the related vertebrae.

1	Conus medullaris	4	Iliohypogastric nerve
2	Filum terminale	5	Ilioinguinal nerve
3	Subcostal nerve	6	Genitofemoral nerve

7	Lateral femoral cutaneous nerve
8	Femoral nerve
9	Obturator nerve

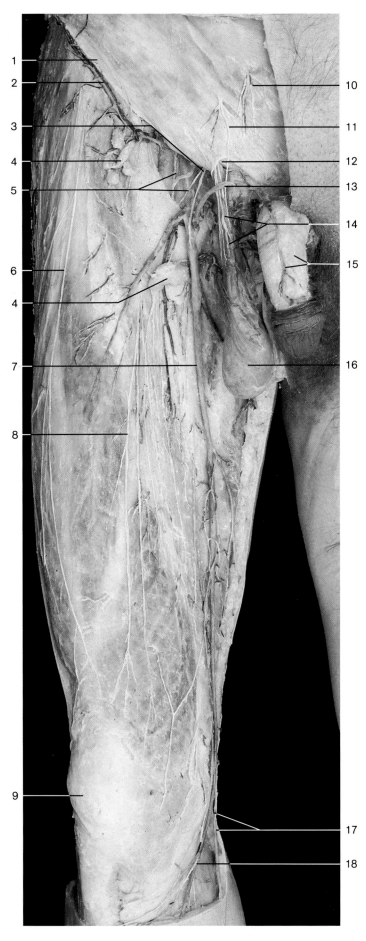

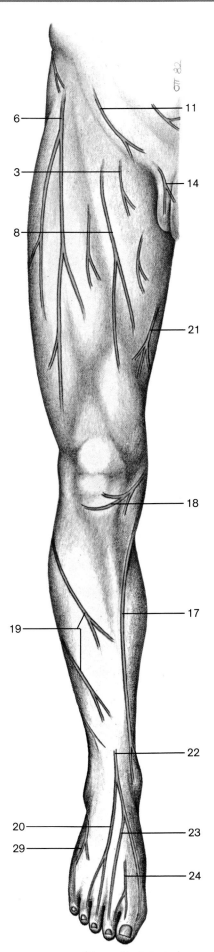

Cutaneous nerves and veins of thigh (anterior aspect).

Cutaneous nerves of lower limb (anterior aspect).
(Schematic drawing.)

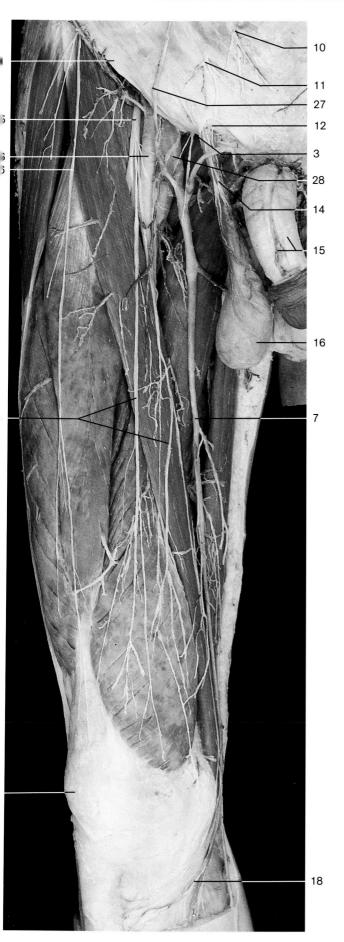

1 Inguinal ligament
2 Superficial circumflex iliac vein
3 Femoral branch of genitofemoral nerve
4 Superficial inguinal lymph nodes
5 Saphenous opening with femoral artery and vein
6 Lateral femoral cutaneous nerve
7 Great saphenous vein
8 Anterior cutaneous branches of femoral nerve
9 Patella
10 Terminal branches of subcostal nerve
11 Terminal branches of iliohypogastric nerve
12 Superficial inguinal ring
13 External pudendal vein
14 Spermatic cord with genital branch of genitofemoral nerve
15 Penis with superficial dorsal vein of penis
16 Testis and its coverings
17 Saphenous nerve
18 Infrapatellar branch of saphenous nerve
19 Lateral sural cutaneous nerves
20 Intermediate dorsal cutaneous branch of superficial peroneal nerve
21 Cutaneous branch of obturator nerve
22 Superficial peroneal nerve
23 Medial dorsal cutaneous branch of superficial peroneal nerve
24 Deep peroneal nerve
25 **Femoral nerve**
26 **Femoral artery**
27 Superficial epigastric vein
28 **Femoral vein**
29 Lateral dorsal cutaneous branch of sural nerve
30 **Inguinal nodes** (enlarged)
31 Lympathic vessels
32 Sartorius muscle

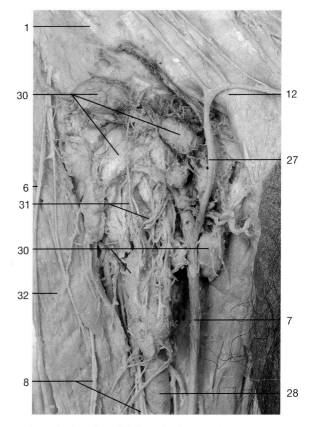

Cutaneous nerves and veins of thigh (anterior aspect).
The fascia lata and fasciae of the thigh muscles have been removed.

Inguinal nodes with lymphatic vessels
(anterior aspect).

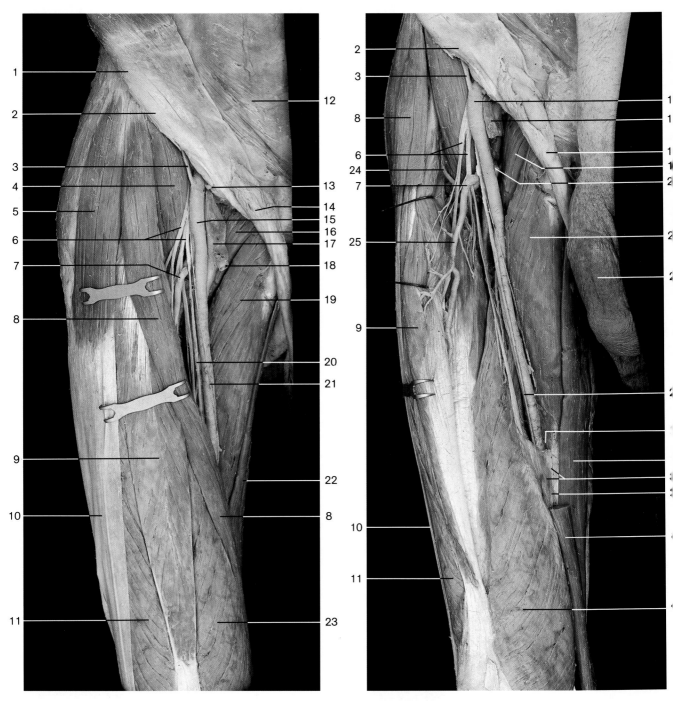

Anterior region of right thigh (anterior aspect).
The fascia lata has been removed, and the sartorius muscle
has been slightly reflected.

Anterior region of right thigh (anterior aspect).
The fascia lata has been removed, and the sartorius muscle
has been divided.

1 Anterior superior iliac spine
2 Inguinal ligament
3 **Deep circumflex iliac artery**
4 Iliopsoas muscle
5 Tensor fasciae latae muscle
6 **Femoral nerve**
7 **Lateral circumflex femoral artery**
8 Sartorius muscle
9 Rectus femoris muscle
10 Iliotibial tract
11 Vastus lateralis muscle
12 Anterior sheath of rectus abdominis muscle
13 Inferior epigastric artery
14 Spermatic cord
15 **Femoral artery**

16 Pectineus muscle
17 **Femoral vein**
18 Great saphenous vein (divided)
19 Adductor longus muscle
20 **Saphenous nerve**
21 Muscular branch of femoral nerve
22 Gracilis muscle
23 Vastus medialis muscle
24 Ascending branch of lateral circumflex femoral artery
25 Descending branch of lateral circumflex femoral artery
26 Medial circumflex femoral artery
27 Adductor longus muscle
28 Penis
29 Entrance to adductor canal
30 Vastoadductory lamina of fascia beneath sartorius muscle

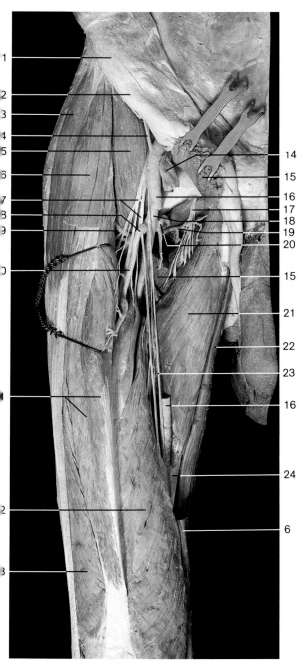

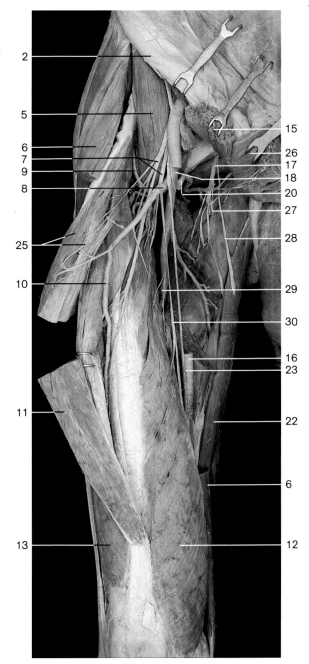

Anterior region of right thigh (anterior aspect).
The fascia lata has been removed. Sartorius muscle,
pectineus muscle and femoral artery have been cut to
display the deep femoral artery with its branches. The
rectus femoris muscle has been slightly reflected.

1   Anterior superior iliac spine
2   Inguinal ligament
3   Tensor fasciae latae muscle
4   Deep circumflex iliac artery
5   Iliopsoas muscle
6   Sartorius muscle (cut)
7   **Femoral nerve**
8   **Lateral circumflex femoral artery**
9   Ascending branch of lateral circumflex femoral artery
10 Descending branch of lateral circumflex femoral artery
11 Rectus femoris muscle
12 Vastus medialis muscle
13 Vastus lateralis muscle
14 Femoral vein
15 Pectineus muscle (cut)
16 Femoral artery (cut)

Anterior region of right thigh (anterior aspect).
The sartorius, pectineus, adductor longus and rectus
femoris muscles have been divided and reflected.
The greater part of the femoral artery has been
removed.

17 **Obturator nerve**
18 **Profunda femoris artery**
19 Ascending branch of medial circumflex femoral artery
20 **Medial circumflex femoral artery**
21 Adductor longus muscle
22 Gracilis muscle
23 Saphenous nerve
24 Distal part of vastoadductory lamina
25 Rectus femoris muscle with muscular branch of
    femoral nerve
26 Adductor longus muscle (divided)
27 Posterior branch of obturator nerve
28 Anterior branch of obturator nerve
29 Point at which perforating artery branches off from
    profunda femoris artery
30 Muscular branch of femoral nerve to vastus medialis muscle

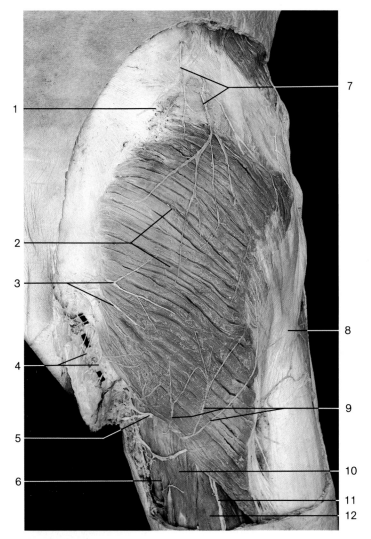

Gluteal region, right side (posterior aspect).

1 Iliac crest
2 Gluteus maximus muscle
3 **Middle cluneal nerves**
4 Anococcygeal nerves
5 Perineal branch of posterior femoral cutaneous nerve
6 Adductor magnus muscle
7 **Superior cluneal nerves**
8 Position of greater trochanter
9 **Inferior cluneal nerves**
10 Semitendinosus muscle
11 Posterior femoral cutaneous nerve
12 Long head of biceps femoris muscle

A **Suprapiriform foramen**
   of greater sciatic foramen

   Superior gluteal artery, vein and nerve

B **Infrapiriform foramen**
   of greater sciatic foramen

   Sciatic nerve
   Inferior gluteal artery, vein and nerve
   Posterior femoral cutaneous nerve
   Internal pudendal artery and vein
   Pudendal nerve

C **Lesser sciatic foramen**

   Pudendal nerve
   Internal pudendal artery and vein

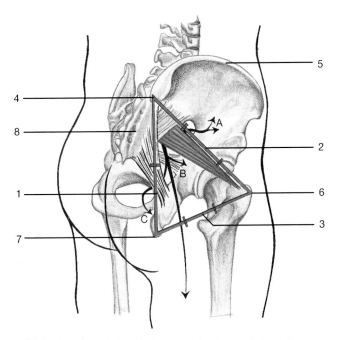

Gluteal region, right side (posterolateral aspect). Location of sciatic foramina in relation to the bones. (Schematic drawing.)

Red lines

1 **Spine-tuber line.**
   In the middle of this line the infrapiriform foramen is situated
2 **Spine-trochanter line.**
   In the upper third the suprapiriform foramen is located
3 **Tuber-trochanter line.**
   Between the middle and posterior third, the ischiadic nerve can be found

Other structures

4 Posterior superior iliac spine
5 Iliac crest
6 Greater trochanter
7 Ischial tuberosity
8 Sacrum

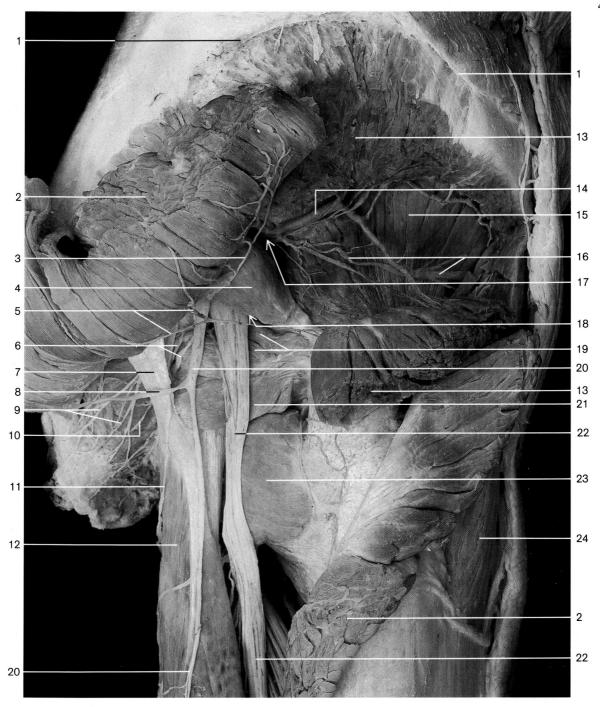

Gluteal region, right side (dorsal aspect). The gluteus maximus and gluteus medius muscles have been divided and reflected. Notice the position of the foramina above and below the piriformis muscle and the lesser sciatic foramen.

1	Iliac crest	13	Gluteus medius muscle (cut)
2	Gluteus maximus muscle (cut)	14	Deep branch of superior gluteal artery
3	Inferior gluteal nerve	15	Gluteus minimus muscle
4	Piriformis muscle	16	Superior gluteal nerve
5	Muscular branches of inferior gluteal artery	17	**Suprapiriform foramen**
6	Pudendal nerve and internal pudendal artery within the	18	**Infrapiriform foramen** } greater sciatic foramen
	lesser sciatic foramen (entrance to the pudendal canal)	19	Tendon of obturator internus and superior gemellus
7	Sacrotuberous ligament		muscles
8	Inferior cluneal nerve	20	Posterior femoral cutaneous nerve
9	Inferior rectal nerves	21	Inferior gemellus muscle
10	Inferior rectal arteries	22	**Sciatic nerve**
11	Perforating cutaneous nerve	23	Quadratus femoris muscle
12	Long head of biceps femoris muscle	24	Tensor fasciae latae muscle

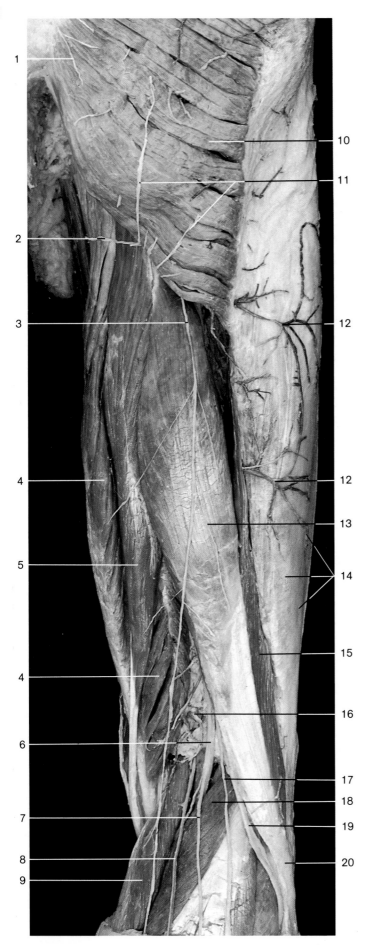

1   Middle cluneal nerves
2   Perineal branch of posterior femoral cutaneous nerve
3   **Posterior femoral cutaneous nerve**
4   Semimembranosus muscle
5   Semitendinosus muscle
6   **Tibial nerve**
7   Medial sural cutaneous nerve
8   **Small saphenous vein**
9   Medial head of gastrocnemius muscle
10   Gluteus maximus muscle
11   **Inferior cluneal nerve**
12   Cutaneous veins
13   Long head of biceps femoris muscle
14   Iliotibial tract
15   Short head of biceps femoris muscle
16   Popliteal fossa
17   Lateral sural cutaneous nerve
18   Lateral head of gastrocnemius muscle
19   **Common peroneal nerve**
20   Tendon of biceps femoris muscle
21   Inferior gluteal nerve
22   Sacrotuberous ligament
23   Inferior rectal branches of pudendal nerve
24   Anus
25   Gluteus medius muscle
26   Piriformis muscle
27   **Sciatic nerve**
28   Inferior gluteal artery
29   Gluteus maximus muscle (cut)
30   Quadratus femoris muscle
31   Sciatic nerve dividing into its two branches: the common peroneal nerve and the tibial nerve
32   Muscular branches of sciatic nerve to hamstring muscles
33   **Popliteal artery**
34   **Popliteal vein**
35   Small saphenous vein (cut)
36   Long head of biceps femoris muscle (cut)
37   **Superficial peroneal nerve**

Cutaneous nerves of thigh (posterior aspect).
The fascia lata and the fasciae of muscles have been removed.

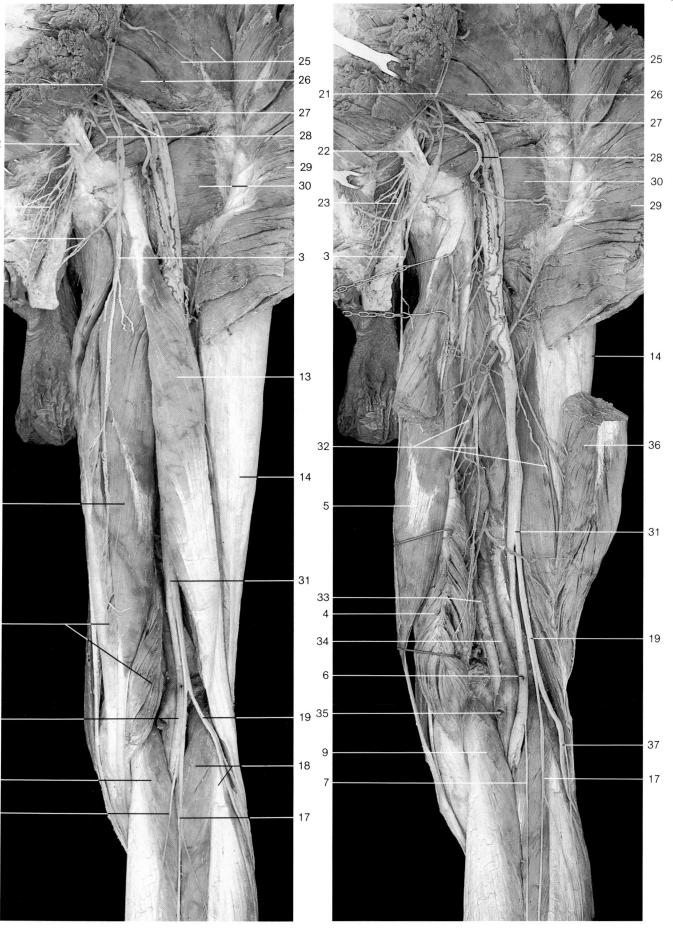

Posterior femoral region and gluteal region, right side (posterior aspect). The gluteus maximus muscle has been divided and reflected.

Posterior femoral region and gluteal region, right side (posterior aspect). The gluteus maximus muscle and the long head of biceps femoris muscle have been divided and reflected.

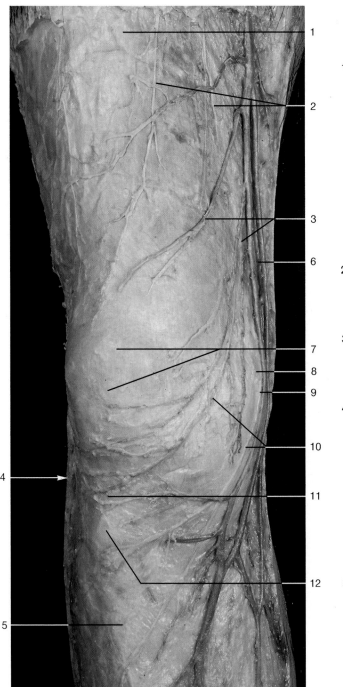

Anterior region of right knee, cutaneous nerves and veins
(anterior aspect).

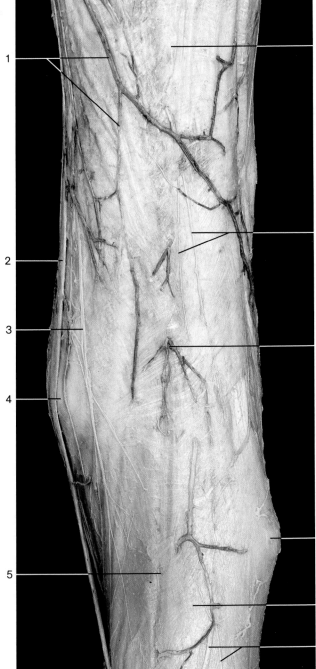

Posterior region of right knee, cutaneous nerves and veins
(posterior aspect).

1   Fascia lata
2   Terminal branches of anterior cutaneous branches
    of femoral nerve
3   Venous network around knee
4   Position of head of fibula
5   Superficial crural fascia
6   **Great saphenous vein**
7   Patella
8   Position of medial epicondyle of femur
9   Saphenous nerve
10 **Infrapatellar branches of saphenous nerve**
11 Patellar ligament
12 Position of tuberosity of tibia

1   Cutaneous veins (tributaries of great saphenous vein)
2   **Great saphenous vein**
3   Cutaneous branch of femoral nerve
4   Position of medial epicondyle of femur
5   Position of small saphenous vein
6   Fascia lata
7   Terminal branches of **posterior femoral cutaneous nerve**
8   Cutaneous veins of popliteal fossa
9   Position of head of fibula
10 Superficial layer of fascia cruris
11 Lateral sural cutaneous nerve

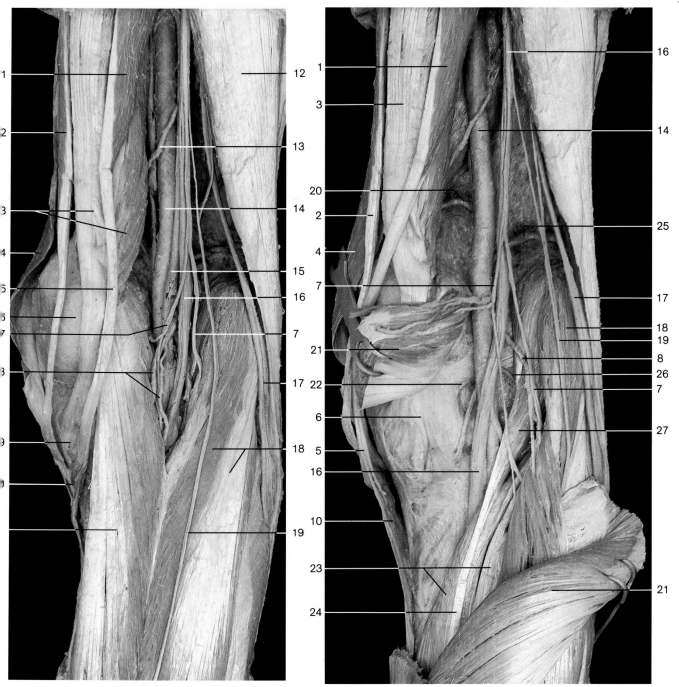

Right leg, posterior crural region (posterior aspect).
The gastrocnemius muscle has been divided and reflected.

Right leg, posterior crural region, deep layer (posterior aspect).
The gastrocnemius and the soleus muscles have been divided and reflected.

1　Semitendinosus muscle
2　Gracilis muscle
3　Semimembranosus muscle
4　Sartorius muscle
5　Tendon of semitendinosus muscle
6　Position of medial condyle of femur
7　Muscular branches of tibial nerve
8　Sural arteries and veins
9　Tendon of semimembranosus muscle
10　Common tendon of gracilis, semitendinosus and sartorius
　　muscles
11　Medial head of gastrocnemius muscle
12　Biceps femoris muscle
13　Muscular branch of popliteal artery

14　**Popliteal artery**
15　**Popliteal vein**
16　**Tibial nerve**
17　**Common peroneal nerve**
18　Lateral head of gastrocnemius muscle
19　Medial sural cutaneous nerve
20　Medial superior genicular artery
21　Medial head of gastrocnemius muscle (cut and reflected)
22　Medial inferior genicular artery
23　Soleus muscle
24　Tendon of plantaris muscle
25　Lateral superior genicular artery
26　Lateral inferior genicular artery
27　Plantaris muscle

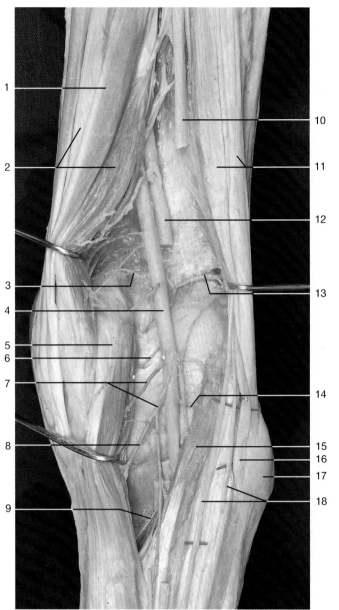

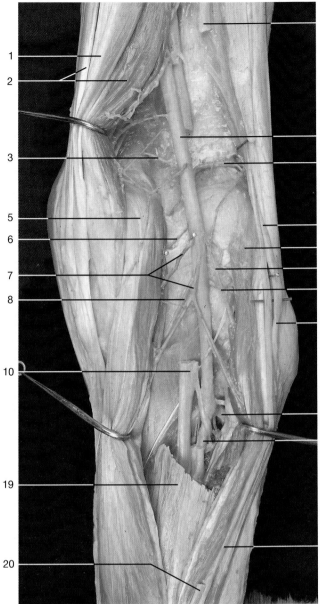

Right leg, popliteal fossa, deep layer (posterior aspect). The muscles have been reflected to display the genicular arteries.

Right leg, popliteal fossa, deepest layer (posterior aspect). Tibial nerve and popliteal vein have been partly removed and a portion of the soleus muscle was cut away to display the anterior tibial artery.

1 Semitendinosus muscle
2 Semimembranosus muscle
3 Medial superior genicular artery
4 **Popliteal artery**
5 Medial head of gastrocnemius muscle
6 Middle genicular artery
7 Muscular branches
8 Medial inferior genicular artery
9 Tendon of plantaris muscle
10 **Tibial nerve** (cut)
11 Biceps femoris muscle

12 Popliteal vein (cut)
13 Lateral superior genicular artery
14 Lateral inferior genicular artery
15 Lateral head of gastrocnemius muscle
16 **Common peroneal nerve**
17 Head of fibula
18 Lateral sural cutaneous nerves
19 Soleus muscle
20 Medial sural cutaneous nerve
21 **Anterior tibial artery**
22 **Posterior tibial artery**
23 Lateral sural cutaneous nerve

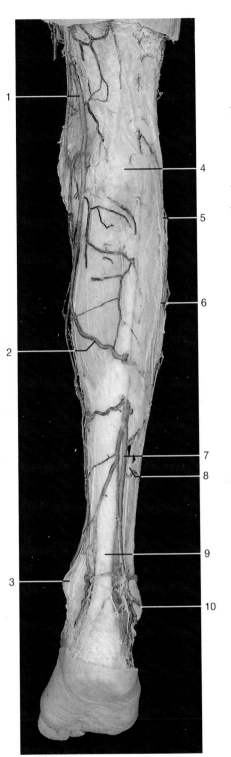

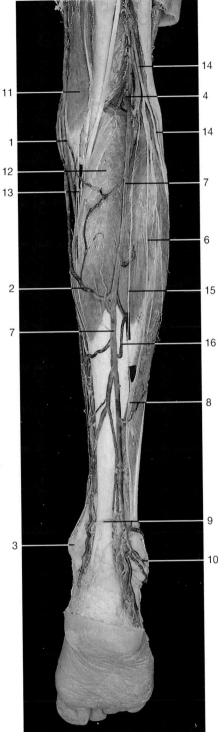

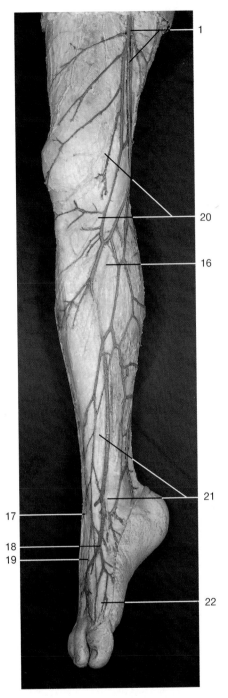

Right leg, cutaneous veins and nerves (posterior aspect).

Right leg, cutaneous nerves and veins (posterior aspect). The superficial layer of the crural fascia has been removed.

Right leg, cutaneous veins and nerves (anterior-medial aspect; veins are colored).

1 **Great saphenous vein**
2 Venous anastomosis between small and great saphenous veins
3 Medial malleolus
4 Popliteal fossa
5 Position of head of fibula
6 Lateral sural cutaneous nerve
7 **Small saphenous vein**

8 **Sural nerve**
9 Calcaneal tendon
10 Lateral malleolus
11 Semitendinosus muscle
12 Medial head of gastrocnemius muscle
13 Saphenous nerve
14 **Common peroneal nerve**
15 Medial sural cutaneous nerve

16 Perforating veins
17 Superficial peroneal nerve
18 Dorsal venous arch
19 Intermediate dorsal cutaneous nerve
20 **Infrapatellar branches of saphenous nerve**
21 Terminal branches of saphenous nerve
22 Medial dorsal cutaneous nerve

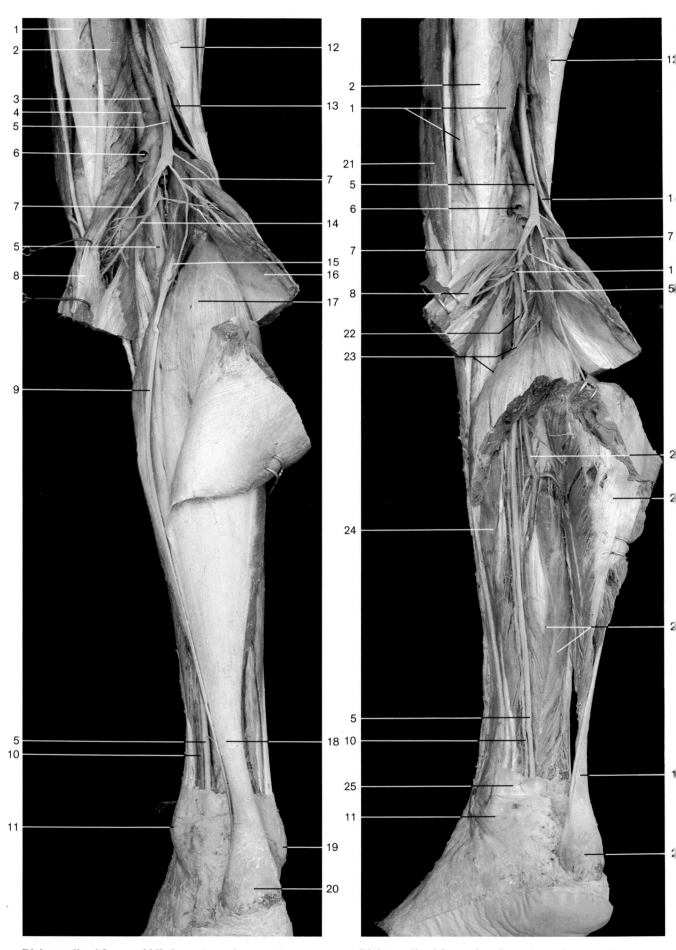

Right popliteal fossa, middle layer (posterior aspect).
The cutaneous veins and nerves have been removed.

Right popliteal fossa, deep layer (posterior aspect).
The medial head of gastrocnemius muscle has been divided
and reflected.

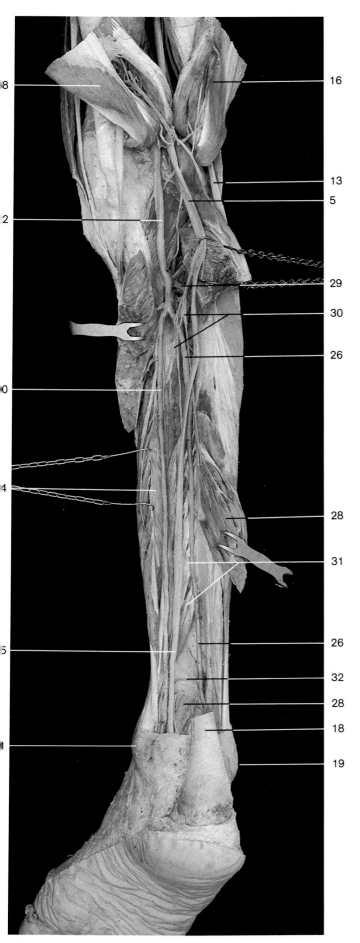

1 Semimembranosus muscle
2 Semitendinosus muscle
3 **Popliteal vein**
4 Popliteal artery
5 **Tibial nerve**
6 Small saphenous vein (cut)
7 Muscular branch of tibial nerve
8 Medial head of gastrocnemius muscle
9 Tendon of plantaris muscle
10 **Posterior tibial artery**
11 Medial malleolus
12 Biceps femoris muscle
13 Common peroneal nerve
14 **Sural arteries**
15 Plantaris muscle
16 Lateral head of gastrocnemius muscle
17 Soleus muscle
18 Calcaneal tendon
19 Lateral malleolus
20 Calcaneal tuberosity
21 Sartorius muscle
22 **Popliteal artery**
23 Tendinous arch of soleus muscle
24 Flexor digitorum longus muscle
25 Flexor retinaculum
26 **Peroneal artery**
27 Soleus muscle
28 Flexor hallucis longus muscle
29 **Anterior tibial artery**
30 Muscular branches of tibial nerve
31 Tibialis posterior muscle
32 Communicating branch of peroneal artery
33 Tendon of tibialis anterior muscle
34 Tibia
35 Tendon of extensor hallucis longus muscle
36 Tendons of extensor digitorum longus muscle
37 Anterior tibialis artery
38 Fibula
39 Tendons of peroneus longus and brevis muscles

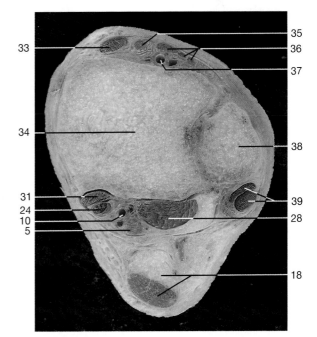

Right leg, posterior crural region, deepest layer (posterior aspect). Triceps surae (gastrocnemius and soleus) and flexor hallucis longus muscles have been cut and reflected.

Cross section of the leg, superior to the malleoli (from below).

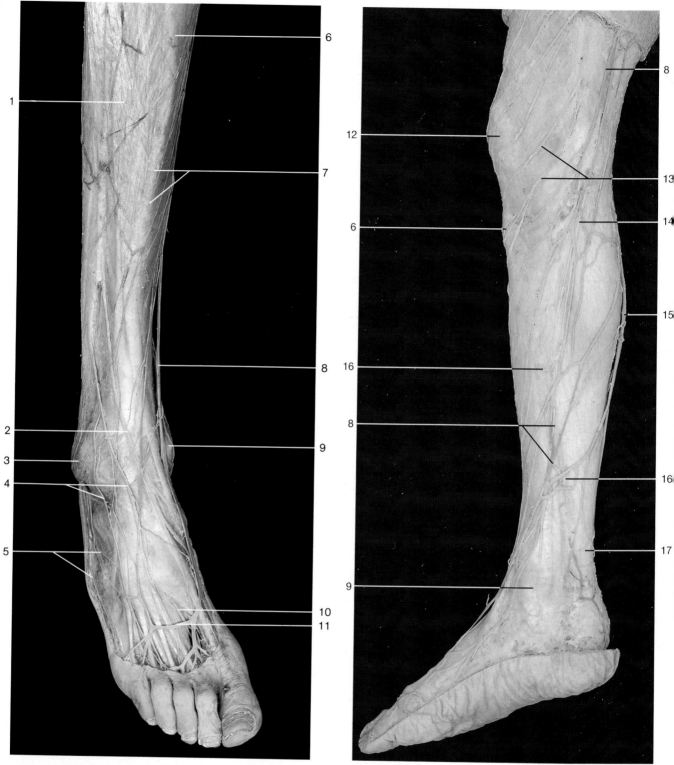

Right leg and foot, anterior crural region and dorsum of foot, cutaneous nerves and veins (anterior aspect).

Right leg and foot, cutaneous nerves and veins (medial aspect).

1   Superficial crural fascia
2   Medial cutaneous branch of superficial peroneal nerve
3   Lateral malleolus
4   Lateral cutaneous branch of superficial peroneal nerve
5   Cutaneous branch of sural nerve
6   Position of tuberosity of tibia
7   Anterior margin of tibia
8   **Great saphenous vein**
9   Medial malleolus

10   Deep peroneal nerve
11   **Venous arch of dorsum of foot**
12   Position of patella
13   **Infrapatellar branches of saphenous nerve**
14   Saphenous nerve
15   Small saphenous vein
16   Perforating vein
17   Calcaneal tendon

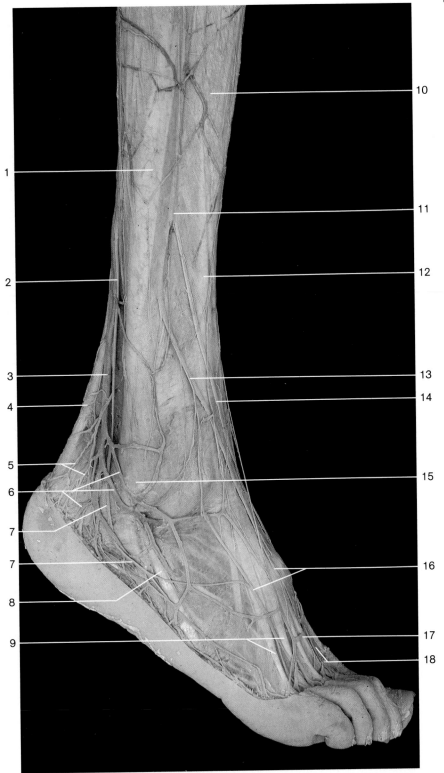

Right leg and dorsum of foot, cutaneous nerves and veins (lateral aspect).

1 Position of fibula
2 **Sural nerve**
3 **Small saphenous vein**
4 Calcaneal tendon
5 Lateral calcaneal branches of
    sural nerve
6 Venous network at lateral malleolus
7 Cutaneous branch of sural nerve
8 Tendon of peroneus brevis muscle
9 Tendons of extensor digitorum
    longus muscle

10 Fascia cruris
11 Superficial peroneal nerve
12 Position of tibia
13 Lateral cutaneous branch } of **superficial**
14 Medial cutaneous branch   } **peroneal nerve**
15 Lateral malleolus
16 Dorsal digital nerves
17 Dorsal venous arch
18 Deep peroneal nerve

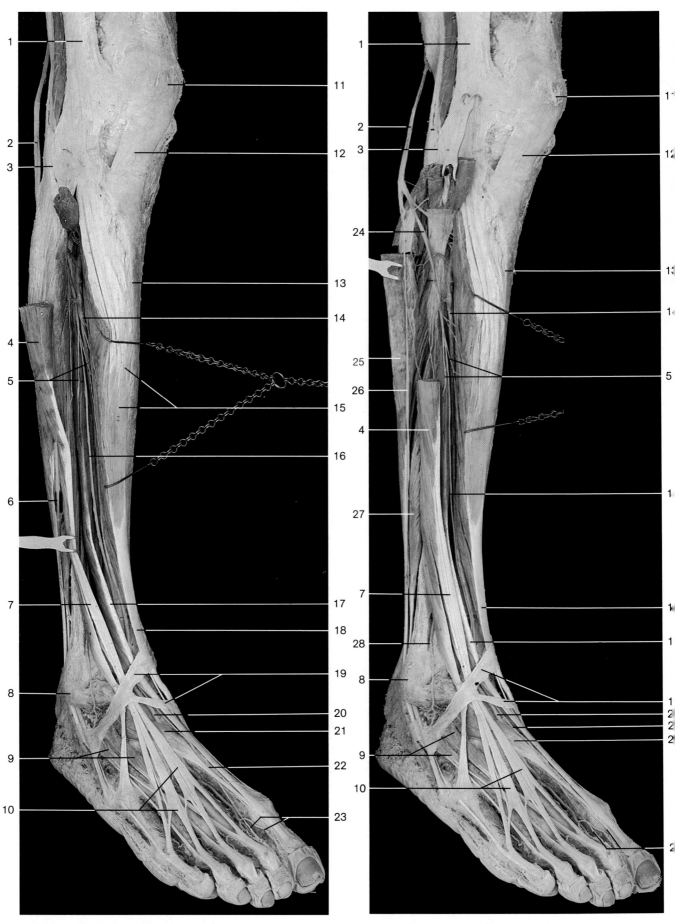

Right leg and dorsum of foot, middle layer (anterior lateral aspect). The extensor digitorum longus muscle has been divided and reflected laterally.

Right leg, deep layer (anterior lateral aspect). The extensor digitorum longus and the peroneus longus muscle have been divided or removed. The common peroneal nerve has been elevated to show its course around the head of fibula.

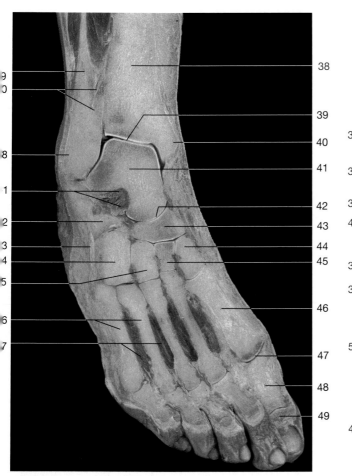

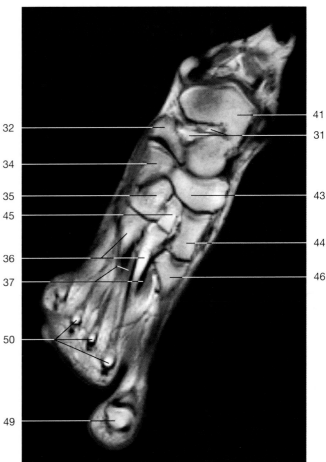

Coronal section through the foot and talocrural joint
(anterior aspect).

Coronal section through the foot
(MRI scan after Heuck A, Luttke G, Rohen JW, 1994).

1	Iliotibial tract
2	**Common peroneal nerve**
3	Position of head of fibula
4	Extensor digitorum longus muscle
5	Muscular branches of deep peroneal nerve
6	**Superficial peroneal nerve**
7	Tendon of extensor digitorum longus muscle
8	Lateral malleolus
9	Extensor digitorum brevis muscle
10	Tendons of extensor digitorum longus muscle
11	Patella
12	Patellar ligament
13	Anterior margin of tibia
14	**Anterior tibial artery**
15	Tibialis anterior muscle
16	Deep peroneal nerve
17	Extensor hallucis longus muscle
18	Tendon of tibialis anterior muscle
19	Extensor retinaculum
20	Dorsalis pedis artery
21	Extensor hallucis brevis muscle
22	Deep peroneal nerve (on dorsum of foot)
23	Dorsal digital nerves (terminal branches of deep peroneal nerve)
24	**Deep peroneal nerve**
25	Peroneus longus muscle (cut)

26	Superficial peroneal nerve (with peroneal muscles laterally reflected)
27	Peroneus brevis muscle
28	Lateral anterior malleolar artery
29	Fibula
30	Distal tibiofibular joint (syndesmosis)
31	Interosseous talocalcaneal ligament
32	Calcaneus
33	Tendon of peroneus brevis muscle
34	Cuboid bone
35	Lateral cuneiform bone
36	Metatarsal bones
37	Dorsal interosseous muscles
38	Tibia
39	**Talocrural joint**
40	Medial malleolus
41	Talus
42	**Talocalcaneonavicular joint**
43	Navicular bone
44	Medial cuneiform bone
45	Intermediate cuneiform bone
46	First metatarsal bone
47	Metatarsophalangeal joint of great toe
48	Proximal phalanx of great toe
49	Distal phalanx of great toe
50	Heads of metatarsal bones II–IV

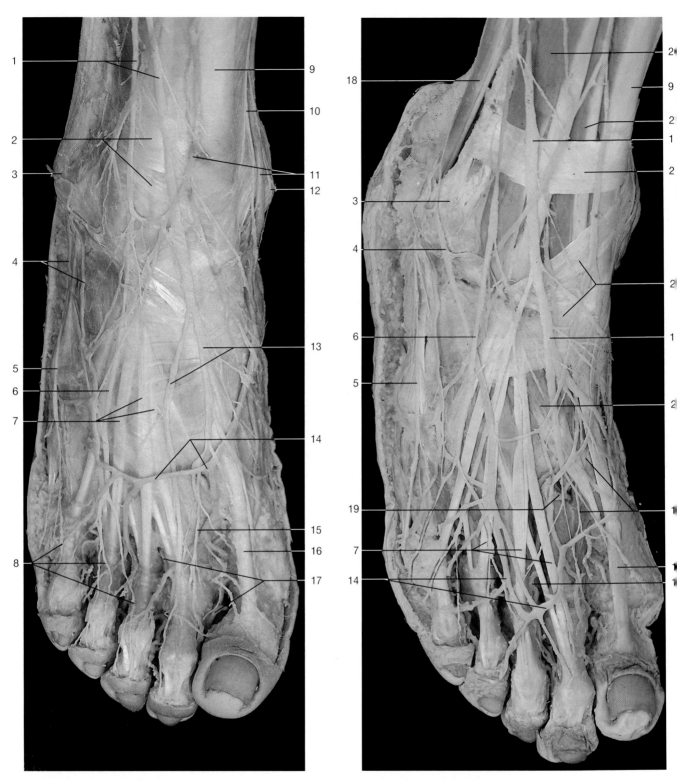

Dorsum of the right foot, superficial layer (anterior aspect).

Dorsum of the right foot, superficial layer. The fascia of the dorsum has been removed.

1	**Superficial peroneal nerve**	9	Tendon of tibialis anterior muscle
2	Superior extensor retinaculum	10	**Saphenous nerve**
3	Lateral malleolus	11	Venous network of medial malleolus and
4	Venous network of lateral malleolus and		tributaries of great saphenous vein
	tributaries of small saphenous vein	12	Medial malleolus
5	Lateral dorsal cutaneous nerve (branch of	13	Medial dorsal cutaneous nerves
	sural nerve)	14	**Dorsal venous arch**
6	Intermediate dorsal cutaneous nerve	15	Dorsal digital nerve (of deep peroneal
7	Tendons of extensor digitorum longus muscle		nerve)
8	Dorsal digital nerves	16	Tendon of extensor hallucis longus muscle

17	Dorsal digital arteries
18	Peroneal muscles
19	Deep plantar branch of dorsalis pedis artery anastomosing with plantar arch
20	Extensor digitorum longus muscle
21	Extensor hallucis longus muscle
22	Inferior extensor retinaculum
23	Extensor hallucis brevis muscle

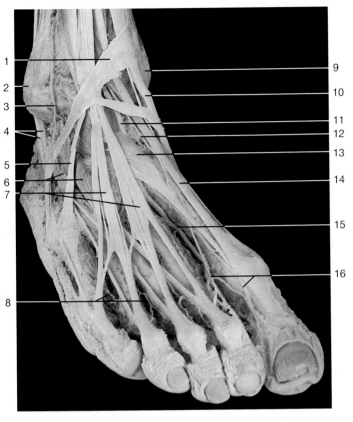

1   Extensor retinaculum
2   Lateral malleolus
3   Lateral anterior malleolar artery
4   Tendons of peroneal muscles
5   Tendon of peroneus tertius muscle
6   Extensor digitorum brevis muscle
7   Tendons of extensor digitorum longus muscle
8   Dorsal metatarsal arteries
9   Medial malleolus
10 Tendon of tibialis anterior muscle
11 **Dorsalis pedis artery**
12 Deep peroneal nerve (on dorsum of foot)
13 Extensor hallucis brevis muscle
14 Tendon of extensor hallucis longus muscle
15 Dorsalis pedis artery with deep plantar branch to
    the plantar arch
16 Dorsal digital nerves (terminal branches of deep
    peroneal nerve)
17 Lateral tarsal artery
18 Extensor digitorum brevis muscle (divided)
19 Arcuate artery
20 Dorsal interosseous muscles
21 **Deep peroneal nerve**
22 Medial cuneiform and first metatarsal bone
23 Tendon of peroneus longus muscle
24 Abductor hallucis and flexor hallucis brevis muscles
25 Medial plantar artery, vein and nerve
26 Fourth and fifth metatarsal bone
27 Adductor hallucis (oblique head)
28 Tendons of flexor digitorum longus muscle
29 Lateral plantar artery, vein and nerve
30 Flexor digitorum brevis muscle
31 Plantar aponeurosis

Dorsum of right foot, middle layer (anterior lateral aspect).
The cutaneous nerves have been removed.

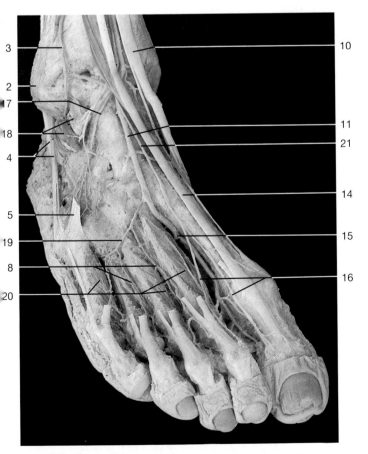

Dorsum of right foot, deep layer (anterior lateral aspect).
The extensor digitorum and hallucis breves muscles have
been removed.

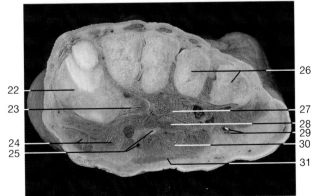

Cross section of the right foot at the level of the
metatarsal bones (posterior aspect).

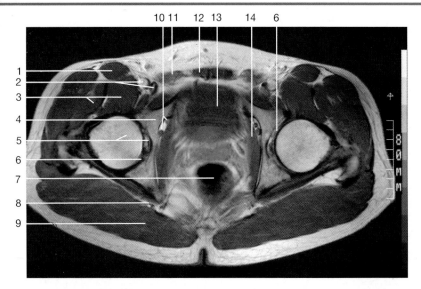

Axial section through the pelvis and the hip joints
(section 1, MRI scan, inferior aspect).

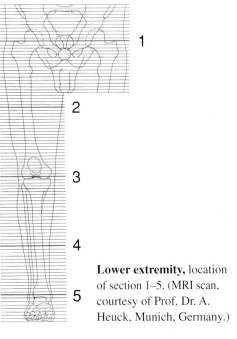

Lower extremity, location of section 1–5. (MRI scan, courtesy of Prof. Dr. A. Heuck, Munich, Germany.)

1   Sartorius muscle
2   **Femoral artery and vein**
3   Iliopsoas muscle
4   Pubis (os pubis)
5   **Femoral head** with ligament of femoral head
6   Articular cavity
7   Rectum
8   **Sciatic nerve** and accompanying artery
9   Gluteus maximus muscle
10 Obturator vessels and obturator nerve
11 Rectus abdominis muscle
12 Pyramidalis muscle
13 Urinary bladder
14 Obturator internus muscle
15 Rectus femoris muscle
16 Vastus intermedius and vastus lateralis of quadriceps femoris muscle

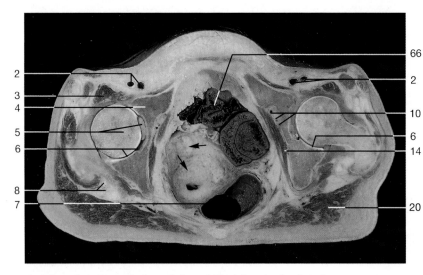

Axial section through the pelvis and hip joints in the female
(section 1, inferior aspect). (Arrows: uterus, myometrium with myoma.)

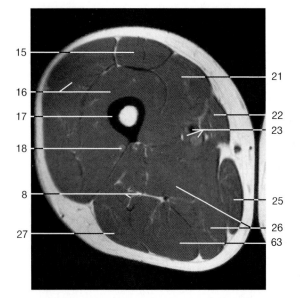

Axial section through the middle of the thigh
(section 2, MRI scan, inferior aspect).

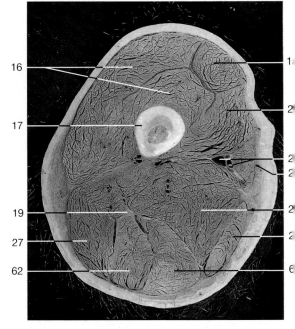

Axial section through the middle of the right thigh (section 2, inferior aspect).

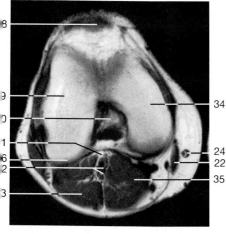

28
6
39
34 29
64
30
34
24 65
22 6
32
35 33

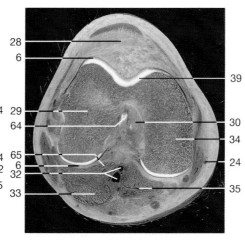

Axial section through the knee joint
(section 3, MRI scan, inferior aspect).

Axial section through the right knee joint (section 3, inferior aspect).

17 **Femur**
18 Perforating artery
19 Sciatic nerve
20 Gluteus maximus muscle (insertion)
21 Vastus medialis muscle
22 Sartorius muscle
23 Femoral artery and vein
24 Great saphenous vein
25 Gracilis muscle
26 Adductor muscles
27 Biceps femoris muscle
28 Patellar ligament
29 Lateral condyle of femur
30 Posterior cruciate ligament
31 **Tibial nerve**
32 Popliteal artery and vein
33 Lateral head of
gastrocnemius muscle
34 Medial condyle of femur
35 Medial head of
gastrocnemius muscle
36 Tibialis anterior muscle
37 **Tibia**
38 Deep peroneal nerve, anterior tibial
artery and vein
39 Patellar surface
40 Peroneus longus and brevis
muscles
41 **Fibula**
42 Soleus muscle
43 Flexor digitorum longus muscle
44 Tibialis posterior muscle
45 Posterior tibial artery and
vein and tibial nerve
46 Peroneal artery
47 Small saphenous vein and
sural nerve
48 Extensor hallucis longus muscle
49 Extensor digitorum longus muscle
50 Tendon of peroneus longus
muscle
51 Lateral malleolus (fibula)
52 Peroneus brevis muscle
53 Tibialis anterior muscle
(tendon)
54 Dorsalis pedis artery
55 Medial malleolus (tibia)
56 Tibialis posterior muscle
(tendon)
57 Flexor digitorum longus muscle
(tendon with synovial
sheath)
58 Flexor hallucis longus muscle
59 Posterior tibial artery and
vein
60 Lateral and medial plantar
nerves
61 Calcaneal tendon
62 Semitendinosus muscle
63 Semimembranosus muscle
64 Anterior cruciate ligament
65 Plantaris muscle
66 Small intestine

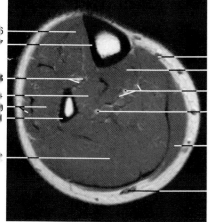

36
37
24 48
43
49
45 44
46 40
41
35 42
33
47

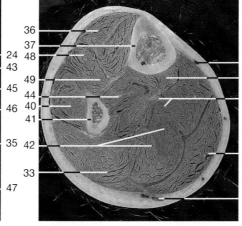

24
43
45
35
47

Axial section through the middle of the leg (section 4, MRI scan, inferior aspect).

Axial section through the middle of the right leg (section 4, inferior aspect).

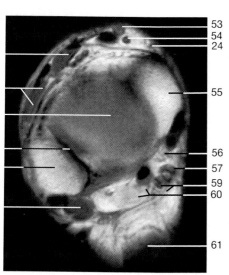

53
54
24
55
56
57
59
60
61

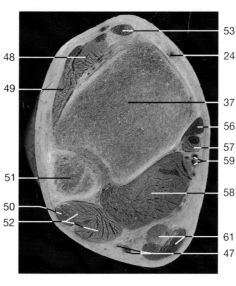

53
48 24
49
37
56
57
51 59
58
50
52
61
47

Axial section through the end of the right leg (section 5, MRI scan, inferior aspect).

Axial section through the end of the right leg (section 5, inferior aspect).

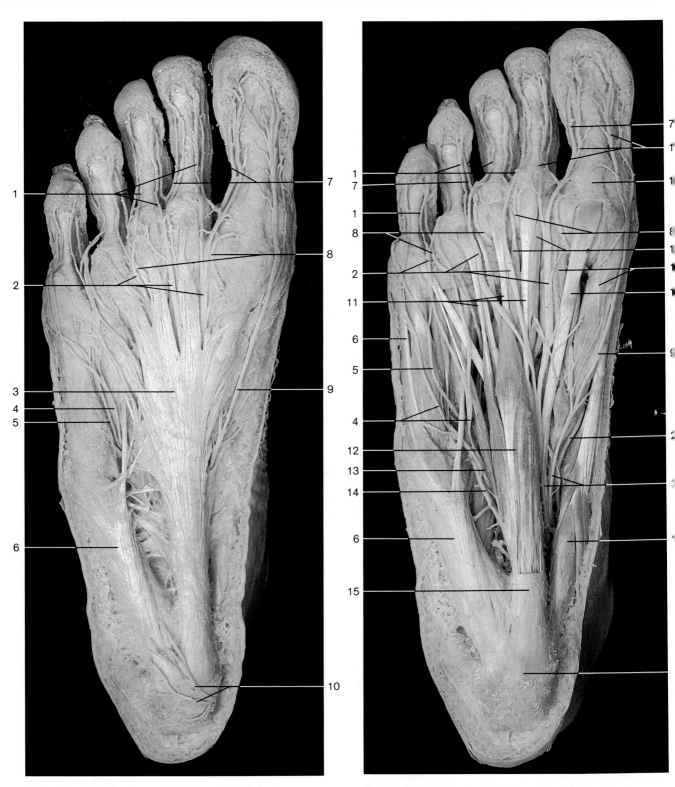

1
2
3
4
5
6

7
8
9
10

1
7
1
8
2
11
6
5
4
12
13
14
6
15

7
1
1
8
1
9

Sole of the right foot, superficial layer (from below);
dissection of cutaneous nerves and vessels.

Sole of the right foot, middle layer (from below).
The plantar aponeurosis has been removed.

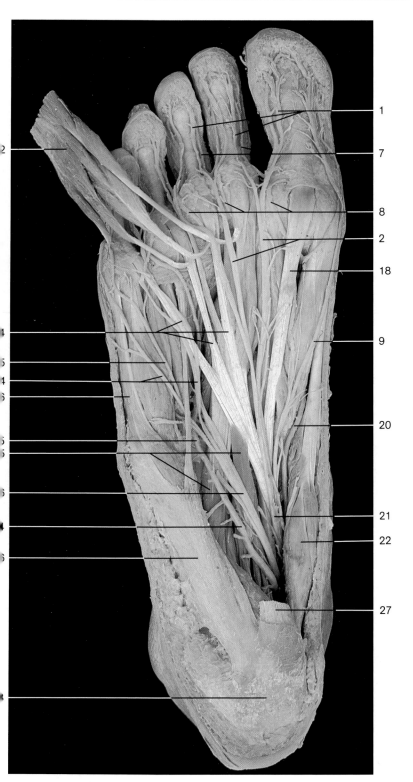

1 Proper plantar digital nerves
2 Common plantar digital nerves
3 Plantar aponeurosis
4 Superficial branch of lateral plantar nerve
5 Superficial branch of lateral plantar artery
6 Abductor digiti minimi
7 Proper plantar digital arteries
8 Common plantar digital arteries
9 Digital branch of medial plantar nerve to great toe
10 Medial calcaneal branches
11 Tendons of flexor digitorum brevis muscle
12 Flexor digitorum brevis muscle
13 **Superficial branch of lateral plantar nerve**
14 **Lateral plantar artery**
15 Plantar aponeurosis (remnant)
16 Digital synovial sheath
17 Lumbrical muscles
18 Tendon of flexor hallucis longus muscle
19 Flexor hallucis brevis muscle
20 **Medial plantar artery**
21 **Medial plantar nerve**
22 Abductor hallucis muscle
23 Calcaneal tuberosity
24 Tendons of flexor digitorum longus muscle
25 Quadratus plantae muscle
26 **Lateral plantar nerve**
27 Flexor digitorum brevis muscle (cut)
28 Synovial sheaths
29 Plantar arch

Sole of the right foot, middle layer (from below); dissection of vessels and nerves. The flexor digitorum brevis muscle has been divided and anteriorly reflected.

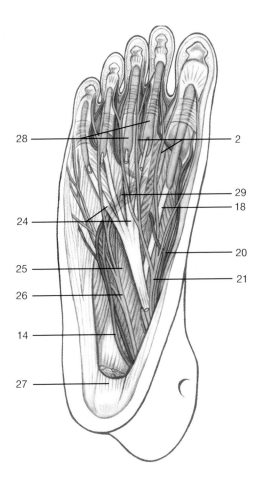

Sole of the right foot. Synovial sheaths of flexor tendons indicated in light blue. (Schematic drawing.)

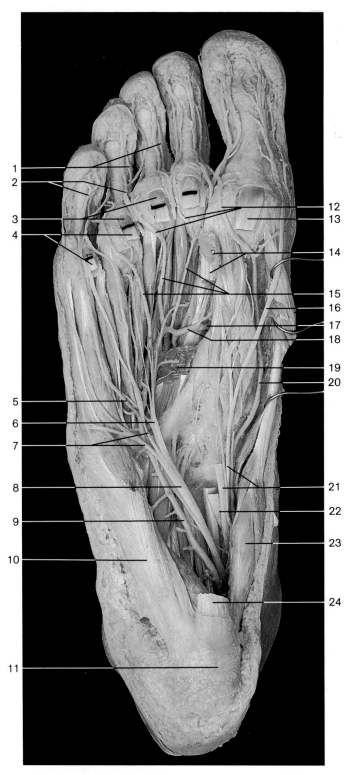

1   Proper plantar digital arteries
2   Proper plantar digital nerves
3   Tendons of flexor digitorum brevis muscle
4   Tendons of flexor digitorum longus muscle
5   Superficial branch of lateral plantar artery
6   Deep branch of lateral plantar nerve
7   Superficial branch of lateral plantar nerve
8   **Lateral plantar nerve**
9   **Lateral plantar artery**
10 Abductor digiti minimi muscle
11 Calcaneal tuberosity
12 Common plantar digital arteries
13 Tendon of flexor hallucis longus muscle
14 Insertion of both heads of adductor hallucis muscle
15 Plantar metatarsal arteries
16 Medial plantar nerve of great toe
17 Deep plantar branch of dorsalis pedis artery
     (perforating branch)
18 **Plantar arch**
19 Oblique head of adductor hallucis muscle (cut)
20 **Medial plantar artery**
21 **Medial plantar nerve**
22 Crossing of tendons in sole of foot (flexor hallucis
     longus and flexor digitorum longus muscles)
23 Abductor hallucis muscle
24 Origin of flexor digitorum brevis muscle

Sole of the right foot, deep layer (from below); dissection
of vessels and nerves. The flexor digitorum brevis muscle,
the quadratus plantae muscle with the tendons of the flexor
digitorum longus muscle and some branches of the medial
plantar nerve have been removed. The flexor hallucis brevis
and adductor hallucis muscles have been cut and portions
removed to show the somewhat atypical course of the medial
plantar artery and deep muscles of the foot.

Index

Page numbers in **bold** indicate
main discussions